Marriage of Convenience

Rochester Studies in Medical History

Senior Editor: Theodore M. Brown
Professor of History and Preventive Medicine
University of Rochester

ISSN 1526–2715

Marriage of Convenience

Rockefeller International Health and Revolutionary Mexico

ANNE-EMANUELLE BIRN

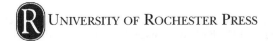 UNIVERSITY OF ROCHESTER PRESS

First published 2006
Transferred to digital printing 2012

University of Rochester Press
668 Mt. Hope Avenue, Rochester, NY 14620, USA
www.urpress.com
and Boydell & Brewer Limited
PO Box 9, Woodbridge, Suffolk IP12 3DF, UK
www.boydellandbrewer.com

ISSN: 1526-2715
Hardcover ISBN: 978-1-58046-222-8
Paperback ISBN: 978-1-58046-444-4

Library of Congress Cataloging-in-Publication Data
Birn, Anne-Emanuelle, 1964-
    Marriage of convenience : Rockefeller International Health and revolutionary
Mexico / Anne-Emanuelle Birn.
        p. ; cm. − (Rochester studies in medical history, ISSN 1526-2715 ; v.8)
    Includes bibliographical references and index.
    ISBN 1-58046-222-7 (hardcover : alk. paper) 1. Public health−Mexico−History−
20th century. 2. Public health−International cooperation−History−20th century.
3. Rockefeller Foundation International Health Division−History−20th century.
4. Mexico. Departamento de Salubridad Pública−History−20th century.
    [DNLM: 1. Rockefeller Foundation. International Health Division. 2. Mexico.
Departamento de Salubridad Pública. 3. Public Health−history−Mexico. 4. History,
20th Century−Mexico. 5. International Cooperation−history−Mexico.
6. Public Health Administration−history−Mexico. 7. Sanitation−history−Mexico.
8. World Health−Mexico. WA 11 DM4 B619m 2006] I. Title. II. Series.
    RA451.B55 2006
    362.10972−dc22

                                                                    2006006563

A catalogue record for this title is available from the British Library.

This publication is printed on acid-free paper.

Front cover image: Rockefeller Foundation officer explaining lifecycle of hookworm to a
rural household, 1927. Back cover image: Mothers and children attending infant hygiene
clinic in Mexico, 1929. Both images are courtesy of the Rockefeller Archive Center.

To my parents

"There is no more important country for our purposes than Mexico."
Frederick Russell to Henry Carr, May 19, 1927, RG 5, Series 1.2,
Box 296, Folder 3753, Rockefeller Foundation Archives.

"The most important point in Mexico is that, using the experience and the teachings of the best health departments from abroad, almost all of them well-established and with many years of trials, successes, and errors, we have not blindly imitated or copied these organizations, but instead have transformed and adapted them to our own circumstances; we have taken into account the scarcity of economic resources, communication and transportation problems, the absence of health education, and the urgency of facing the problem and beginning to resolve it."
Miguel E. Bustamante, *Gaceta Médica de México* (1934), 200.
Translated from Spanish by Anne-Emanuelle Birn.

Contents

Illustrations

Figures

Tables

Introduction

The Fever of International Health

In January 1929, just a few months after he returned to Mexico from his doctoral studies at the Johns Hopkins School of Hygiene and Public Health in Baltimore, Maryland, Rockefeller Foundation (RF) fellow Miguel Bustamante penned a heartfelt letter to his former dean, William Howell. Peppering his progress report with words of gratitude, Bustamante wrote of his new appointment as chief of the Port of Veracruz sanitary unit, Mexico's first attempt at "cooperative and systematic work for the improvement of the Public Health conditions in our Cities." He relayed the "real effort" his country was expending and hoped that he would be "doing something good with the cooperation of our people." Bustamante concluded, "Of course I recognize how much I own [*sic*] to our School and the Foundation and hope not to disappoint any of you."[1]

This missive, written by one of Mexico's most esteemed public health doctors, embodied the characteristics of the relationship between revolutionary Mexico and the RF: multifaceted interaction. Bustamante conveyed a mixture of national pride and know-how, the challenge of collaborating with the public, a reliance on modern public health methods, and his indebtedness to international patronage.

The principals in this three-decade public health partnership were the RF's International Health Division (IHD; International Health Board until 1927) and the Mexican government's Department of Public Health (Departamento de Salubridad Pública; DSP). In addition, numerous other parties—ranging from traditional healers to national leaders, elite physicians to rural health officers, foreign philanthropists to small townsfolk—would also be involved. Different ideas would appear, some homegrown, some imported, some local, some international, some traversing back and forth. In the course of this complex involvement, there would be times of productive cooperation, appropriation, disdain, rejection, outright hostility, and bona fide accomplishment, making the survival of the relationship an achievement in and of itself.

This interaction took place between 1921 and 1951 through a series of projects centered in a handful of Mexican states and administered from Mexico City, New York, and several regional capitals. The RF-Mexico liaison began with a large-scale yellow fever campaign based along the Gulf Coast and extending into the Yucatán peninsula. In 1924, the yellow fever effort was converted into a lower-cost but intensive hookworm campaign that reached hundreds of thousands of people in small towns, mostly in the state of Veracruz, and, later, in Oaxaca and Chiapas. By the late 1920s, mutual DSP-IHD interest in developing permanent local health services led to the establishment of a series of cooperative health units in large and small towns in Veracruz and Oaxaca, as well as a statewide demonstration project in Morelos that lasted through the 1930s. In the 1940s, the collaboration included small-scale malaria research projects in five states and scattered support for health units in northern states.

During this period, the IHD and DSP were also engaged in a far-reaching educational and professional placement initiative, one that enabled Bustamante's graduate studies in the United States and his leadership role upon his return to Mexico. Overall, the RF sponsored sixty-eight Mexican public health fellows to pursue advanced degrees in North America and arranged public health tours to the United States for thirty-six high-level DSP officials. Starting in the 1930s, the DSP and IHD jointly organized half a dozen training stations in Mexico, by 1950 having prepared almost two thousand doctors, sanitary engineers, nurses, midwives, and other health workers.

What kind of relationship was this and how did it last for thirty-plus years amidst binational tensions, domestic turmoil, institutional soul-searching, and a history of suspicion and resentment? A marriage of convenience is contracted for practical reasons, usually involving social, economic, or political gain. Such a union is formed in the absence of mutual affection but does not preclude moments of appreciation. In the case of the Rockefeller Foundation and revolutionary Mexico, the two entities shared a coinciding mission: improving human well-being and modernizing society. Yet they did not always agree on how to carry out this project or on what and whom to involve, and they brought different concerns and capabilities to the table. Each party was path-breaking in its own way and held many interests outside the relationship.

For the RF, Mexico could have been just another country in its stock philanthropic approach, whereby modest investments were carefully structured to generate the largest impact possible. Disposing of financial capital and scientific expertise, the foundation partnered with national and colonial governments—which marshaled their own resources and experts—in order to spread its public health gospel. By 1920, the RF was already playing a leading role in the planning and administration of public health programs, research, and education in dozens of locales around the globe, including virtually every Latin American country.[2]

Latin America served an important role in the RF's international strategy. Allocated between one fifth and more than one third of the IHD budget depending on the year—and far outstripping the attention allotted to other underdeveloped regions—Latin America offered a clear example of what public health philanthropy could achieve in scientific and economic terms in the region of the world over which U.S. interests held the most sway. In many ways, it was behemoth Brazil that was the prize of Latin America: the IHD devoted more time and money to Brazil than to any other country in the region, spending ten times more than the $10.7 million (estimated in 2004 dollars) disbursed during its three decades in Mexico.

Yet Mexico was also special to the RF, as demonstrated by the IHD's staying power through good times and bad. In geopolitical terms, Mexico's trajectory had great bearing on stability and prosperity in the Americas due to its proximity to the United States, its importance in the realms of trade and investment, and its violent revolution of 1910–20. Mexico's economic potential and its influence within Latin America as the most populous Spanish-speaking country—together with its large indigenous population, sovereign pride, and accomplishments in many fields—made it a natural leader for the region and ripe for RF cooperation.

In health and disease terms, Mexico represented both promise and threat. Epidemic diseases could cross borders, threaten commerce, and generate social unrest, while endemic diseases lowered productivity and stymied modernization. The promise came in the form of the RF's ability to parade newfound U.S. expertise in disease control to Mexico, other recipient countries, and European competitors.[3] While yellow fever eradication campaigns in a number of Latin American countries were used to this end, the disease's elimination in the Gulf Coast region of Mexico—where European and North American interests operated oil companies—was particularly significant. Mexico could serve as a showcase for successful public health development from the Rio Grande to Tierra del Fuego.

Over time, Mexico's place on the RF's world stage shifted. It began as an important locus of yellow fever efforts. It then became an example of the modernization and extension of public health services in a revolutionary context. In the 1930s, Mexico tested the RF's claims of neutrality and the United States' "Good Neighbor" policy through populist–socialist politics and the nationalization of oil. Following the outbreak of World War II, Mexico, together with other Latin American countries, enjoyed additional RF resources diverted from Europe. Throughout these changes the RF always categorized Mexico, in social and economic terms, within North America rather than Latin America and compared it to the South of the United States at an earlier stage of development.

From a Mexican perspective, collaboration with the RF—even as an endeavor to advance human welfare—was at the start highly suspect. Since Mexico's independence from Spain in 1821, Mexican dealings with both public and private U.S. interests had proven problematic, notwithstanding extensive social and economic ties between the countries. Large-scale U.S. economic investment—while furthering Mexican industrial development—allowed few resources for local needs or redistribution. Repeated U.S. invasions of Mexico had ended in massive territorial seizure, countless deaths, and deep resentment. Subsequent humanitarian gestures on the part of U.S. organizations could not counteract the memories of these aggressions and typically—as in the case of the sanitary campaign following the U.S. invasion of Veracruz in 1914—met with disparagement and distrust.

As the revolutionary fighting began to subside, Mexican professionals and the bureaucratizing state sought to address the nation's growing social demands by combining domestic expertise with international knowledge and experience; in the health arena, there was no partner more ready, willing, and able than the RF. The RF's interest coincided with Mexico's postrevolution modern state-building effort: the creation of national political and cultural institutions, the consolidation of Mexico's medical elites and other professionals, and rapid advancements in education and other social sectors all aimed at extending the sense of national citizenship.[4] In 1920 the still shaky Mexican leadership recognized RF cooperation as the right move for the time. In short order, Mexico's DSP forged a useful, ongoing—if occasionally discordant—relationship with the RF that went beyond professional and political purposes to meet a range of national and local needs and circumstances.

Above all, the relationship between the RF and Mexico was marked by constant interplay between and among the official partners and an assortment of local and transnational players, from traditional midwives to modern microbiologists to consummate politicians to foundation officers. Though not in a romantic marriage, Mexico and the RF managed to live with one another—sometimes distantly, sometimes intimately—through decades of ups and downs.

The RF-Mexican collaboration was much more than a neighborly affair: it was an ambitious enterprise in international health, one whose failure might bear considerable consequences for future health cooperation and whose success might leave a legacy of operating patterns and principles. The story of the RF in Mexico thus opens a window to the story of international health in the twentieth century in which the reach of public health was extended, albeit under often complicated, contested, and even chaotic circumstances.

The Birth of International Health

Today we take the "globalization" of "public health" to be an obvious pairing of terms,[5] but a century ago this was a new notion that emerged at the intersection of economic and scientific internationalization and involved, at one and the same time, local, national, international, public, and private interests. The making of this modern commitment to international public health stemmed from a confluence of factors. Large-scale immigration from Europe and Asia to the Americas and the explosion of industrial capitalism and trade—enabled by a revolution in transportation and shipping routes—heightened the threat of epidemic disease throughout the world. No longer were outbreaks of plague, yellow fever, cholera, and other ailments solely a matter for local concern, binational disputes, or colonial managers. The now globalized economic system meant that a real or threatened epidemic in one part of the world could impede production, trade, and consumption elsewhere and on a fast timetable.[6] Of course, international disease control measures necessarily rested on local and national attention to public health.

Imperial powers had long paid heed to the role of public health in protecting conquering armies and settlers, improving the productivity of workers, and reinforcing the stratification of colonizers and colonized, and they eventually trained local experts to carry out disease control activities in colonial territories in Africa, Asia, and other regions.[7] Heightened economic interdependence both magnified the potential dangers of disease and made its control a far trickier political affair involving settings within and beyond existing imperial structures.

Manufacturers, merchants, transporters, and other industrial parties feared the interruption of commerce provoked by disease outbreaks. Measures designed to stem epidemics, especially the quarantine of ships, people, and goods, proved extremely costly. Municipal authorities, particularly in port cities, met with their own practical responsibilities. The disastrous experiences of nineteenth-century cholera and yellow fever epidemics in ports as far flung as Naples, New Orleans, and Buenos Aires, where local governments were typified by lack of authority, disorganization, corruption, and sabotage by commercial interests, long remained fresh memories. Furthermore, the rapid urbanization of the period, accompanied by "disruption, deprivation, disease, and death,"[8] demanded that municipalities pay increasing attention to their "medical police" roles, including sanitation, proper burials, public hospitals, and disease control. Public health measures—ranging from housing codes to food hygiene—also offered prospects for improving workplace productivity thanks to reduced sick days and overall urban prosperity. As Munich's health officer Max von Pettenkofer argued in 1873, "the value of public health to a city" was evidenced through benefits that far outweighed the costs.[9]

The public frequently protested the authoritarian measures imposed during nineteenth-century epidemics; by the early twentieth century such opposition began to be replaced by increasing claims on the state for better health conditions. In some settings these claims were mediated by social reformers—often middle-class women—motivated by an almost religious zeal for melioration; in other places, it was political and social activism—particularly working-class movements—that directly demanded state action. At the same time, public health served as an opportunity for a burgeoning state apparatus to build bureaucratic power, often resulting in increased control over the population.

Undergirding these developments was the increasing scientific and technical potential of public health and medicine spawned by the germ theory of disease; bacteriological and parasitological findings by the likes of Louis Pasteur, Robert

Koch, Carlos Finlay, and Patrick Manson; laboratory-based verification of disease; and a small but growing armamentarium of disease control measures, such as diphtheria antitoxin treatment, deriving from work by Emile Roux, Emil von Behring, and others. This powerful explanatory framework and the accompanying interventions began to displace public health's existing community-oriented activities. The "new" public health found itself at the vortex of clashing constituencies: scientific experts striving to assert their status, reformers seeking to increase social order, liberal industrialists eager for steady economic growth, and bureaucrats looking to increase their purview, as well as socialists, feminists, and laborites fighting for better working and living conditions.

The very advances of the transformed field of public health raised increasingly complex questions. Was public health a technical or a social endeavor? Should health be a right of citizenship, a responsibility of industry, or a burden on the individual to resolve in the marketplace? Should health investments and resources be under political or expert control? Arriving at a consensus over the nature, funding, and scope of these measures was far from automatic. Public health became embroiled in the political and social struggles of the day, at certain times offering a justification for an activist state, at others suffering from a backlash against such interference, and at still other times, paradoxically, given its public mandate, serving private interests.

By no means did the late nineteenth- and early twentieth-century convergence of the need and ability to protect nation, industry, and populace through public health measures lead to uniform structures, ideologies, or practices. Different political contexts, traditions, institutional cultures, historical trajectories, configurations of power relations, and geo-epidemiological conditions made the concepts, the delivery, and the objectives of public health look rather different in different countries.[10] Germany's commitment to aggressive public health policies, such as compulsory vaccination and quarantines, was rooted in the need to fend off epidemics from the East, as well as to fashion a domestic politics of power—in large part to reduce worker unrest—in a state that was late in forming.[11] In the Soviet Union, public health was centralized from above, with local level medical societies and health initiatives abolished after the 1917 Revolution.[12] Britain's more laissez-faire approach drew from a long history of local and voluntary governance and a belief that its island geography protected it against epidemics (as well as its reluctance to disturb lucrative trade with India and its other colonies).[13] In China, the political fragmentation following the 1911 Revolution meant that public health problems received only isolated and disorganized attention.[14]

In most Latin American countries, the sanitary authorities that had been mobilized periodically to combat epidemic outbreaks during centuries of Spanish and Portuguese colonialism were transformed into permanent health and hygiene boards beginning in the late nineteenth century.[15] Infused with the new ideas and practices of the day, national health agencies sought to centralize power, implement modern public health measures, and increase the reach of the state over social welfare, which was historically dominated by the Catholic Church. These efforts took place mostly in leading cities, with water and sanitation systems catering to urban elites, child health activities (often carried out by charitable organizations) focused on poor and working-class communities, and food, beverage, and housing regulation monitored unevenly. As the number and range of public health tools—from Wasserman tests to mosquito larvae control—increased after 1900, new public health ministries and medico-civic professionals throughout Latin America advocated greater attention to endemic problems. Still, health authorities in many settings were hampered by limited state capacity and low responsiveness to popular needs: the region's large rural populations were typically allotted few systematic health improvements beyond vaccination campaigns and epidemic disease control.

Given the impediments to local and national efforts, international sanitary agreements—not to mention the establishment of international agencies involved in cooperative public health activities—posed an even greater challenge.

Philanthropy and Health: A U.S. Model

In the United States, a different configuration of factors formed the contours of public health. While the pragmatic and symbolic benefits of modern public health could not be disregarded, the decentralization of political power thwarted national efforts at public health organization until the fourth decade of the twentieth century. Except for a few activities protecting the nation's borders through the medical inspection of immigrants, limited bacteriologic and infectious disease research, military public health organization, and a short-lived National Board of Health (1879–83)—responsibility for public health remained largely in the hands of jealous state and local governments until the Great Depression,[16] when dire social and economic conditions and the associated popular mobilizations pressured the federal government to provide support for the most marginal populations.[17] There was thus room and a cultural affinity for private and voluntary agencies, such as insurance companies and philanthropic foundations, to mount public health activities. Public health was also part of the Progressive Era's agenda of rationalization, bureaucratization, and social betterment, particularly at the level of the municipality.

If the implementation of public health measures necessarily took place on a national or local level, public health's international dimensions emerged at the forefront of its new scientific underpinnings. The expansion of social, scientific, and economic relations between countries enabled public health specialists to meet at congresses and publish in international journals. Health problems began to be identified with greater consistency, facilitating the worldwide diffusion and implementation of standard interventions.

But international agreement was not automatic. In Europe it took more than half a century to transcend inter-imperialist jealousies and resolve concerns over national sovereignty in order to establish a uniform system of disease notification, ship inspection, and maritime sanitation. A treaty was finally signed in 1903, the culmination of 11 international sanitary conferences held since 1851. Its institutional counterpart, the Office International d'Hygiène Publique (OIHP) established in Paris in 1907, was charged with organizing periodic conferences, regulating quarantine agreements, and conducting studies on epidemic diseases. It was only with the founding of the League of Nations Health Organization (LNHO) after World War I that a bona fide system of international health cooperation was started in Europe.[18]

In the Americas there were fewer impediments to international sanitary agreement: in contrast to the multiple centers of power in Europe, the United States was the dominant economic force in the region. The 1881 international sanitary conference held in Washington, D.C. opened the door to regionwide sanitary agreement, bolstered by several South American meetings in the 1870s and 1880s and an 1887 Sanitary Convention signed by Brazil, Argentina, and Uruguay detailing quarantine periods for ships bearing cholera, yellow fever, and plague. By the 1890s growing trade and immigration heightened fears of epidemic disease throughout the Americas. The United States' imperial expansion to Cuba, Puerto Rico, and the Philippines following the 1898 Spanish-American War brought the potential of outbreaks even closer to home. In 1902 the United States—stimulated by an earlier meeting in Mexico—led a group of seven governments in the region to found the Pan American Sanitary Bureau (PASB; initially the International Sanitary Bureau) in Washington, D.C. under the aegis of the U.S. Public Health Service (USPHS). Most Latin American republics soon joined and were represented at quadrennial conferences. Within a few decades the Bureau had developed a hemisphere-wide sanitary code, a disease-reporting system, a widely disseminated public health journal, and an incipient system of technical cooperation. Its agenda remained focused on sanitary and commercial concerns into the 1930s.[19]

All of these endeavors—in the Americas and throughout the world—required resources to pay for research, personnel, and infrastructure. On one hand, governments were gaining new taxation powers over citizens and industry; on the other, the enormous profitability of transportation and commerce, natural resource extraction, manufacturing, and the oil that literally greased the wheels of industry resulted in surpluses of colossal magnitude. If business and political authorities in many European countries came to realize that public health spending was an important investment in civic efficiency, the pervasive individualist ideology in the United States delayed the recognition that public health improvements could lead to increased productivity and consumption. Private industry's stance against social spending—coupled with political reluctance to dedicate new federal revenues to nonmilitary pursuits—left a vacuum in national and international health activities, one most notably filled by Rockefeller philanthropy.

Founded in 1913 "to promote the well-being of mankind throughout the world," the RF had, by the time its International Health Division was disbanded in 1951, carried out scores of hookworm, yellow fever, malaria, and other public health campaigns in the U.S. South and almost one hundred other settings around the world. Over the same period it founded a series of schools of public health in North America, Europe, Asia, and Brazil, and sponsored thousands of foreign health professionals to pursue graduate study, mostly in the United States.[20] The goals of the foundation transcended public health per se. The potential to stimulate development, stabilize nation-states by helping them meet the social demands of their populations, improve diplomatic relations, expand consumer markets, and encourage overall economic vitality combined with the more direct activities of diffusing and internationalizing scientific, bureaucratic, and cultural values. Through this arrangement, national elites were linked to elites of the world's great economic powers, enabling "backward" countries to join "world culture."[21]

If the earlier inspiration for international health organization was the need to protect trade from epidemic-induced interruption—launched through the sharing of information about disease outbreaks and an agreed-upon system for the control of epidemic disease in port cities—the RF took international health to a new level. The IHD was instrumental in turning existing efforts of colonial health and a budding spirit of medico-commercial cooperation into an international health system that generated its own demand through the creation of new national bureaucracies, programs of aid and development, and rural public health activities around the world.

All the while, the RF was also focused on garnering popular acceptance for public health activities at the local level. Its work patterns included carrying out focused disease campaigns, maintaining a missionary zeal in its own officers, nudging government commitment to public health through programs heavily cofinanced by national and local entities, and using graduate fellowships to mold a worldwide cadre of public health leaders. Perhaps the RF's most influential ideology was and has been international health's specific disease control approach, which—if it does not entirely disregard social understandings of disease—decidedly privileges technological over social measures. As the RF discovered with hookworm, diseases with a clear, technical solution, regardless of their epidemiological importance, could demonstrate accomplishment in terms of outreach and treatment over a short period of time and at low cost, allowing the RF to claim success and permitting it to work in a large number of settings simultaneously. In a sense, the RF's own institutional needs and continuity superseded the goal of improving health conditions in particular locales. Because the RF was accountable to no one beyond its own carefully selected board members, it exhibited the flexibility and audacity to experiment in a way that a governmental or supragovernmental agency could not. These characteristics were key to its diplomatic, technocratic, and scientific appeal and to its success.

Undoubtedly, the extensive institutionalization of public health was a vital concomitant to the rise of international health. If only a handful of countries had ministerial-level public health departments in 1900, today virtually all national (and many local) governments have an executive public health agency. Although the RF claimed a role in this institutionalization in the almost one hundred countries where it operated and beyond, the reality was far more complicated. In Mexico, for example, the federal government was already poised to build its public health bureaucracy when the RF arrived in the early 1920s. The RF aided and accelerated this process in certain regards but surely did not instigate it; indeed, the IHD's resource-hungry disease campaigns may even have slowed institutional expansion. It would thus be a gross overstatement to attribute to the RF the Mexican Secretariat of Health's current institutional capacity and longevity, its form of organization, and its professional and technical orientation. Yet the interaction around the IHD's programs in Mexico shaped a persistent debate about the scope, ideology, and practices of international health.

A Framework for International Health

Evaluation of the international medical and sanitary work of the RF has ranged from adulation for the agency's contribution to improvements in medical research, diffusion of technology, disease eradication, public health organization, and health status,[22] to skepticism about the actual impact of the foundation's activities in settings where such transformations were already occurring,[23] and to contempt for Rockefeller complicity in the promotion of capitalist medicine and public health that at once commodified health, generated medical dependency, re-created hierarchical distinctions within the health sector, advanced a reductionist paradigm, favored cure over prevention and technological rather than social measures, and promoted values that denigrated local approaches to health improvement.[24] The history of the RF's public health programs in Mexico might find some merit in each of these explanations, but individually—or even all together—they remain incomplete.

In recent years, more nuanced assessments of Rockefeller medicine and health have emerged, attempting to document the various forms of invitation, accommodation, negotiation, co-optation, interpretation, adaptation, reluctance, and refusal expressed by societies "receiving" Rockefeller programs.[25] No longer can so-called host countries be seen as unitary actors; instead a variety of players and agents interacting with one another and the RF must be recognized. The RF too has been re-examined for its sociological complexity—the differences among founders, board members, New York administrators, and officers working at the country level—and the tensions between the foundation's unified vision and mission and its sometimes inconsistent practices.[26] Like any institution, the RF changed over time; perhaps uniquely in the first half of the twentieth century, it was at once a national, bilateral, multilateral, international, and transnational agency.

Similarly, we cannot understand the 1920s and 1930s in Mexico as a single, cohesive effort at progress, nationalism, and organized patron-client systems. Mexico's revolutionary era—and the role of the social and political protagonists of the day—has undergone renewed scrutiny that challenges the official ideology and portrays a diversity of revolutionary experiences by region and sector.[27] A recent renaissance of work in the history of medicine, public health, and social welfare in Mexico has provided a rich tapestry of local and nationwide institutions, movements, and ideologies that, until the early 1990s, were little remembered or appreciated.[28]

In view of the multiple dimensions of the main players in this story, we need to examine their interaction in a similarly complex fashion. One of the challenges of this "multiple players" approach is nomenclature: both RF men and their Mexican counterparts referred to the IHD (and, until 1927, the International Health Board or IHB) and RF interchangeably, rarely distinguishing one entity from the other. This conflation existed when the IHB operated as a semi-independent board and persisted after it was reined in as a division under a new organizational structure. Here we will seek consistency, referring to the IHB or IHD when the matter pertains to the International Health Board or Division and the RF when it refers to the foundation; nonetheless, in remaining true to the language of the original sources, we may not always be able to avoid the overlapping use of institutional names.

Because of the RF's highly bureaucratic documentation system, clear trajectory of personnel and programs, and well-preserved archives, it is tempting both to focus on the RF's version of the story and to overstate its role. However, such a portrayal would be sorely deficient: even in a mere shell of a nation with few professionals, bureaucrats, or institutions to speak of, RF programs could not be studied in a vacuum. Nor can the relationship between the RF and Mexico be considered a one-sided penetration process whereby local actors simply fell into line as long as their own interests were met.

The RF's influence on Mexican public health might be further attenuated on at least three fronts. First, the geographic scope of its operations was limited, with most activities taking place in three states and the replication of RF initiatives in other locales being somewhat circumscribed. Second, the DSP and numerous states and municipalities around the country were already active in a variety of public health efforts—disease campaigns, growing infrastructure, and experimentation with new models of public health delivery—some of which were purposely avoided or even disdained by the RF. Third, Mexican medicine and public health were influenced by other international medical and public health traditions, movements, and institutions. The development of vital statistics capacity, for example, was consistent with the proliferation of international standards in the late nineteenth century. Until the 1920s, most elite physicians studied in the leading medical universities of France and Germany. Maternal and child health drew from pre-Columbian traditions, the Latin American feminist movement, and French and other European influences in puericulture and eugenics. Mexico's 1926 sanitary code was based upon the PASB's model of consensual region-wide (if U.S.-led) norms on disease reporting and control measures. The new Soviet approaches to public health and social welfare also entered into Mexican discussions and developments. By no means was the RF the only game in town.

What emerges, then, is a portrayal of a far more intricate and evolving dance involving multiple partners who interacted in and around the institutions, ideologies, politics, and practices of public health. Several of these dancers—most notably the RF home office and key officials in the Mexican host agency, the DSP—sought to be the lead partner without always succeeding, but each dancer taught the other new steps and affected the overall performance. Thus, this story incorporates a sometimes confusing mix of elements—conspiracy, charity, mutual interest, repudiation, resignation—ultimately revealing a relationship of dynamic continuity.

What did Mexico and the RF really want from this marriage of convenience? Was the RF seeking to create a sanitary-economic empire, using local politicians to leverage its entry and influence? Was Mexico using the RF for free technical expertise, political and professional opportunism, diplomatic gains, and the resolution of internal conflicts? Was this a purely charitable enterprise on the part of "do-gooders"—yes, generating binational friendship—but with no ulterior motives? What, then, do we make of the RF's reluctance to tackle Mexico's most pressing causes of illness and death? What accounts for the shared faith in the ability of science-based public health to resolve social problems? And why did the RF set up a complex challenge and reward system to govern its programs? Or was this whole effort largely chaotic, with countless rivals putting their hands into the philanthropic pot to no specific ends?

As an illustration of the possibilities, dilemmas, and limits of international health, there are few examples more instructive than the collaboration between the RF and revolutionary Mexico. Here we explore these issues before a backdrop of institutionalization, political turmoil, social change, health advancement, and problematic diplomatic relations. Miguel Bustamante, upon returning to Mexico from his RF fellowship, was quick to recognize the complicated give-and-take between his patron and his *patria*. This motif of interaction remains ever present in the story of how Mexico and the RF took, gave, shared, rejected, owed, and survived one another through a remarkable relationship.

A Road Map

The focus of this study is the relationship of RF public health activities to ongoing and new institutional and ideological developments and an array of national, local, and transnational actors in Mexico. We explore these questions by tracing the footsteps and interactions of many parties through the course of RF-Mexico public health cooperation from 1921 to 1951. At times, we focus on day-to-day goings-on, at times on larger policies and politics, at times on the two simultaneously.

In chapter 1 we examine the origins of the RF and its interest in international health; the social and political background of the Mexican Revolution and the Mexican state's renewed interest in public health; and the way in which the RF courted Mexico through an expensive yellow fever campaign in the early 1920s. Centered in the pivotal Gulf Coast state of Veracruz, the large-scale operation helped eliminate the threat of a frightening disease, dispelled Mexican suspicions of the RF, quieted some of the national government's political rivals, and killed household bugs.

Chapter 2 witnesses the interaction among Rockefeller public health men, Mexican health department officials, local healers, and townsfolk as a jointly funded mobile hookworm campaign was deployed in 1924 to introduce sanitary principles to government and populace alike. Under challenging political conditions and with occasional clashes of medical opinion, RF and DSP officers traveled to numerous towns in Veracruz, and later Oaxaca and Chiapas, seeking to convince local authorities to invest in public health and to persuade townsfolk and peasants that they were worm-infested, required treatment, and needed to learn how to defecate differently. Above all, this undertaking against a relatively minor ailment served to consolidate the relationship between Mexico and the RF.

Chapter 3 explores the cooperative development of local health units in provincial towns beginning in the late 1920s, the most important and challenging aspect of the RF-Mexico partnership. Appearing at a time when Mexico had stabilized sufficiently to begin to focus on the provision of permanent government services, local health units became the subject of competition between the RF and Mexican public health officials over their authorship, design, and operation. Unlike elsewhere in Latin America—where RF-sponsored health units appeared later or were greatly overshadowed by disease campaigns—in Mexico the units served as the fulcrum of RF activity for more than a dozen years.[29] We analyze the circumstances under which the local health units were born, the continuing interplay between the RF and the Mexican government over their management and multiplication, the general terms of their engagement with the public, and their various forms of interaction with women as patients, healers, and intermediaries.

In chapter 4 we move from this incipient process of public health organization to an era of tumultuous institutionalization. During the presidency of

Lázaro Cárdenas in the 1930s, the relationship between the RF and Mexico was marked by alternating intervals of coyness and pursuit. Initially, it was the RF that was reluctant to invest in a socialist-talking Mexico, though the Cárdenas government beseeched the RF for assistance in its grand plans for health development. As the reach and range of the DSP grew and gained visibility, the RF shifted gears, emphasizing professional training over joint projects as a means of engaging its partner. This ambitious program to educate government health leaders, public health specialists, and rank and file health workers intersected with national health policymaking and institutional developments, though not always in the expected fashion. By the late 1930s it was the RF that was anxious to stay in Mexico: the radical organization of collectively controlled rural health services and Cárdenas's controversial oil nationalization were met with barely a whimper from the RF home office. Mexican RF fellows and RF officers—focused on operational questions—were caught in the middle of these larger political struggles. All the while, the marriage continued, if at times inconveniently.

In chapter 5 we seek to identify the ingredients of this mutual survival. We follow the RF's final years in Mexico, for the end of a relationship may be as enlightening as its beginning. We discuss particular RF strategies, such as why certain significant health issues were never addressed by the RF in spite of their importance to Mexico and multiple requests for cooperation. Malaria, for instance, was recognized by RF field men, Mexican health officials, local doctors, and the public as the country's leading disease problem, yet the RF paid scant attention to it. Finally we turn to the relationship as a whole, assessing the range of interactions over time as an illustration of international health cooperation.

The epilogue returns to this question from a contemporary perspective, tracing the long-term imprint of RF-Mexican cooperation and the legacy of the RF for the larger system of international health. It suggests that the principles of RF practice—as played out in Mexico—have enabled international health's bureaucratic continuity amidst shifting international politics, at the high price of an overly technical orientation of health cooperation that avoids tackling the underlying determinants of health and disease.

Chapter One

A Match Made in Heaven?

Public health, foreign capital, social revolution, modern state-building: perhaps nowhere did these forces so vividly coalesce, captivate, and challenge one another than in the interactions between the Rockefeller Foundation and Mexico. For the RF, public health represented an appealing sphere of action for its domestic and international philanthropic investments, one that—consistent with its motto—could widely benefit mankind. For Mexico, public health offered a concrete, feasible area through which the state could enlarge its authority by meeting revolutionary expectations for improved social conditions, build a sense of citizenship—particularly among rural populations—and tether science and scientific professionals to renewed national goals. Beyond this shared attraction to public health, bringing together Mexico's revolutionary state and Rockefeller dollars through cooperative health activities required mutual confidence. As a civilian stand-in for U.S. foreign development policy, the RF was well attuned to Mexico's role as trade partner, investment locale, and source of laborers and well aware of its bitterness toward repeated U.S. aggressions. The RF agreed that public health could help in the building of modern Mexico, with diplomatic by-products of reduced political, social, and disease threats to the U.S. and much-needed binational goodwill. If Mexico could trust the RF's professed independence from the U.S. government, the International Health Board's (IHB) ability to support—and perhaps accelerate—Mexico's public health modernization made it a potentially palatable associate.

During the first half of the twentieth century, no agency was as far-reaching or as active in promoting international public health as the RF. Virtually every facet of public health's early twentieth-century revolution—the scientific breakthroughs in bacteriology and parasitology; the advances in epidemiology and vital statistics; the training of professionals; the awakening of public health consciousness; the building of institutions; the application of these developments to the health of populations around the world; and the very model of scientific public health—involved the foundation in some dimension. The Rockefeller family, the foundation trustees, and powerful foundation administrators and officers were in a position to channel Rockefeller capital to a bewildering array of activities, but they also recognized that public health was not always an end in itself. While RF projects were narrowly focused, the RF's executives understood the attendant value of international public health in improving productivity and fomenting economic development, stabilizing social and political conditions, protecting trade, and enabling countries to enter into the global capitalist system.

Similarly, various parties in Mexico recognized international health's relevance to multiple agendas. The 1910–20 Mexican Revolution—complex, brutal, and in many ways ambiguous—laid the groundwork for a new country, one in which the national state gained greater presence and purpose in education, economic activity, public health, and other arenas. The building of the new state responded to claims put forth by groups far beyond the nineteenth-century social, intellectual, and landholding elites who had previously ruled independent Mexico: these included new industrialists and professionals, war-hero politicians and soldiers, a growing urban working class, and the rural masses of mestizo and indigenous peasants—temporary laborers, small and communal landowners, and sharecroppers—who sacrificed the most for the revolution.

The rallying cry of sovereignty from foreign economic and politico-military interference unified Mexico, yet social and scientific priorities blurred the meaning of sovereignty. Most medical elites welcomed RF public health, employing the prestige of the RF to help institutionalize health and medicine and to legitimize their growing role over the nation's well-being. Some local healers saw professional advantages in working with RF projects while others resisted these efforts. Organized movements in key states made use of the RF's presence to leverage resources from and access to Mexico's federal government. At different times, national and regional leaders refused RF cooperation; more typically politicians harnessed RF activities to their own stock and power.

With international public health collaboration appealing to many groups, it was also interpreted and refashioned by them all: the RF's model of public health was no more uncontested than it was neutral. The RF's cooperative efforts underwent a complex and changing process of adaptation, digestion, regurgitation, and refusal between and among RF executives, Mexican leaders, and various transnational parties—including RF officers on the ground and Mexican professionals who obtained advanced public health degrees in the United States. Although these complicated interchanges occasionally flared into disputes, the relationship between the RF and Mexico was mostly marked by continuity and reciprocal, if contrasting—or even contradictory—satisfaction.

This chapter traces how the RF and Mexico each came to public health and then to one another through their first cooperative health program. The encounter itself—a "big bucks" yellow fever campaign in the early 1920s— proved to be the high-flown launching of what would become an enduring relationship, but the staging of the initial meeting between the two parties was tortuous.

Rockefeller Philanthropy and International Health

Unlike the international health efforts that preceded it, Rockefeller public health hailed neither from government nor from charity. Moneymaking, American-style, spawned this new system of social melioration. The rapid expansion of the United States' free market economy in the second half of the nineteenth century produced a new, extraordinarily wealthy class, one delineated not by heredity, as in older European societies, but by leadership in the world of business. The so-called robber barons constituted an American royalty born of opportunism in highly profitable arenas such as railroads, shipping, oil, manufacturing, and finance.

During the same period, the lure of employment in these very industries undergirded the arrival in the United States of millions of immigrants, particularly from southern and eastern Europe, and the internal migration of rural southerners to industrial cities in the Northeast and the Midwest. Explosive and unruly urban growth and miserable living conditions fueled the militancy of laborers who were producing but not profiting from the new American wealth. By the end of the nineteenth century, working-class resentment of the robber barons was joined by the voices of middle class reformers who railed against deplorable social conditions and sought secular—often governmental—solutions to such problems.[1]

Business leaders were distressed by these populist and radical impulses and by their own inability to rely on government to further their interests as in the past. A few of the capitalists began to recognize in this situation new outlets for investing their accumulated millions. In 1889, Andrew Carnegie, whose fortune sprang from steel manufacturing, published an article in the *North American Review*, entitled "The Gospel of Wealth," which outlined his belief that rich individuals were only the trustees of their amassed riches and had a responsibility to channel their wealth to the public good by supporting hardworking, ambitious individuals rather than charity cases.[2] For Carnegie, this duty led to a concrete legacy of several thousand libraries and public baths around the country as well as major research and cultural organizations.[3]

John D. Rockefeller, whose great and growing prosperity derived from oil and finance, admired Carnegie's efforts and wanted to go even further. A devout Baptist, Rockefeller had contributed a portion of his earnings to charity since his youth. By the 1890s, he became dissatisfied with his pattern of donations to churches, schools, and hospitals. Instead, he sought to put his money to work in a more systematic and effective manner that would advance society and resolve social problems through scientific and educational initiatives.[4] In 1891, Rockefeller gave $1 million to found the University of Chicago, after having been courted for several years to support this project by fellow Baptist Frederick Taylor Gates, executive secretary of the National Baptist Education Society. The same year, Rockefeller invited Gates to become part of his staff. Gates became the mastermind of the Rockefeller philanthropies, soon to be joined by Rockefeller's firstborn, John D. Rockefeller Jr.[5] Under Gates's influence, Rockefeller Sr. began to support the fields of science and medicine, and in 1901 he pledged $200,000 (almost $5 million in 2004 dollars)[6] over a ten-year period to the Rockefeller Institute for Medical Research in New York City. The subsequent year he gave $1 million to launch the General Education Board to promote public education of both blacks and whites in the South and other regions of the country.[7]

The Birth of Rockefeller Public Health

What Rockefeller's separate donations to higher education, medical research, and public schools did not do, however, was directly apply new scientific findings to the public good. In 1909 this situation was addressed when Rockefeller was convinced to sponsor his first public health venture—a five-year hookworm campaign in the South of the United States. The brainchild of an ambitious medical zoologist, an influential advisor, and a bold southern educator—respectively, Charles Wardell Stiles, Frederick Gates, and Wickliffe Rose—the Rockefeller Sanitary Commission for the Eradication of Hookworm Disease marked the beginning of a long association between Rockefeller philanthropy and scientific public health.

Hookworm—the so-called germ of laziness—was believed to be a key factor in the South's lower productivity; its eradication, these men believed, would pave the way for the region's industrialization and advancement. Hookworm disease (also called uncinariasis or anquilostomiasis)—prevalent in a tropical and subtropical belt around the globe—was first identified in humans in the 1830s.

According to a century of medical understanding,[8] hookworm is caused by the infection of hookworms (*Necator americanus* in North and Central America, *Anchylostoma duodenale* elsewhere) in the human digestive tract, especially in people with malnutrition. Hookworm infection results in anemia, stunted growth, fatigue, and weakness—hence the designation "germ of laziness." Other symptoms include yellowed skin and swollen legs and bellies. Hookworm larvae enter the body where the skin is tender—often between the toes—then migrate through blood vessels to the lungs, where they are coughed out and then swallowed into the alimentary tract. There, the nourished larvae grow into half-inch long worms, cling to the intestinal walls, and reproduce, expelling thousands of eggs with the stool. If the conditions are right—warm, moist, shaded soil—the eggs will hatch and develop into larvae: transmission typically occurs when people going barefoot are exposed to infected feces or swallow contaminated soil. Misery and lack of sanitation serve alongside topographical, climatological, and helminthological factors as determinants of the distribution of hookworm disease.

What made hookworm control feasible at the turn of the twentieth century was the combined power of diagnosis and cure: (1) hookworm ova could be detected in the feces under microscopic examination and (2) hookworm disease could be treated through thymol crystals and an Epsom salt purgative (later replaced by oil of chenopodium and other drugs). The first hookworm campaign to employ these techniques took place in the U.S. possession of Puerto Rico beginning in 1903 at the urging of U.S. Army physician Bailey Ashford, who claimed to have discovered the New World hookworm parasite. The worm was also described and named by his competitor Wardell Stiles as *Necator americanus*.[9] A few years later the Costa Rican government conducted a similar campaign, and several other countries, including Mexico, identified the ailment and undertook hookworm surveys in this period.[10]

But it was the Rockefeller Sanitary Commission, headed by Wickliffe Rose, that perfected the hookworm campaign as a tool of public health. The commission's teams of physicians, sanitary inspectors, and laboratory technicians joined with churches, agricultural groups, and existing local health authorities in a bid to educate poor southerners about hookworm, administer hundreds of thousands of treatments for the disease, promote the wearing of shoes, and convince inhabitants to build and use latrines to avoid the future spread of the disease.[11]

Hookworm's underlying causes—poverty and the absence of sanitary infrastructure—were sidestepped by the commission's evangelical approach but generated no discernible consternation among commission members or the target population. The campaign was generally respectful of southern whites—particularly medical and civic authorities—but far less sensitive to African Americans, who were often compelled more than persuaded to participate in the hookworm effort, and who were excluded from some educational activities.[12] The commission's only hitch was some suspicion that the Rockefellers were using the campaign to peddle shoes (which they were not), an impression that was subsequently dispelled by keeping the Rockefeller name in the background of campaigns. Between 1910 and 1914, the commission led a veritable sanitary revival, reaching more than a million southerners in countless rural communities in eleven states at a cost of approximately $800,000 ($15.5 million in 2004 dollars). Almost half showed evidence of hookworm infection.

The magic of the hookworm campaign stemmed from quick identification of the disease under the microscope, the ease of cure, the almost immediate visibility of results—with those treated feeling more energetic (or less lazy!) just a day after swallowing the medication—and its low cost, eventually less than 50 cents per person treated. That hookworm was not a lethal disease was no hindrance to its usefulness as propaganda; news of the rapidity of treatment encouraged greater attendance at hookworm clinics. The bacteriological revolution had spawned the idea of specific disease-causing germs for a panoply of ailments, but it may have been hookworm treatment—far more than smallpox vaccine or diphtheria antitoxin—that was able to put this notion into practice for rural populations in the South of the United States.

One persistent question was whether hookworm needed to be eradicated or only controlled in order for the campaign to demonstrate success. Eradication was certainly the stated aim, and the doctors who worked with the campaign believed in the possibility of hookworm's elimination. But even Stiles, the campaign's zoological father, had serious doubts from early on about the possibility of eradication. Over time other objectives dislodged the aim of eradication. The commission's men discovered that weekly doses of antihelminthics combined with health education measures—delivered through newspaper articles, pamphlets, inspiring lectures, cartoons, school shows, fair exhibits—offered a highly effective means of stimulating popular interest in public health. The paucity of public health infrastructure in the South hampered any ready response, but the needs were duly noted. Thus, even though it was ultimately unable to eradicate hookworm disease, the Sanitary Commission alerted its funder to a range of public health priorities, including popular health education, professional training, and the organization of permanent health departments. Meeting these priorities—at home and abroad—would become a central occupation of Rockefeller philanthropy for half a century.

Institutionalizing Philanthropy

In 1909—the same year that he funded the Sanitary Commission—Rockefeller decided to formalize his philanthropic efforts. Under the guidance of a handful of trusted advisors, he earmarked $50 million (over $1 billion in 2004 dollars) worth of his Standard Oil Company's shares for a trust devoted to the development of science, education, and religion. Anxious to give permanence and stature to his new venture, Rockefeller attempted to obtain a U.S. Senate charter similar to those acquired by other associations, including his own General Education Board. However, Progressive Era antimonopoly sentiment aimed at Rockefeller business interests (which famously led to the 1911 breakup of the Standard Oil Trust) also channeled suspicion of Rockefeller "charity." Such hostility resulted in an extended congressional fight and the ultimate rejection of the philanthropic charter.

In 1913, the Rockefeller Foundation was finally incorporated under New York State law.[13] At their first meeting, the trustees decided that extending the Sanitary Commission's work overseas would be "one of the most productive lines of activity."[14] The Sanitary Commission was folded into the RF and rapidly reincarnated as the International Health Commission (re-christened the International Health Board in 1916 and then reorganized as the International Health Division, or IHD, in 1927).[15] The RF's motto was "to promote the well-being of mankind throughout the world." Its own well-being came first—in the form of an enormous endowment. By 1930 the foundation had received close to $250 million ($2.8 billion in 2004 dollars) from the Rockefeller family. In addition to the General Education Board and the IHB, the foundation's early decades saw the launching in 1914 of the China Medical Board, which supported the Peking Union Medical College; in 1918 of the Laura Spelman Rockefeller Memorial Fund, which funded the social sciences and humanities; in 1919 of the Division of Medical Education; and in 1923 of the International Education Board, which focused on the natural sciences.[16] Until the late 1920s, each board had its own trustees and operated semi-independently.

Most of the RF boards concentrated on one or two areas of the world, reflecting a set of priorities that their trustees and administrators attached to each region. The General Education Board was devoted to the United States, with activities divided into basic and technical education and advanced scientific training at elite universities. The China Medical Board had a singular focus, while the International Education Board paid much of its attention to interwar Europe (in the 1920s, for example, funding refugee scholars from the Soviet Union). Both the Spelman and the Medical Education divisions operated mainly in Europe and North America, although small grants were occasionally provided to Latin American institutions in the fields of medicine, social sciences, and the humanities.

The IHB was the least geographically bound RF entity, funding rural health initiatives throughout North America, disease campaigns in Asia, Africa, and Latin America, and health administration and education activities in Europe, North America, and scattered settings in Asia and Latin America. In general, RF trustees held that colonial and economically underdeveloped settings such as Latin America benefited most from the foundation's contribution to meeting basic "human needs," largely through the IHB. Accordingly Latin American countries were deemed too "backward" to be part of the "uniform advance of knowledge" that characterized RF activity in North America and Europe.[17]

Although the RF was legally independent of Rockefeller business interests, in the early years both were managed by an overlapping set of individuals, including John D. Rockefeller Sr. and his son John D. Rockefeller Jr.—the foundation's first president—as well as Frederick Gates, Starr Murphy, Jerome Greene, and Charles Heydt. Gates moved easily between managing philanthropic and business matters, and he served as Rockefeller's right hand man for both spheres of activity. Murphy was Rockefeller's lawyer and a foundation trustee. Greene was the first secretary to the RF as well as John D. Rockefeller Jr.'s private secretary, and Charles Heydt also served as both board and staff member to JDR Jr. RF trustees in turn overlapped with members of the IHB, with the latter entity accented by medical men such as Johns Hopkins University Medical School Dean William Welch, U.S. Surgeon-General William Gorgas, and Rockefeller Institute Director Simon Flexner. Other early board members represented the worlds of education—Wickliffe Rose, University of Chicago President Harry Pratt Judson, retired Harvard President Charles Eliot—and business, including banker A. Barton Hepburn.[18]

By the 1920s the RF—like other foundations—began to hire professional managers. Though they were given considerable independent decision-making powers, the perspectives of these managers usually sat comfortably with those of board members. The IHB/D was run by particularly strong-minded leaders ("medical barons," in Robert Kohler's sobriquet),[19] who were successful in maintaining the IHB's large budget within the foundation and in shaping its activities, often independently of the trustees. Rose, a college administrator from Tennessee, was the first and only nonmedical director of the IHB, serving from 1913 to 1923. More than anyone else, he shaped the IHB's mandate to institutionalize public health throughout the world, going well beyond the disease eradication vision articulated by Gates. His successor, Frederick Russell (1923–35), a long-term military physician and laboratory scientist, oversaw the IHB's transition to the IHD in 1927 and turned its emphasis from field applications to research. Wilbur Sawyer (1935–44), a midwestern-born, Harvard-trained physician and long-term RF man with both field and laboratory experience, solidified the IHD's research orientation. The IHD's last director, George Strode (1944–51), was a career IHD field officer and administrator who was unable to forge a renewed direction for the IHD following the founding of the World Health Organization (WHO).[20] The technical personnel placed in field positions around the world were an eclectic bunch. Ambitious doctors turned public health professionals, they generally hailed from less urbane backgrounds than the administrators in New York. Adventurers, do-gooders, old-fashioned town doctors, new believers in scientific public health, many of them were from rural areas in the United States and understood the value of public health campaigns from firsthand experience.

RF philanthropy was initially conceived as a conciliatory mechanism between men of business and the public, without the encumbrances of government. In contrast to the experiences of European states, where working-class activism generated an expanded role for government in social welfare, the U.S. context favored private efforts at social melioration. Whether philanthropy "at its best had an important and creative role to play in supplementing the state as an agent for social well-being" in areas in which government was "reluctant to experiment,"[21] or whether it served to supplant or even preempt such government involvement[22] remains subject to debate.[23] Indisputably, philanthropy—no matter how many people it reached—was a most undemocratic institution, reflecting the concerns of wealthy elites (typically mediated through professionals), who were becoming captains of the nation's social and scientific policymaking as well as of its industry.

The contradictions of socially-oriented philanthropy funded by private industry profits were quickly revealed. In April 1914, a protracted strike by Colorado coal miners protesting poor working and living conditions, and challenging the mineowners' refusal to recognize their organization of the United Mine Workers of America, ended with a state militia attack on the Ludlow mining camp. More than twenty people were killed, including

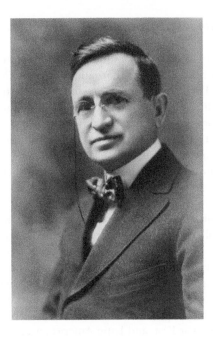

Figure 1.1. Wickliffe Rose, first IHB director (1913–23), Courtesy of the Rockefeller Archive Center.

thirteen women and children who burned and suffocated to death when the militia torched their tents. As the controlling interest in Colorado's largest coal producer, the Rockefeller family was blamed for the deaths, and met with widespread outrage. Public criticism was also aimed at Rockefeller philanthropy, which was accused of being both dangerous and hypocritical. According to Barry Karl and Stanley Katz, "philanthropy by individuals who seemed the very agents of the evils they were trying to overcome was bound to be suspect. The chief criticism was that such philanthropy was a way of acknowledging guilt without being obliged to reform the system that had made these crimes possible." Militant laborites argued that spending on scientific research, housing, and education became "ways of assuring a healthy and contented work force—one devoted nonetheless to serving capitalism."[24]

The Rockefellers were both hurt and confounded by the continued animosity toward their charitable ventures. As a result, in 1917 John D. Rockefeller Jr. recommended concentrating on medicine, "a field in which there can be no controversy, so that I think the possibility of criticism as regards the use of the fund or its potential dangers would be almost nothing."[25] Medicine and public health became safe and effective ground for the philanthropy's active footsteps.

Rockefeller Health Goes International

Following the Sanitary Commission's southern campaign, its director, Wickliffe Rose, became head of the RF's new International Health Commission (referred to hereafter as the IHB, the abbreviation for its post-1916 name), and was charged with expanding hookworm work overseas. Rose and his colleagues had strategized a worldwide hookworm assault as early as 1911, when they enlisted the State Department to send out questionnaires about the presence and severity of hookworm disease to dozens of U.S. consular officers stationed overseas.[26] Rose began his new mission in 1913 by consulting British colonial authorities in London, and then traveled to the Middle and Far East, as well as to the English Caribbean. Although he relied on his staff for initial site visits to Central America, there was little doubt that Latin America and the Caribbean—long a focus of U.S. political and economic interests—would be a key locale for hookworm activity.

The IHB's first foreign undertaking was a small-scale hookworm campaign in British Guiana in 1914, designed to minimize publicity should this trial run prove problematic. Although colonial administrators were reluctant to build privies and improve sanitation, the campaign was deemed a success and extended to other Caribbean settings, the Far East, and Latin America, eventually reaching fifty-two countries and twenty-nine islands.[27]

Unlike the Sanitary Commission—which bypassed local government authorities that lacked capacity—the IHB adhered to a "policy always to work with Governments."[28] This cooperative arrangement, based on the "conviction that public health is essentially a function of government,"[29] meant that the RF pledged its role as a "partner, but not a patron."[30] From early on, RF initiatives began with surveys of local conditions, consultations with U.S. envoys, and preliminary discussions with government authorities.[31]

The pragmatic Rose articulated the IHB's operating principles, as developed in its formative years, in a 1922 memo. First, for reasons of efficiency, IHB projects were to work with "agencies that are grounded in the life and traditions of the people." Second, if new agencies were necessary, they should be "made to graft" onto existing ones, giving them "official standing," power, and responsibilities. Third, all efforts were made to focus attention on local agencies—not the IHB—so that they "may be made to grow into strong permanent agencies for the cure and prevention of all preventable diseases." Finally, host countries should "in the end assume the burden of responsibility" for disease eradication activities, with the IHB helping to organize and give prominence to local forces.[32]

These principles differentiated the IHB from colonial health agencies in conveying greater sensitivity to existing institutional cultures and giving credit and support to local agencies.[33] The principles also presumed a direct and colossal influence for the IHB. If the experience on the ground demonstrated a far more intricate and coequal process of give-and-take, the early diplomatic benefits of the RF's international philanthropy—which helped improve the image of the United States across the globe[34]—entrenched a semi-mythic status for the RF's operating principles.

Public health proved an ideal area for Rockefeller philanthropy. Aimed at the larger good, involving professional elites, government authorities, and impoverished communities, and applying the fruits of scientific knowledge to social problems, public health allowed John D. Rockefeller Sr. and his close circle of advisors to fulfill multiple goals at once: advancing developing economies, promoting international goodwill, improving productivity, and preparing the state and professionals for modern development. While no grand plan existed in the minds of these philanthropists, the new public health was, as Elizabeth Fee has argued, "largely shaped by a small number of men in a position to marshal considerable social, intellectual, and financial resources."[35]

In conceptualizing public health in disease terms, the RF model gave preference to medical and technical measures to prevent and treat the biological dimensions of health problems, at the expense of socio-political explanations and solutions. Based on the germ theory of disease and on findings from the new fields of bacteriology, parasitology, and helminthology, this narrowed framework emphasized the control of individual diseases, with particular microorganisms causing particular diseases and specific tools designed to combat them. In other contexts, especially in Europe, a more social understanding of public health, prevalent before the advent of germ theory, became integrated with the new sciences of public health. Vaccines could thus be employed in a broader effort to improve housing, hygiene, sanitation, employment, and overall living conditions. But the RF's advocacy of public health advancement disease by disease meant that social understandings and approaches were secondary to technical and biological ones.

Hookworm control, for example, entailed drug treatment and education stressing personal responsibility for prevention through shoe-wearing and latrine construction. That the disease was rooted in rural poverty and could be permanently addressed through improved living conditions, including indoor plumbing and an adequate sewage system, did not form part of the Rockefeller credo. The role of government health authorities, according to this formulation, was to oversee the dissemination of public health's technical tools, not to participate in social reform efforts.

Upon the creation of the RF in 1913, Rockefeller confidant Gates had proposed that the new IHB's mission be tripartite: extending to other countries the work of eradicating hookworm and other ailments, promoting public sanitation, and spreading the "knowledge of scientific medicine,"[36] and each IHB activity served a specific purpose in reaching these goals. Because reducing the overall burden of death and disease was not its highest priority, the IHB chose diseases that had a rapidly demonstrable, technical, inexpensive cure or "correction" and that served, in Rose's words, "as a means to a greater end" of awakening grassroots interest in disease control and enlisting government participation in public health.[37] In this scheme, the hookworm campaign worked as a "preliminary survey" of health and disease conditions, a "demonstration of cure and prevention," and an introduction to the role and value of public health.[38] This role for hookworm differentiated it from campaigns that might have required years of investment in underlying living and working conditions, as for example, the prevention of tuberculosis.[39] Costly projects necessitating construction of water and sewage systems, such as diarrhea control, were likewise not considered to offer the effective public health publicity that hookworm campaigns garnered.

Under Rose, hookworm work became the hallmark Rockefeller international health activity, not because of hookworm's epidemiological importance but because of the campaign's simplicity and utility. Rose pointedly proposed nearly a dozen steps through which a hookworm campaign could modernize a nation's health system. One step was setting up "demonstration" projects in a particular area as a competitive spur to action in other areas, as had been attempted in the United States. Another was to train locals and place them in positions of responsibility "as fast as warranted." Yet another step was ensuring that hookworm activities were "cooperative," requiring contributions from local, regional, and national governments as well as the RF.[40] Hookworm infestation rates were no longer the yardstick of effectiveness; instead, the host country's commitment to public health became the philanthropy's gauge of success.

Belief in the hookworm campaign as a tool to excite interest in public health and enable international cooperation did not even require belief in its importance as a disease, let alone belief in its eradicability. Hookworm cheerleader Rose barely mentioned the disease when setting the IHB's goals of extending hookworm work to Latin America in 1915:

> The work for relief and control of [hookworm] . . . is to be regarded merely as an entering wedge toward a larger and more permanent service in the medical field. It will lead inevitably to the consideration of the whole question of medical education, the organization of systems of public health and the training of men for the public health service. . . . [T]he South American people have come to know us mainly as a people interested in our own business advancement. Such service as the Foundation has to render will tend to counteract the effect of the purely mercenary spirit and to establish a basis of real cooperation.[41]

Hookworm control, so important in engaging the participation of governments across the tropical belt—and in securing John D. Rockefeller's own interest in public health—was far from a pressing international health priority in an era when infant mortality rates soared as high as 500 deaths/1000 live births, and a range of infectious diseases raged. But it was hookworm that paved the way for the broader ends of Rockefeller philanthropy at home and abroad.

Hookworm was the first—and in many ways the ideal—Rockefeller disease campaign, but it was not the only disease pursued by the IHB. Beginning in 1915, the IHB was involved in several small malaria studies in Arkansas and Mississippi that evaluated the effectiveness of quinine medication and mosquito control measures such as window screens and swamp draining. With the adoption of Paris green as mosquito larvicide in the early 1920s, IHB malaria programs quickly expanded throughout the U.S. South and to Puerto Rico, Central America, Brazil, the Philippines, Palestine, and elsewhere, by this time focusing almost exclusively on mosquito control.[42] These efforts emphasized field research and training activities, with large-scale disease control measures in the background.[43]

Two campaign locales served as dramatic exceptions to this characterization. In Italy, the IHB (then IHD) joined pre-existing malaria control efforts in the 1920s and early 1930s.[44] After World War II, the RF returned to Sardinia with the United Nations Relief and Rehabilitation Administration to organize an antimalaria army of thousands of Sardinians to literally soak their island with the new insecticide DDT, effectively eradicating malaria (and communist political power) but not the *Anopheles* mosquito.[45] A similarly militaristic effort took place in Northeastern Brazil in 1939–41 where Dr. Frederick Soper—famed director of the IHD's yellow fever operations in Brazil, subsequently head of the PASB, and proponent of the WHO's Global Malaria Eradication campaign—joined with national authorities to eradicate the *Anopheles gambiae* mosquito which had been introduced from West Africa.[46] The extreme difficulties in fulfilling Soper's dream of species eradication through larvicides and insecticides (other than on islands and in places where particular mosquito species were newly resident) revealed the limitations of the RF's technical approach to malaria.[47]

By far the most visible and costly of the IHB's international health efforts was its campaign against yellow fever, begun at almost the same time as the malaria effort. A deadly mosquito-borne virus, in its urban form transmitted via the domestic mosquito vector *Aedes aegypti* (known at the time as *Stegomyia fasciata*), yellow fever had paid ominous visits to North and South American ports for hundreds of years, killing up to half of its victims—typically new migrants, who had no acquired immunity to the virus—from a painful hemorrhagic fever. [48] In 1878, Cuban physician Carlos Finlay had proposed that yellow fever was transmitted by the *Stegomyia* vector, a theory confirmed in 1900 in Havana by U.S. Army Surgeon Walter Reed and his associates.[49] These findings became the basis for a massive sanitary campaign by U.S. Colonel William Crawford Gorgas, chief sanitary officer for the Department of Cuba under U.S. occupation. Gorgas claimed responsibility for successively ridding occupied Havana and then the Panama Canal construction zone of yellow fever and malaria through fumigation, quarantine, isolation, and demolition.[50]

In 1914, Gorgas, by this time army surgeon-general, convinced Wickliffe Rose that the soon-to-be opened Panama Canal might facilitate the spread of yellow fever. Gorgas—who had contracted yellow fever at a Texas army base early in his career—believed that eradicating yellow fever would be a most promising task for the RF. Regarded as a grave threat to world commerce and offering a chance for Rockefeller scientists to showcase their expertise internationally, yellow fever served as an expensive exception to the IHB rule of reasonably priced programs with a ready cure. It was Rose's recognition of the global—not just local—implications of yellow fever eradication that led to this exception.

Rose took up Gorgas's challenge with gusto, innocent of the difficulties ahead.[51] Yellow fever's possibilities as a disease campaign were recognized beyond medical and commercial quarters. A Harvard archaeologist working in southern Mexico in the early 1920s shared Rose's enthusiasm, noting that the "great glory for [yellow fever's] reduced state belongs to the United States" and that the RF's "splendid organization" meant that "we may confidently await the final announcement that yellow fever has been stamped out forever. It will not be long in coming."[52]

Initially, the RF had considered that private companies, such as the United Fruit Company, might support yellow fever work, "which offers an immediate and direct benefit" to them.[53] Instead the RF decided to keep itself separate from U.S. business interests in Latin America once it became clear that an efficient campaign could be based on the destruction of mosquito larvae breeding sites. In 1916, the IHB constituted a Yellow Fever Commission headed by Gorgas to make a yellow fever reconnaissance trip through South America. The commission included Dr. Henry Rose Carter, who helped to develop the "key centers" theory, which led the RF to concentrate eradication efforts on cities that harbored endemic yellow fever, so-called seed beds of the disease. Despite the observations of Colombian and Brazilian doctors that yellow fever also existed in a sylvan form (known as "jungle yellow fever"),[54] Carter's theory focused the commission's travel—and subsequent eradication efforts—on urban locales suspected of being endemic yellow fever loci in Ecuador, Peru, Colombia, Venezuela, and Brazil. Following this criterion, the commission found that only the port of Guayaquil, Ecuador harbored yellow fever, and in 1918—after a delay due to the United States' entry into World War I—the IHB began a two-year disinfection campaign. Notwithstanding requests from both Guayaquil officials and commission observers that the IHB's efforts include the improvement of water supply and sewage, the campaign was aimed solely at mosquito extermination.[55]

With equal single-mindedness, the IHB's yellow fever campaign moved on to Colombia, Peru, and Central America, as well as to Brazil, where epidemic yellow fever was initially believed to be more problematic in the north than the south. The disease's unexpected reemergence in Rio de Janeiro in the late 1920s—combined with a new government committed to modernization—resulted in a massive two-decade long RF–Brazilian yellow fever campaign that eventually extended into rural areas.[56] But in 1920 the principal remaining focus of yellow fever—and the one that posed the greatest danger to the United

States due to its proximity and the volume of migration and trade—was believed to be Mexico.

The Role of Training

By the early 1920s, the IHB was running hookworm, yellow fever, and malaria campaigns throughout Latin America and the Caribbean and in the Far East, and expanding its research and application capacities in several other areas. Closely linked to these public health campaigns was the RF's role in graduate public health education, a realm of training which the RF itself had essentially founded. The lessons of the Sanitary Commission had been clear: there existed no pool of health officials prepared to garrison the front lines of public health in the South of the United States. Rose had found that most local health officers were untrained, part-time political appointees who were primarily concerned with curative medical care. He concluded that for the IHB to operate successfully, it needed to create a new profession of public health with institutions that were independent from those of clinical medicine.

In the 1910s, the RF had begun funding the modernization of medical training in the United States, acting on the findings of the 1910 "Flexner Report." Southern educator Abraham Flexner (brother of Rockefeller Institute scientist Simon), in a report written for the Carnegie Foundation for the Advancement of Teaching, had called for a transformation of medicine following the principles of a full-time, research-oriented faculty, close ties to a university and hospital, adequate laboratory facilities, and a scientifically prepared student body.[57] The RF offered generous grants to so-called A-schools, such as Harvard and Johns Hopkins, to adapt to these principles, leaving many other medical schools to wither.

In late 1913, Abraham Flexner, who served as secretary of the RF's General Education Board, was asked to head an RF committee on public health education. After several years of debate and discussion among Flexner, Rose, and a handful of other leaders in the fields of sanitation, preventive medicine, and philanthropy, including Dr. William Welch, dean of Johns Hopkins Medical School and an IHB trustee, in 1916 the RF chose to back the Johns Hopkins University as the site of the first school of public health in the U.S. RF donations enabled the founding of similar schools at Harvard in 1922 and the University of Toronto in 1925 (opened in 1927). These three schools trained the vast majority of IHB/D officers as well as hundreds of Latin American public health and nursing fellows whom the RF sponsored over the decades.

Despite Rose's intention to separate and elevate the status of public health, its role relative to medicine remained ambiguous, and the organization of both the RF and the new schools of public health reflected these tensions. The flagship Johns Hopkins School of Hygiene and Public Health—like the schools that followed—emphasized medically-oriented research rather than combining the social and medical sciences; early on, more practice-based units in areas such as health education, epidemiology and public health administration were far outnumbered by laboratory-oriented pathology and physiology departments which emphasized disciplines such as helminthology, parasitology, bacteriology, and chemical hygiene. This organization along medical science specialties seemed to suggest that public health was subsidiary to medicine.[58]

The relationship between medicine and public health was ill-defined in both the RF's New York office and in the field. The IHB/D relied on the existence of "trained medical men" in the countries where it operated, yet it was organizationally separate from the RF's Division of Medical Education until 1951 when the two entities were merged into the Division of Medicine and Public Health.[59] As evidenced in Latin America, field officers often complained about the dearth of well-trained medical graduates, but the IHB/D sought to distance itself from medical education concerns, concentrating instead on those competent graduates eligible for its own fellowships.[60] Still, at least some RF leaders held that receptivity to public health measures "might be stabilized through improvements in medical education" in Latin America.[61]

Beginning with RF officer Richard Pearce's survey of Brazilian medical schools in 1916, visiting RF experts made periodic assessments of medical education in a variety of Latin American countries.[62] Although officers Pearce, Alan Gregg, and their colleagues wrote detailed accounts of their visits—critiquing heavy reliance on clinicians as medical school faculty members, overcrowded classrooms, excessive French influence, and an insufficient role for experimental research—the RF's involvement in Latin American medical education remained circumscribed until after World War II. The only Latin American medical school that the RF deemed worthy of assistance before this time was São Paulo's. Because São Paulo was, according to RF President Raymond Fosdick (1936–48), "progressive," likely to maintain improvements, and blessed with able leadership, it received a grant of nearly $1 million ($5.3 million in 2004 dollars) in the 1920s to carry out Flexnerian reforms.[63]

The RF's limited engagement was justified *ex post facto* by RF officer Robert Lambert's 1943 assessment that Latin Americans were already "universally" accepting of Western medicine and needed only to improve their medical schools' quality of teaching, facilities, and institutional affiliations. There was no need to eliminate proprietary, "diploma mill" medical schools because these were virtually nonexistent in Latin America.[64] Lambert was implicitly comparing the situation in Latin America to China, where the RF invested $45 million (well over $600 million in 2004 dollars) in the Peking Union Medical College between 1915 and 1949 to "introduce" Western medicine to a "pre-scientific" country.[65] Though no other institution in the world reached the same level of support, many North American, European, South Pacific, and Southeast Asian medical schools received RF funding while most Latin American schools were neglected.

Lambert's line of reasoning might have led the RF to invest in Latin American schools of public health instead of medical schools, but it supported only one such effort (although it did provide support to schools of nursing in Venezuela and Brazil).[66] Of the twenty-one schools of public health the RF sponsored outside North America, almost all were in central and western Europe (including the London School of Hygiene and Tropical Medicine, which trained health professionals from throughout the British Empire),[67] with São Paulo again selected as the lone Latin American site.[68] Marcos Cueto has argued that Brazil was selected over the more scientifically advanced Argentina because the RF preferred a country where there were fewer obstacles to the implementation of public health measures and where government institutions and medical elites would be most receptive.[69] RF officials also hoped that strengthened medical and public health schools in some Latin American countries would serve as magnets for students from neighboring countries; however, it soon became apparent that most students pursuing advanced training chose to go to the United States (where fellowships were available) rather than to neighboring countries.[70]

But the RF did not ignore Latin American public health training: it oriented its investment to individuals rather than to institutions. Each year it awarded dozens of public health fellowships to Latin American doctors, sanitary engineers, and nurses to study in the United States and return to their home countries to fill key positions. Between 1917 and 1950, 2,500 public health and nursing fellows were sponsored (including approximately 650 U.S. fellows), with some 450 fellows from Latin America and the Caribbean, including 68 Mexican public health fellows.[71] It turned out that this *was* a multimillion-dollar investment in Latin American public health education (to Mexico totaling several hundred thousand dollars—almost $3 million in 2004 dollars), and various observers from both the U.S. and Mexico considered the RF and other fellowship programs to be the most successful component of U.S.–Latin American cooperation.[72] As we shall see, it was these fellows who managed the relationship between the RF and Mexico, variously serving as marriage counselors, interlocutors, loyal offspring, rebels, and mature admixtures of these roles.

By the time of the IHD's dismantling in 1951, it had operated in over ninety countries with activities to combat diseases, educate professionals, and modernize and institutionalize government commitment to public health. It had organized campaigns and carried out research on hookworm, malaria, yellow fever, tuberculosis, typhus, influenza, yaws, schistosomiasis, and other ailments in the field and the laboratory. It had posted scores of its own health personnel in dozens of countries for years at a time. It had helped to educate tens of thousands of health workers at training stations throughout the world and through fellowships to the United States. It had supported numerous local health efforts by running rural health demonstrations and investing in local institutions. It had been an active participant in scientific conferences and international organizations. In sum, the RF was involved in all aspects of public health: ideas, theory, research, professional training, practice, implementation, organization, and institution building. As the only health agency truly operating internationally until the founding of the WHO in 1948, it helped to shape global public health to a greater extent than any other organization of its day.

The United States and Public Health's International Stage

The RF was by no means the only international health player of the early twentieth century, but it had by far the widest purview. Colonial health agencies restricted their work to colonial possessions; prestigious medical institutes, such as France's Institut Pasteur and the Liverpool School of Tropical Medicine, for the most part followed these colonial routes (in both cases the exception involving research activities in Brazil).[73] The PASB (founded in 1902) spent its first decades focused on sanitary agreements in the Americas. The OIHP (1907) served mostly as a clearinghouse for health statistics and epidemiologic surveillance.[74] The LNHO (1923), founded out of an effective postwar epidemic commission, worked mainly in Europe. Major North American philanthropies founded in the 1920s and 1930s, such as the Ford, Guggenheim, and Kellogg Foundations, had neither the reach nor the scope of the RF until much later. The RF was little accompanied in its worldwide enterprise, but it risked association with U.S. economic and political interests, which might have limited its international operating theater.

One of the reasons the RF escaped significant controversy internationally was precisely its assertion of independence from U.S. business and government.[75] While public health activities undoubtedly played a role in securing the United States' economic and political foothold overseas, the RF's modus operandi differed markedly from that of other U.S. interests.[76] Until World War II and well beyond, the U.S. government's overseas health efforts were closely tied to military occupation—for example, the U.S. Army Board's attempts to keep its men healthy in the Philippines[77] and ridding occupied Havana and the Panama Canal Zone of yellow fever and malaria[78]—and protecting commerce, through the USPHS's instrumental role in the founding and leadership of the PASB's early focus on sanitary treaties to prevent the epidemic interruption of trade.[79] All the while, more pressing—and endemic—problems for local populations were overlooked.[80]

During the early twentieth century, U.S. enterprises in Latin America and elsewhere—such as the United Fruit Company—also employed public health measures in order to maximize profits[81] by reducing absenteeism, improving worker productivity, protecting investments, and staving off unrest.[82] The limits to this self-interested approach are exemplified in the career of tropical nutrition specialist Dr. William Deeks, originally from Canada. Deeks bridged the worlds of military and company medicine, spending almost a decade as clinic director for the Ancon Hospital—which treated employees of the Panama Canal Zone— and then serving as general manager of the United Fruit Company's Medical Department for fifteen years.[83] Deeks found that an adequate diet was instrumental in preventing tropical diseases such as malaria and hookworm. However, he considered malnutrition a problem of bad individual choices rather than a consequence of poor living conditions and low salaries, circumstances that United Fruit was in a position to improve but did not.[84]

Though RF administrators interacted with the medical officers of U.S. companies operating internationally, they were careful to keep their activities separate. When in 1923 Deeks requested 2,000 reprints of the IHB's hookworm prevention pamphlets suitable for "our employees in the Tropics," the IHB office sent only one copy, requiring United Fruit to print the pamphlets under its own name.[85] Deeks complimented the IHB as the "most reliable source of information . . . [for] the class of people with whom we have to deal,"[86] but the IHB director remained mindful of not appearing to work with, or for, the company.

Though the RF shared many of the same concerns and worldviews with both government and private industry, their interests were not identical. Although its own trustees included powerful businessmen, the RF sought to transcend the private sector's preoccupation with improving the health of laborers and safeguarding trade, and distanced itself from U.S. military efforts.

The RF took skillful advantage of the ease with which it could pioneer and experiment with new projects, sometimes over the course of many years. It always worked through national governments, but the RF and IHB remained accountable to only a handful of trustees, and its officers had the ability to negotiate, quickly assign funds, and launch work in new fields, suffering few public repercussions in cases of failure.

Of course the RF's claim of independence did not preclude collaboration with the U.S. government. From early on, RF administrators consulted with the State Department, U.S. ambassadors, and American military doctors before they began projects in new countries, and U.S. consuls and military officers often served as public health informants to the IHB in far-flung places. State Department officials sometimes facilitated the IHB's contact with foreign government officials and, in turn, asked to be kept closely apprised of the IHB's work.[87] At times, RF representatives served as ersatz U.S. envoys, accomplishing, according to one American retiree in Mexico in 1922, "more than all our diplomacy."[88]

The RF mindfully limited these associations, at least publicly. In 1925, U.S. Ambassador to Mexico James Sheffield urged RF President George Vincent to expand health activities in Mexico since its government was unable to "cope wisely or effectively." Moreover, RF work "would add to a better feeling between the U.S. and Mexico."[89] While Vincent assured Sheffield that the RF was "anxious at all times to have the representatives of our Government familiar with what we are doing," it would be embarrassing to both if the RF appeared nationalistic.[90] In reply to Sheffield's insistence that RF efforts should be widely publicized to temper Mexican anti-Americanism, Vincent explained that this was not the way the RF operated.[91]

In later years the RF and government collaborated more directly. Before and during World War II, for example, the U.S. State Department invited philanthropic organizations to further cultural ties with Latin American countries in order to secure support for the Allied Powers, a sphere of activity the RF took to heart.[92] The RF's Mexican Agricultural Program—which launched the Green Revolution—began in 1943 largely at the urging of U.S. Vice President Henry Wallace.[93] These ties between government and philanthropy served the purposes of both entities, furthering the RF's reach and promoting U.S. interests.

Public health offered a new opportunity for a young power like the United States to showcase itself internationally, generating goodwill in place of gunboat diplomacy and demonstrating a new American scientific expertise in disease control to recipient countries and European rivals.[94] Washington was not disposed to do this. Notwithstanding its involvement with the PASB, the U.S. government paid little heed to the cooperative dimensions of international health until the 1940s.[95] In the 1920s—though hardly isolationist in economic and military terms—the United States refused to join the League of Nations, giving ample room for the RF to serve as both liaison and patron to the LNHO and to substitute for the League in the Americas. Even in the 1930s, when President Franklin D. Roosevelt pursued a "Good Neighbor" policy with Mexico and the rest of Latin America, the U.S. government was not yet prepared to involve itself in public health abroad. The RF easily filled this space. Indeed, it served as the United States' international health arm for almost thirty years.

The Mexican Revolution and Public Health

Mexico, the first country to undergo a revolution in the twentieth century, represented an enormous opportunity for the fostering of public health in the "developing" world. By no means did the country require a partner for this endeavor, nor was the RF the obvious choice. The decades preceding the 1910–20 Revolution had laid the groundwork for modern public health. In the late nineteenth century, a new scientifically oriented class receptive to European knowledge and practices backed the introduction of sanitation, the systematic control of epidemic outbreaks, and related activities. This was a self-serving effort, with public health measures applied in cities and specific neighborhoods where civic elites chose to mobilize resources. But the rest of the population

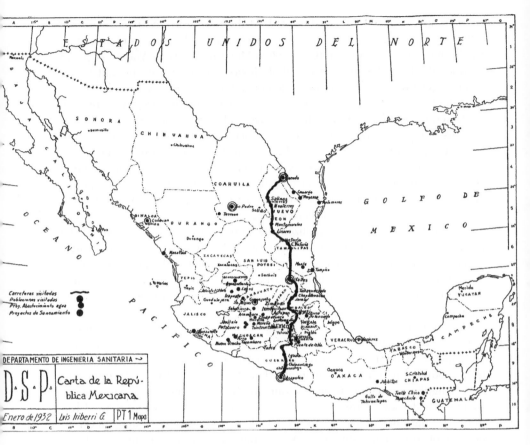

Figure 1.2. Map of Mexico, Department of Sanitary Engineering, DSP, 1932. From José Siurob, *Memoria del Departamento de Salubridad Pública 1935–1936* (México, D.F.: DSP, 1937). Courtesy of the Secretaría de Salud, Mexico City, Mexico.

could not remain ignored indefinitely. Repeated outbreaks of typhus, yellow fever, cholera, malaria, smallpox, and other diseases revealed the deplorable health and social conditions in which the majority of Mexicans lived.[96] Growing public and professional demand for improved health conditions pushed both federal and local governments to act, and late nineteenth- and early twentieth-century Mexico witnessed the beginnings of public health campaigns, legislation, and infrastructure. The Revolution interrupted but did not overturn these developments, and by 1920 public health efforts resumed.

Mexico's modern state began to emerge some sixty volatile years after it obtained its independence from Spain in 1821.[97] In the 1820s, Mexico lived through almost continuous warfare and an aborted return to Spanish control, followed by a string of rapid presidential successions in the 1830s and near anarchy in the 1840s. Then came the so-called Mexican-American War of 1846–48 in which the United States seized half of Mexico's territory.[98] In the mid 1850s, a liberal government came to power, led by Benito Juárez, Mexico's first Indian (Zapotec) president (1857–63 and 1867–72). The country's 1857 Constitution weakened the Catholic Church, the military, and regional powerbrokers. These reforms were interrupted by the puppet dictatorship of Emperor Ferdinand Maximilian Joseph (1863–67), Archduke of Austria, who was installed by France to recover Mexico's debts to Europe. After Maximilian's assassination, the liberals returned to power, and were faced with economic problems and the stalling of reform. Juárez sought to replace the country's long tradition of Catholic charity with the public provision of social services; however, this effort resulted in an arrested centralism that marginalized the Church more than it extended the reach of the state. It was the dictatorial reign of Porfirio Díaz—the Porfiriato—which lasted from 1876, when Díaz was initially elected to the presidency, until 1911, when he was ousted from office, that at one and the same time provided continuity for Mexico's economic and institutional modernization and set the stage for its violent revolution.[99]

Though Díaz professed belief in Mexico's economic sovereignty, his administration's policies and the stability of his regime encouraged sizeable foreign investments in mining, railroads, oil, real estate, banking, and other industries.[100] Sovereign ground was maintained not by excluding foreign investors but by forcing them to compete against one another for markets and concessions. By the first decade of the twentieth century, foreign capital represented two thirds of total investment in Mexico, with U.S. interests comprising almost 40 percent of foreign investment.[101] Almost half of all U.S. investment in Latin America went to Mexico, the only country in the region in which U.S. investment exceeded that of the British.[102] Foreign investment concentrated on the export of raw materials. Between 1877 and 1911 Mexico's manufactured goods never exceeded 5 percent of exports, while gold and silver comprised between ⅓ and ½ of exports, trailed closely by agriculture and livestock exports.[103] In total, the value of exports during the course of the Porfiriato increased by some 600 percent, with tremendous profits accruing to foreign and domestic investors. Oil became particularly attractive in the late Porfiriato, with a major oil discovery in Veracruz in 1910 and exports climbing steadily during the Revolution. These developments had little bearing on the structure of the labor force. From the mid 1890s through the early 1920s, industrial workers stayed at approximately 15 percent of the total labor force and agricultural workers at just under 70 percent.[104]

The Porfiriato's economic and social policies were shaped by a new technocratic intellectual class. Díaz surrounded himself with a group of "positivists" (in Spanish, *científicos*)—young scientists, engineers, and educators—who believed that

Mexico's scarce resources should be concentrated on the country's rational and productive Spanish-descended elite. As prosperity came to this appointed set, the *científicos* believed, it would gradually extend to mestizos (those of mixed European and indigenous descent) and eventually to the indigenous population. Influenced variously by evolutionism, eugenics, and statism, the positivists argued that liberal democracy would evolve simultaneously to economic modernization.[105] Such confidence raised the expectations of Mexico's small but growing middle and industrial classes who eagerly awaited Díaz's promises.

Under the Porfiriato, record economic growth translated into almost 15,000 miles of railroad tracks, a communications network, and new public works and cultural institutions for the urban elite, while social conditions were deteriorating in diverse ways. Though Mexico's social, economic, and political inequalities—characterized by tremendous polarization between landholding elites of mostly European descent and land-tied mestizo and indigenous peasants—originated in the era of Spanish colonialism, new configurations of social stratification developed in the late nineteenth century.

The Díaz government oversaw large-scale expropriation of communally owned free villages in central and southern Mexico, typically involving land which had increased in value following the construction of railroads. As a result, the economic circumstances of agricultural laborers worsened markedly, though not uniformly. In densely populated central Mexico, most former communal landowners were forced to become tenant sharecroppers and temporary laborers on large haciendas, where they experienced sharp declines in the real value of their wages over the course of the Porfiriato. In the south, the former owners of expropriated land were joined by displaced laborers from the north and center of Mexico as debt peons and forced laborers, subject to extremely repressive hacienda owners. While those communal landowners who retained their village property were better off in relative terms, they were also subject to increased prices for food and necessities imposed by hacienda owners, mine companies, and local bosses. In the north and center of the country, free laborers had a greater opportunity for mobility as hired technicians and supervisors, but their employment prospects became more precarious after 1900.[106]

Over the same period, along the country's northern border, frontiersmen and indigenous communities lost not only their property but also the political independence they had enjoyed before railroads and industrial development integrated the region into the larger Mexican economy. By the late Porfiriato, material and political deprivation extended further to the middle and industrial classes, when investment-driven inflation and tax increases began to cut into wages—further exacerbated by the 1908 depression—and Diaz's regional bosses began to restrict access to political patronage. Economic modernization came at a steep price to diverse segments of Mexican society.

Disease and death rates reflected these economic trends. According to contemporary data—which were collected almost exclusively in urban areas and

Table 1.1. Death rate/1000, 1911, cities with 400,000–700,000 inhabitants

Madrid	Amsterdam	Baltimore	Mexico City	Madras	Cairo
23.00	12.40	18.52	42.30	39.51	40.15

Source: Alberto Pani, *Hygiene in Mexico: A Study of Sanitary and Educational Problems*, trans. Ernest L. de Gogorza (New York and London: Knickerbocker Press, 1917), table I, 4–5.

which undoubtedly captured only a portion of deaths among the poorest sectors—Mexico's infant mortality increased after 1900, a period during which many countries experienced declines in infant mortality.[107] In 1900, more than one third of the population was estimated to be seriously ill in the course of a year.[108] In 1902, Mexico City's overall life expectancy at birth was twenty-eight years,[109] among the lowest recorded in the world, and its crude mortality rate was higher than that of almost every city that collected vital statistics, including Madras and Cairo (see table 1.1).[110] The published—albeit flawed—mortality statistics of the day cited Mexico City's leading causes of death from 1904 to 1912 as digestive diseases (causing one third of deaths), respiratory diseases (one fifth), and general diseases (one fifth); these included tuberculosis, typhus, smallpox, measles, whooping cough, and syphilis.[111] While the disease rates themselves are unreliable, we may take greater stock in the ailments that concerned contemporary observers: gastrointestinal and respiratory diseases were preventable through known measures aimed at improving nutrition, sanitation, and dwelling conditions, measures which were increasingly viewed as the duty of the state.

Urban living conditions were deplorable for all but the most privileged classes. Díaz and his *científicos* had passed the country's first sanitary code in 1891 mandating indoor plumbing and sewage for new buildings, and in March 1900, Diaz himself proudly inaugurated a modern water supply and drainage system for Mexico City designed to stem flooding and cesspools. But only wealthy districts enjoyed such benefits.[112] In working-class areas, people typically lived in crowded, poorly ventilated, unfinished, windowless, one-room shacks or tenements and slept on straw mats on the ground. Sewage waters, food waste, animal and human corpses, and other sources of filth combined into a putrid stew that traveled the streets of Mexico City, worsened by continuous flooding during the rainy season.[113] As Alberto Pani, an engineer, bureaucrat, and businessman friendly with Standard Oil who later became finance minister, put it, Mexico City in the early twentieth century was "assuredly, the most unhealthful city of the whole world."[114] While Pani may not have had evidence at hand to substantiate such an assertion, his statement probably seemed accurate to anyone familiar with the streets of Mexico's capital.

Deteriorating social conditions, foreign exploitation, and decades of favoritism under the Porfiriato were the main factors leading to the Mexican

Revolution, according to many classic accounts.[115] Some scholars suggest that the revolution was not so much social as political, sparked more by struggles for power and favor within the upper and middle classes than by conflict between the lower and upper classes.[116] Others recognize a combination of these factors: Diaz's alienation of domestic forces as varied as dispossessed landholders, northern frontiersmen, and small-time entrepreneurs was exacerbated by his policy of pitting U.S. investors against Europeans, which backfired, particularly angering U.S. investors.[117] All, however, have agreed that the revolution mobilized the middle class, industrial laborers, and large numbers of peasants from distinct regions. Cross-class alliances and enormous sacrifices put these distinct sectors in a position to make legitimate claims on the revolutionary state. Whether the revolution fundamentally transformed Mexico or marked a substantial continuity of its prerevolution capitalist economy, the state that resulted had to answer to a wider range of domestic players than before the conflict. In terms of Mexico's economic relations with foreign parties, revolutionary rhetoric of economic nationalism long preceded its realization.[118]

The conflict itself began in 1910 with Francisco Madero's aborted and then successful overthrow of Díaz, followed by Madero's election to the presidency in October 1911. Confronted by various pro-Díaz mobilizations, Madero, in turn, was ousted and murdered in February 1913. In all, the revolution lasted over a decade, witnessing multiple leaders, assassinations, and a complex geography of bloody warfare. Among the most notable commanders were the colorful Pancho Villa with his northern division and, in the south-central region, Emiliano Zapata, who mobilized his fellow Morelos peasants with the Plan de Ayala's call to reclaim expropriated village lands from haciendas.

The ongoing contest for power left some places intact, others in utter ruin. Both the railroad and monetary systems were hit hard. Mexico City enjoyed periods of normalcy, especially under President Venustiano Carranza around 1916 when plans for the new government began to be organized in line with a series of concrete policy proposals. However, much government activity was all but suspended for a decade, and the federal government remained vulnerable long after the officially marked end of the revolution in 1920. In 1923–24, an uprising that threatened the presidency was quelled in Veracruz, later that decade the religiously inspired *Cristiada* rebellion in a group of central-western states was costly in terms of lives and resources, and regional skirmishes continued into the 1930s. In total, almost one million of Mexico's approximately 15 million inhabitants died in the conflict.

International rivalries added drama to the hostilities. *Caudillos* played foreign interests off one another, and various Mexican leaders used U.S. political and private business support to bolster their positions. The U.S. military invaded Mexico twice. The first time was in 1914 when U.S. forces occupied Veracruz as a pretense at mediation, claiming that Germans were supplying Mexico with munitions through this port of entry. U.S. President Woodrow

Wilson rationalized the invasion as good for both the "populist aspirations of the revolutionaries" under Carranza and for U.S. business, though undoubtedly the decision was anchored by U.S. business motives to protect Veracruz.[119] Veracruz was the hub of Mexican oil production and a key component of the flourishing export economy of the revolutionary years.[120] The second invasion was in 1916, when U.S. General John Pershing headed a 6,000-man army to chase vengefully after Pancho Villa after Villa and his men sacked Columbus, New Mexico.[121] This time, Wilson held that securing the southern border of the United States was more than enough justification for military action against Mexico. If he had not been running the risk of fighting two wars simultaneously—the United States' entry into World War I was partially incited by the March 1917 interception of German Foreign Minister Zimmerman's telegram calling for a Mexican-German alliance—Wilson's incursions might have turned into long-term U.S. intervention and occupation. The constant menaces and short-term encroachments were sufficient reminders of the United States' historic treatment of Mexico, fueling anti-Americanism and serving to unify most of the parties to the revolution around a pro-sovereignty rallying cry.[122]

The revolution involved shifting alliances of peasants, industrial workers, militant Catholics, landed gentry, and the industrial and petite bourgeoisie. Bourgeois groups may have ended up as the greatest beneficiaries of the revolution, but it was Mexican peasants—day laborers, sharecroppers, and debt peons who had seen their land expropriated—as well as small landowners who comprised the largest fighting force under a variety of *caudillos*. Zapata's famous cry for land and liberty, for example, rallied tens of thousands of Mexican men and women to take up arms in Morelos and adjacent regions.[123] Once they were armed, peasants, whether viewed as the main motor or only adherents to the revolution, wielded new power and made new demands on the state that could no longer be disregarded.

At the Constitutional Convention in Querétaro in 1917, both peasants and the middle classes sought to defend their interests, and the new Mexican constitution held promise for political democracy, land reform, education, improvements in social and working conditions, and economic sovereignty. The constitution also laid the groundwork for the development of public health, social security, and social welfare measures.[124]

The apparent losers were the agrarian gentry—whose land was slated for return and redistribution to the former peasant landowners—and foreign oil and mining companies, which were subject to Article 27's prohibition on the foreign ownership of subsoil rights. This measure called for a return to pre-Porfirian ownership conditions, when the subsoil had belonged first to the Spanish crown and subsequently to independent Mexico (it was only in 1884 that Porfirio Díaz had altered this tradition and invited foreign investment in oil).[125] Given oil's profitability—Mexico had become the world's second largest producer in 1920—and the support for sovereignty of most parties to the revolution, the oil-producing region of Veracruz would remain politically critical until the late 1930s when the international dispute over Article 27 reached a climax.

The revolution and new constitution marked a mixture of continuity and change in the areas of medicine and public health. The constitution's formulation of the principle of state responsibility for health with universal access to occupational and public health came with a particular mechanism for implementation: Article 73's creation of a new federal Department of Public Health,[126] with executive authority to implement decisions without the prior knowledge or consent of the president. The state's commitment to public health was clear: how and how quickly this commitment would be realized remained uncertain.

Medicine and Public Health before, during, and just after the Revolution

Many of the features of public health and the structure of medical practice in early twentieth-century Mexico had roots in the colonial era. The Spanish invasion and imperialist system had a devastating demographic impact on indigenous populations, with between one third and one half of inhabitants killed in the sixteenth century by warfare, forced labor, and disease. Epidemics of measles, smallpox, and other contagious diseases were enabled by the military, economic, and social aspects of the conquest.[127] While pre-Columbian societies in Mesoamerica experienced significant mortality from violence, occasional famine, and infectious diseases,[128] the conquest stood out because of the magnitude of death as well as the mortality differential between invaders and invaded.

There is also evidence that sanitary and living conditions—and the associated gastrointestinal and respiratory mortality—worsened markedly under Spanish imperialism. The Mexica (Aztecs), for example, kept the streets, markets, and plazas of their capital Tenochtitlán conspicuously clean through regular refuse collection and extensive sanitary and hygienic measures; waste water was carefully separated from the clean sources of Lake Texcoco, which surrounded the city.[129] After Tenochtitlán was destroyed and rebuilt as Mexico City under Spanish rule, Lake Texcoco was transformed into a giant cesspool: landfill projects, heavy canal commerce, and inadequate sewage disposal led to frequent flooding and contamination, with damaging health consequences.[130]

The colonial Spanish administration—together with the Catholic Church—carried European medical practices to the territories of New Spain, building over one hundred twenty hospitals, at which physical and mental ailments were treated.[131] The colonists imported the Spanish hierarchy of medical practitioners consisting of titled physicians serving urban elites; surgeons, phlebotomists, and apothecaries providing hands-on care to townsfolk; Catholic hospitals providing charity care; and traditional healers and unlicensed midwives attending the majority of the population. European healing practices—based on Greek and Roman teachings (particularly those of Hippocrates and Galen)—were designed to restore the balance of the body's fluids through adjustment of the four "humors": blood, yellow bile, black bile, and phlegm. Indigenous healers began to meld local traditions with humoral and herbalist practices from Europe.[132]

A fragmented and overlapping set of health authorities emerged in colonial Mexico. The three-member Protomedicato (medical board) was charged with issuing medical licenses and rooting out irregular and "racially impure" practitioners. The viceroy and religious agencies assumed medical authority during epidemic times.[133] In the late eighteenth century important cities, such as Veracruz and Mexico City, began to implement environmental and sanitary measures that were somewhat effective in controlling yellow fever and other disease outbreaks.[134]

These arrangements outlasted Spanish colonial rule. Between Mexican independence in 1821 and the revolution, the central government had a limited but growing role in the provision and regulation of health and welfare services. Formal responsibility rested in the hands of local governments, which exercised their powers unevenly, leaving most care to a range of healers. Traditional practitioners—men and women—continued to see the popular classes. European-style allopaths and homeopaths served mainly the wealthy classes of *criollos* and urban mestizos, although demand for their services, particularly in cities and towns, arose from all sectors.[135]

Elite physicians in the late nineteenth and early twentieth centuries studied at the National School of Medicine (now the Faculty of Medicine of the National Autonomous University of Mexico) and a handful of intermittently functioning regional universities. University-trained physicians founded the national journal, *Gaceta Médica de México*, in 1864 and the Mexican Academy of Medicine in 1870 and were active in the flourishing scientific societies of the period.[136] Regional medical associations were subsequently founded in Jalisco, Michoacán, and other states. The Mexican Medical Association was founded in 1919, offering professional prestige without addressing vocational matters.

Mexico, like most of Latin America, followed a French model of medical education well into the twentieth century. Indeed, starting with the founding of the Medical Sciences Establishment—precursor to the national Faculty of Medicine—in 1833, Mexican medical schools employed French texts and methods, and the medical community discussed and adapted French understandings of the medical themes, discoveries, and practices of the day.[137] The most brilliant and financially able students traveled to Paris for graduate training and returned as leading researchers and medical authorities. In the late nineteenth century, other influences, including German bacteriology and British, Danish, and U.S.

tropical medicine, gained a foothold,[138] though French ideas and practices retained their influential role in medicine and social welfare for several decades after the revolution.[139] For example, infant health and welfare services founded in the Porfiriato and the 1920s borrowed and adapted heavily from French notions of puericulture and eugenics.[140] As late as 1928, a prestigious new medical journal named *Pasteur* was founded in Mexico by the Franco-Mexican Medical Association, offering extensive coverage of French medical developments and French visitors to Mexico, as well as of the leading national public health and medical developments.[141]

Beginning in the colonial period and through the nineteenth century, physicians appealed to the state and sought the authority of their growing medical knowledge to squeeze out competing healing professions, including midwifery.[142] Notwithstanding the Porfiriato's support for scientific elitism, this effort met with little success.[143] Still, by the early twentieth century, titled physicians had gained more power, acceptance, and diffusion among popular sectors than before.[144] In 1910, there were some 2,500 allopaths (or one physician per 5,900 persons); this number rose to almost 7,000 (one physician per 2,900 persons) by 1940.[145]

Continuing their role from the colonial period, Catholic charity hospitals, together with a limited number of new municipal institutions, served the poor. Their concentration in Mexico City and other urban settings and their unfavorable reputation often made them a last resort for care. In times of illness or pregnancy, most of the urban and rural population relied upon traditional healers and midwives who resided in most communities. Depending on the setting, whether the inhabitants were mestizo or indigenous, and local customs and cultures, this popular medicine might include a mix or fusion of ideologies and practices, such as spiritism, magic and divination, herbalism, hot and cold influences (such as food and drugs that might induce fever or chills), natural and supernatural therapies, evil air healing, and home remedies.[146]

Health authorities in Mexico—as elsewhere in the nineteenth century—had few specific tools at their disposal beyond smallpox vaccination and environmental sanitation. It was principally during major epidemics, such as the 1833 cholera outbreak, that quarantine, fumigation, and isolation were carried out in the capital as well as in Guadalajara and other provincial cities.[147] National legislation passed in this period expanded state control over hygiene and morality[148]—as in an 1864 law mandating the inspection of prostitutes—but for the most part public health functioned locally or on an ad hoc basis. Appointed sanitary commissions were responsible for monitoring housing conditions, cemetery hygiene, and street and market cleanliness, following some of the practices of Aztec, Maya, Toltec, and other pre-Columbian cultures. While doctors began to discuss the local application of international medical developments, and several jurisdictions passed extensive health legislation long before the nation's first sanitary code in 1891, public health officials were rarely given the resources or the authority to utilize these tools to redress health problems.

By 1900, the larger towns began to employ some of the new bacteriologically based public health tools: sanitation, food and milk inspection, and diphtheria anti-toxin, as well as the sporadic collection of mortality statistics. These measures did not supplant more traditional functions such as housing reform and enforcement of wet nurse and prostitute regulations.[149] Public health officials in key ports, most notably Veracruz, who were particularly concerned with outbreaks of plague, yellow fever, cholera, and other epidemic diseases, wielded substantial implementation powers, and in turn faced considerable popular resistance.[150] While a handful of state-level authorities also assumed such responsibilities, public health in rural Mexico received little routine attention, although certain national campaigns against smallpox and plague were able to reach even remote villages.[151] For the most part, it was Mexico City and a few provincial capitals that experienced incipient public health efforts.

At a national level, responsibility for public health resided in the Superior Council of Public Health, founded in 1841 as a consulting agency to the federal government.[152] The council's permanent jurisdiction covered only Mexico City; even during epidemics, the council was not empowered to act outside the capital except in response to requests for assistance. The 1857 Constitution restricted the council's authority so that it would not infringe upon the sovereignty of states and municipalities, many of which had their own public health councils.[153] The 1891 sanitary code expanded the federal purview to include ports and borders, but it was unable to overturn the decentralized structure of routine public health functions.[154] While President Díaz praised his administration's public health accomplishments, the press repeatedly mocked the council as ineffectual and recommended that it be disbanded.[155]

Nonetheless, as Ana María Carrillo has abundantly demonstrated, over the course of the Porfiriato the purview of the Superior Council of Public Health expanded considerably. From 1885 to 1914 its president was Dr. Eduardo Liceaga, a revered public health leader, who reorganized the council's responsibilities to include routine vaccination, the study of epidemics, and urban sanitation, and who oversaw the nation's first sanitary census.[156] By 1904, the council had six permanent members and over 6,000 employees, many of whom had received specialized training.[157] The federal government organized a bacteriological laboratory along European lines and supported Liceaga's extended visit to Europe in 1887 to study urban sanitation systems and to learn about Louis Pasteur's rabies vaccination (announced in 1885) at the Institut Pasteur in Paris. Upon his return to Mexico, Liceaga oversaw the implementation of Pasteur's methods, and within just a few years thousands of Mexicans had been vaccinated in the capital's anti-rabies institute.[158] After 1900 the council increased the enforcement of measures such as mandatory smallpox vaccination, the firing of employees with tuberculosis, and the isolation of schoolchildren with infectious diseases. All of these efforts took place mainly in urban settings.[159]

The council's direct assistance in the control of epidemics also expanded in this period. An outbreak of plague in the port of Mazatlán in 1902 induced state authorities to cede full control to the council for the first time in its history; the campaign inaugurated the application of new bacteriological and tropical medicine findings, and the council's success in combating plague made this a model for future federally led epidemic campaigns.[160] Liceaga was lauded throughout the Americas for overseeing the elimination of yellow fever from Veracruz after a 1903–4 epidemic through a combination of sanitary measures, isolation of the sick, disinfection, and petrol-based insecticides.[161] By 1914, even the *New York Times* had to recognize that "authorities of Mexico have given considerable attention to the study of sanitation and preventive [*sic*] medicine." Reflecting longstanding U.S. fears about Mexico's health conditions, the article lamented, "less progress has been made in obtaining the co-operation of the people in the enforcement of health laws than in almost any other part of the civilized world."[162]

An area in which prerevolutionary Mexican public health authorities were particularly active was international health organizations, most prominently in the Americas. Mexican professionals participated in virtually every Latin American and international congress on scientific and social matters starting in the late nineteenth century, frequently hosting such conferences. Mexico joined the American Public Health Association in 1892, Eduardo Liceaga became the Association's first Latin American President in 1896, and the association held its annual meeting in Mexico City in 1892 and again in 1906.[163] The call for the American republics to organize along sanitary lines took place at the Second International Conference of American States held in Mexico City in January 1902, and under Liceaga's representation, Mexico became one of seven founding members of the International (Pan American) Sanitary Bureau in December of that year. Liceaga was a confidant of the head of the bureau (U.S. Surgeon-General Walter Wyman), and he was closely involved in shaping the PASB's direction in its first decade. Liceaga's words held significant sway in Washington, and he was instrumental in pressuring the United States to sign the 1905 Sanitary Convention of the American Republics.[164] In the early twentieth century, Mexico was also active in European-based efforts. It was a frequent presence at nineteenth-century international sanitary conferences and an early signatory to the Paris-based OIHP.[165] In medical matters, too, Mexico was eager to sign onto international developments. Mexico became one of the first countries to formally adopt Jacques Bertillon's system of disease classification with national representation at the 1900 meeting in Paris to revise the International Classification of Diseases.

On the eve of the revolution, then, Mexican public health was a study in contrasts. Elites and a small middle class had begun to enjoy the fruits of new medical and sanitation developments, particularly in urban settings. But most of the population lived under public health conditions comparable to those they had endured during the colonial period. Outside of the capital, implementation of routine sanitary measures was left largely in local hands: some municipal governments took these responsibilities very seriously; most, however, had few resources and little power to act. National authorities in the late Porfiriato strongly supported modern medicine and public health,[166] but other than in a handful of locales, these activities reached most of the populace only sporadically in the form of campaigns against epidemics. While Mexico exhibited leadership in international health matters, at a national level few legally enforceable sanitary mechanisms existed.

During the years of the revolution, health conditions only worsened, exacerbated by famine, untreated epidemics, and deteriorating sanitary conditions. The 1917 Constitution raised expectations for addressing such problems. The new Department of Public Health (Departamento de Salubridad Pública; DSP) reported directly to the president. It federalized responsibility for public health and enabled health authorities to act independently, unlike its precursor, the Superior Council of Public Health (which continued in existence until 1925, largely as a research body).[167] Dr. José María Rodríguez, a military general, advisor to Presidents Madero and Carranza, and vocal advocate of the new department, was named its first director.[168] Almost immediately, Rodríguez—who had succeeded Liceaga as director of the Superior Council of Public Health— expanded the federal government's activities by organizing a series of mobile health brigades to meet pressing concerns over smallpox, typhus, malaria, rabies, and other problems, as well as the devastating influenza pandemic of 1918–19.[169] Routine administration of vaccines, infectious disease control, clean water and sanitation, and food hygiene initially remained under local authorities, who, for the most part, were short of resources.[170]

Despite the optimism generated by the new constitution and the waning of the most unstable and bellicose period of the revolution, Mexico in 1920 was a war-devastated land, plagued by internal divisions strapped for funds, diplomatically unrecognized by its largest trading partner, the United States, and faced with the immense psychological and physical task of reconstruction.

Beyond creating the DSP, the revolution poised the country for more progress than it could pledge according to a specific timetable or set of services. National control of health meant the possibility of sanitary improvement and the development of public health institutions and services, as well as obligatory smallpox vaccination and other features of a "sanitary dictatorship."[171] The immense loss of life during the revolution focused attention on the urgency of public health measures, particularly those aimed at reducing infant mortality. The needed expertise, personnel, and resources began to materialize in the early 1920s, when the DSP benefited from a budget increase, launched an ambitious training effort for public health personnel, and created offices of infectious and tropical diseases, school and infant hygiene, sanitary engineering, food and beverage control, among others.[172] But these changes did not arrive overnight,[173] and the

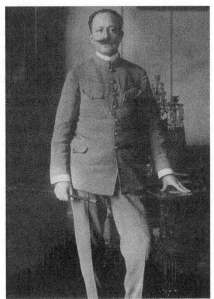

Doctor y general José María Rodríguez. Archivo familiar.

Figure 1.3. Dr. José María Rodríguez, first DSP chief (1917–1920). From Miguel E. Bustamante, *Cinco Personajes de la Salud en México* (México, D.F.: Grupo Editorial Miguel Angel Porrúa, 1986). Courtesy of Rodríguez Family Archive and Grupo Editorial Miguel Angel Porrúa.

form that revolutionary public health and medicine would take was far from established.

First Engagement:
The Yellow Fever Campaign

Even before the passage of the 1917 Constitution, which specified a heightened role for Mexico's government in the provision of public health, the RF had expressed an interest in Mexico as a locale for an international health mission. Revolutionary warfare and political instability did not stop it from trying. Numerous arguments might have compelled this insistence. Beginning in the late nineteenth century, newspapermen and medical authorities articulated fears that Mexico's physical proximity to the United States meant that its unfavorable health conditions could directly and indirectly affect the health of the U.S. population and the U.S. economy.[174] In the late 1870s, the U.S. Marine

Hospital Service (precursor to the USPHS, as it was renamed in 1912) had begun monitoring epidemic outbreaks in its weekly bulletins, as reported by a worldwide network of informants.[175] An 1893 U.S. presidential act obliged all immigrants and cargo ships to present certificates of health signed by the U.S. consul and a medical officer in the departing port, and the Marine Hospital Service stationed a number of its own officers in key ports around the world to inspect ships for disease and to enforce quarantine.[176] For decades Mexico figured prominently in the weekly bulletins, with frequent reports of cholera, plague, typhus, and other disease outbreaks emanating from a chain of ports and border towns; however, the Mexican government was reluctant to allow U.S. medical inspectors to be posted in its territory.[177]

Amid the tensions of the revolutionary years, the RF was ready to offer assistance in the control of epidemics without the involvement of the less than welcome U.S. government.[178] Given the conflictual history between Mexico and the U.S., RF men considered the potential goodwill to be generated by a philanthropic health endeavor all the more valuable. By the late 1910s, the IHB was already operating campaigns in numerous countries throughout Central and South America and the Caribbean: in the view of the RF home office, the political and social restructuring launched by the Mexican Revolution made the timing for the RF's entry into Mexico propitious. Wickliffe Rose himself may have viewed Mexico as a natural candidate for the IHB's standard hookworm campaign.

Notwithstanding the RF's eagerness to work in Mexico, this attitude was not reciprocated. Much as the RF proclaimed its independence from the U.S. government, Mexican authorities—most notably President Carranza—do not seem to have been prepared to disassociate the two. Since the 1823 declaration of the Monroe Doctrine, the United States had justified its military occupation of Mexico and other Latin American countries in the name of maintaining continental stability and protecting business interests. Mexicans were deeply resentful of the United States' repeated violations of their sovereignty. The revolutionary years continued to be marked by U.S. invasion, threats, and political manipulation.

Nor did Mexicans consider public health cooperation to be a neutral activity: the U.S. military occupation of Veracruz from late April to November of 1914 (which resulted in 126 Mexican deaths and the seizure of millions of dollars in customs receipts) was accompanied by a repressive sanitary invasion. Following several days of a brutal offensive on Veracruz, the USPHS and the Red Cross joined the military forces in a massive public health campaign. U.S. army planning for such a sanitary occupation seems to have begun soon after the outbreak of the revolution,[179] in an effort to avert the disastrous troop losses due to yellow fever and other infectious diseases that had occurred when U.S. forces invaded Cuba in 1898. In Veracruz, too, the U.S. military's most urgent objective was to protect its men from disease, but the campaign also cleaned up the destruction left by ruthless shelling and a citywide sweep of armed resisters. One thousand U.S. marines, assisted by hundreds of local hired hands, collected and burned refuse, inspected

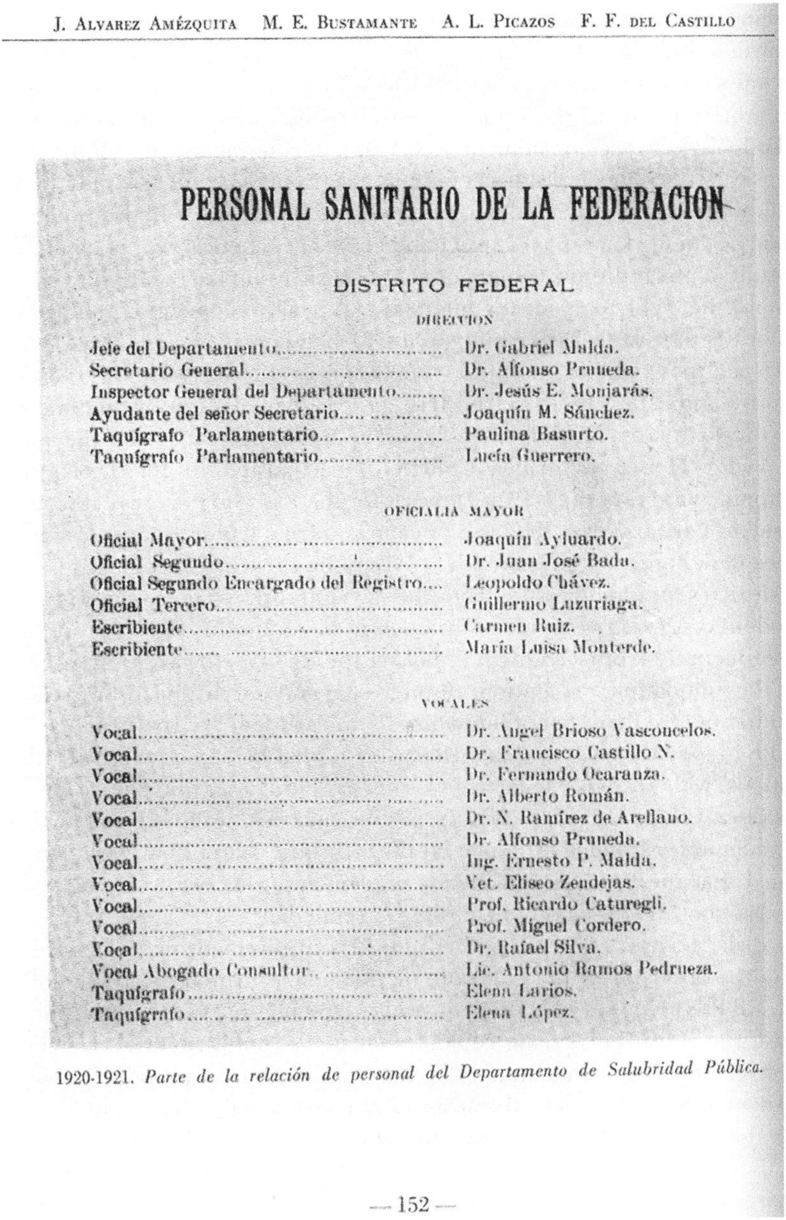

J. ALVAREZ AMÉZQUITA M. E. BUSTAMANTE A. L. PICAZOS F. F. DEL CASTILLO

PERSONAL SANITARIO DE LA FEDERACION

DISTRITO FEDERAL

DIRECCION

Jefe del Departamento	Dr. Gabriel Malda.
Secretario General	Dr. Alfonso Pruneda.
Inspector General del Departamento	Dr. Jesús E. Monjarás.
Ayudante del señor Secretario	Joaquín M. Sánchez.
Taquígrafo Parlamentario	Paulina Basurto.
Taquígrafo Parlamentario	Lucía Guerrero.

OFICIALIA MAYOR

Oficial Mayor	Joaquín Ayluardo.
Oficial Segundo	Dr. Juan José Badu.
Oficial Segundo Encargado del Registro	Leopoldo Chávez.
Oficial Tercero	Guillermo Luzuriaga.
Escribiente	Carmen Ruiz.
Escribiente	María Luisa Monterde.

VOCALES

Vocal	Dr. Angel Brioso Vasconcelos.
Vocal	Dr. Francisco Castillo N.
Vocal	Dr. Fernando Ocaranza.
Vocal	Dr. Alberto Román.
Vocal	Dr. N. Ramírez de Arellano.
Vocal	Dr. Alfonso Pruneda.
Vocal	Ing. Ernesto P. Malda.
Vocal	Vet. Eliseo Zendejas.
Vocal	Prof. Ricardo Caturegli.
Vocal	Prof. Miguel Cordero.
Vocal	Dr. Rafael Silva.
Vocal Abogado Consultor	Lic. Antonio Ramos Pedrueza.
Taquígrafo	Elena Larios.
Taquígrafo	Elena López.

1920-1921. *Parte de la relación de personal del Departamento de Salubridad Pública.*

— 152 —

Figure 1.4. DSP central staff, 1920–21. From José Alvarez Amézquita, Miguel E. Bustamante, Antonio L. Picazos, and F. Fernández del Castillo, *Historia de la Salubridad y de la Asistencia en México*, vol. 2 (México, D.F.: Secretaría de Salubridad y Asistencia, 1960). Courtesy of the Secretaría de Salud, Mexico City, Mexico.

dwellings, drained stagnant water, sprayed petroleum as an insecticide, built public latrines, and washed city streets. To the occupiers and the supportive U.S. press, this was a successful effort to "civilize" degenerate Mexicans who overlooked the filth around them. To the Veracruzanos, the sanitary campaign was both risible and offensive, an accompaniment, not an antidote, to the brutality of the military offensive.[180] U.S. medical officers were unable to understand why most Mexican medical personnel either fled or refused to work with them.[181] In this atmosphere, public health work was seen as just another face of American imperialism, hardly the stuff of philanthropic cooperation. For Mexico—unlike the RF—it was decidedly *not* the right moment for international health cooperation, and national authorities repeatedly barred entry to the RF between 1915 and 1920.

Despite these various "political complications," the RF persevered, pursuing various approaches. In 1915, the IHB gave a small amount of funding for an abortive Red Cross mission to Mexico. The following year it sent the assertive Dr. Victor Heiser, a former USPHS officer posted in the U.S.-occupied Philippines and now the IHB's "Director for the East," to negotiate directly with President Carranza over IHB assistance to combat a typhus outbreak. This time hopes were higher, as U.S. President Wilson had recently recognized Carranza as Mexico's president. Rose laid the groundwork by meeting with Eliseo Arredondo, Mexico's consul to Washington, in advance of Heiser's trip. A State Department desk officer sought to bolster the RF's case by assuring Arredondo that the foundation was "entirely disinterested and purely philanthropical" with no other motive than that of humanity."[182] In early January 1916, Heiser cabled the RF in New York, via the State Department, that he had established "friendly relations" with Mexico's de facto government.[183] But after initially accepting the RF's offer, Carranza backtracked, in part because his health advisor (and head of the Superior Council of Public Health), Dr. José María Rodríguez, rightfully argued that the Council was already implementing its own campaign against typhus under the direction of Dr. Alfonso Pruneda.[184]

Not all Mexican officials opposed the RF's involvement in Mexico. In early 1919, the governor of the gulf state of Tamaulipas invited the IHB's cooperation. RF President George Vincent—while agreeing that a demonstration project for the control of disease could "stimulate . . . public interest in sanitation and hygiene around the country"—refused the invitation, explaining that such activity needed to be under the auspices of the national government.[185]

By this time it had become clear that the RF's compelling interest in Mexico was also disease-specific: Mexico was among the last countries in the hemisphere to harbor yellow fever. As RF yellow fever efforts in South and Central America were starting to bear fruit, Mexico was a problematic holdout: yellow fever was a continuing menace to commerce if it persisted and a boon to the RF's scientific prestige if eradicated. As early as 1915, an RF officer had calculated that quarantine in a secondary port in Mexico could cost $60,000 (well over $1 million in 2004 dollars) in trade losses in a single year.[186] Mexico's epidemiologic surveillance had deteriorated during the years of the revolution, and the IHB kept a close eye on newspaper reports of yellow fever cases.

In July 1918, Rose advised the State Department of the importance of combating yellow fever in Mexico, citing the assessments of U.S. Surgeon General Rupert Blue and Army Surgeon General Gorgas that endemic yellow fever in Mexico was "a constant menace to Cuba" and the U.S. and that the IHB ought to "undertake the eradication of yellow fever in this seed-bed of infection."[187] Rose attributed Mexico's repeated refusal of the IHB as the reflection of broader suspicion of the role of foreign economic interests, including Rockefeller-owned Standard Oil, in Mexico's political troubles, lamenting, "Any organization therefore bearing the Rockefeller name would not be kindly received by the present government authorities."[188]

In December 1919, Rose sent Dr. Theodore C. Lyster—the IHB's yellow fever point man in Central America—to Mexico City to try again to convince Carranza to invite the IHB, this time to combat yellow fever. While some Mexican doctors, this time including DSP chief Rodríguez, were keen on the yellow fever collaboration, Carranza once more rebuffed the IHB, in Lyster's frustrated words, due to "Just a case of pride."[189]

But in 1920 the situation changed. Carranza was assassinated in May, and Adolfo de la Huerta, Governor of the northern state of Sonora, was installed as interim president. In September Alvaro Obregón—one of the revolution's leading generals, who had denounced Carranza and initiated the revolt against him—was elected president, and he took office in December 1920. Just as these events were unfolding, yellow fever reappeared in the port of Veracruz in June 1920 after an absence of more than a decade.[190] In an abrupt turnaround, Alfonso Pruneda, now secretary-general of the DSP under de la Huerta, invited RF cooperation against yellow fever a few weeks before Obregón was sworn in. Pruneda—who would keep his post under Obregón—stressed that Mexico had the personnel for a "fruitful campaign" and had already initiated activities to combat mosquito-borne diseases. Even so, he continued, yellow fever was a problem "of international importance, and especially in our case where it is a question of contiguous countries with so many interests in common, and at present happily united by a cordial friendship."[191] At almost the same time, Dr. Francisco Castillo Nájera, an envoy of Mexico's Military Medical Corps, met with Lyster in New York and also invited him to Mexico to cooperate with sanitary authorities.[192] At last a rendezvous was arranged.

In December 1920, Lyster met with the new president and drafted a campaign plan,[193] and on January 19, 1921, Obregón signed a yellow fever agreement, appropriating 50,000 gold pesos (over $250,000 in 2004 dollars) for the first year's effort, approximately one fifth of what the RF would spend that year.[194] Under the guidance of DSP Chief Dr. Gabriel Malda, the president decreed the creation of a "Special Commission for the Yellow Fever Campaign" with Lyster as its director.[195] Lyster's December plan called for two IHB men to serve as sub-directors with Mexican assistance from representatives of the DSP, the Bacteriologic Institute, and the Secretariat of War, but Obregón had other plans. Dr. Angel Brioso Vasconcelos—an esteemed DSP man and editor of the *Gaceta Médica de México*, the nation's foremost medical journal—was named the campaign's subdirector.[196]

What might explain Mexico's sudden change of heart? Certainly, President Obregón—who had for a time organized military medical services during the revolution—was quick to recognize that the country could benefit from aid in addressing the yellow fever outbreak, and the RF appeared to be a good risk. The RF's offer to foot much of the bill undoubtedly sweetened the deal. Not only would RF cooperation help build the new DSP, but a highly visible health campaign could also serve to solidify Obregón's shaky hold on power.

The DSP's invitation was both daring and calculated: Washington was withholding its recognition of Obregón's government due to the impasse over Article 27's prohibition on foreign ownership of subsoil resources, most importantly oil,[197] and the RF was linked—at least by association and overlapping board membership—to the Standard Oil Company, one of the main parties to Mexico's oil reserves.[198] Obregón may have considered his support of the joint yellow fever campaign to be a gesture of good faith to a hostile U.S. government and to angry oil companies. Perhaps, too, as was the case in a parallel accord between the RF and Soviet Russia in the early 1920s,[199] the yellow fever agreement may have been prompted by DSP officials who saw cooperation with an RF campaign as a possible means of facilitating U.S. diplomatic recognition of Mexico.

Still another factor was at play. Outside the country, Alvaro Obregón's election signified the end of the Mexican Revolution. However, armed opposition to Obregón's government persisted, and Veracruz was one of the states where his power remained tenuous. The new president was thus particularly agreeable to the RF's interest in targeting the state of Veracruz and other Gulf of Mexico locales.

Veracruz's defiance was entwined with its history of peasant, tenant, and labor mobilization, its ongoing nurturing of powerful regional leaders and organized rebel movements, and its strategic location around the country's largest port.[200] The state's agricultural and oil riches augmented its importance. Before the Revolution, Veracruz was noted for producing two thirds of the country's coffee.[201] With the 1910 oil discovery in Veracruz, the state was transformed into a leading economic engine: by 1920 Mexico had passed Russia to become the world's second largest petroleum producer after the United States.[202]

The national government's reliance on the federal army to consolidate its power, the army's hostility to revolutionary demands for land redistribution,[203] and its ongoing conflicts with peasants also turned elements of the Veracruz state government and regional *caudillos* against President Obregón, who was accused of corruption, stonewalling agrarian reform, and accommodation to foreign interests. Because many Veracruz elites also despised the foreign ownership of

Mexican oil, sugar, coffee, and tobacco industries, they formed strategic alliances with various groupings of peasants and workers opposing the president.[204]

In the face of this unrest, the IHB was intrepid, a sign of the importance of eradicating yellow fever—and the importance of Mexico—to the RF. Armando Solórzano has argued that Mexico did not really need a yellow fever campaign;[205] the last large outbreak had been in 1903, and the 505 cases and 249 deaths reported in 1920 in Veracruz, Sinaloa, Yucatán, and a handful of other states[206] were more the result of a wartime breakdown in the sanitary measures that had been enacted two decades earlier under the Superior Council of Public Health's leader, Eduardo Liceaga, than a consequence of Mexico's inability to combat the disease. Indeed, the DSP had proven highly capable of controlling disease outbreaks even with slender resources. Almost at the same time as the yellow fever epidemic, in late May 1920 Mexico's Gulf Coast experienced an outbreak of plague, likely brought by a ship from New Orleans. The DSP quickly mobilized an isolation effort—poorly received by the Veracruz public—and then a far more popular de-ratting cleanup effort that successfully combated the disease by mid-October.[207] The thirty-seven plague deaths paled before the yellow fever count, but even at its peak, yellow fever did not appear on the country's list of leading causes of death. Nevertheless, yellow fever's high and frightening case fatality rate, the threat of quarantine, the potential suspension of trade, and the political importance of Veracruz and other Gulf Coast ports to Mexico City— together with the high price tag of controlling the disease—served to justify Mexico's invitation to the RF.

In February 1921, the Special Commission for the Eradication of Yellow Fever in Mexico dispatched a cadre of four senior and six junior IHB officers, four senior and seven junior DSP officials, and numerous military doctors from forces loyal to Obregón, and it began to hire hundreds of local assistants. Initially the country was divided into two regions, one centered in Yucatán, the other in Veracruz. The country was further subdivided into six zones after the discussions of the First Yellow Fever Convention (the first ever held in Mexico and the first such meeting in which the RF participated), organized by Lyster and DSP chief Malda, held in Mexico City in October 1921.[208] Operations concentrated in the state of Veracruz and reached as far north as the port of Tampico in the state of Tamaulipas, as far west as Colima, Sinaloa, and other Pacific states, and as far south as Quintana Roo and Chiapas, eventually joining with the IHB's campaign in Central America.

The Special Commission adhered to a strict set of rules agreed upon by the IHB and the DSP.[209] Since 1915, the IHB's yellow fever campaigns had assigned top priority to Henry Rose Carter's dictate: "Get rid of the yellow fever mosquito. Disregard the human host—the man sick of yellow fever—and concentrate on the control of the insect host—the mosquito."[210] Based on the IHB's experience in Brazil and other South American settings, this approach entailed inspecting and treating water-filled household receptacles and local swamps and ponds, any of which might harbor mosquito larvae, with petroleum or larvicidal fish. This did

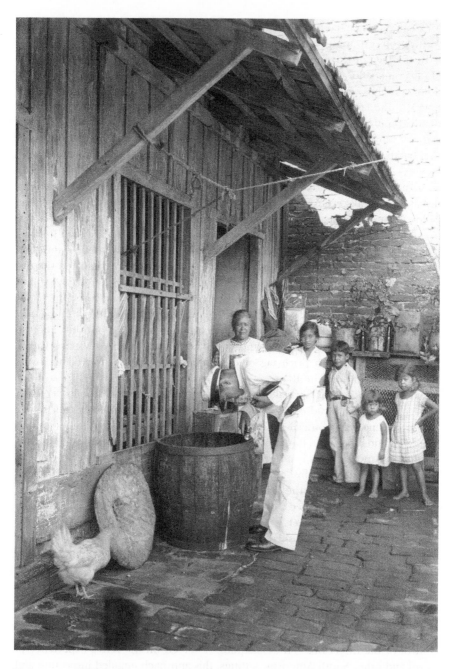

Figure 1.5. Yellow fever campaign officer inspecting and treating household water sources. Courtesy of the Rockefeller Archive Center.

not preclude the isolation of yellow fever cases or even the recognition of the role of an unclean water supply in facilitating the spread of the disease.[211] But the IHB philosophy—and the organization of the country into divisions, zones, regions, districts, blocks, and so on—gave the yellow fever campaign a clear combat-like strategy and an unequivocal target: the larval form of the *Aedes aegypti* mosquito.[212]

Hierarchically organized mobile brigades—consisting of a chief inspector, four sanitary inspectors, several assistants, and five to seven laborers—went from dwelling to dwelling and swamp to pond in search of *Aedes aegypti* larvae. Over the course of three years, the almost 500 members of the Special Commission inspected several million houses, treated over 12 million household water receptacles, applied oil (purchased directly from oil companies drilling in Mexico) to millions of stagnant water sources, and deposited countless larvicidal fish into *Aedes aegypti* breeding sites. The campaign generated publicity through handbills, circulars, announcements, and newspaper articles about the spread of yellow fever authored by prominent local doctors. The most effective health education and propaganda was achieved through the daily rounds and anti-larval activities of the inspectors.[213] As noted by Dr. Genaro Angeles, one of the numerous DSP officers engaged in ongoing yellow fever efforts, health propaganda aimed at persuasion was far less successful than visible antilarval measures.[214]

The RF's anti-yellow fever approach differed from that of Mexico's Liceaga, who twenty years before had combined eradication measures with sanitation—street cleaning and the establishment of potable water and sewage systems. This approach eliminated the household need for collecting water in the first place and thus prevented the proliferation of breeding sites.[215] In the early 1920s, U.S. Surgeon General Hugh Cumming echoed Liceaga, suggesting to IHB Director Frederick Russell that though targeting mosquitoes could result in the "quick elimination of yellow fever," what were truly needed were "improvements of a permanent nature."[216] The RF did not consider such long-term investments to be either efficient or necessary for the control of yellow fever.

The specific terms of the Mexican yellow fever campaign, as set under its first director Lyster (replaced after one year by RF yellow fever officer Dr. Joseph White), stipulated that the DSP serve as the campaign's "supreme authority," with U.S. personnel to regard themselves as representing DSP Director Malda rather than the IHB. Lyster—who himself required the services of a translator—stressed, "The more intimate and direct this relationship the better." Close links with local authorities were also to be maintained. While the DSP would be encouraged to cooperate financially and would be expected to pay the salaries of its own employees, IHB funds were to be "available any time, any place" so that lack of funding would "not be an excuse for worklag."[217]

At the same time, the IHB directed the campaign to employ punitive—and even coercive—methods to ensure that antilarval measures were not jeopardized. A month after the campaign was launched, Lyster called upon Secretary-General Pruneda to authorize fines of 5 to 500 pesos for breeding site violations.

While the Special Commission distributed larvicidal fish for use in appropriate water containers, the owners of these receptacles were held responsible— subject to fines[218]—for maintaining the fish and for informing the DSP of their death. This ruling also allowed campaign officers the right to enter any premises to inspect for breeding sites.[219]

In more than a dozen towns along the Gulf Coast, the commission joined ongoing antilarval efforts by the DSP, which for the most part had already brought the disease under control before the commission was even launched. At times the two groups unified their labors, but there was also overlap or even repetition of the other's work. Commission Subdirector Brioso Vasconcelos, who had been at the helm of the DSP's yellow fever activities since the beginning of the outbreak in 1920, criticized this duplication as unnecessary, costly, and unproductive. Not willing to fully integrate the two yellow fever campaigns, Lyster promised virtual carte blanche financing for the commission.[220] Brioso Vasconcelos was satisfied with this solution and requested that "Dr. Rose be told that this was one of the best means of helping the DSP."[221]

In some settings, the Special Commission continued the work of local authorities, such as city of Veracruz health officials, who had effectively stamped out yellow fever between September and December of 1920 through sanitary inspection and petrolization efforts.[222] In other places, such as Tampico, the commission replaced larvae control campaigns financed and overseen by the Associated Oil Managers, services which IHB officers believed were deficient and "egoistical . . . never prompted by altruistic motives."[223] The Military Medical Corps collaborated fully with the yellow fever campaign, delighting in the strict organization of vaccination and antilarval efforts.[224] In all instances, yellow fever personnel engaged in a detailed accounting exercise—with each larvicidal fish and liter of oil tallied and every inspected receptacle and home counted—following the IHB's detailed data collection methods for measuring productivity, outreach, and yellow fever cases.[225] Along with suspected and verified yellow fever cases and deaths, the commission's main indicator of concern was the percentage of houses that had *Aedes* larvae. Below an index level of 5 percent (i.e., fewer than 5 percent of households found to have larvae), according to the commission, yellow fever reinfection could be prevented.[226]

The Gulf Coast, Yucatán Peninsula, and Central American campaigns were also used by Rockefeller Institute scientist Hideyo Noguchi as key locales to test his yellow fever vaccine, even before the RF's official involvement in the campaign. In October and November 1920, one third of Túxpam's 6,000 residents were vaccinated, as were almost all troops traveling to yellow fever zones. By 1922, some 2,000 doses per month were being adminstered to Mexican troops. Vaccination was an important feature of the campaign in spite of the skepticism of various DSP and IHB officers—as well as other Latin American doctors—regarding the vaccine's efficacy.[227] Though it ultimately proved a failure, Noguchi's yellow fever vaccine set a precedent for the use of IHB campaigns as field trial opportunities.[228]

The prominent role assigned to the Noguchi vaccine acts as a reminder that the grandiose Mexican campaign was part of the RF's effort to garner an international reputation for controlling yellow fever through new technologies as well as serving as a cooperative health initiative in a particular country.

According to the RF's own men, the general reception of the campaign by the public—from housewives to merchants—was extremely favorable,[229] though widespread "support and encouragement" did not preclude frequent disputes and difficulties.[230] For example, many people removed the larvicidal fish from drinking water cisterns, and housewives reportedly resisted covering laundry water receptacles due to the inconvenience.[231] RF officers reported great satisfaction with "the conscientious and faithful service of the personnel of our brigades entirely made up of Mexicans. . . . Better men cannot be found in any other country." RF officer Bert Caldwell wrote admiringly to the DSP, which "has done everything possible in order to crown our work with success," stating that civil authorities were "kind, courteous, with generous and friendly help."[232] These assessments were corroborated by the numerous petitions of support sent to the commission and the DSP by ordinary townsfolk, local shopkeepers and hoteliers, soldiers, laborers, and oil companies in Veracruz.[233]

Yellow fever cases and deaths plunged by over 70 percent before the end of 1921 and by 90 percent the following year (in 1921 there were 123 reported cases and in 1922 there were forty-one reported cases and twenty-five deaths). The number of home inspections—together with the number of receptacles treated with oil and larvicidal fish—more than doubled in 1922 and tripled in 1923 to reach over 2.5 million houses, covering almost half the population in inland towns and even more along the coast.[234] With uncertainty about the length of time needed to ensure an area was free of yellow fever and concerns that migrant sugarcane workers from inland states constituted new pools of "susceptibles," these extensive measures were believed by the IHB to be vital to ensuring the permanent disappearance of yellow fever.[235] But they also marked the Herculean efforts of a persistent courtship.

The close contact between RF officers and the Mexican public in Veracruz and other states through house-to-house visits—and the campaign's secondary effect of decreasing the number of pesky household insects[236]—also appeared to reduce anti-U.S. sentiments. That a young RF doctor, Howard Cross, died of yellow fever in Tuxtepec, Veracruz, in December 1921 heightened local admiration for the RF's efforts. President Obregón ordered that Cross be given homage as a "hero of humanity" and, after a wake in Veracruz, his corpse was transferred to Mexico City, where it was received by DSP chief Malda and other health officials.[237]

Only in the port of Túxpam, Veracruz, located at the mouth of a major river with access to rich oilfields, did Commission men report that the brigades were "merely tolerated" with no assistance from local officials or the public. During the first year of the campaign, inspectors were blocked from entering homes,

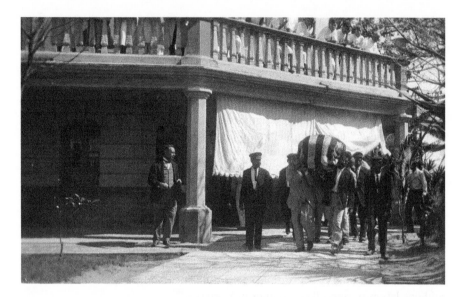

Figure 1.6. Funeral procession for RF yellow fever officer Dr. Howard Cross, with coffin draped in U.S. and Mexican flags, 1921. Courtesy of the Rockefeller Archive Center.

insulted, and even physically threatened. In the 1920 yellow fever outbreak, Túxpam had the country's second highest number of cases at 187, and the highest number of deaths—ninety-seven—of any Mexican locale.[238] DSP delegate Dr. Leonides Guadarrama attributed the high mortality to late diagnosis of yellow fever, poor sanitary conditions, civil authorities' refusal to cooperate with the DSP, and opposition to quarantine measures by merchants and laborers alike, with the press inflaming the distrust of popular sectors.[239] According to RF officer Emmett Vaughn, many locals, who were "more than tainted with Bolshevistic doctrines," suspected that the yellow fever work was a prelude to U.S. invasion. This region, he sympathized with President Obregón, would cause the Mexican government "no end of troubles."[240]

Part of the localized opposition to the yellow fever campaign may have stemmed from the alliances Obregón had forged in Veracruz. The populist state governor, Adalberto Tejeda (1920–24 and 1928–32), who had tied his fortunes to Obregón, built his political base by installing his own supporters in local level political bodies—typically bypassing and challenging the power of existing leaders. Túxpam was one of a handful of localities where ousted politicians and their supporters vehemently protested Tejeda's maneuvers,[241] and the yellow fever campaign became caught up in this rivalry.

The DSP, while actively collaborating with the IHB, seemed to hold its enthusiasm in check. From the perspective of Brioso Vasconcelos, the IHB's cooperation was important, offering opportunities for scientific research (although campaign-based publications in the *American Journal of Tropical Medicine* were authored only by RF staff) along with the campaign activities. Many staff members relished the new attention being paid to their work by the press.[242] The DSP's officer in Yucatán—where no yellow fever cases were reported after December 1920—expressed an enormous debt to the RF for helping to restore the state's yellow fever service.[243] Others warmed to the IHB only after seeing the yellow fever teams in action. Dr. Juan Graham Casasús, head of the DSP's Antilarval Service in the state of Veracruz before the creation of the Special Commission, initially resented the RF's overshadowing of the ongoing—and encouraging—work of Mexican brigades. Indeed, despite his position, he appears to have been shunned by Lyster and the organizers of the Yellow Fever Convention in 1921.[244] But according to M. E. Connor—Lyster's IHB deputy— by 1924, Graham Casasús held that the campaign had "favorably impressed the Mexican people and [had] been [a] factor in causing the average Mexican to see the [United] States from other than a Washington viewpoint."[245]

For DSP officers, the Special Commission served as an added partner in ongoing Mexican efforts, rather than as a new initiative: other than the flawed Noguchi vaccine, the IHB doctors brought no new control methods and knew nothing more than Mexican doctors.[246] Several DSP officers noted that the commission paid no attention to the lack of a piped water supply, a problem that inevitably led to mosquito breeding sites due to household needs to store water.[247] Dr. Alfredo Cuarón, who had only reluctantly taken on the post of DSP representative in Tampico,[248] confidentially complained to Brioso Vasconcelos that the IHB officers were disdainful and "do not take our opinions into consideration."[249] Perhaps in an effort to counter the IHB's taking credit for the yellow fever campaign's success, Brioso Vasconcelos reiterated to his superiors that the "intelligence and patriotism of the [Mexican] government which has generously promoted the campaign"[250] could not go unnoticed.

What the IHB did bring was enormous resources, which it deployed— together with the DSP—at a scale and level of organization with little precedent. By the end of 1923, the IHB reported just a single case of yellow fever and no fatalities. The commission continued small-scale monitoring activities with inspection visits by IHB officers for two more years, with no more cases reported.[251] Yellow fever had all but disappeared from Mexico at an expense to the RF of more than $400,000 (approximately $4.5 million in 2004 dollars). While the DSP would continue the commission's antilarval work for many years,[252] and though U.S. consuls and the USPHS continued to monitor the yellow fever threat to the U.S. from Mexico,[253] the IHB considered its objectives and mission accomplished.

The Special Commission had not only laid claim to eliminating the menace of yellow fever in Mexico (and to international commerce), it had given a marvelous boost to the popular reputations of both the RF and the DSP. RF officers served as friendly emissaries at the very time when U.S.-Mexican diplomatic relations were suspended over the question of foreign ownership of subsoil rights.[254] President Obregón and other government officials were pleased with the outcome of the campaign—which helped to increase local support for the President in the Veracruz region—and he urged a continuation of the relationship between the RF and Mexico.

The local medical establishment also appeared satisfied. After having shunned U.S. sanitary efforts during the invasion of Veracruz, many Mexican doctors involved in the yellow fever campaign allied themselves with the IHB, became avid readers of IHB publications on yellow fever, and began to use their connections to North American public health to increase their "reputation and power within the emerging Mexican State."[255] The IHB believed that the campaign had had a positive impact on DSP officials who, according to IHB officer Connor, recognized "the advantages to be gained from co-operation" and hoped that the IHB "would maintain contact with the Departamento for years to come or until the Departamento was well on its own feet."[256] If a small number of health officials disliked the RF intrusion, others remastered the yellow fever campaign as a single element of the DSP's packed agenda.

For Mexican politicians, the yellow fever campaign was a proposition too good to refuse in financial, policy, and patron-client political terms. The various parties to the campaign—local authorities, public health officials, IHB men, health workers, and the targeted populace—all agreed on the enormous potential of the local provision of public health services. The RF's optimism that a cooperative public health program could help dispel Mexican bitterness toward the U.S. seemed to have been borne out. Success, goodwill, and the prospect of future cooperation was generated on behalf of all parties.

Still, the yellow fever campaign was more of an elaborate mutual introduction of Mexico and the RF than a real taste of the relationship that lay ahead. On one level, the RF's campaign in Mexico was part of its larger aspirations for eradicating yellow fever in the Americas. On another level, the campaign's militaristic style and high price tag represented an atypical courting of a country initially reluctant to invite the RF. In a sense, the IHB was countering its own dictum—serving as patron as well as partner. To be sure, Mexican politicians and doctors also claimed credit for the campaign's positive outcomes, but the tumultuous timing of the campaign left little room for local adaptation. That would have to await the next campaign.

Chapter Two

Hooked on Hookworm

Because the RF's first public health campaign in Mexico had been funded and organized on a scale both to satisfy the RF's larger yellow fever eradication ambitions and to woo its hard-to-get Mexican counterpart, it was the campaign that followed yellow fever that would better define the terms of the relationship. At the most pragmatic level, the IHB's stock campaign against hookworm disease offered a compromise collaboration. It would both keep the RF in Mexico at a lower expense and extend the reach of the DSP, albeit for an ailment that was not a high epidemiologic priority. The claims on Mexico's federal government stemming from the revolution demanded far more public health infrastructure than the hookworm campaign could provide, yet the campaign's very existence in a key region served as a powerful demonstration of the institutionalization of health services to come.

In locating the campaign in and around Veracruz, where unrest continued to threaten Mexico City, the Mexican government and the RF shared the view that popular public health efforts could help stabilize the region. As during the yellow fever campaign, the IHB sought to play both sides against the middle, courting Mexico City officials and Veracruz leaders at the same time. The DSP made use of the IHB campaign to heighten its presence in Veracruz during a politically thorny period, distancing itself from the RF as necessary. This was a dangerous game for all parties, and the RF-Mexico collaboration at times seemed to be tempting fate.

The hookworm agreement sought to establish a balance of power between the DSP and the IHB, in which the IHB maintained the upper hand in the selection of the disease and in decisions over the financial obligations of all parties. In addition, RF officers were given considerable latitude in day-to-day operations, even when the campaign faced controversy over treatment regimes and preventive measures.

But the DSP was no *tabula rasa* waiting to be inscribed upon from afar. At the time when arrangements for a new cooperative endeavor were being crafted in 1922–23, the DSP was expanding its role in areas such as health education, child hygiene, and professional training.[1] The hookworm campaign served as an extra activity that could help the DSP make headway in extending its services to small towns and rural populations. Though Mexican health officials were afforded little day-to-day administrative control over the campaign, they were in a position to interpret campaign goals and structure them in the context of other DSP activities. It soon became apparent that local forces were just as astute as the DSP in using the hookworm campaign to advance political and social agendas without bending to the public health approach that the RF was advocating.

Amidst these concerns, the hookworm campaign itself might have become lost. Instead, it served to solidify the mutual commitment of Mexico and the RF as long-term partners.

The Bait

From Yellow Fever to Hookworm

With the yellow fever campaign in sight of completion by late 1922, the RF had to decide if it would remain in Mexico and if so, which public health campaign might be a worthy successor. The challenge for the RF resided at the very heart of the organization's modus operandi: how to devise and bring to fruition public health activities that would become financially and institutionally stable and garner permanent commitment by the host country—all without breaking the RF bank.

Whether to stay hardly seemed an issue. The RF did not want to lose the good favor of Mexicans nor miss the opportunity to help shape Mexico's revolutionary public health system. *Which* campaign to offer likewise required little deliberation.

A campaign against hookworm—after all an endemic rather than an epidemic disease and not a big killer—might seem a poor selling point to a country with so many pressing public health needs. But in the early 1920s, hookworm remained the IHB's most important tool for introducing the principles of hygiene and awakening government and popular interest in the provision of public health services. If anything, the hookworm campaign was even more technically feasible than a decade earlier, given the availability of more powerful and less toxic antihelminthic drugs—chenopodium and carbon tetrachloride. The combination of the IHB's longtime experience with hookworm, its satisfaction with other international campaigns from both technical and political standpoints, and Mexico's apparent interest made the decision to launch a hookworm initiative unproblematic.

Following the scientific and cooperative accomplishments of the yellow fever campaign, Mexican officials had similarly high expectations for a subsequent endeavor. Although Secretary of Health Gabriel Malda and DSP Secretary-General Alfonso Pruneda seem to have been loath to indicate priorities to the IHB, Angel Brioso Vasconcelos, subdirector of the yellow fever commission, was less reticent. He complained that Mexico was one of the countries that had "least benefited" from RF monies and activities,[2] and he blamed the United States for Mexico's slow progress in health matters.[3] Brioso Vasconcelos emphasized to Pruneda that malaria—as one of the nation's leading problems—merited urgent attention.[4] The DSP implicitly endorsed this position by folding the yellow fever commission into a DSP campaign to combat both yellow fever and malaria. The IHB's own yellow fever officers in Mexico received various local appeals for a campaign against malaria.[5] But the IHB home office ignored these appeals and criticisms, assuring Brioso Vasconcelos that a joint hookworm endeavor would "assist you in your admirable efforts to build up in the minds of the public a belief in and support of public health measures, hookworm disease being particularly well-suited for educational and demonstration work."[6] Brioso Vasconcelos insisted that hookworm had been designated a priority by unnamed "authorized persons,"[7] rather than by national health officials, but his concerns fell on deaf ears in Mexico City and New York alike.

By the time hookworm was proposed for Mexico, RF hookworm campaigns had been carried out in numerous settings in the Americas, Asia, and the Pacific.[8] These efforts—many realized in British colonies—were typically proclaimed great successes by the IHB. As cited in official reports, the campaign in the West Indies had cured 76 percent of the infected population in only three years, with just 6.3 percent of the population opposing treatment.[9] According to longtime RF man Victor Heiser, the hookworm campaign begun in the Fiji Islands in 1915 had miraculously transformed inhabitants from "a dejected, downcast, docile, uninterested people" into one that was healthy, alert, and mentally progressive.[10] The Jamaica Hookworm Commission made evident the monetary value of eradicating hookworm: laborers were "healthier and capable of performing harder work," with a 25 percent increase in "average working time."[11] Some Jamaican workers reported salary increases of 200 percent following treatment.

But an apparent hitch had emerged by 1920: although the IHB had begun to require that its hookworm campaigns—which increasingly emphasized treatment—be preceded by sanitation and latrine-building efforts, neither political authorities nor plantation owners in settings from the Caribbean to South Asia were willing to take on this responsibility.[12] Still, a focus on hookworm's treatment achievements enabled the IHB to confirm its mantra that "prudent spending on public health constituted an investment, not a drain on resources."[13]

Mexico's campaign would prove more challenging than IHB men might have imagined based on experience elsewhere. Beginning with a survey that seemed to discredit the very selection of hookworm, the campaign faced a host of problems: political turmoil within Mexico, bilateral tensions, discrepancies between the field and the IHB home office over treatment regimens, popular reluctance to participate in certain aspects of the campaign, the reproaches of some Mexican physicians who disagreed with the IHB's methods, and periodic differences between the IHB and the DSP on how best to pursue the campaign. Still, if measured against IHB Director Rose's longtime aims of strengthening the commitment of government and populace to modern public health, the Mexican campaign had great potential.

The Agreement and Its Terms

With Mexico and the RF having entered into a relationship through the yellow fever campaign, a replacement initiative no longer required persistent RF entreaties for Mexican participation. In December 1922, Rose sent a short letter to DSP Secretary-General Pruneda, soliciting the country's participation in a hookworm campaign. Rather than proposing that a plan be jointly devised from the outset, however, the IHB insisted that Mexico request its help. Rose wrote, "We shall be glad to receive a communication from the Departamento de Salubridad Pública inviting the Board's co-operation in a program for the control of hookworm disease. Such an invitation will receive sympathetic consideration."[14] Two months later, Pruneda extended an invitation to the IHB, optimistic that "goodwill and affection towards Mexico" would continue to yield "such satisfactory results."[15] Dr. Frederick Russell, who replaced Rose as IHB director in early 1923, proposed a more equal relationship, vowing that "we also hope to learn Mexican methods and apply them to the U.S."[16]

President Obregón, pleased with the outcome of the yellow fever campaign, the opportunity to distribute plum public health posts, and the prospect of counteracting repeated threats to his government from Veracruz, strongly supported the agreement. That the U.S. had not yet recognized his government does not appear to have been an impediment to the initial drafting of plans for a joint hookworm campaign. By August 1923, the diplomatic impasse was resolved through the signing of the Bucareli Street agreements by Obregón and U.S. President Calvin Coolidge. The accords—which temporarily resolved the bilateral dispute in the U.S.'s favor by awarding compensation for wartime damage to U.S. property owners and making Mexico's constitutional prohibition on foreign ownership of subsoil mineral rights nonretroactive—may have eased any concerns about Mexico–U.S. relations from the RF's New York office. On November 12, 1923, the IHB's Executive Committee approved a joint hookworm campaign in Mexico (known in Spanish as the "Lucha contra la Uncinariasis").

Typically, after the IHB had answered a specific government invitation, it carried out a survey of health, social, and political conditions to settle on the scope and location of the initiative. Unlike the yellow fever campaign, the hookworm campaign was subject to all standard IHB policies: (a) the host government would assume financial responsibility for program administration at the outset; (b) the RF's contribution would diminish and that of the host government would increase each year until the latter assumed the entire financial burden; and (c) until the program's termination (or beyond that time), the RF would oversee the program

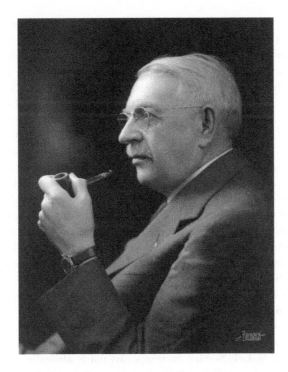

Figure 2.1. Dr. Frederick Russell, second IHD director (1923–35). Courtesy of the Rockefeller Archive Center.

through its representatives stationed in the country and via periodic visits by IHB officials.[17]

In Mexico, as elsewhere, the publicity-shy RF was adamant that the host government receive recognition for program accomplishments. As RF President George Vincent put it in 1925, "After all, we are trying to help the government and we want government authorities to get all the credit. In this way we are able to give the greatest help."[18] In this way the RF also avoided controversy and accusations of interference.

When the IHB converted its campaign from yellow fever to hookworm, its annual spending in Mexico dropped by almost 90 percent, going from over $100,000 per year (in total the equivalent of approximately $4.5 million in 2004 dollars) between 1921 and 1923[19] to an average of one tenth this amount in subsequent years.[20] In contrast to the limitless budgets of the yellow fever years, the IHB set an annual ceiling on its own spending for the hookworm campaign. As important, the new co-funding arrangement established Mexico's financial responsibility from the beginning of the campaign. The five-year operating budget, which averaged combined DSP-IHB annual spending of $45,000 dollars

($490,000 in 2004 dollars), began with 80 percent financing by the IHB and 20 percent by the DSP. Each year the IHB's contribution was cut by 20 percent, and the DSP's contribution was increased by a corresponding 20 percent, until the final year, when the Mexican government was slated to pay 100 percent of the budget and fully incorporate the hookworm campaign into the DSP.[21]

The operating budget reflected only part of the DSP's financial support. While the IHB was to furnish the salary and expenses of one officer (to serve as program subdirector), occasional fellowships for Mexicans to study in the U.S., and an initial supply of equipment and drugs, the Mexican government was expected to cover virtually all overhead costs—a well-equipped central office in Mexico City, regional offices as necessary, secretarial services, free franking and telegraph privileges, discount railroad passes for all employees of the campaign, a chauffeured car for the IHB representative, exemption from customs fees for campaign materials and the personal effects of IHB officers, and the salary and travel costs of the campaign's director and other commissioned doctors.[22] The Mexican government quickly found that its "invitation" to the IHB would obligate it to pay lavish expenses. At the same time, virtually all budgeting, personnel, and planning decisions were in the hands of the IHB representative, even once the Mexican government was funding the entire hookworm campaign.[23]

In an attempt to institutionalize its international health work in Mexico, the IHB agreed that the DSP would designate the director of the new Hookworm, Yellow Fever, and Malaria Service (its temporary name while the yellow fever campaign was winding down). Brioso Vasconcelos went from being subdirector of the yellow fever campaign to acting director of the new initiative.

The campaign's subdirector—who managed virtually all day-to-day decisions and often superseded the authority of the director—was to be an IHB officer, Dr. Andrew Warren. In contrast to the urbane Brioso Vasconcelos, Warren was from a farming family in North Carolina. In 1920, following his graduation from medical school, he joined the IHB and spent several years setting up demonstration health units in rural Kansas and Oregon before being assigned to Mexico. After a long career as an RF officer, he became director of the RF's Division of Medicine and Public Health in the 1950s. As Warren later recalled, he had been posted to Mexico in 1923 to show "sick people out in the bush" that "something could be done for their health and [this] helped develop national interests and responsibilities."[24] His actual role was far more specific: the young Warren was vested with the power to hire and fire personnel, assign responsibilities to the entire campaign staff, and allocate program funds for the joint IHB-DSP hookworm campaign; he laid out ambitious plans for the hookworm campaign emphasizing discipline and popular support.

Governance of the campaign was shared by the DSP leadership: Secretary-General Pruneda proved a determined—if gracious—partner to his IHB counterparts during both yellow fever and hookworm campaigns. Having run the country's antityphus program since 1915, Pruneda understood the clinical,

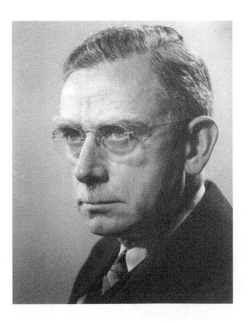

Figure 2.2. RF officer Dr. Andrew Warren. Courtesy of the Rockefeller Archive Center.

epidemiological, and political aspects of public health campaigns. With a career committed equally to education—he was the first rector of Mexico's "Popular University" established in 1913, later serving as rector of the National University of Mexico—and medicine, as pathologist and professor, Pruneda's vision transcended disease-control concerns. As DSP secretary-general from 1920 to 1924, he is credited with furthering school hygiene and health education efforts, launching the country's infant hygiene network, and founding the DSP's graduate school of public health.[25] Pruneda was as keen to cultivate good relations with the IHB as he was to leverage its efforts in Mexico to address rural health needs as part of the nation's social hygiene and social medicine agenda. The hookworm campaign would engage multiple facets of Pruneda's savoir-faire.

The Site and the Survey

In Mexico, not only did the decision as to *what* campaign to pursue predate a survey of local conditions, but the decision of *where* to conduct the campaign was also made before the actual survey was carried out. Veracruz, the focus of the yellow fever campaign, remained vital to President Obregón's government, the DSP, and the RF in overlapping ways. In the early 1920s, Veracruz was the nation's leading economic engine: as a hub of oil, commerce, and agriculture,

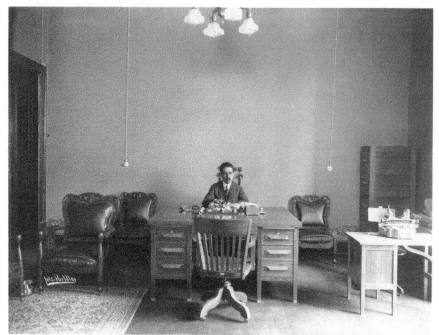

Doctor Alfonso Pruneda, General Secretary of the Department and also of the Board of Health.

Figure 2.3. Dr. Alfonso Pruneda, secretary-general of the DSP (1920–24). Courtesy of the Rockefeller Archive Center.

the state generated significant export revenues and was a major destination for U.S. and European investors.[26] From a political perspective, Veracruz carried enormous strategic importance. Ongoing tensions over foreign drilling rights meant that oil companies and oil workers were continuously at odds, even after the signing of the Bucareli Street agreements. Health work—which could temper unrest as well as keep morale and productivity high, trade flowing, and investors satisfied—became a partner to economic prosperity.

Veracruz's importance also stemmed from its position as a leading center of political mobilization and peasant radicalism in the mid 1920s. Several powerful *caudillos*, who were variously friend or foe of President Obregón's, were based in Veracruz, heightening the role of Governor Adalberto Tejeda (1920–24, and 1928–32) in consolidating Obregón's authority.[27] In his first term, Tejeda lessened restrictions on political activism, encouraging political movements in both urban and rural areas.[28] Long a site of industrial labor activity and a point of entry for anarchist ideologies and activists, Veracruz in the late revolutionary period began to witness growing rural mobilization. In the late 1910s and early 1920s, the Regional Confederation of Mexican Workers (Confederación Regional de

Obreros Mexicanos CROM; the national labor organization, created in 1918) and the Veracruz section of the Communist Party (founded in 1919) played a central part in peasant organizing around questions of literacy, higher wages, and the establishment of formal work contracts. In spite of the Comintern's interest, Veracruz's agrarian movement was never a direct arm of the Communist Party.[29] Rural activism was also influenced by the urban labor movement,[30] with many of the state's agrarian leaders having sharpened their organizing teeth as industrial workers in larger towns and cities before returning to the countryside.[31]

Meanwhile, Tejeda armed "agrarian committees" as a paramilitary dependency of the state's civil guard, seeking to secure his own power base and challenge the forces of General Guadalupe Sánchez, a former ally of Obregón's and now the spokesman for the state's hacienda-owning and commercial elites. While labor organizations were plagued by factionalism, it was Tejeda who urged the creation of a statewide peasant league in 1923 to further strengthen his agrarian support. Amidst this rural turbulence, the state's leading municipalities—the port of Veracruz, state capital Jalapa, agricultural center Córdoba, and others—were marked by ongoing unrest in the form of rent and labor strikes. These protests were in part motivated by deplorable health conditions.[32] In 1923, the turmoil virtually paralyzed the port of Veracruz, alarming Tejeda's one-time patron Obregón and fueling further clashes among Tejeda's supporters, the federal army, General Sánchez's forces, and others. Beset by political infighting, labor uprisings, the opposition of landowner and commercial interests, and rural violence, Tejeda's first administration was chaotic, limiting his ability to govern and frustrating his efforts at land redistribution.[33]

The yellow fever campaign—which had concentrated on ports and oil towns—avoided much of the strife, but a more rural hookworm campaign could become embroiled in both local and national politics. Obregón's government recognized the need to increase its rural profile in order to gain wider popular support and legitimacy and thus counter opposition—particularly in the state of Veracruz. Education might have played the most obvious role in this effort. In 1921 Obregón's dynamic education minister, José Vasconcelos, had launched an ambitious and widely supported expansion of federal schools to complement state educational systems. However, despite Tejeda's support, Veracruz initially saw little improvement in either primary school enrollments or in the overall proportion of educational support provided by the federal government.[34]

Public health was an area where the federal government might have a more effective presence. Although longtime endemic problems—such as dysentery, respiratory diseases, and malaria—posed far larger health problems, both the DSP and the Veracruz state government supported the hookworm campaign. A visible health initiative—even one patronized and organized via the federal government—could only help Tejeda's cause. For the DSP, which was expanding its work on many fronts simultaneously, a hookworm campaign offered a convenient cooperative effort in a difficult locale. The RF may have been playing an even trickier game: it recognized the importance of maintaining contact with both the federal government and Veracruz leaders should there be a power shift on the national political scene.[35] Given this volatility, the arrangements over where to organize the hookworm campaign were made at the highest levels—between the RF home office and the Obregón government—even before the hookworm survey was carried out.

Although actual epidemiological conditions were evidently a secondary consideration, DSP officials and IHB officers in Mexico agreed that a hookworm survey was necessary. The survey would require considerable technical expertise and, if done well, would offer useful information about the general sanitary and social conditions of rural Mexico. That the hookworm campaign was slated to begin in early 1924[36]—at the same time as the survey—did not diminish the belief on the part of Mexican and U.S. doctors in the survey's role in shaping the campaign.

DSP Secretary-General Pruneda was eager that the *joint* hookworm campaign likewise be launched by a *joint* hookworm survey. He suggested that the survey be conducted by an experienced IHB physician with two Mexican assistants.[37] One of the proposed Mexicans, Dr. Angel de la Garza Brito (subsequently Dean of Mexico's School of Public Health), had already carried out his own hookworm survey in Mexico City and earnestly shared with IHB director Russell a hookworm pamphlet he had penned.[38]

But Russell had other plans, assigning neophyte IHB officer Dr. Henry Pardee Carr, a recent Harvard medical school graduate from rural Georgia, to help Warren with the survey. Even after Russell's decision, outgoing IHB yellow fever officers endorsed Pruneda's idea, reasoning that a competent Mexican physician might serve as a better survey assistant to Warren than the inexperienced Carr.[39] This proposal was promptly rejected by the RF home office. Instead, Russell pictured the "place" of the two doctors assigned to campaign director Brioso Vasconcelos as being in the "office doing routine campaign work . . . so they can take it over when we leave." Meanwhile, the IHB director gave Carr most of the responsibility for the survey, keeping Warren focused on initiating the campaign. Russell insisted that Carr be given rigorous instruction, arguing that it would be "good for Carr and he will do it properly."[40]

In April 1924, Carr set out to examine the geographic distribution of hookworm in Mexico, the demographic makeup of the infected population, living and working conditions, the severity of the disease, the source of the infection, the species of hookworm implicated, and the overall "effect of the disease upon the individuals involved."[41] Only superficially alerted to dangerous regions, Carr vowed to survey troubled states as soon as they were free of conflict.[42] He was warned that he would likely be asked to provide medical care beyond hookworm treatment; his refusal could jeopardize cooperation with the survey, but the excessive provision of free care would inhibit his progress. Carr would need to exercise his epidemiologic and diplomatic skills simultaneously, for, as IHB officer Emmett Vaughn (who remained in Mexico to help with the transition from yellow fever to hookworm campaigns in Veracruz) stressed to him, "you are responsible for success or failure."[43] A few months later, Russell echoed this point. All officers had to adjust to "the difficulties of being an investigator in a new field," just as Russell himself had done in his early days in Puerto Rico. Advancing the IHB's program to effectively organize rural health agencies, he argued, would afford Carr the opportunity to contribute "to knowledge of disease and public health methods."[44]

Cognizant of Mexico's "remarkably varied climatological characteristics," which distinguished it from "most other tropical countries,"[45] Carr divided the country into regions of likely or unlikely hookworm infestation based on altitude and rainfall. Using the preliminary information Warren had amassed, Carr expected to find significant hookworm infestation in lowland, high rainfall coastal areas but not in mountainous inland regions toward the Mexico City valley, in the desert north, or in low rainfall regions of the Pacific Coast. Based on these assumptions, most of his survey was concentrated in the wet coastal regions of the states of Veracruz, Oaxaca, and Tabasco along the Gulf Coast and the southern Pacific region of Chiapas, though several other states that fit hookworm's geographic criteria, such as Tamaulipas and Campeche, were not included in the survey. Carr also surveyed small areas in the mid-Pacific state of Colima, arid Yucatán, and the highland state of Tlaxcala, which represented low hookworm topographical regions, in order to verify that his assumptions were correct.

In other countries, surveys had estimated only the number of persons with hookworm disease, but the Mexican survey was to calculate the density of infection as well as the clinical manifestations of the disease.[46] This modification was in response to IHB officer Wilson G. Smillie's work in Rio de Janeiro, which had demonstrated that quantitative "before and after" surveys of the number of persons infected and the level of infestation showed improvements due to hookworm campaigns, while qualitative surveys—which carefully considered both clinical symptoms and the social and geographic representativeness of surveyed populations—did not.[47]

Carr's quantitative and clinical mandate required him to employ a new way of measuring hookworm infection. Up to that time, most IHB officers had used the Willis-Molloy salt-flotation technique, which determined the general presence or absence of hookworm ova in the stool. The home office instructed Carr to use a newer egg-counting method, developed by Norman Stoll of Johns Hopkins, because it gauged not just the existence of infection but also its severity through careful study of fecal matter.[48] Testing whether the Stoll method—which estimated the relationship between the hookworm ova count and the number of worms in the feces—could provide a more accurate picture of hookworm infection was a considerable responsibility for Carr.

Admitting to his "limited experience," Carr faced the challenge boldly. He found that the exact volume of worms in a person's intestines was a less valuable measure of infection than were hemoglobin levels, which could indicate

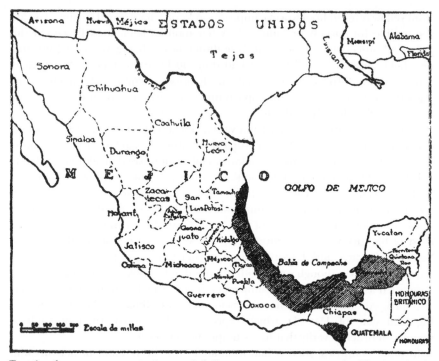

Fué hecho un reconocimiento del País que mostró que la Uncinariasis está limitada a una zona definida. El mapa indica, en la parte sombreada, los límites de esta zona.

Figure 2.4. Map of hookworm survey results indicating the limits of the hookworm zone. From Bernardo Gastélum, *Memoria de los Trabajos Realizados por el Departamento de Salubridad Pública 1925–1928*, tomo 1 (México, D.F.: Ediciones del DSP, 1928). Courtesy of the Secretaría de Salud, Mexico City, Mexico.

anemia. With the help of a single assistant and a few instruments in rough field conditions, Carr set out to demonstrate that low hemoglobin levels (indicating severe anemia) were correlated with high egg counts, and he developed a rough scale to gauge the level of severity. Although he noted the potential confounding factor of malaria infection (which also depresses hemoglobin levels), he was able to carry out malaria diagnosis through spleen examination in only a small number of children. For the most part, therefore, he relied on his own judgment as to whether an area was "probably free of malaria,"[49] a poor indicator of a highly under-reported disease with which Carr had had little experience. An additional confounder would have been nutritionally related anemia. Carr made reference to infrequent meat consumption among the "laboring classes"[50] but did not pursue this issue further. Based on egg counts and hemoglobin analyses of 1,120 persons surveyed in eight locales in four states where hookworm was known to exist, Carr identified severe hookworm infection in less than 9 percent of men and boys and only 4 percent of women and girls. According to his hemoglobin scale, some 40 percent of the population had a "significant grade of severity," yet this did not uniformly translate into clinical manifestation of the disease[51] (likely due to the confounding factors of malaria and low iron consumption), and he subsequently specified that he had found hookworm in only 10 to 20 percent of the population in the affected region.[52]

Although Carr reported his findings to be significant for many of the locales he visited, his survey revealed considerably lower levels of hookworm infection than in other locales where the IHB was working, such as Puerto Rico, India, and Ceylon.[53] In Jamaica, for example, 80 percent of the population in rainy mountainous districts was found to be infected, and the Dutch Indies (Indonesia) had a 98 percent hookworm infestation rate.[54] Given that only six of Mexico's then thirty states and territories were found to harbor the disease, hookworm was indeed a circumscribed problem.[55]

Notwithstanding these limited findings, Carr remained eager to participate in the hookworm campaign itself. If the political and military situations stabilized, he saw "great opportunities" for hookworm control, and he believed that his survey work would make him more effective in Mexico than elsewhere.[56] Nevertheless, the IHB home office, perhaps considering Carr too inexperienced for the volatile situation in Mexico, transferred him back to Georgia in the fall of 1924 to conduct scientific research in RF tropical disease specialist Samuel Darling's malaria laboratory. Russell then sent him to pursue graduate studies at the Johns Hopkins School of Hygiene and Public Health.

Regardless of hookworm's actual prevalence or importance, the IHB was determined to carry out a hookworm campaign;[57] because Mexicans were barred from the survey team and initially not privy to its results, the selection of hookworm could not be contested by the DSP either. Indeed, neither IHB officers on the ground nor DSP officers were able to question the survey results to propose an alternate disease campaign. Nor could these parties challenge the DSP's and the IHB's joint pinpointing of Veracruz as the desired campaign site.

Flapping Around

The False Start

Almost as soon as the ink had dried on the hookworm agreement, the audacity of locating the campaign in Veracruz became evident. In early December 1923, Veracruz was the seat of an attempted overthrow of Obregón's government, when his finance minister, Adolfo de la Huerta, arrived in Veracruz and declared himself in opposition to the president. Persuaded to revolt by General Sánchez

of Veracruz and other *caudillos* in Jalisco and Oaxaca, de la Huerta and his fol-
lowers claimed that Obregón's army reforms were unfair, that his agrarian policies were too radical, and that his maneuverings to ensure the election of
Interior Minister Plutarco Elías Calles constituted a fraudulent presidential succession. De la Huerta named a provisional replacement for Veracruz Governor
Tejeda, and fighting broke out around the state of Veracruz and along a wide
path to Mexico City. Sánchez's forces, joined by federal troops stationed in
Veracruz, rapidly captured the region's main cities, taking state and federal officials by surprise. The rebels vainly sought the backing of at least some peasant
forces; but the agrarian movement rallied to the support of Tejeda and
Obregón.[58] The U.S. State Department was initially divided over whom to support; only in January 1924, after Obregón employed threats and cajoling to
obtain the Mexican Senate's ratification of the Bucareli Street agreements, did
Coolidge organize a blockade at the oil port of Tampico to counter the rebels
and arm Obregón's forces.[59]

With wire, steamer, and train service suspended, the IHB's men were stranded in
Veracruz; fruit boats en route from Central America to the U.S. were the region's
only means of communication. Despite the danger and uncertainty, the IHB home
office remained optimistic, holding that its work was "appreciated by both parties
to the controversy and that either of them would probably support the program."[60]

From the perspective of IHB officers in Mexico, however, it was politically prudent—not to mention safer—to delay the campaign's debut in Veracruz. IHB
yellow fever officer Vaughn was deeply troubled at the possibility that the RF's
accomplishments could be lost. He explained to newcomer Warren: "The Latin-
American is suspicious of all foreigners and the Mexican, in particular, of his
northern neighbors." Thanks to the yellow fever campaign, "I feel sure that no
foreigners in Mexico ever achieved our standing in the eyes of the people and
government." Vaughn worried that the IHB's reputation was imperiled by the
many U.S. citizens in Veracruz who were "openly sympathizing" with the de la
Huertistas and because Juan López, a yellow fever Special Commission
employee, was an active member of the rebel movement. As a result, Vaughn
believed it would be "natural" for the Mexican government to become "suspicious of our most innocent activities."[61]

Vaughn proposed that at least one IHB officer go to Mexico City for the remainder of the crisis in order to stay in close contact with DSP officials. This plan would
enable the RF to keep counsel with both the Obregón government and the de la
Huertista rebels in Veracruz. If the opposition won, IHB programs were safe since
the "staff is all known personally to the revolutionary chiefs and has their confidence." If the federal government won and IHB representatives had neglected
relations with Mexico City, Vaughn feared, President Obregón could:

> consider all Americans more or less persona non grata and this would materially inter-
> fere with the programme I have laid out. A distrust on the part of the Obregón

government might eventually spread to Central America and impair a record built up after years of untiring effort and an expenditure of hundreds of thousands of dollars.[62]

Vaughn's plans were followed to the letter. The U.S. consul advised Warren to evacuate his family from Veracruz and relocate in Mexico City, traveling via New Orleans. On February 10, Carr and Vaughn also arrived in Mexico City. DSP officials, for their part, were embarrassed that the Veracruz unrest was affecting the campaign and distressed at the potential impact on the Mexico-RF relationship. Pruneda gladly welcomed the officers to the capital, concerned that the IHB might abandon the country altogether.[63] The acting hookworm director, Brioso Vasconcelos, apologized to Russell for his country's "turbulent politics," hoping it would not discourage the RF. Assuring that normality would return "little by little," Brioso Vasconcelos used the occasion to make an unsuccessful petition for an increase in funds.[64] (Several DSP men later remembered the problem with Veracruz as climatological rather than political. There is no evidence, however, that the rainy season impeded hookworm work in Veracruz at any time.[65])

De la Huerta's rebellion was put down by the end of January 1924, but turmoil continued in Veracruz for many months. DSP and IHB officers watched and waited from Mexico City, planning the campaign from afar. In March 1924, Brioso Vasconcelos—who had expressed repeated skepticism of Mexico's need for a hookworm campaign—left to become head of fumigation and public baths for the DSP. The campaign's new director was Dr. Juan Solórzano Morfín, previously the chief quarantine officer for Veracruz, who had overseen the port's antiplague efforts and had been extremely supportive of the yellow fever campaign. Solórzano Morfín was one of the best regarded physicians in Mexico, a brilliant lecturer, committed to public health and scientific research, founding editor of the *Revista Médica Veracruzana (Veracruz Medical Journal)* and a close associate of President Obregón's.[66] The selection seemed astute. Solórzano Morfín was at once a technical man, an IHB fan, and politically connected both locally and federally. Outgoing yellow fever officer Vaughn considered him ideal for Mexico's hookworm campaign, "probably one of the most important the IHB has ever undertaken."[67]

The question of further hiring was made complicated by the Veracruz situation. The IHB was concerned about filling high-level posts with persons who might prove controversial pending political outcomes. There was certainly no shortage of interested parties. Soon after the inception of the hookworm campaign, Mexican doctors began making inquiries about obtaining jobs. Some even wrote to the IHB's New York office, praising the success of the yellow fever measures, lauding Rockefeller efforts around the world, and requesting positions with the campaign.[68] Over the short term, the IHB decided to maintain several of its own experienced staff members in Mexico as a precautionary measure. During this time the IHB also discouraged the hiring of Mexican physicians other than

GACETA MEDICA DE MEXICO

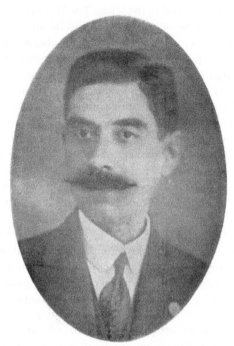

DR. JUAN SOLORZANO MORFÍN.

Figure 2.5. Dr. Juan Solórzano Morfín, hookworm campaign director (1924–26). From *Gaceta Médica de México* 58 (1927): 632. Reproduced by permission from the *Gaceta Médica de México*.

those who had already proven themselves with the yellow fever campaign, initially employing only lower-level assistants to work with the hookworm brigades.

In April 1924, with hookworm staff trained and supplies ready, both the Mexican government and the IHB home office pressured campaign officers to begin action somewhere and soon. Yellow fever hand Vaughn worked closely with Warren to relocate the campaign to the highland state of Tlaxcala. Months before the campaign started, Warren guessed that because Tlaxcala was very poor, agricultural, and populated by "pure-blooded" Indians, "There is every reason to believe that hookworm infection is general in this state as the inhabitants still live in the most primitive manner."[69] But this claim was soon negated by Carr, who found that Tlaxcala's high, arid plateau was "not involved in the hookworm problem of Mexico."[70] Indeed, the state's dry, mountainous enclaves topographically inoculated the population against hookworm. Tlaxcala's selection indisputably disregarded the standard IHB criterion of significant disease prevalence. In Tlaxcala's favor, however, was its location along major rail lines midway from Mexico City to the Gulf of Mexico. Although Carr's hookworm survey estimated the states of Tabasco, Oaxaca, and Chiapas to have far higher rates of hookworm, they were more distant from Mexico City and less accessible to Veracruz during times of unrest: uncertain transportation made these states undesirable candidates for a temporary campaign.

Thus, the first phase of the IHB-Mexican hookworm campaign was carried out in a region the IHB determined to be outside the hookworm zone. Working alongside Carr, the hookworm team merely repeated his negative survey results, showing that only eight of 1,232 persons examined had hookworm. Further, the campaign's health education efforts at local silver mines appeared to be duplicating existing activities carried out by mine owners.[71] Although Tlaxcala ranked among the neediest states in terms of public health according to the prevalence of other ailments,[72] the campaign quickly moved on, predictably unable to demonstrate the value of hookworm treatment on a large scale.

In June 1924, Veracruz was still not sufficiently pacified, so the campaign moved from Tlaxcala to the nearby mining district of Pachuca, Hidalgo, to see if it merited a campaign. Here, rates were somewhat higher, with 17.7 percent of 1,367 Pachucans and 25 percent of miners exhibiting hookworm. Miners tended to work barefoot, with hookworm infection exacerbated by unsanitary latrines and moist conditions in the mines.[73] The IHB decided *against* staying in Pachuca, however, given that mine latrines, even if deficient, were already universally used and "under excellent medical supervision. They have been doing and are doing anti-hookworm work and they do not especially appreciate our appearance upon the scene."[74] Once again, the campaign moved on as soon as it could because, as Warren subsequently noted: "the demand for a more respectable showing in order to justify the campaign, necessitated that the scene of activities be transferred from the Mesa Central where Uncinariasis did not exist, to a more favorable area."[75]

The Real Start in Veracruz, in Dosefuls

By mid 1924, IHB administrators in New York were losing their patience. With the stops in Tlaxcala and Hidalgo further delaying a bona fide inauguration of the campaign, the home office reiterated that Veracruz was the locale most in need of hookworm sanitation.[76] In July 1924, Veracruz was finally deemed sufficiently safe, and the campaign was initiated in the uplands town of Córdoba (population 12,000), located in the heart of Veracruz's coffee, sugar, and fruit-growing region. Ironically, Carr cited the Córdoba area as showing "the lightest infestation . . . within the entire hookworm area,"[77] but at the time it was one of the safer parts of the state.

Warren, accompanied by a brigade of assistants and by now without either Vaughn or Carr, was eager to get started. Through campaign director Solórzano Morfín—who traveled between Mexico City, the hookworm campaign site, and the port of Veracruz—the DSP was in contact with the brigades but prudently maintained its distance while the situation in the state remained unstable. Warren seemed oblivious to all but hookworm. His frustration at the ambivalent reception accorded the campaign in Tlaxcala and Hidalgo rapidly melted. Within a matter of weeks he reported that "our initial efforts have been enthusiastically received by all classes of people," and that hundreds of local inhabitants seeking treatment had "mobbed" the Córdoba unit each day.[78]

Like the IHB's efforts in the South of the U.S., the hookworm campaign in Mexico pursued a three-pronged approach of treatment, education, and latrine-building. Hookworm treatment was administered by uniformed officers to dozens of townsfolk each day. On the prevention front, the campaign brigades constructed model latrines and carried out household and community level health education measures to convince peasants to wear shoes, use the model latrines, and then build their own. The brigades—consisting of one doctor, four assistants, and one or two sanitary inspectors—carried out these activities simultaneously. Treatment, which showed immediate results, was generally emphasized over prevention, which was considerably slower to take hold.

Based on experience elsewhere, the IHB had developed detailed hookworm control guidelines, with a special focus on treatment methods and the role of diagnosis. By 1920, Samuel Darling and his colleagues working with the Rockefeller Uncinariasis Commission to the Orient had demonstrated the effectiveness of an oral dose of oil of chenopodium (initially set at 3 cc. per treatment) in removing hookworm ova from the stool, repeated as warranted in subsequent weeks.[79] Because the treatment provoked aftereffects including nausea, burning skin, headache, gastric pain, vertigo, deafness, and diarrhea, a lower dose (1.5 cc.) and a purge of magnesium sulphate were adopted to mitigate some of these side effects. In 1924, RF officer Robert Lambert showed in Fiji that carbon tetrachloride was also effective in eliminating worms, and, when it was taken with a purgative, there were virtually no side effects. If the patient had consumed alcohol before the treatment, however, there could be toxic aftereffects. IHB officer Smillie's studies in Brazil in the early 1920s determined that chenopodium and carbon tetrachloride could be combined to a maximum dose of 3 cc., but this was soon cut in half to reduce the risk of poisoning. A minimum of three weeks was needed between treatments, and it was believed unsafe to give more than two treatments in total. Patients were to be treated on an empty stomach to prevent nausea; treatment contraindications, which usually went undetected, included alcohol consumption, pre-existing pulmonary and heart problems, and calcium deficiency.[80]

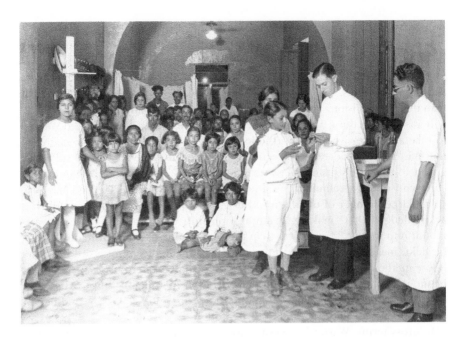

Figure 2.6. Hookworm dispensary. Courtesy of the Rockefeller Archive Center.

Warren was given considerable leeway in flouting these guidelines. As soon as he arrived in Córdoba, Warren adopted Darling's method of "mass treatment" of hookworm at dispensaries. Mass treatment forewent the preliminary diagnosis: anti-hookworm medication was administered to the entire population regardless of whether they had hookworm disease. The IHB generally advocated mass treatment only in areas of high infection—over 75 percent—where lower per capita expenditures could be obtained and many more people reached through this strategy. But in Córdoba, under 60 percent of the population surveyed was infected with hookworm, and less than 5 percent had very severe infestation. Warren held that the long delays in the hookworm campaign's Veracruz inauguration demanded this dramatic method.

Warren also admitted to using treatment doses "not advocated by the Board." He justified a higher dose of chenopodium (2 cc. at one time, instead of 1.5 cc. divided into two doses) on the grounds of its efficiency despite "the possibility of intoxication." Because the entire dose (though not the purgative) was taken in front of unit personnel, he argued, its correct administration was assured. Even after a man almost suffocated under Warren's care, he viewed the absence of "distressing consequences" as an encouraging sign.[81]

When Warren informed the RF home office of his activities, he was given only generic counsel. The IHB's assistant secretary, Florence Read, advised Warren to proceed slowly, starting new Veracruz units only if the area had been surveyed, "sanitated," and a successful education program on the value of treatment and sanitation had been implemented. New staff members were not to be added without DSP guarantees, for the "wisdom of slow and sound growth" had been proven many times. When Warren solicited specific advice, however, Read was firm that the decisions and responsibility went to the "man on the ground."[82]

It was perhaps these mixed messages from the New York office that led Warren to take an aggressive and unorthodox approach to treatment. He recognized that the "rate and degree of infection in the area probably was not of sufficient gravity to absolutely justify" mass treatment, but he believed that by eliminating "time-consuming preliminary examinations," the campaign could quickly provide a large number of treatments, thus gaining popular recognition.[83] Warren acknowledged that "making an impression with the campaign" was of "paramount importance," far greater than the actual value of the treatments. Ideally, he held, mass treatment was to be conducted through the intensive house-to-house method rather than at the hookworm dispensaries, so that patients could be monitored closely throughout the day of their treatment.[84] If the drugs were entirely harmless, Warren reasoned, the mass "shotgun" method would be less objectionable, an assumption that turned out to be erroneous.

In gross terms, Warren's cocksure approach quickly paid off. By the end of 1924, over 20,000 people from the larger Córdoba region (including most of the town's inhabitants) had received hookworm treatment. The latrine-building campaign, by contrast, was far less popular, and the campaign staff resorted to building three hundred latrines with little local cooperation. In his first year-end evaluation, Warren recited the campaign objectives as they had been directed from New York: diagnosis and treatment of hookworm, community sanitation, and distribution of information on the cause and prevention of hookworm.[85] Only later did he understand that the numeric results of the first year of work did not automatically translate into the campaign's goals of "chang[ing] the intimate habits of a race of people" and improving their economic lot. Achieving these tangible outcomes required "as the foundation the people and their convictions," and "The community must be convinced that the project is first practical, second beneficial, and third the cost must be within the means of the tax-payers."[86]

These caveats notwithstanding, Warren deemed the Córdoba campaign a success. He attributed the positive reception of the hookworm campaign in Córdoba to the "hearty cooperation" of civil, church, and military authorities, a feat unimaginable during the early part of 1924 when the same parties had joined in an "attempt to overthrow the constitutional government."[87] Conditions in many parts of the state had been unsafe when the IHB entered Córdoba in the summer of 1924; even at the end of the year, the political situation in Veracruz was volatile.

In early 1925, the hookworm campaign left Córdoba for the town of Alvarado, a fishing port along the south-central Veracruz coast. Warren would have preferred to stay in Córdoba, both for safety's sake and to enable the hookworm campaign to attain greater coverage and recognition. But his superiors in New York pressed him to move on as soon as it was clear that the community had understood the campaign's public health message. For Warren, general community acceptance of hookworm activity was assured only through universal treatment and demonstrated local commitment. From the perspective of the RF in New York, popular approval of public health was sufficient; guaranteeing coverage and enabling local implementation would be the responsibility of the Mexican government.

Warren pushed for a permanent unit to take over the brigade's work in Córdoba under the direction of one of the campaign's men, so that hookworm treatment and sanitation would continue along the same lines. The DSP agreed to appoint a sanitary inspector, but "unfortunately the [local] politicians received notice of the impending appointment and our suggestion was not followed. A woman was appointed to the position."[88] With his plans foiled by what he deemed to be patronage politics—more likely the result of women's increasing labor organization and growing civic networks in the Córdoba region[89]—Warren lamented that prospects for further sanitary activity were dismal.

The campaign's moves were orchestrated by Solórzano Morfín so that the IHB neither aggravated local authorities nor jeopardized its relationship with the DSP. Given the turmoil of 1924, the DSP's initial hands-off stance proved effective. But with Obregón's term coming to an end, the hookworm campaign found itself embroiled in battles between local Veracruz officials and the federal government in Mexico City. In late 1924, Warren was instructed by the New York office to move his base to Mexico City, traveling back and forth to Veracruz as needed, while keeping in frequent contact with all parties.

By the end of the year, the situation had calmed. In December 1924, Obregón's anointed successor, Plutarco Elías Calles (1924–28)—a one-time schoolteacher turned first revolutionary, then landowner and financier—became president. Early in his term, Calles solidified the state's partnership with organized labor, and he named Luis Morones—the head of the umbrella union CROM—as his minister of industry, commerce, and work, giving CROM hegemonic control of labor. In September 1925, Calles signed a measure granting temporary ownership of planted fields to communal landowners with eventual conversion to individual family property, intensifying agrarian reform, albeit more along the lines of private initiative than of collective ownership.[90]

With federal power now stabilized, Russell asked Warren to shift his office from Mexico City back to Veracruz so that he could save money on travel and keep a closer eye on hookworm activities. Amidst these changes, the hookworm campaign was off to a steady start.

In its first year and a half, the campaign did not venture beyond central and southern Veracruz, a region with sufficient hookworm to allow the campaign to make a positive impression despite the risk of unrest. State health officer Agustín Hernández Mejía now joined Solórzano Morfín in helping Warren plan

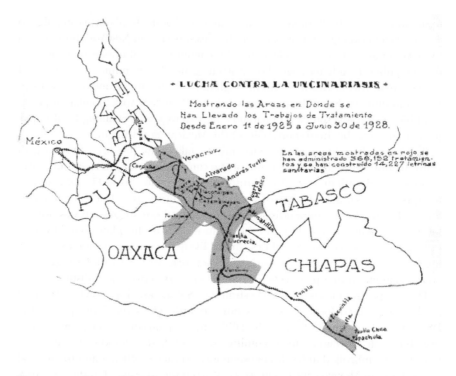

Figure 2.7. Map of hookworm campaign locales, 1925–28. From Bernardo Gastélum, *Memoria de los Trabajos Realizados por el Departamento de Salubridad Pública 1925–1928*, tomo 1 (México, D.F.: Ediciones del DSP, 1928). Courtesy of the Secretaría de Salud, Mexico City, Mexico.

the movements of the brigades to places where the agrarian movement was strong[91] and where a public health campaign might make the best showing. In 1925 the hookworm brigades reached only five towns, but in 1926 they worked in fourteen sites, including, for the first time, a Oaxacan locale near the Veracruz border. As with the yellow fever campaign, the day-to-day contacts made by the hookworm brigades were at the heart of the appoach.

Finding the Disease

It was not only Henry Carr who hunted for hookworm in his survey but also the hookworm brigades, who struggled to convince Mexican peasants that this previously unfamiliar disease was a problem that merited their understanding. Beyond the counting of hookworm lectures and of persons attending them, Warren and his successors barely discussed health education efforts in their

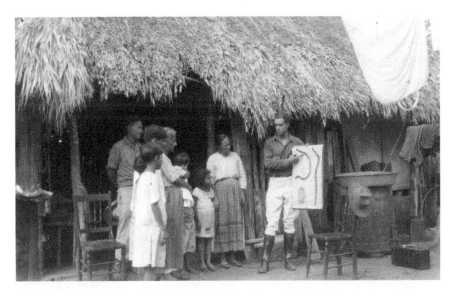

Figure 2.8. RF officer explaining the life cycle of hookworm to a rural household, 1927. Courtesy of the Rockefeller Archive Center.

correspondence with the home office, even though education was a stated pillar of the campaign. Both small and large group health education strategies were used to explain how hookworm disease was transmitted and to try to persuade rural Mexicans to wear shoes, build and use latrines, and undergo treatment. Historian John Ettling has noted that before the RF "could set about the business of destroying" hookworm in the South of the U.S., it had to expend energy and money to "create the disease in the minds of the people."[92] In Mexico, as in the southern U.S. campaign, people with hookworm-induced weakness, fatigue, or distended bellies may have considered these conditions to be unavoidable circumstances of subsistence and plantation farming, perhaps not unlike periods of hunger, rather than as an illness requiring special attention.

Traditional medical beliefs adhered to in much of Mexico in the early twentieth century typically did not distinguish physical symptoms from spiritual well-being, though they did separate natural from supernatural illnesses. In the case of an unusual or chronic illness, an initial course of action might include prayer and home remedies to frighten away evil and supernatural forces, followed by a visit to one of several resident *curanderos*—locally renowned healers who might administer an amalgam of herbal remedies, tonics, sacrifice, ritual bathing, and sorcery.[93] Only if these therapies failed might allopathic practitioners be consulted.[94] Traditional healers undoubtedly would have been present in all of the locales where the hookworm campaign worked. For example, the town of San

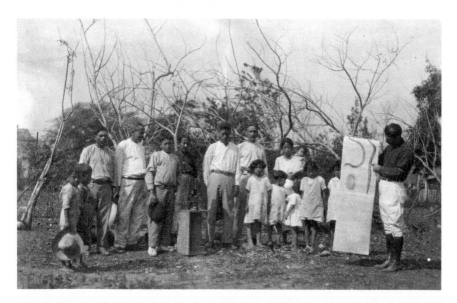

Figure 2.9. Hookworm campaign officer giving field lecture during house-to-house census, 1927. Courtesy of the Rockefeller Archive Center.

Andrés Tuxtla, where the hookworm brigades spent several months in 1926, was the home of a number of famous healers.[95]

Yet IHB men—seemingly oblivious to local medical beliefs, low levels of schooling and literacy in rural Mexico at the time, and widespread poverty— expected their public lectures and illustrated, house-to-house seminars on hookworm transmission to replace popular conceptions of sickness and to lead the audience to build their own latrines and wear shoes.

Perhaps the best evidence of the incompatibility of the medical ideas and practices of the IHB officers with the setting of rural Mexico comes from a series of photographs included with the IHB hookworm campaign reports in the 1920s. Although staged by IHB officers to depict the successful outreach efforts of the Mexican hookworm campaign, the photographs reveal a distance between the public health officer and the peasants placed around him. In one instance, a woman and her family stand outside their straw-roofed hut, squeezed in a semi-circle around an IHB officer who is using poster illustrations to demonstrate the life cycle of *Necator americanus* from egg to larva to full-grown worm. The bewildered faces and tense limbs of the Mexican peasants are in sharp contrast to the tall, confident officer, who uses "simple language" to discuss hookworm symptoms, treatment, and prevention. Another photo depicts a similar scene, this time in the woods behind a group of houses, an area that might otherwise be used for defecation. Here, a group of adults and bedraggled, barefoot children stare at the camera, while the officer, his white pants tucked into knee-high boots—displaying perhaps the ultimate foot protection against soil-happy hookworms—remains fixed on his hookworm poster.[96]

IHB officers were slow to understand why their efforts to promote shoes did not take hold; they do not seem to have understood the economic and cultural factors that limited the use of closed shoes. Anthropologist Oscar Lewis's study of a Morelos town in the 1940s, for example, found that less than 8 percent of the population wore shoes, with older people more likely to wear sandals or go barefoot than younger people. Notwithstanding some improvements in the standard of living since the 1920s, persistent deprivation of all but the most basic needs meant that—other than for those whose occupations demanded it—shoe-wearing remained out of the reach of the majority of the population.[97] Even so, the IHB campaign conceptualized shoe-wearing in terms of individual enlightenment, not social conditions. When Warren finally encountered a shoe-wearing community, he gloated that "It is the culture and intelligence that causes the people to wear shoes,"[98] overlooking his own observation that the village's local black, sticky, and hot soil demanded foot protection unlike the sandy soils of most locales.

The dual problem of "disease not perceived" by the target population and of "local circumstances not understood" by IHB officers made the hookworm campaign considerably more challenging than the yellow fever campaign had been. Peasants and townspeople were asked to accept disease where it did not seem to exist and to submit themselves to unfamiliar treatments and healers in spite of the apparent absence of recognized symptoms. One IHB officer estimated that 90 percent of people tested for hookworm would not ordinarily go to the physician for this condition. Given wide participation in the hookworm campaign—and subsequent village-level demands to local and national authorities for further sanitation—these communities appear to have appreciated the new health activities.[99] But, according to Mexican doctors of the day, few, if any, became new subscribers to modern medicine thanks to the hookworm campaign. Moreover, the campaign's aggressive pursuit of patients and autocratic treatment modalities were at odds with existing norms of healing,[100] in which *curanderos* and their communities worked together in the healing process and held to a unified concept of spiritual and physical well-being.[101] Popular bewilderment was no impediment; instead the campaign became more assertive, particularly on the treatment front.[102]

The hookworm campaign's strong presence in the communities where it operated—and the large pool of treated persons, including schoolchildren, who recounted their experiences to their families—facilitated its local reception. That hookworm was not understood as a problem a priori did not preclude the value of the physiological changes induced by treatment. Indeed, the empirical orientation of traditional medicine made its adherents open to certain allopathic medical practices perceived as successful, enabling a pluralism—sometimes uneasy—of various forms of healing.[103]

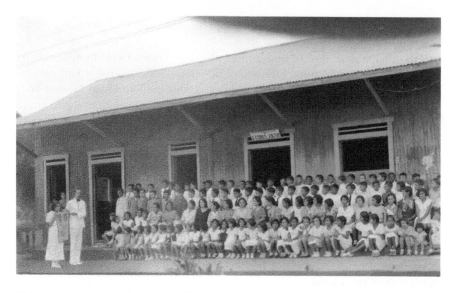

Figure 2.10. Hookworm lecture to schoolchildren, Puerto México, 1934. Courtesy of the Rockfeller Archive Center.

Treatment and Its Dangers

Since hookworm campaign subdirector Warren kept in closer touch with the IHB home office than with the DSP, it was sometimes difficult for the DSP to keep watch over the details of the campaign, even with Solórzano Morfín's involvement. In 1925, the campaign discontinued the use of the dispensary method, which required the population to come to the doctor at a hookworm clinic, because treated individuals could not be supervised during the hours after they took the medicine and many failed to return to the clinic for subsequent treatments. The replacement intensive method required the hookworm brigades to travel from house to house to administer treatment. By this time Warren had changed the antihelminthic dose to .75 cc. of chenopodium in combination with 1.50 cc. of carbon tetrachloride. The drugs were swallowed under the eye of a trained inspector in the home of the individuals being treated, but the inspector did not wait to make sure that the magnesium sulphate purgative was taken. Assistants returned during the course of the day to monitor the condition of those treated. Preliminary fecal examinations were administered only to individuals who refused treatment. Positive results gave, according to Warren, "an added weight to [the inspector's] already heavy argument, and the individual usually takes the medicine."[104]

The combined use of mass treatment and the intensive method meant that the hookworm campaign reached almost the entire population of each community visited. Even though inspectors now administered the antihelminthics directly, the zeal behind the mass method caused the dangers of treatment to multiply. Nevertheless, the IHB home office continued its laissez-faire approach to Warren's treatment methods, expressing little concern about the not infrequent instances of poisoning. Over the five-year campaign, there were at least four deaths and dozens of recorded intoxications. Most of the fatalities were in young children, who died within hours of antihelminthic administration. Though poisonings were communicated to the home office through mandatory reports, these episodes were not always shared with the DSP: IHB men did their best to muzzle publicity, lest the hookworm campaign be jeopardized.

While candid, the IHB incident reports offered extremely defensive interpretations of events that might put the competence of officers into doubt. In the first months of the campaign, Warren reported that "We have had a very unusual experience that involves the question of the advisability of allowing non-technical men of limited secondary education to administer highly toxic drugs."[105] After receiving oil of chenopodium and carbon tetrachloride, ninety-three people became ill, thirty severely so. Warren identified the probable cause not as the antihelminthics, but rather as *pulque*, a homemade alcoholic drink made from the fermented *maguey* plant and consumed in large quantities, he maintained, by the majority of the population. Warren shifted between blaming his Mexican assistants and blaming Mexican drinking habits for the disaster, leaving the treatment methods themselves beyond reproach. Because of the difficulty in changing the popular *pulque*-drinking custom, Warren's safeguard was to end the use of carbon tetrachloride, which caused adverse effects when mixed with alcohol. Russell recommended that, instead of discontinuing the use of carbon tetrachloride, patients be advised to eat starchy food before treatment in order to protect the liver.[106] Warren does not seem to have heeded this suggestion.

Warren also failed to reveal that he had hired nonmedical assistants to save money. Russell had requested that Warren maintain annual spending at $45,000 so as to "keep the work within the capacity of the Mexican government to take over."[107] Warren worried that spending caps would be "at the expense of thoroughness,"[108] but budget rules were one parameter he would not violate. He had promised that he could sustain the campaign at a cost of less than $1 per treatment (almost $11 in 2004 dollars) as long as there were no interruptions due to unrest.[109] The fact that Russell did "not feel competent at this distance to advise [Warren] regarding the method of treatment" and wrote that "you will be able to arrange this yourself"[110] only seems to have reinforced Warren's haughty attitude.

In early 1926—at the height of the campaign—several poisonings turned fatal. Hookworm treatment "should not have killed," a nine-year-old girl from Tlalixcoyan, Veracruz, according to Warren, but she suffered from malnutrition and a previous bout of malaria. Instead of admitting that the hookworm team ought to have recognized her condition and adjusted the dose, Warren denied responsibility.[111] (Another RF officer in Mexico later found that a castor oil purge made the chenopodium less toxic, especially for children).[112] He accused the *ayudantes* (assistants) of failing to follow instructions and noted that the Mexican hookworm campaign director, Solórzano Morfín, was the doctor in charge. Normally, Warren asserted, the hookworm staff was both well paid and well trained, attracting high-quality men. However, he claimed, the unavoidable hiring of lower-salaried, less-educated *ayudantes* had led to the deaths of this child and others. The *ayudantes*, Warren insisted, could "not be trusted. . . . When a $100.00 peso indian [*sic*] tells me he has done something I do not believe him until I have seen the results."[113]

Around the same time, Warren reported that a seven-year-old boy from San Andrés Tuxtla had died, but he claimed that the death was due to intestinal obstruction, not from the antihelminthics the boy had been given. In his own defense, Warren claimed that the child could not have died from the treatment because his entire family was infected with hookworm and all the others had survived the treatment. Warren then contradicted himself, suggesting that had he been in charge of the case—instead of hookworm team member Bernardo Peña, a Harvard-trained doctor—he would have administered a smaller dose of carbon tetrachloride and chenopodium.[114]

This time, however, Solórzano Morfín stepped in. He had a different interpretation, complaining that the "medically ignorant" Warren had attempted to increase the number of treatments administered with little supervision. In seeking to quickly expand the work of the hookworm brigades, Warren had approved the hasty hiring of *ayudantes* who were assigned a minimum quota of weekly treatments and left to work with little supervision by brigade doctors.[115] Warren was also met with criticism from local doctors who decried the dire consequences of hookworm treatment. Warren claimed these stories were "originated by charlatans and the few we have encountered who were not in sympathy with the work."[116] He continued, "it is well known that some of our men resign and advertise themselves as specialists"; Mexico's "lax" medical practice laws permitted "almost anyone" to practice, and, for example, an "ignorant mozo [errand boy] is treating people for ten pesos a shot."[117]

Whether the deaths were directly Warren's fault or not, his cavalier style and unwillingness to take responsibility were met with surprising indifference from the IHB home office and silence from the DSP, which was not always informed of campaign casualties. That the local population appeared convinced of the importance of undergoing hookworm treatment in spite of mishaps and fatalities fueled Warren's audacity. After two years running the campaign, he boasted that "the confidence of the people is such that we can kill a member of the family with chenopodium and the other members will demand that they continue to receive their treatment. And to throw this bouquet does not cause me the slightest embarrassment."[118]

Latrine-Building and Its Discontents

The hookworm campaign in Mexico was organized after the IHB had learned that it could not rely on local authorities in most parts of the world to enact sanitary measures before campaigns were begun; as such it included a significant latrine-building component. Indeed, the campaign's long-term success required popular participation in its latrine effort so that people who were treated for hookworm would not become reinfected. By far the most challenging part of the campaign for IHB officers, the building and promotion of latrines were slow to take hold. From the inception of the campaign in Córdoba, Warren grumbled, "no type [of latrine] suits the needs of the people here. On account of the poverty and the lack of intelligence, the septic tank, the septic privy, the chemical closets, the bucket types, and the concrete dry vault types may be immediately dismissed as being types that are not practical."[119] Even Warren's own experience as a native of rural North Carolina—where the RF had pursued a similar campaign—was of little use to him.

Warren was greatly concerned about the low number of latrines constructed even though his superiors in New York advised that "Mexico needs a preliminary period of education" before a large area could be sanitized.[120] Warren reported that the need for latrines was absolute—only 20 percent of houses in most towns had *excusados* (outhouses), and virtually no homes in villages had them. Members of the hookworm brigade proposed that only the common earth pit was economically feasible for the local population, but these calculations did not take into account the trade-offs that most subsistence-level peasants had to make. Warren despaired that for a "peon" to spend a large sum for the "construction of a place to defecate when he and his ancestors have for hundreds of years used the open spaces without apparent cost, is almost too much for us to expect him to comprehend."[121] Over the long term, Warren argued, the cost of the *excusado* would be far smaller than the costs of disease and death, but this was not a "tangible thing" to "peons."

Warren finally decided on a pit latrine as the "simplest, the cheapest, the most practical" solution. He designed an inclined platform for squatting rather than sitting, since, he noted, even North Carolina farmers "could not defecate when sitting . . . upon the seat of a water closet." Forced to sit on a wooden platform or not, few rural Mexicans used the latrines built by the brigades in Córdoba. Warren sought to explain this refusal by comparing peasants to rabbits, which were not attracted to brightly colored hutches because they were so different from the rabbits' customary quarters. He believed that Mexican "peons" failed to use the sleek, new pit latrines because they were "much better than the houses in which they lived."[122] Under Warren's direction, campaign staff downgraded the quality of construction, building rudimentary pit latrines surrounded by wobbly walls in an attempt to increase their acceptability.

The latrine-building enterprise revealed the crudest judgments of RF personnel. Warren and other officers undoubtedly reflected their own social origins

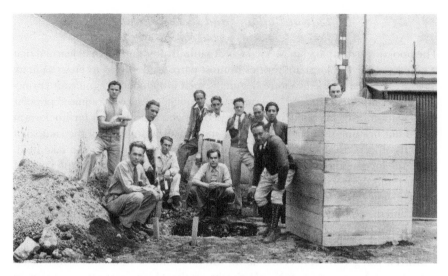

Figure 2.11. Student sanitary inspectors constructing a pit latrine, with RF health officer demonstrating the privacy provided by outhouse walls. Courtesy of the Rockefeller Archive Center.

and the prejudices of North American culture.[123] Some officers reportedly failed to learn Spanish.[124] Most made negative generalizations about the populations targeted by the IHB—principally mestizo and indigenous peasants and towns-folk—believing them to be morally and scientifically backward. The officers assumed that notions of sanitation, disease control, and personal cleanliness were unfamiliar. In Pachuca, for example, IHB representative Vaughn described "natives" who:

> exhibited a peculiar psychological reaction. They were willing to take the medicine and even demanded it . . . [but] when it came to submission of a fecal specimen they were very reluctant. In so doing they felt ashamed; that their dignity was being lowered. And yet it is not an uncommon sight to see natives defecating in the principal streets of the smaller towns.[125]

Warren expressed "disbelief" that rural Mexicans were "afraid of fresh air" but not of their own bodily waste, even though they bathed in, laundered with, and drank from the same river waters. With no reference to the role of clean water and sewage systems, Warren complained that peasants "do not seem to under-stand how a bucket of river water that seems to be reasonably free of solid mate-rial could produce typhoid fever and dysentery; nor that mosquitoes can inoculate them with malaria."[126] A decade later, another RF officer similarly blamed the inhabitants of hookworm and malaria infested areas for being "ignorant of the causes," since "suffering from these infections is the normal state of life. They are indifferent toward health and welfare, due in a large measure to ignorance of the constant danger they are in of germ and parasitic infection."[127]

But Warren went even further in assigning malevolent motives to Mexican peasants. He objected to offering material support to peons in building latrines because "they are a tricky, trifling lot and they will do nothing they can make some one else do."[128] Peons could be instructed to build latrines, but if supplied with wood, Warren argued, they would sell it rather than build latrines for their families. Because the building of latrines could not guarantee their use, Warren encouraged the Veracruz governor and state health officer Hernández Mejía to mandate latrine use. This was a necessary step, Warren held, as "The people here are so accustomed to doing things only when they are compelled to." While a latrine use decree was readily issued by these officials, the Veracruz state health department did not dispatch personnel to verify compliance, perhaps because local health workers better understood the economic barriers to latrine-building for most rural families.

Though he shared few of his woes with his Mexican counterparts, the frustrated Warren was not without support. Russell backed his efforts, agreeing that convincing peons to use latrines would solve the hookworm problem in Mexico. Russell suggested a psychological trick the IHB had used in Jamaica, where the government sold the wood at cost to the people instead of providing it for free, thus interrupting resale for profit. Russell also reminded Warren that unless he could get state inspectors to supervise the construction and maintenance of the latrines, the project would fail in the long run. For now, rather than rely on the state health department to monitor the latrine effort, Russell urged Warren to thoroughly train the members of his own staff to inspect latrines and to organize their transfer to government service. He pointed out that Warren was probably better at training than was the DSP, and he could "weed out" the incompetent inspectors and assure compliance.[129] Russell's praise continued unabated. Warren's building of a model latrine deserved congratulations, for Russell knew that there was "a crisis at every step."[130]

The tribulations Warren and the brigades faced in promoting latrine construction and use suggest that even coercion could not easily change the economic constraints and defecating habits of rural Mexicans. At the same time, Russell's constant comforting of Warren indicates the high priority placed on preserving the IHB's own staff's faith in the hookworm campaign's doctrines.

For Warren, this faith was anchored by the notion of individual rather than employer responsibility for latrine construction. When he found that hookworm existed among residents of the small port of Alvarado, Veracruz—where there was little agricultural employment—he mistakenly assumed that agricultural labor was "not important at all" as a determinant of hookworm disease.[131] Warren failed to understand that hookworm's classification as an occupational ailment did not preclude its presence under certain other conditions, even in an "urban community" such as Alvarado. Warren's generalization contradicted the findings of Mexican doctors, including campaign director Solórzano Morfín, and the IHB's Smillie in Brazil, who concluded that hookworm was an occupational disease of barefoot agricultural workers who became infected in the fields.[132] But the home office agreed that Warren's stance corroborated evidence from William Cort in Puerto Rico and from Carr's initial survey in Mexico, both of which found foci of human pollution near homes to be the most important factor in hookworm infection.

In de-emphasizing hookworm's relation to the work environment, Warren highlighted the centrality of individual households in reducing their infection. Because hacienda owners were losing money as the Veracruz uprisings continued into 1925, Warren held that it would be impossible to convince them to build *excusados* on their property for their laborers.[133] Instead, the campaign assigned the responsibility for latrine-building to each rural family (many of which lived in hacienda-controlled housing), thus minimizing the obligations of landowners. Warren failed to note that this policy was based on faulty—if not ironic— economic reasoning. Subsistence farmers, plantation employees, or town craftsmen could barely afford the basic necessities of life—food, clothing, water, and shelter—but Warren argued that it was hacienda owners, not laborers, who were unable to meet the expense of latrines.

In transferring the costs of prevention—via latrine-building and shoe-wearing—to the public, the hookworm campaign ignored the seemingly dubious cost-effectiveness of these activities to a poverty-stricken population. After all, the IHB had long known hookworm was a disease of poverty. By overlooking the realities of rural misery, the IHB avoided the politically and ideologically divisive issue of land reform in Mexico. It also implied that the state's responsibility for public health could be defined more in curative terms—through delivery of treatment—than in preventive terms. The prevention of disease in turn became a question of changing individual attitudes and household priorities rather than addressing underlying social conditions. In the years to come, the DSP and the IHB would struggle over which of these paradigms of public health was best suited to the needs of Mexico's rural population.

The Personnel and the Political

As a cooperative international health initiative, the hookworm campaign derived authority from stable institutional relations. With ongoing disturbances in Veracruz, Secretary-General Pruneda spent the first year of the hookworm campaign fretting that the IHB would pull its men out of Mexico,[134] even as he monitored and adjusted the DSP's profile in Veracruz based on political circumstances. In this atmosphere the IHB and the DSP remained steady partners, while the larger relationship between the RF and revolutionary Mexico was more flexible, enabling the Americans to interact with both national and regional politicians.

The actual hookworm work was by and large protected, owing to Solórzano Morfín's careful campaign choreography. Warren was certainly aware of the turbulence, and for the most part he refrained from discussing the political situation by mail, fearing that his letters could be censored or "construed as a defamation against the Country and result in serious difficulty for me . . . [or] seem to be an excuse for my work."[135]

Moreover, because he claimed no investments in Mexico and had only a "casual interest in politics," Warren wrote only about those troubles that presented direct obstacles to the IHB's labors. Since the de la Huertista defeat in early 1924, Warren reported, federal soldiers had routinely supervised the activities of the IHB and other foreign operations in Veracruz. Because the campaign typically worked in towns where there were army garrisons, it had thus far avoided conflict. For the most part, hookworm activities were confined to safe areas near railroads, though Warren warned that this did not afford full protection: "On two different occasions, trains on which my men were traveling in connection with their work were assaulted, [although] none of my staff were injured."[136] In 1925, several hookworm campaign assistants were assaulted and robbed while traveling on horseback between two towns in Veracruz. All of their possessions and clothing except underwear were stolen, causing them to suffer "considerable inconvenience." Replacement clothing could not be purchased locally, and "on account of the condition of the territory through which they were compelled to travel, the return journey was made in the day, and being without clothes, one of the men suffered severe sunburn."[137]

After Calles was inaugurated as president in late 1924, Pruneda assured Russell that the new leader would follow the policies of Obregón's government by improving living conditions through "education, solving agrarian problems, . . . and stimulating sanitary work."[138] By directly courting the allegiance of the rural population, the Mexican government hoped to divide the Veracruz opposition forces and stave off future rebellion.[139]

This time Warren did not refrain from discussing politics. He perceived the central government's decision to arm "peons who are to receive the land of their former employers" as a potential danger. These "unsettled conditions" had forced the hookworm brigades out of the Veracruz towns of Alvarado, Naranjal, and Tlacotalpan, but Warren was "most depressed" by economic circumstances, "now the most serious handicap to peace and happiness." Once the peasants received land, according to Warren, their salaries were terminated, and they faced starvation because they lacked the "intelligence to use the land." The hookworm brigades were able to maintain harmony only because health personnel explained to the agrarian population that the "work was inaugurated for their benefit." He added—perhaps revealing the IHB's pro-Calles partisanship—"This is a bit of a deception."[140]

Shielded though it was, the IHB could not remain entirely above the fray. During the January 1924 revolt in Veracruz, Juan López—a yellow fever Special Commission worker—had joined the de la Huertistas and was forced to temporarily resign from the IHB staff. While serving as treasurer-teneral with the rebels, López had purportedly extracted forced loans from various Veracruz merchants, who two months later succeeded in blocking his nomination to become the director of the Hookworm Service (the appointment went to Solórzano Morfín). Warren wished to hire the administratively skilled López in another position, but the IHB resisted budgeting an extra salary. Russell told Warren to follow his own judgment on the López case, warning, "since he has aligned himself with the revolutionary cause he has forfeited special consideration."[141]

As soon as it was clear that federal forces had triumphed, Russell was willing to abandon old allies, such as López.[142] In a bid to clear his name, López praised Warren's "honesty, tact, and enthusiasm" to RF administrators in New York and described his personal popularity among townsfolk and cabinet ministers alike.[143] López ultimately secured a job, but several years later, the DSP secretary-general insisted that both López and a physician who headed one of the hookworm brigades be severed from DSP employment due to their participation in the de la Huerta rebellion.[144] Warren's successor was quick to declare the two "persona grata" and to rehire them. Throughout the controversy, the IHB officer insisted that "I was careful that I should not be guilty of going over the heads of the Departamento."[145] Yet he did just that, by now confident that the IHB could teach Mexico City a lesson about prizing technical expertise over political loyalty.

In the autumn of 1925, violence again erupted in and around the port of Veracruz. After municipal voters elected anti-Calles leaders, federal troops invaded the opposition "Rojo-Negro" headquarters, killing fourteen people and injuring dozens more. Labor leaders responded by organizing a boycott against the twelve leading commercial houses. With human barricades blocking the entrance to stores and warehouses, and no imported goods arriving at the harbor, many businesses closed down and food supplies began to run low. Meanwhile, strikes had broken out against El Aguila and Huasteca oil companies for refusing to meet labor demands, leaving water and sewage plants without fuel.[146] Tejeda's successor as governor, Heriberto Jara (1924–28), supported the strikers, demanded that the oil companies pay back taxes they owed, and proposed expelling all foreign merchants. This position infuriated the president, eventually leading to Jara's downfall. With only lukewarm support from the agrarian movement, which considered Jara less committed to land reform than his predecessor, and due to Jara's strained relations with the labor movement, Calles was eventually able to arrange a successful military coup against the governor.[147]

Russell was initially concerned that turmoil in Veracruz might jeopardize Warren's work. On a site visit to Veracruz in September 1925, during the buildup to the autumn violence, Russell—a friendly acquaintance of Governor

Jara's—wrote to his colleagues back in New York that it was the "disturbed conditions" of other states, not Veracruz, that "makes our work impossible."[148] Warren seemed to share this view, assuring in October that "work is progressing despite the rains,"[149] even as the turbulence persisted. Veracruz was one of the main foci of unrest in Mexico until at least 1926, when the *Cristero* rebellions began in the central-western region of the country.

It is possible that Russell was misinformed during his trip, but, more likely, he saw with his own eyes that the conflict in Veracruz was not imperiling the RF's goals; indeed, given the DSP's detachment, the IHB's role was magnified. Still, according to Carr's survey, hookworm infestation was more severe in Chiapas and Tabasco than in Veracruz; these two states were relatively calm. The campaign could have shifted location, but the IHB was not immediately interested in this possibility. Veracruz remained strategically important both to the RF and to Mexico's federal government, leaving other infected areas ignored during the early years of the campaign. By the end of 1925, Russell justified the decision to stay in the state, satisfied that the hookworm campaign had been "little affected by the difficult conditions in Veracruz."[150]

Notwithstanding the attitudes of Russell and Warren, the RF's presence in Veracruz was both politic and daring. On one level, it was hedging its bets, maintaining friendly relations with both federal and regional politicians and *caudillos*, should there be a change in regimes. Facing such risks, the hookworm campaign began small and expanded slowly; more time in Veracruz would be needed to reach more people. On another level, the RF recognized the important part the IHB could play in overturning anti-American sentiment in the heart of oil country. This too was a gradual process, and there was no need to hurry out of the state. Admiring the value of the Veracruz work during his visit, Russell optimistically remarked that Mexico had become much more pro-U.S. since the revolution. "During the next ten years," he promised, "we will have an opportunity to do pioneer work, and one can reasonably expect big results in that time."[151]

Through its hookworm campaign, the IHB also believed itself able to counteract Veracruz's radical agrarian politics by offering social improvements within the context of capitalist state-building. Russell ventured:

> It may be that public health work will help to clarify . . . a new relationship between the peon and the state and federal governments, and help the peon to understand and appreciate the duties and responsibilities of government to the people and convince him that the government has a real interest in his welfare, health and happiness.[152]

Russell—like Mexican revolutionaries—recognized that public health services could instill values of citizenship in the rural population. Rather than viewing this as a collective process, however, Russell marked the civic progress of the "peon" by individualizing his relationship to the state, implicitly separating him

Table 2.1. Hookworm campaign activities, 1924–28

Year	Number of Persons Treated	Number of Treatments	Number of Latrines Built	Joint Spending in Constant Dollars*	Approximate Spending in 2004 Dollars
1924[1]	21,529	28,763	337	43,836	481,300
1925[2]	44,917	79,228	631	35,694	380,600
1926[3]	53,527	97,660	6,328		
1927[4]	61,877	126,799	5,179		
1928[5]	32,557	78,420	2,768	45,000	492,500
Total	214,407	410,870	15,243		

*Includes U.S. and Mexican contributions. *Note:* empty boxes indicate missing data.
1. Warren, "First Annual Report of the Activities of the Hookworm Campaign for Mexico during the Year 1924," RG 5, Series 3, Box 143, RFA. The per capita cost of the hookworm campaign was $1.03 ($11.20 in 2004 dollars), including both persons who received treatment and persons not infested with hookworm (and not receiving treatment) in the denominator.
2. Warren to Russell, December 31, 1925, RG 5, Series 3, Box 144 RFA. By the second year of the program, the per capita cost dropped by more than half, to 43 cents.
3. Carr, "Annual Report of the Lucha Contra la Uncinariasis, Section for Tropical Diseases of the Departamento de Salubridad Pública, for the Year 1926," RG 5, Series 3, Box 144, RFA.
4. Carr, "Annual Report of the Lucha Contra la Uncinariasis, Section for Tropical Diseases of the Departamento de Salubridad Pública, for the Year 1927," RG 5, Series 3, Box 144, RFA.
5. Carr, "Annual Report of the Lucha Contra la Uncinariasis, Section for Tropical Diseases of the Departamento de Salubridad Pública, for the Year 1928," RG 5, Series 3, Box 144, RFA.

from social and political movements. In ideological terms, he was claiming a transformation that differed markedly from that advocated by Veracruz's agrarian organizations. In the end it was Mexico's federal government—which responded to both capitalist and socialist interests—that would instill a sense of national belonging through health services.

The Scatological and the Political

In the short term, the success of the cooperative hookworm endeavor was judged not by state-society relations but by the activities of the campaign. By January 1926, with the latest Veracruz crisis having passed, the hookworm brigades proved themselves more capable than before. In 1925, the number of persons treated had more than doubled to 44,917 at a cost of only 27 cents per treatment ($2.82 in 2004 dollars) and by 1927, 61,877 people were reached (see table 2.1).

The most notable turnaround was in regard to latrines. Whether or not Warren recognized it, the brigades had learned from townsfolk across Veracruz state a better way of promoting latrine use. After Warren's initial rigidity on the question of household responsibility for latrine-building backfired in 1925, the brigades themselves took on the task of latrine construction, amounting to literally hundreds of latrines built per community and thousands per year. Moreover, instead of demanding that every home have its own latrine, the brigades began building collective latrines for clusters of households. In 1925 the brigades built 631 latrines and inspected 6,371 buildings, 5,141 of which were without latrines.[153] The following year the brigades constructed 6,328 latrines, a tenfold increase.[154]

After the hookworm brigades had spent several months in the municipality of San Andrés Tuxtla, Veracruz, in 1926, for example, 90 percent of homes had access to decent latrines with seats made of suitable lumber. Warren boasted to Russell that, thanks to the accompanying educational effort, the local people "know [the latrines] will protect against reinfection." Although, according to Warren, "one half the Indians in the good agricultural area don't speak Spanish, they can see an improvement," a sign of the campaign's "excellent propaganda."[155]

How did this "excellent propaganda" make the hookworm campaign popular in spite of lack of familiarity with the ailment, the potential dangers of treatment, and the cost of recommended preventive measures? Annual hookworm reports of course gave credit to the campaign itself, in addition to repeatedly acknowledging the cooperation of the DSP and the Veracruz state government.[156] Successful campaign outreach in Mexico also required fruitful interaction with local institutions, just as it did in the South of the United States, where schools, churches, agricultural societies, and other civic groups became involved in the hookworm work. Other than the early work in Córdoba—where, as Warren had noted, "The participation of the local municipal authorities, the military authorities, and the Church authorities have made possible the success attained so far"—the campaign left few records of its relations with these entities or of the role of local organizations in shaping the campaign. Though many of the campaign stops were brief, the brigades generated ample publicity through their activities. Still, Mexico's hookworm campaign, while aimed at sparking popular and government interest in public health services, was initially less involved in institution-building than the southern U.S. campaign.

In all likelihood, another factor was at play in Veracruz and beyond: years of radical agrarian politics and labor mobilization had resulted in a public primed for improved living conditions and attention to social needs. The campaign's effectiveness in San Andrés Tuxtla, for example, might be at least partially attributed to the Communist Party's control of municipal politics. With a membership that included a wide range of rural and urban laborers, artisans, and shopkeepers, the party would have been a useful partner to the hookworm campaign. Although it was unable to significantly raise the "socioeconomic condition of the peasantry,"[157] the Communist Party and red politics may have helped the campaign's outreach efforts and enabled the popular acceptance of latrines in a variety of settings. Such left-wing political preparation for the hookworm stops was unlikely to be included in official reports, but it was probably a valuable element of the campaign's popularity.

In June 1926, the growth and stability of the campaign led the IHB, with the DSP's approval, to place Mexican doctors at the head of each of the hookworm brigades, in conjunction with the campaign's long-awaited expansion into the states of Oaxaca and Chiapas along key railroad lines. The new brigade chiefs were Dr. Gabriel Garzón Cossa, who had studied at the Johns Hopkins School of Hygiene and Public Health, Dr. Bernardo Peña, who had been working with the campaign in Veracruz, and the recent medical graduate Dr. Pilar Hernández Lira, who would continue his affiliation with the RF for some twenty-five years. Each man headed lab units and teams of four or five assistants, who carried out house-to-house censuses, hookworm lectures, treatments, and latrine construction. Under this more efficient arrangement, 27,579 treatments were administered and 1,117 latrines were built in the second quarter alone, and even more later in the year.[158] Warren was certain that this increased role for Mexican physicians would improve the work of the brigades, combat criticism, and boost public confidence in the campaign.[159]

This change also motivated the resignation of Solórzano Morfín, the campaign's formal director and principal liaison between the campaign and the DSP. Solórzano Morfín was displeased with the administrative arrangement requiring Mexico to contribute most of the resources (which rose substantially with the new responsibilities of Mexican doctors) but yield technical control to the RF.[160] While others may have shared his frustrations, Solórzano Morfín's resignation appears to have been an isolated event. Indeed, the RF's managerial function persisted even after the Mexican government had officially taken over the hookworm campaign at the end of 1929, with the RF representative to Mexico advising the campaign well into the 1930s.[161]

The Mexican Medical Elite

By the late 1920s, the elite academic wing of the Mexican medical profession had established important ties with the hookworm campaign. Several leading Mexican physicians had served in the DSP position of campaign director. The placement of Mexican doctors at the head of the hookworm brigades generated ever more participation in the campaign[162] and launched these doctors' careers in the DSP. These doctors also formed part of the first generation of Mexicans to receive RF fellowships to study public health in the U.S., and they served as effective ambassadors for the RF and its programs in Mexico.

At the same time, however, several Mexican doctors inside the campaign sought to dissociate themselves from the IHB regarding various aspects of combating hookworm. Certainly the reports produced by Mexican doctors working with the hookworm campaign reflected greater appreciation of the cultural norms surrounding healing, shoe-wearing, and defecating in Mexico. But this was not only a matter of sensitivity: the Mexican understanding of hookworm's etiology and underlying causes was more involved than that of Warren. By posing the question of who was the expert in the hookworm campaign, Mexican doctors also challenged the IHB's authority.

An example of this local professional interpretation of the determinants of disease was provided by Dr. Bernardo Gastélum, a worldly physician, academic, energetic public health leader, and civil servant, who had served as Mexico's ambassador to Uruguay and secretary of education before being named DSP chief by Calles.[163] Gastélum had been involved with anti-yellow fever activities in his native Sinaloa in the early 1920s, and not long after he assumed the DSP leadership, he spent a brief period with the hookworm campaign. In a May 1925 report on hookworm in coastal Alvarado, Veracruz, Gastélum demystified the age, gender, and occupational patterns of exposure to the disease. He explained that, although girls typically defecated in only one place, they began wearing shoes around the age of ten, which reduced their infection rate from that age onward. Young boys always defecated in a new place, but by ten years of age, they concentrated their excretions in one place. Because they did not customarily wear shoes, older boys had higher infection rates than girls. Many of the young men of the area became fishermen and, given that they spent most of their days on boats, they were less exposed to hookworm infection. As they returned to work in their villages as net-menders, however, older men once again contracted hookworm at higher rates.[164] Warren sought to counteract Gastélum's findings two months later with a simplistic analysis that claimed to debunk the association between hookworm and agricultural occupation.[165] As we have seen, not only did Warren's assertions fail to prove his point, they did little to illuminate hookworm's epidemiology.

In contrast to Warren's report, Gastélum's anthropological observations were extremely useful from the standpoint of a public health campaign, for they identified the origins of the hookworm problem and the best points of intervention for various groups in the community. But as chief of the DSP, Gastélum had little chance to pursue this avenue. Instead, he concluded his report with an assessment not dissimilar to Warren's: "breeding sites would be avoided if each town had two public latrines and citizens were obliged to use them instead of defecating on the ground without realizing what they are doing."[166] Though the more culturally and class-grounded approach advocated in Gastélum's report contested the IHB's framing of the problem as one of individual behavior, the DSP was then too busy to intervene in the day-to-day operations of the hookworm campaign. Under Gastélum, the DSP expanded health education efforts, issued new regulations governing milk and food hygiene, rebuilt the Institute of Hygiene, enacted internal

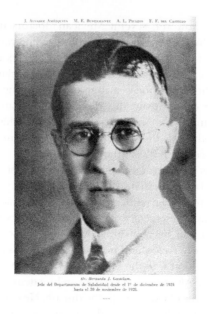

Figure 2.12. Dr. Bernardo Gastélum, director of the DSP (1924–28). From José Alvarez Amézquita, Miguel E. Bustamante, Antonio L. Picazos, and F. Fernández del Castillo, *Historia de la Salubridad y de la Asistencia en México*, vol. 2 (México, D.F.: Secretaría de Salubridad y Asistencia, 1960). Courtesy of the Secretaría de Salud, Mexico City, Mexico.

regulations and a new sanitary code, carried out campaigns against childhood diseases, malaria, smallpox, meningitis, venereal diseases, and tuberculosis, and trained hundreds of health professionals.[167] As long as the IHB helped out by building much-needed latrines in rural areas, the DSP kept its distance.

Some doctors in larger towns could not tolerate such a hands-off position: they viewed the activities of the hookworm campaign as unfair competition. These local physicians complained that the IHB was generating demand for modern technology (microscopes and medicines) at the same time as it was reducing the burden of disease. As such the campaign was making local doctors look bad while lowering patient interest in their services.[168]

Many more Mexican doctors welcomed the RF as a boost to medical prestige and salaries and a sure route to increasing the state's recognition of the importance of health services. If European—particularly French—influences in Mexican medicine were indirectly exhibited through local diffusion of foreign medical ideas, technology, publications, choice of medical school textbooks, and study abroad, the physical presence of IHB doctors began to enhance the U.S.'s influence in the public health arena.

Only a handful of elite physicians regarded the hookworm campaign as an explicit menace to Mexican medical sovereignty. As documented in a series of articles published in the *Gaceta Médica de México*,[169] Dr. Juan Solórzano Morfín, the former director of the hookworm campaign, made a public presentation on hookworm diagnosis and treatment to the Mexican Academy of Medicine as part of his bid for membership in 1927. He attributed the awakening interest in this "silent and draining plague on tropical countries" to government efforts, preventive and curative measures put in place by doctors working for mining and agricultural firms, and the collaboration of the IHB.[170] According to the author, modern medicine had triumphed in its scientific understanding of the epidemiology, prevention, and treatment of the disease, but the great task of eradication remained.

While Solórzano Morfín acknowledged the role of foreign investigators and the RF in hookworm research and control, he emphasized the large part played by Mexican doctors since the turn of the century. In 1902, Dr. Ricardo Manuell, a prominent military physician, had discovered a group of soldiers suffering from hookworm in the Military Hospital of Mexico City. Subsequently, hookworm was encountered in a number of coastal and mining states. In 1912, another physician had conducted a meticulous survey of the nation's doctors to determine the extent of hookworm infection among their patients, and, over the years, more than a dozen Mexican physicians had published articles about hookworm. Solórzano Morfín ranked a long list of locally developed anti-helminthic treatments (all of which were less toxic than chenopodium), including traditional medicinal plants, which had not been tested by the RF.[171]

He also condemned pharmaceutical manufacturers for failing to provide a medicine chest to help treat adverse reactions to their drugs. This was a case the RF had not made, despite field officers' complaints that their budgets did not cover such remedies. While Solórzano Morfín accepted the biological explanation of hookworm, he was concerned that the IHB's hookworm campaign paid scant attention to the likelihood that hookworm infection would increase susceptibility to tuberculosis or malaria and other parasitic ailments. Solórzano Morfín was also highly critical of the unnecessary deaths caused by hookworm treatment. He blamed these problems on the poor management of the campaign, which, he said, was entirely in the hands of the IHB representatives, even though by this time the DSP furnished the bulk of the budget. Solórzano Morfín was particularly unhappy about the IHB's naming of Andrew Warren, only a "post-graduate medical student," as head of the campaign instead of a more competent and experienced yellow fever officer.[172]

Solórzano Morfín was awarded a prize for his presentation, but his assessors at the Mexican Academy of Medicine—apparently reluctant to publicly pass judgment on the RF—did not acknowledge his disputes with the RF, and they criticized his ranking of hookworm treatments.[173] In a subsequent article, Solórzano Morfín was more conciliatory. He optimistically pronounced that the arrival of microscopes in the humblest of rural clinics marked the "splendid future of scientific medicine in Mexico."[174] This time the article's evaluator declared that accepting Solórzano Morfín "into the bosom of the National Academy of Medicine has been an act of justice, rewarding he who deserves."[175] Then, in late 1927—before his second article was published—Solórzano Morfín suddenly died.[176]

A few months later, Solórzano Morfín's critique formed the basis of a detailed analysis of hookworm treatment in the regionwide *Boletín* of the PASB,[177] but his work had little resonance in the Mexican context. In the end, Solórzano Morfín was advocating Mexico's therapeutic independence to a physician elite for the most part willing to forego medical sovereignty in the interest of professional success. The lure of the IHB was too great. Not only did Mexican physicians gain scientific contacts, specialized training, and technical armamentaria thanks to the RF, its very presence in Mexico helped expand the purview of medicine, leading both the public and the government to accept a wider societal role for medical practitioners. At the same time, Mexican doctors found that RF programs could be retrofitted and harnessed to local needs.

Reeling It In

Courting Mexico City

After the mid 1920s uprisings subsided, unrest in Veracruz began to pose less of a threat to national stability, although it remained a regional concern. Around the same time, the hookworm campaign was gradually facing fewer operational problems and began building a track record. These factors enabled the IHB to pay more attention to public health's state-building aspects, while advocating for a politics-free "scientific commitment" to public health. In the midst of the de la Huerta rebellion in January 1924, IHB chief Russell had told the then Mexican hookworm director, Brioso Vasconcelos, "It is a comfort to realize that politics do not any longer play an important part in public health work, and that leads us to hope that some day politics may be entirely divorced from public health so that campaigns against disease can go forward systematically and regularly regardless of political conditions."[178] More a misguided advisory than an assessment of the state of affairs in that tumultuous year, some twenty months later this stance was echoed in the words of Dr. Angel de la Garza Brito, a hookworm advocate and rising public health official: "Our sanitary work is improving day by day and we hope in two or three years we will have such a fine Health Service as yours. Our motto by now is the words you told us 'Better health and less politics' and it runs quite well."[179]

With the RF's promotion of U.S.-style values as a backdrop, the Mexican hookworm campaign became a vehicle for reaching multiple and simultaneous ends: diffusion of scientific medicine; federal, state, and local government commitment to public health; household responsibility for health; better social conditions; increased productivity and economic development; and improved relations between the two countries. These competing goals reflected the differing power and priorities of a series of actors: the RF home office, the Mexican government, IHB officers in Mexico, officials in the DSP, the local hookworm campaign staff, hacienda owners and other employers, peasants, and local community leaders.

From New York and on his field visits, Russell sought to parlay the campaign's achievements in Veracruz into greater institutional support in Mexico City. After the federal government had consolidated its military superiority over rebels in much of the country in 1926, Russell again asked Warren to spend more time in Mexico City to revitalize the IHB's relationship with the government and to secure support for IHB projects. Russell emphasized that showing the new secretary-general of the DSP, Roberto Medellín Ostos, the hookworm campaign in action was "a very important matter," just as it had been with his predecessor Alfonso Pruneda: once Pruneda saw with his own eyes the work of the brigades in Córdoba "all difficulties [with the DSP] disappeared."[180]

Warren resented having to repeat the groundwork that had been laid in Mexico just a few years earlier. He complained that Dr. Gastélum "seems to have just realized that we are a vital part of his organization and that we are in a position to be of further service to him and to his people."[181] The DSP chief certainly mentioned the RF in various reports on DSP activities. In the 1928 *Memoria* describing the overall accomplishments of his administration, for example, he dedicated a chapter to the hookworm campaign, complete with RF maps and charts. But the text of the chapter was less than two pages long, and followed much lengthier accounts of efforts against yellow fever and malaria, described as the country's most important infectious disease campaigns.[182] Warren's frustrations may have derived from a sense that Gastélum was showcasing the hookworm campaign without sufficiently deferring to the IHB's interpretation of its impact on the DSP.

Warren's return to Mexico City coincided with renewed federal attention to the social welfare arena. The energetic, demanding, and efficiency-minded Gastélum[183] reorganized the DSP, changing it from a group of offices that operated almost entirely in Mexico City to a set of agencies—including an infectious disease service and sanitary delegations—that began to have national scope. But, as he himself claimed at the end of his term, Gastélum had garnered insufficient resources, little acclaim, and attacks from the press. Even the most optimistic assessments credited his administration with organizational advancements in administrative and legal terms, but not in implementation per se.[184] Perhaps Gastélum's larger challenge of "refining the Treasury's understanding of public health activities"[185] led him simultaneously to ignore the IHB on a day-to-day level and to appropriate its work as one of a few demonstrations of major outreach to a population outside the capital.

Gastélum's stance toward the IHB had its counterpart at the presidential level. Although Warren considered his April 1926 meeting with President Calles to be

ORGANIZACION DEL DEPARTAMENTO DE SALUBRIDAD:

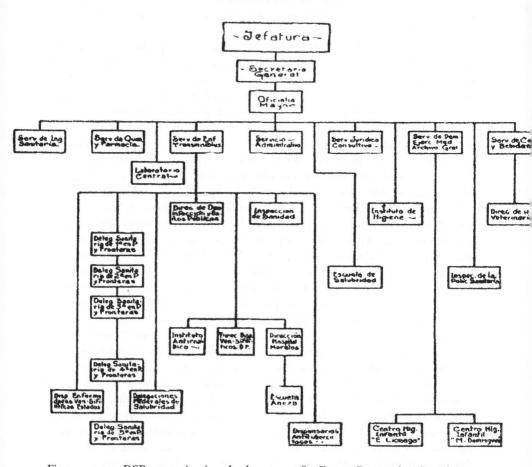

Figure 2.13. DSP organizational chart, 1928. From Bernardo Gastélum, *Memoria de los Trabajos Realizados por el Departamento de Salubridad Pública 1925–1928*, tomo 1 (México, D.F.: Ediciones del DSP, 1928). Courtesy of the Secretaría de Salud, Mexico City, Mexico.

"most encouraging," the well-informed leader noted enviously that the IHB's activities were more extensive in other countries, especially Brazil. As instructed from New York, Warren reassured Calles that the decline of turbulence made the RF much more "kindly disposed" to Mexico.[186]

Though outspoken, Calles was also careful to moderate the somewhat hasty decisions of his health chief regarding the RF. On his visits to Mexico, Russell was struck by "how completely the Mexican medical profession had been shut off from recent progress,"[187] and he charged Warren with finding Mexican medical graduates worthy of RF fellowships to the U.S. When Warren had initially broached the subject of fellowships in January 1926, Gastélum said the DSP preferred to train its men without RF assistance. Warren believed that this was not an indication that they "wish[ed] to be independent of IHB advice and guidance," and more a matter of "national pride not to accept money."[188] President Calles reversed this decision, immediately offering ten qualified young physicians as RF fellows. Thereafter, Warren worried, "every time I give a Johns Hopkins or Harvard catalog it's an invitation" to the Mexican government to ready more fellows.[189]

If Calles and Gastélum seemed to deal with Warren unperturbedly—even when countering his decisions—Warren was more excitable. Notwithstanding Russell's assurances, Warren struggled with his peacetime gatekeeper role, both proud of his accomplishments—that the campaign had become more scientific and had achieved "extraordinary co-operation between State and National health departments"[190]—and annoyed at his inability to dispel the suspicions of some Mexican officials and doctors. Faced with promoting North American values in foreign lands, he wished that Mexican leaders could reside in the U.S. for a period to make "bitter feelings between the countries . . . disappear. . . . I fully understand that I am not here on a diplomatic mission, but our success is so dependent upon the good will of the people that I must of necessity be interested in the question."[191] Warren, it seemed, was more effective dealing with local crises and running mobile health brigades firsthand than he was at balancing the many competing roles of an RF country officer stationed in the capital.

The IHB undoubtedly had its reasons for sending the brusque Warren to the difficult setting of Veracruz. Although he was not the ideal man to interact with Mexico City authorities, his persistent and maverick qualities enabled the hookworm campaign to survive challenging circumstances in the field. Whether or not prompted by Warren's prickly relations with federal officials, Russell recalled Warren to the U.S. in the autumn of 1926. Like the other field-based officers, Warren was to obtain a master's degree in epidemiology at the Johns Hopkins School of Hygiene and Public Health. He would complement his fieldwork with classroom learning just as the first crop of RF fellows from Mexico was returning from the U.S. to put their training to practice.

Carr's Return and the Perfecting of the Hookworm Campaign

Warren's successor was none other than his junior officer from several years earlier, Henry Carr, who returned to Mexico after completion of his graduate studies in public health at Johns Hopkins University. Though he had been

removed from the campaign following his 1924 survey, Carr remained enthusi-
astic about hookworm work. Before leaving for Mexico, Carr assured Russell that
hookworm was "capable of solution . . . and then [there is the] entirely virgin
field of malaria control."[192] Carr oversaw the geographic extension of the campaign, but he also narrowed its focus to concentrate on treatment.

After several years on the campaign trail, Carr acknowledged that persons
with an "adequate and balanced diet could resist a higher number of intestinal
parasites." But like William Deeks of the United Fruit Company (see chapter 1),
he held that nutritional status played a "secondary role to the actual number of
parasites present and the symptoms exhibited by each individual."[193]
Administration of chenopodium, according to this reasoning, was a far better
answer to the hookworm problem than was improving the nutritional status of
people in high prevalence areas.

This conviction reflected Carr's newfound advocacy of a curative approach to
disease control. Hookworm, Carr believed, "depends upon the insanitary habits
of night soil disposal and these customs are very firmly fixed in the instincts of
the people." He considered the more than 6,300 latrines built in the year he
took over the campaign to be a "definite sanitary accomplishment" that
reflected the "tactful insistence" of brigade inspectors. At the same time, Carr
recognized that rapid change in defecation practices was a huge challenge and
thus turned to treatment as the IHB's "best sort of propaganda for good health."
Each cure of hookworm was "a very obvious and dramatic occurrence," which
became "an advertisement for better hygiene." [194] Carr's resurrection of the dispensary method—which required townsfolk to line up for treatment at a hookworm clinic—augmented the publicity surrounding hookworm treatment. He
believed that curing hookworm would serve as an inducement to pay for and
build latrines in order to prevent the disease in the future. That there was no
follow-up to see if this was actually the case—indeed the number of latrines built
in conjunction with the campaign dropped to 5,179 in 1927 and 2,768 in 1928
(see table 2.1)—seems to have had no effect on his views.

Carr was fully backed by the home office. Only a few months after he had
taken over the directorship of the hookworm campaign, Russell complimented
him on the "revolution you have brought about in sanitation" and on the "good
co-operation from district peons," which Russell jointly credited to Carr and the
DSP.[195] Even after two youngsters died from carbon tetrachloride treatment,
Russell only gently recommended that it was contraindicated in persons with calcium deficiency, especially malnourished children.[196]

Rather than facing the social, economic, and health implications of this problem, Carr concentrated on technical solutions, ever varying the dosage, drug mix,
and interval between hookworm treatments. Under Carr, the doses administered
by the Mexican brigades—1.25 cc. of chenopodium for eighteen-year-olds, gradually reduced for each younger age group until reaching a minimum of .10 cc.
for children of three or four—were now lower than those used elsewhere.

However, after recovering specimens from several people undergoing treatment each day, Carr learned that chenopodium did not have a uniform effect on worm count, and he began to experiment with different combinations of drugs.[197] Even with such changes, Carr admitted, "we have some toxic reactions which are right worrisome."[198] In 1927, Russell asked Carr to conduct a study of the purgative sodium sulphate as a substitute for magnesium sulphate, which was partially absorbed in the intestines, upset the body's calcium balance, and increased the likelihood of intoxication.[199] Unfettered by patient consent standards and with little awareness by DSP authorities, Carr later made a field trial of tetra-chloroethylene—without informing the local population. Finding it less toxic and more efficient than chenopodium, Carr recommended the drug's use.[200]

Carr, like Warren before him, was not always in accord with his superiors regarding campaign policies. One such difference revolved around the question of when to end the course of hookworm treatment. Russell had advised Warren that the word "discharged" was to be used in place of "cured" because the latter term could be misleading and hard to define. Tropical disease authority Samuel Darling had recommended the disappearance of clinical symptoms or the absence of hookworm ova in the feces as appropriate endpoints.[201] Carr believed that the variable efficiency of antihelminthics justified making a microscopic examination of the worm count before ending treatment. In several countries, the RF was careful to evaluate the effectiveness of its campaigns by measuring infection levels after it had left an area.[202] But the hookworm campaign in Mexico paid little attention to the issue of reinfection, and Russell advised Carr that it was senseless to "treat people to a cure" when a small number of parasites "do no real damage."[203]

Not only would remaining worms continue to feed off the intestinal wall, but expelled worms were likely to lead to new infections. The former campaign director, Solórzano Morfín, had argued that his concerns about reinfection were summarily ignored by the campaign despite the obvious money-saving and persuasive value of the prevention of reinfection.[204] From a medical standpoint, Carr concurred with Russell that reduction of hookworm to a light infestation was "For all practical purposes" a cure. But Carr also agreed with Solórzano Morfín that preventing reinfection by eliminating worms built legitimacy among the members of the public. Neither of the two was able to convince New York on this question. The RF home office's indifference regarding reinfection underscored the notion that it was using the hookworm control program for ends other than eradicating, or even permanently diminishing, hookworm disease in Mexico. It was only in the early 1930s, when the DSP was fully in charge of hookworm control, that educational efforts to increase latrine use and prevent ground contamination were specifically tied to the risk of reinfection through the continuous monitoring of hookworm infestation rates.[205]

On the administrative front, Carr experienced ongoing battles over Mexico's hookworm payments, which had been increasing each year of the campaign by 20 percent until they were slated to become the complete responsibility of the

Mexican government in 1928. That year Carr had trouble collecting the monthly installments of funds for the campaign, even when he told Mexican Treasury officials that theirs was an "international obligation."[206] The RF home office was adamant that the Mexican government take the "entire financial responsibility for continuing" the hookworm campaign, yet it urged Carr to prevent interruption of the work.[207] From the DSP's perspective, it was one matter to support an outside-patron-sponsored rural health effort where none existed, and an entirely different matter for the Mexican government to fund this as a priority. Carr pushed the DSP to incorporate the hookworm campaign into its regular budget, but the higher salaries that the IHB had used to recruit candidates made it difficult to reintegrate the hookworm personnel.[208] The stalemate on this issue lasted well beyond the planned termination of the RF's role in the hookworm campaign. Finally, in June 1930, Carr wired the home office that the DSP would increase the budget for the campaign by 20,000 pesos ($105,000 2004 dollars), "in spite of budget cuts to many dependencies."[209] Unconcerned by the DSP's sacrifices as the Great Depression began to unfold, the home office was pleased that the work of the RF "continues to merit the confidence of the officials of the Mexican government."[210] Given hookworm's low epidemiological priority in Mexico, this was not necessarily a happy result, but in terms of the DSP's desire to carry on its relationship with the IHB, there was reason for the RF to celebrate.

Hooked on Hookworm?

Two decades after the joint RF-Mexican hookworm program ended, the Secretaría de Salubridad y Asistencia (SSA; the DSP's successor) launched a second crusade against intestinal parasites. Unlike the first effort, which was a one-time campaign in each community with little follow-up to determine reinfection rates, this time the SSA aimed for long-term control. Hookworm brigade director Dr. Pilar Hernández Lira (who was an RF fellow and involved with a variety of IHB initiatives before becoming director-general of the SSA) observed in 1949 that:

> Experience acquired over twenty years has taught us that hookworm clinics alone cannot significantly reduce rates of intestinal parasites, because treated individuals who return to their former environment which has not been appropriately sanitized are subject to levels of reinfection that make the results of the hookworm clinics' work look very poor.[211]

If evaluated according to a standard of hookworm disease control through scientific methods, then, the RF hookworm campaign in Mexico was a marked failure. Paradoxically, if evaluated according to the goals of promoting public health more broadly and maintaining good relations between the RF and Mexico, this international health endeavor was far more successful. Although the hookworm campaign gained momentum only slowly, by the late 1920s it had reached several hundred thousand people across a band of south-central states (see table 2.1).

From the perspective of national political leaders, the campaign helped stabilize the tumultuous region of Veracruz: just as significant, its provision of rural health services enabled both federal and local politicians to begin to meet state-building demands. At the level of the DSP internally, hookworm became a big hit, greatly exceeding its planned role as seductive "entering wedge." The DSP's Communicable Diseases Section decried the drainage of family resources caused by persons with hookworm. This "misery can only be attributed to the ignorance of personal hygiene measures."[212] Thanks to the sanitary units, the report boasted, alongside gruesome photographs of ailing youngsters and shots of gleaming new outhouses, "little by little this ignorance is corrected." Indeed, the report went on, the photographed persons would soon die if not treated. Well into the 1930s, DSP reports emphasized the contribution of hookworm to Mexico's excess morbidity and mortality rates. The first was an exaggeration (given hookworm's limited geographic extension and moderate prevalence) and the second a misrepresentation (given the low mortality associated with the ailment), but years of hype had convinced health officials themselves that hookworm's control was among the nation's most valuable public health crusades.

A hallmark of the campaign was its persistent focus on the disease at hand, even if hookworm's elimination was not the ultimate goal. The DSP, various IHB officers, Mexican public health doctors, and the public all emphasized that malaria was a more important disease than hookworm in Mexico and frequent requests for malaria cooperation were made by all of these parties. Nevertheless, the IHB resisted diverting its attention away from hookworm.[213] Almost as soon as he arrived to head the campaign in 1926, Carr reported that "Although the Lucha does not consider the treatment of general diseases as a part of its function, it is occasionally necessary, where no practicing doctor is available, to give preliminary treatment (gratis) before antihelminthics," most frequently for malaria.[214] Under Warren, too, the brigades had provided several hundred malaria treatments per year, with quinine furnished free by the DSP.[215] But through the 1920s campaign, and even though both the DSP and Carr had prioritized malaria (Carr himself hoped to carry out a survey of the disease), Russell repeatedly thwarted any project that would distract from the hookworm work.[216] None of the principals held this against the RF.

Certainly the popularity of the campaign, its simplicity, and its value in promoting public health—all features of the hookworm campaign that had made it attractive to Rockefeller philanthropy for some twenty years—made it appealing to the DSP as well. Moreover, hookworm's health education and social outreach components afforded host countries the possibility of molding the campaign to suit domestic needs and in a format shaped by the local milieu.

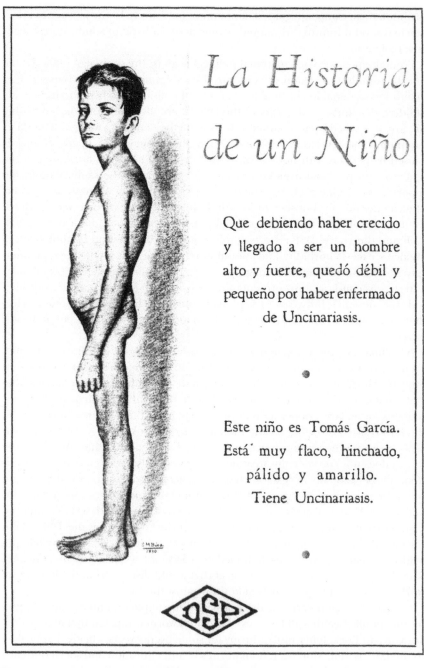

La Historia
de un Niño

Que debiendo haber crecido
y llegado a ser un hombre
alto y fuerte, quedó débil y
pequeño por haber enfermado
de Uncinariasis.

Este niño es Tomás García.
Está muy flaco, hinchado,
pálido y amarillo.
Tiene Uncinariasis.

Figure 2.14. Outside cover of DSP pamphlet, *The Story of a Boy*, 1930. Courtesy of the Rockefeller Archive Center.

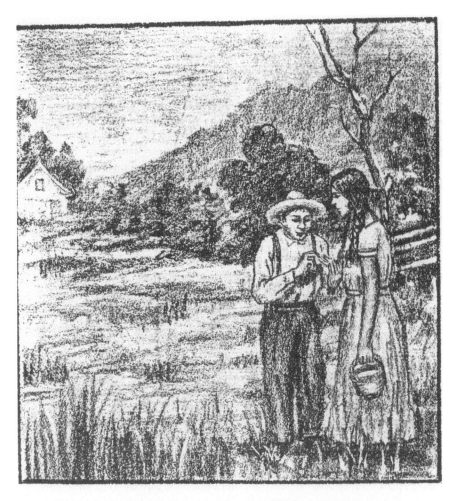

Tomás y Elena ya crecidos. Está sacando una
espina del dedo de Elena.

Figure 2.15. Inside of DSP pamphlet, *The Story of a Boy*, 1930. Courtesy of the
Rockefeller Archive Center.

Once hookworm work was nationalized in Mexico, the DSP tailored health
education to specific audiences. Young men were encouraged to seek preventive
treatment in a culture in which men visited healers principally for acute ailments
and women were more likely to seek care in the case of chronic ailments. A 1930
DSP pamphlet entitled *La Historia de un Niño—The Story of a Boy*—for example,
played on the stereotypes of Mexican machismo. On the front cover of the pamphlet

was Tomás García, a "skinny, swollen, pale, and yellow" boy with a girlish physique. Tomás "should have grown up to be a tall and powerful man but was left weak and small because he had hookworm." The inside of the pamphlet revealed a recovered Tomás who nonetheless had failed to reach his expected manly size and strength. His younger sister Elena, cured from hookworm at an earlier stage, had grown up to be a beautiful and healthy young woman, taller and stronger than her older brother.[217] The DSP employed a gendered cliché to feminize sickness and to cajole young men into undergoing hookworm diagnosis and medical treatment lest they lose their masculine demeanor.

As for the Mexican public, a few detractors made waves but were quieted. In June 1927, the Veracruz newspaper *El Istmo* published an article complaining that the IHB campaign had been poorly managed, causing several people to die at the hands of charlatans. Sent to Carr via Russell in New York, the article accused Carr of not supervising the hookworm clinics and of entrusting Juan López, "the one who is not a doctor," with patient care. The newspaper promised to investigate further and "fight for humanity."[218] Russell was not concerned by the accusations, attributing the views to a single individual rather than to wide displeasure with the RF. Carr identified the article's author as a drunken physician who had been turned down for a job with the campaign. While ignoring the source of the "untrue charges," Carr controlled further damage by entertaining the newspaper's editor and his family, who promptly published "two nice, sensible articles commending our work."[219]

The RF's critics were outnumbered by its fans. A number of Mexican businessmen wrote to the RF in New York, expressing admiration. Mexican drug companies mentioned the Rockefeller name in advertisements for their remedies. Scientists were even more effusive, in one instance appealing to "God that all the benefits that this noble Institution has spread throughout the entire world may be converted into blessings on behalf of the great North American people."[220] Praise was taken to a higher level by some foreign doctors, who posed as Rockefeller employment representatives and offered fraudulent positions with the IHB for a hefty fee.

The Meanings of Success

For the RF, success was unmistakable now that its foot (shoed or not) was in Mexico's door. As evidenced by DSP chief Gastélum's work and the evolving institutional context, Mexico was committed to public health and seemed eager to continue cooperative activities. For campaign officers, combating hookworm— through more than 400,000 hookworm treatments, over 15,000 latrines built, and thousands of health education lectures—perfecting treatment modalities, stabilizing program financing and administration, and engaging the participation of small-town and rural Mexicans were all signs of a job well done. In 1927, the future seemed to hold only more promise. The RF home office held—consistent with Wickliffe Rose's initial vision—that state and local authorities need only be exposed to the hookworm campaign in order to "create . . . a desire for a local health service capable of dealing with the more pressing public health problems."[221]

In a process that was just as important, the RF had converted its own officers and fellows into true believers. Carr, for example, maintained that mass treatment was helping to "alleviate the suffering of the working class."[222] He acknowledged that the campaign worked slowly, but he attributed this to its newness and to the "inertia in people's habits." The cure of even a single case of hookworm, said Carr, was "positive evidence . . . and as advantageous for the person's neighbors as for himself." This served as the best propaganda for "people who are incapable of doing anything for so many diseases," by proving that disease results from "poor hygiene and that public health work can alleviate the suffering of the people."

While the RF home office stressed that the hookworm campaign's chief purpose was to demonstrate the value of public health, IHB officers in Mexico could not remain sufficiently detached from their work to regard this long-term aim as more valuable than the immediate role. Seasoned officers soon forgot that hookworm was not a leading cause of disease and death. Carr, who himself had documented the circumscribed epidemiologic impact of hookworm in Mexico in his 1924 survey, became committed to the merits of controlling hookworm. After two years as the IHB's hookworm officer in Mexico, Carr had become so convinced of the value of hookworm control that he contradicted his own findings, judging it "more important than malaria."[223]

Warren, meanwhile, had conflated the scientific and political ends of the hookworm program, predicting a great future for the hookworm-free individual. More productive due to his improved health and physical condition, his newfound earning power would:

> result in more money in his pocket with which to buy better food, better clothes, better homes, and better schools. With better schools there will come enlightenment. Intelligence will displace ignorance and with intelligence there will come a true social revolution and a better understanding between all classes of men.[224]

Warren had inverted revolution in Mexico: he believed that hookworm eradication would lead to the social transformation of society instead of the Mexican Revolution setting the stage for improvements in social welfare.

But it *was* revolutionary demands for better living conditions and an expanded role for the national government in obtaining them that provided the underpinning for the hookworm effort and ultimately enabled the campaign's realization. Despite the international record of IHB hookworm activities and the prior IHB-DSP achievement of yellow fever control, the hookworm campaign in Mexico was a trying experience. Both the RF and the Mexican government were keen on

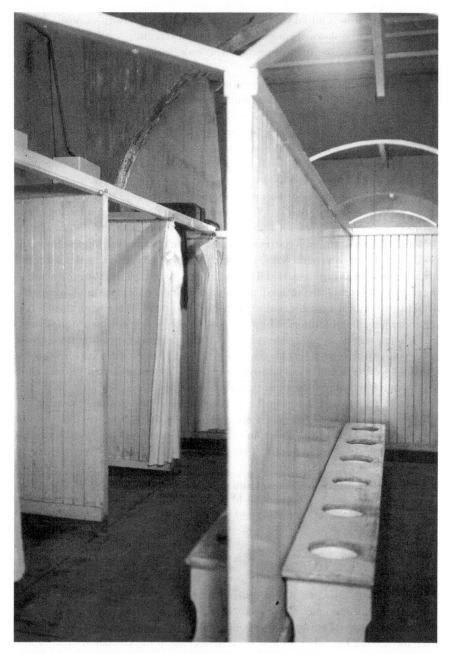

Figure 2.16. Separate men's and women's sanitary facilities in hookworm dispensary for use by persons who stayed until the purgatives took effect, 1929. Courtesy of the Rockefeller Archive Center.

working in Veracruz; political and military activity delayed the campaign and generated personnel problems. IHB officer Warren clashed with Mexican health officials, hookworm treatment resulted in poisonings and deaths, RF administrators paid scant attention to the question of reinfection, and few Mexican peasants built their own latrines. These difficulties gradually faded from attention, leaving in their wake support for the hookworm campaign on the part of government officials, most physicians, and small-town and rural Mexicans, some of whom were witnessing the delivery of routine state-sponsored health services for the first time.[225] Indeed, by the end of the campaign, the DSP claimed credit for the hookworm initiative with a grateful nod to the RF but a victory that seemed its own.

The RF's tendency to see all of its efforts as successful[226] belied an overlapping reality: institutionalizing public health was a complicated dance among various and sometimes changing partners. The hookworm campaign set the terms of the relationship between Mexico and the RF, which persisted, as we shall see, through subsequent programs including the development of a network of local public health departments. The IHB maintained administrative control even though its representatives were officially placed in subordinate positions within the DSP; it set budget incentives that assured Mexico's commitment to the endeavors launched by the RF; it promoted a public health orientation that favored the control of diseases amenable to individualized medical interventions; and it helped to stimulate the professional training and full-time commitment of health personnel. At the same time, IHB men were shaped by their field experiences and adapted local needs and practices—such as communal instead of individual latrine-building—into their modus operandi. While this fulfillment of Russell's 1923 promise that the IHB would learn from Mexico does not seem to have been acknowledged, such two-way learning was increasingly evident as the hookworm campaign evolved.

Ultimately of course, the elimination of hookworm disease was neither the goal nor the result of the hookworm campaign. Instead, it offered a dramatic means of igniting interest in public health among rural Mexicans, interest that had already been awakened through irregular federal and state disease campaigns and revolutionary demands. National and local leaders and health officials soon recognized the political benefits of hookworm control, gaining credibility for bringing an inexpensive, popular program to the people. Once hookworm control was accepted, few health activities could surpass its popularity.

Yet much as the IHB believed the campaign to be influential among diverse Mexican publics, ample evidence demands a more measured evaluation. First, the reach of the campaign was limited, with the south-central region of a single state being the center of much of the campaign's labors. Though rural inhabitants in Veracruz and a few other states indeed embraced hookworm control, this hardly constituted a national movement. The limited dissent among doctors was perhaps because local physicians in other parts of the country were unaware of the campaign.

For the DSP's personnel, the campaign's influence was also smaller than the IHB believed, in part because it competed with so many other initiatives, but mostly because they already advocated an expanded public health purview, if not through hookworm per se. The middle and late 1920s marked a period of considerable activity in the DSP, with a large increase in staff and expansion into new areas of infectious disease control, maternal and child health, sanitary engineering, inspection, and training. These efforts reflected many public health currents of the day, from Britain, France, Germany, the USSR, and elsewhere. For example, President-elect Calles—on a European study trip to gather ideas about how best to address Mexico's social and administrative needs—was allegedly very impressed with Hamburg's Institute of Tropical Diseases and the research carried out on malaria, onchocerciasis, leprosy, and other leading problems of Mexico. DSP administrators exchanged health education materials with their Soviet counterparts beginning in the mid 1920s. The resonance of European science continued for many more years.[227]

Unlike the Europeans, however, the IHB was working in Mexico, and Mexico—heavily engaged in a project of national reconstruction—had little reason to reject this opportunity for cooperation in rural areas. The visibility of the hookworm campaign garnered it local importance, even if hookworm itself was not a significant Mexican concern. Notwithstanding missteps and misunderstandings, the difficult setting of Veracruz, and binational problems, the RF and Mexico recognized that they had something to offer one another. The complicated interplay of RF ideas and approaches and Mexican needs and methods was already evident in the hookworm campaign. But it was in the subsequent cooperative endeavor—the development of local public health units—that the stakes of institutionalization would rise, and the influence, local translation, and selective appropriation of international health would fully play out.

Chapter Three

Going Local

In March 1930, Dr. Francisco de P. Miranda, the DSP's director of the Office of International Exchange, published a speech he had recently given to the visiting "Committee of Cultural Relations between the U.S. and Latin America."[1] Commending the "pioneering American spirit" that had led the group to "learn the truth about Mexico," he noted that Mexico—in the midst of reconstruction—had much to learn from the public health field in the U.S.

But this address, appearing on the front page of the *Boletín de la Oficina Sanitaria Panamericana* (*Bulletin of the Pan American Sanitary Bureau*), was no sycophantic display: Miranda aimed to teach his North American visitors "nothing new except the manner in which we are seeking to resolve our special problems."[2] After tracing the roots of Mexico's involvement in public health to the late nineteenth century, Miranda deftly showcased the DSP's recent burst of activities—from vaccine distribution to food inspection to child health measures—that renewed this commitment. He mentioned the friendly relations that had been established with the RF through the yellow fever campaign, when Mexican and American doctors had worked "arm in arm" and cited continued cooperation in the control of hookworm as well as other activities. As he looked to the future, however, Miranda focused on the areas of tuberculosis, occupational health, malaria, and clean water, none of which involved the RF. Indeed, both the Committee of Cultural Relations—and the *Boletín*'s readership—were likely left with the impression that the RF's efforts were on the margins of a "vast program, hopefully to be realized."[3]

A quick nod of thanks was decidedly *not* what the RF was seeking in its Mexican venture. As the IHB-DSP hookworm agreement was nearing its expiry date in the late 1920s, the RF found itself at a crossroads in Mexico. In some countries, its presence was purposely short-lived, especially once public health activities had gained a solid footing. In Mexico it was precisely because of public health's institutional takeoff that the RF was not ready to leave. Parlaying IHB cooperation into a deeper contribution to Mexican public health, however, required more than another standard disease control campaign.

Separately and at almost the exact same time, the DSP and the IHB became interested in establishing permanent health services in small-town and rural

Mexico. This shared goal of advancing local public health presented an oppor-tune—and at times contested—project for continued collaboration. Far more than the preceding campaigns, the local health units would become embroiled in debates over how best to institutionalize public health, how to balance national and local powers and responsibilities, and how to interact with local health workers, including nurses, midwives, and traditional healers. The devel-opment of the units also reflected competing models of the nature and practice of public health, with the IHB promoting technically oriented and medicalized services while the DSP favored a more socially oriented, comprehensive array of services. Amidst these differences, the partnership did not splinter. Instead, the ongoing interchange between the DSP and the RF generated mutual imitation and learning.

As Miranda's article indicates, Mexico was also re-surfacing on the interna-tional health scene following the turmoil of the revolution. With the country en route to stability and the national public health infrastructure and budget grow-ing, the DSP began to publicize its new efforts in international venues. Whilst these endeavors were widely featured in hundreds of articles in Latin American, North American, and European journals and at numerous conferences, Mexican public health leaders were also searching for relevant public health developments from around the world. Indeed, as the RF-Mexico relationship matured, its nonexclusivity became more apparent. This openness magnified the intensity of the interaction between the two partners, with the local health units now serving as the fulcrum of the collaboration.

Conception

Mexican Beginnings

Prior to the revolution, public health was largely a local responsibility. Although the national government gradually increased its role in infectious disease control, activities were concentrated in a handful of cities and larger towns; beyond these settings and in rural areas, public health was at best a sporadic affair. Still, under the Porfiriato Mexico's public health budget had grown, and advocates sought to renew this commitment during the revolutionary years. After the DSP's founding in 1917, the extension of services beyond the capital was hampered by two main factors: limited resources and possible infringement of state and local jurisdiction over public health. Notwithstanding the new Constitution, the country was still governed by a prerevolutionary Sanitary Code issued in 1902.

The DSP sought to circumvent these constraints by organizing both mobile brigades—which began as an effort to combat epidemic outbreaks of smallpox and malaria under the first DSP chief, Dr. José María Rodríguez[4]—and longer term (though geographically confined) disease efforts, such as the DSP's

Antilarval Service, plague control, and vaccination efforts, as well as the yellow fever and hookworm campaigns cosponsored by the RF. By the early 1920s, dozens of DSP brigades were traveling from village to village, administering smallpox and typhoid vaccines, providing treatment for intestinal parasites, and administering general medical exams to rural and small-town populations.[5] While these activities were generally well-received, insufficient infrastructure and personnel, continuing unrest in many regions, and struggles over resources and recognition among local, state, and federal governments limited the reach of the brigades and delayed the expansion of permanent health services outside urban areas.

In the mid 1920s, these obstacles began to be removed. In 1924, at its quadrennial conference in Havana, the PASB called for standardized legislation to govern commerce and health.[6] Two years later Mexico issued a new Sanitary Code, published in full in the *Boletín de la Oficina Sanitaria Panamericana*,[7] giving primacy to the DSP on health matters. Derived from the provisions of the 1917 Constitution, the 1926 Sanitary Code subordinated local and state health organs to federal authorities for the first time and cleared up ambiguity over the DSP's role. The code delineated three categories of responsibility for health: federal, joint federal and state, and joint state and local. The federal government controlled maritime and air sanitation, migration, medications, alcoholism, and infant hygiene. Federal and state governments were granted joint authority over the prevention of transmissible diseases and the regulation of prostitution, medical practice, and industrial hygiene. The new code gave state and local governments regulatory powers over sanitary engineering, food and beverage hygiene, and transportation health. The DSP named thirty-two health delegations—each composed of three doctors (including a bacteriologist), one pharmaceutical inspector, five sanitary agents, one nurse, and support staff—to state capitals and other leading cities. Charged with carrying out the federal government's new functions, these delegations added to the existing cadre of federal health officers in major ports and border towns.[8]

At first, there was widespread opposition to the new Sanitary Code and scattered jurisdictional disagreements materialized: discord arose when national authorities began to encroach upon areas that state and local health departments claimed as their own.[9] As the DSP began to marshal new resources in the late 1920s, the code became more and more accepted.[10]

With its hands now legally untied, the DSP was eager to expand its public health reach into the hinterland. On February 11, 1927, DSP chief Bernardo Gastélum, backed by President Calles, called upon state governments to work in conjunction with federal authorities to improve the nation's health conditions, given the "urgency of addressing the country's social and economic welfare."[11] Central to this effort was the promotion of municipal (roughly equivalent to county) health units, composed of at least one doctor, one nurse, and one sanitary inspector and equipped with the tools necessary for attending to local health needs as defined by the 1926 Sanitary Code: quinine (as a malaria prophylactic and remedy), petrol (as an insecticide), salvarsan (to treat syphilis), and iodine (to prevent wound infections). The units were to receive federal technical assistance and training to improve the knowledge base of personnel, drawing from the expertise of the new federal health delegates named by the DSP. Beyond technical support, however, the federal government made no provisions to fund the units. Instead—operating as dependencies of either the town doctor or the mayor—the units were to be funded locally or privately, with either paid or voluntary medical personnel, depending on local capacity.

Lacking designated funding, this attempt to jumpstart local health services through voluntary and local government efforts did not succeed. First, municipal authorities did not wish to cede control of a potentially popular service to private hands. Then, few medical personnel were disposed to offering their services to municipal governments for free. In less populated settings, there was little administrative or technical capacity to run local health services, and neither political authorities nor private interests were inclined to take on work that was unlikely to generate income.[12] Indeed, the entire voluntary model of public health—as advocated by the fifth International American Conference and proposed by Gastélum—was inconsistent with the 1926 Sanitary Code's designation of a heightened federal role in public health.

The Sanitary Code itself was also to blame: in devising an administrative division of labor between federal and local responsibilities, it stimulated overlapping functions and offices. Federal and local authorities established health departments virtually simultaneously in some state capitals: their separate responsibilities were clear in juridical terms; however, in practice the differences were not as obvious, for example, in the case of an infectious disease outbreak that crossed jurisdictional boundaries. As a result of these problems and the failure of the voluntary units, the federal government began to rethink its model of local health development. Where necessary, a single person was named as both the state's sanitary delegate and the chief of public health. But the DSP did more than tinker. If this opening effort to extend public health services throughout the country at private or local expense yielded little in concrete terms, it set the stage for a more ambitious and potent successor—the organization of publicly financed cooperative local health units throughout the country.

A Space for International Cooperation

The RF's interest in cooperative sanitary units emerged amidst these national developments. Having remained flexible on the question of federal versus state and local responsibilities during the hookworm campaign, the RF now sought an active role in the DSP's nascent organization of local health services.

This interest was nurtured in New York and Mexico simultaneously. In 1926, IHB officer Henry Carr had acknowledged that, notwithstanding the popularity of the hookworm campaign, its mobile brigades did not address the multiple ailments and ongoing needs in rural Mexico.[13] He envisioned the conversion of the hookworm brigades into permanent, modern health units with exclusive and full-time trained staffs of physicians, nurses, sanitary inspectors, and office clerks. These professionals would be hired according to merit instead of cronyism or political patronage and would receive attractive salaries. At the heart of his plan was administrative and fiscal cooperation among the DSP, the state, and the municipality in order to prevent the duplication of functions and minimize intergovernmental friction. Carr deemed the involvement of state and local authorities to be especially important, in order to "awaken them to their obligation to assume part of the responsibility for the improvement of the health conditions."[14]

These ideas were not unique to the RF and DSP: by the 1920s, cooperative local health organization was advocated by public health professionals around the world. In 1931 the League of Nations' International Conference on Rural Health recommended a model of district and regional health centers.[15] Local health units were established (or re-organized) in societies as varied as the United States—as exemplified by Charles Chapin's much-emulated Providence, Rhode Island Health Department[16]—Spain,[17] and the Soviet Union.[18] All were seeking to expand the reach of public health services using a combination of new bacteriologically based tools—such as the pasteurization of milk and the use of the Schick test to detect diphtheria—and older sanitary measures, including housing codes and piped water and sewage systems.

If the local health principle was widely shared in public health circles, the RF provided a rare private stimulus to its implementation. Following its hookworm campaign in the U.S. South, the RF had begun to sponsor county health units in Alabama, Mississippi, North Carolina, Georgia, and other largely rural states, as well as in Puerto Rico in the mid 1920s.[19] The counties selected were "above average in wealth, population, schools, roads, and progressive spirit, and should be able and willing . . . to appropriate approximately 50 cents per capita."[20] The units received support only for new activities and were financed half by the counties themselves, with the state and the RF splitting the other half. A model health organization in a well-off county, IHB administrators believed, would subsequently be imitated by nearby counties eager to keep up with their neighbors.

The RF saw its experience in the development of local health units in the U.S. as an appropriate example for Mexico, even though many U.S. counties, especially small and weak ones, could not meet financing or performance goals. Fewer municipal resources and little inclination for local government authorities to copy one another's initiatives without state or federal government backing made this scheme potentially even less workable in Mexico than in the U.S. The RF paid little mind to these impediments.

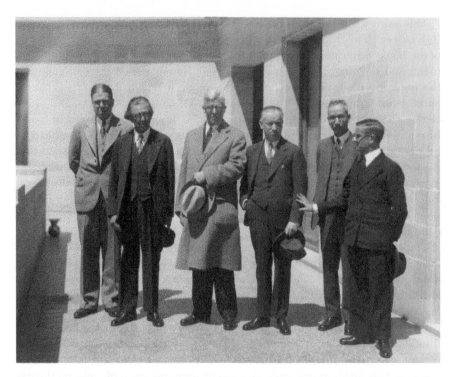

Figure 3.1. RF officer Dr. Henry Carr (far left), IHD Associate Director Dr. John Ferrell, (3rd from left), Veracruz Health Officer Dr. Agustín Hernández Mejía (2nd from right), and colleagues, 1929. Courtesy of the Rockefeller Archive Center.

In the spring of 1927, IHB Director Russell sent his deputy, Dr. John Ferrell, to Mexico to lay the groundwork for a new phase of cooperation. Ferrell—a North Carolina native who was a rural teacher, then a practicing doctor before heading the Rockefeller hookworm campaign in his home state—served as associate director of the IHB from 1913 to 1944. In this post he was responsible for the RF's worldwide hookworm effort, and, especially, for the development of full-time county health units in North America.[21]

On his trip to Mexico, Ferrell was the consummate envoy, relaying contrasting messages to host and patron. To Russell he expressed concern that "The idea of co-operation between federal, state and municipal governments in health work . . . has not gained headway";[22] to his hosts he extolled the public health efforts of the Mexican government. To the home office, Ferrell complained that Mexico's president was "virtually a supreme ruler," and to Mexican officials, he praised the "brilliant young physicians" who had been sent to the U.S. as fellows, the "remarkable wisdom" of DSP personnel, the accomplishments of the School of Public Health, and the "demonstration of brotherhood" in scientific research. To DSP men, Ferrell expressed confidence that their course of action would "bring glory and distinction to the health department and those identified with it,"[23] but he shared with New York colleagues his apprehension about the "many uncertainties which may influence the continuity of health service" in Mexico.

Ferrell set the diplomatic table for further cooperation and gave a sense of the challenges ahead, but it was Carr who would attempt to bring the cooperative local health project to fruition. Following Ferrell's trip, Russell instructed Carr to develop and supervise a local health unit initiative after the hookworm agreement formally expired at the end of 1928.[24] Though he "gladly relied" on Carr's judgment throughout the process,[25] Russell also advanced a political agenda, pushing for the establishment of units close to Mexico City so that Mexican officials would visit them more regularly, and the RF could expand its purview beyond the Veracruz, Oaxaca, and Chiapas locales where the hookworm campaign operated.[26]

Carr's initial proposal would commit the Mexican government to contribute a significant proportion of its budget to the health units. From the start the RF was to provide only 10 percent of the local health units' budget—far less than the 80 percent portion at the beginning of the hookworm campaign—yet RF personnel would delineate the units' range of activities and oversee their management, considerable control for a small budget incentive. Carr also sought to maintain the hookworm campaign—set to be absorbed into the DSP's budget and program—as before, because "backwardness and poverty" impeded the rapid creation of permanent units.[27] Carr suggested that as the number of health units multiplied, a separate hookworm campaign would no longer be necessary.

With Calles preoccupied on other fronts, the DSP was left to decide on its own whether or not to continue the relationship with the RF. Though the RF was clearly eager to remain in Mexico, and despite the country's ongoing interest in local health, the DSP was not willing to commit itself to Carr's plans. Well aware of the RF's disproportionate control over the hookworm campaign, the DSP stalled on a written agreement.

Besides, DSP doctors had their own ideas. Parallel to Carr's efforts and following the failure of the voluntary initiative, the DSP had begun to develop its own extensive plan to replace the country's mobile brigades with permanent health departments.[28]

A principal architect of this endeavor was Dr. Miguel Bustamante, a returned RF fellow and a major figure in Mexican public health for over sixty years. From a prominent Oaxaca merchant family that saw its fortunes decline following the Mexican Revolution, Bustamante was the oldest of fifteen siblings.[29] After completing his medical studies in Mexico City, Bustamante—the nephew of former yellow fever and hookworm campaign director Dr. Angel Brioso Vasconcelos—received an RF fellowship to study epidemiology and public health at Johns Hopkins University from 1926 to 1928. There he was a classmate of RF officer

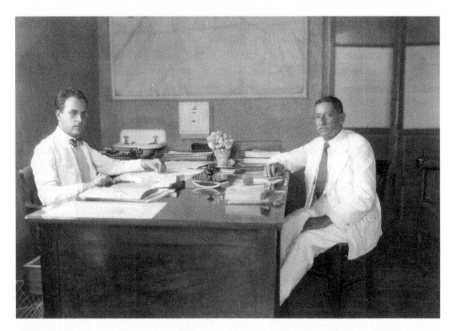

Figure 3.2. Dr. Miguel Bustamante (left), head of Veracruz health unit, with staff member. Courtesy of the Rockefeller Archive Center.

Andrew Warren, who as Mexico representative had selected Bustamante for the fellowship. After receiving his degree, Bustamante returned to Mexico with skills that matched his ambitions. Bustamante's role in the expanding DSP grew concomitantly, and he founded and directed a variety of key agencies, including the Office of Coordinated Health Services in the States, the Xochimilco Public Health Training Station, and the Department of Infant Welfare. He subsequently rose to become secretary-general of the PASB in Washington, DC, and deputy secretary of health in Mexico.[30]

Both the RF and the DSP claimed credit for the cooperative health unit proposal, which was no surprise, given that both proposals drew from ideas developed at Johns Hopkins, through the IHB's county health initiative in the U.S., and at international health agencies.[31] While the models developed by Carr/IHB and Bustamante/DSP overlapped considerably, Bustamante favored a centralized network of units and a broader range of activities for the health units in an effort to address the underlying causes of high death rates, including unfavorable economic and social conditions and poor sanitation.[32] As with the RF's disease campaigns, Carr's plan remained fixed on those ailments that could be combated most economically and most dramatically. But it was in the implementation rather than the design of the health units that the contrasting priorities of the respective parties fully emerged.

Competition over authorship of the plan was the first of several collisions between Bustamante and the RF. Even though Bustamante went on to hold many positions connected to local health administration and the RF, he periodically clashed with a succession of RF representatives, who resented his ideas and influence over Mexico's public health system. These policy differences were portrayed as personality problems by various RF officers, who (typically) complained that Bustamante was "capable but he has a strange character and an unhappy faculty of making enemies and frequently is unscrupulous to obtain his aims."[33]

Though criticism of Mexico's local health plans was aimed at Bustamante, it seemed to reflect a more generalized disregard by the RF of Mexican health developments. Long-standing RF policy called for extensive surveys of local disease prevalence and social conditions to precede each new initiative.[34] When the focus of IHB work in Mexico shifted from hookworm to local health departments, however, no such survey was even suggested. Perhaps the controversy surrounding who should conduct the 1924 hookworm survey soured the RF on repeating the experience, or a new survey may have been deemed redundant given the wide agreement on the need for local health units. But Carr did not even gather information on existing health offices in ports and state capitals,[35] implying that the U.S. experience in local health was the only model for Mexico.

Another point of contention was whether the local health units should be placed in truly rural locales or oriented first to medium-sized municipalities capable of furnishing financial and infrastructural support. If the RF and DSP could agree that the health units should be established outside of Mexico City, the RF tended to think of the units in rural terms—much as it did in the U.S.— even though it typically took a good-sized town to meet the minimal conditions of cooperation. The DSP, on the other hand, understood that services were needed throughout the country, including urban and semi-urban areas. Nonetheless, the DSP eventually agreed to the designation "Rural Hygiene Service" (Servicio de Higiene Rural), since it suggested a focus on the peasant population, which was not receiving government attention as quickly as perennially promised by revolutionary politicians.

In the end, Mexican officials agreed to RF collaboration in the development of local sanitary units, but the DSP also prevailed in framing the initiative as an ongoing national endeavor.[36] The DSP recognized that RF involvement risked intrusion on its public health strategy. It also knew that the RF's cooperation could speed the development of health services. This joint effort staked out a more prominent role for the RF in the design of Mexico's public health system than had been intended by Bustamante and his colleagues. The experience also fueled Bustamante—and others—to develop and defend a national approach to public health. Indeed, within a short time, who was learning from whom, influencing whom, and copying whom would become difficult to untangle.

Politics of Every Variety

While the DSP and RF were deliberating over how to organize cooperative local health services, a series of diplomatic, political, economic, and institutional factors surfaced that would shape—and could potentially jeopardize—the initiative.

When Plutarco Calles took over the presidency, he began to reverse the conciliatory politics of his predecessor; Mexico-U.S. relations took a turn for the worse. Calles championed the constitution's prohibition on foreign ownership of petroleum, refusing to adhere to the Bucareli Street agreements (preventing the retroactive application of Mexico's exclusive subsoil rights), which Obregón had signed with the U.S. The U.S. government—displeased with Calles's stance on oil—repeatedly threatened to invade Mexico and blocked almost all trade between the two countries for several years. Finally, in late 1927, in large measure thanks to new U.S. Ambassador Dwight Morrow's diplomatic savoir faire, the two countries agreed on oil legislation that gave Mexico subsoil rights but barred the retroactive implementation of the ban on foreign holdings.[37] This "gentleman's agreement" satisfied the oil companies and Mexico's national reconstruction imperative, saved face for Calles, and managed to stave off further crisis for the time being. The compromise also lessened the risk of operational disruptions to RF-DSP projects: prior difficulties between the two countries had not caused the RF to abandon Mexico at any time since its arrival in 1921, but both the RF and the DSP preferred to work without diplomatic tensions.

A second set of factors threatening the joint public health programs had to do with economic and political problems on Mexico's domestic front. In the mid 1920s, after several boom years, oil and then mineral exports began to drop precipitously. By 1926, the country was facing an economic crisis, followed by banking and financial crises. Although the Calles government had resumed payments on the foreign debt, the Treasury was soon unable to meet its financial obligations, and within a few years Mexico suspended its debt payments indefinitely.[38]

In the midst of these troubles, Calles was met with both an army insurrection in 1927 and the *Cristiada*—an explosive rural rebellion lasting from 1926 to 1929. Centered in five states in the middle-western region of the country, the *Cristeros*—tens of thousands of peasants, guerrilla fighters, and militant ranchers opposed to the constitution's separation of church and state and aggravated by Calles's anticlericalism—organized violent uprisings against the government. The government responded with repression and massacres carried out by the army. The costs of the war were high: the federal army sustained losses of up to 60,000 men, while the *Cristeros* lost some 30–40,000; a large proportion of the federal budget was spent on the conflict; and significant harvest shortfalls in affected regions led to famine, epidemics, and migration northward.[39] Only in 1929 did the parties reach a compromise—also partially shepherded by Ambassador Morrow—which allowed the Church to resume its affairs.

Faced with these problems, Calles became increasingly authoritarian, ridding himself of once trusted advisors and reneging on promises to jumpstart the redistribution of land to peasants. If Calles had joined the revolutionary-strongman-with-a-social-agenda tradition upon assuming office, he had long ceased moving the country along a progressive and sovereign trajectory.[40]

In spite of strained coffers, government-led institution-building continued. Even with limited attention to social policy, the Calles period oversaw a doubling of the DSP's annual budget[41] and concomitant growth in its staff and activities, as called for in the 1926 Sanitary Code. Moreover, owing to the multiple pressures on Calles, he allowed considerable autonomy to the DSP and other government agencies. Obregón had seen RF programs as instrumental to the solidification of his power, particularly in the Veracruz region; a few years later Calles regarded them as useful but less pressing. As a result, he granted the DSP flexibility and independence to negotiate directly with the RF.

As Calles's term was coming to an end in 1927, the constitution's "no re-election" provision was modified—permitting multiple, but not successive, presidential terms. Former President Obregón mobilized his supporters, ran, and won. The day after the election, Obregón, now a threat to the forces supporting Calles, was assassinated, either by a *Cristero* militant or by an agent of Calles's Labor and Industry Minister Luis Morones[42] (popular lore implicates a Calles operative more directly).[43]

Initially, Calles—whose credibility had already taken a beating due to the *Cristero* conflict—saw his prestige diminish even further.[44] But he was also able to take advantage of a power vacuum in the wake of Obregón's death. First he had his own designee—Emilio Portes Gil—installed as president. Then in early 1929, Calles helped to "institutionalize" the postrevolutionary political system through the organization of a dominant political party—the National Revolutionary Party (Partido Nacional Revolucionario; PNR).[45] Although regional parties were invited to join the PNR under a confederation arrangement, in reality the party quickly became centralized and authoritarian, basing itself on individual membership and thus minimizing the role of regional political organizations. The party itself—rather than rival regional leaders—became the ascendant source of political power in Mexico. At the same time, the party was financed through civil servant payroll deductions and thus depended on the state.[46]

The new system enabled Calles to remain the power behind the Presidency without actually holding office. This so-called Maximato was a quasi-monarchical setup in which Calles exercised supreme influence through the PNR well after his formal term as president ended.[47] He continued to control and bully the three presidents who succeeded him (Portes Gil, Pascual Ortiz Rubio, and Abelardo Rodríguez), each of whom served for just two years. Only after General Lázaro Cárdenas—also a Calles protégé—won the presidency in 1934 did Calles finally become politically emasculated and then exiled in mid 1935.

With these political developments entrenching Calles's authoritarianism, the U.S.-Mexico relationship improved. The Maximato was favorably regarded by the U.S., for despite Calles's nationalism, by the late 1920s he represented political and economic moderation. Though some U.S. politicians compared the Mexican situation to revolutionary Bolshevism in the Soviet Union, these views had little bearing on dealings between the U.S. and Mexico. Indeed, the "gentleman's agreement" that had been engineered between Calles and Morrow promised U.S. noninterference in Mexican affairs as long as Mexico was stable and the southern flank of the U.S. remained secure. This arrangement—beneficial for elites of both countries—allowed for Mexico's experiments with a mixed economy and an independent foreign policy, at least for a time.[48]

The Great Depression could also have put in jeopardy the cooperative RF-DSP programs. Mexico's economic woes predated the Depression; after 1929, government spending was under even more strain. For its part, the RF had adroitly shielded its assets from the stock market crash,[49] but it was reluctant to expand activities in order to avoid having to suddenly suspend funding. When Carr proposed a program expansion in 1930, Ferrell stressed that the RF had a stronger obligation to scientific projects than to administrative efforts and that its expenditure in Mexico for administration "far exceeds what has been customary elsewhere."[50] On Mexico's side, RF-DSP programs were spared the worst of Mexico's belt-tightening, initially growing, then sustaining 10 percent cuts compared to a one-third reduction in the total DSP budget.[51] Ferrell considered it "admirable if the [Mexican] government, even in the face of economic difficulties, will enlarge its program of health work."[52] Though a hardship, the Depression was only one in a series of political and economic problems weathered by the DSP-RF relationship.

A final factor affecting the future of RF programs in Mexico took shape at the RF's home office in New York. On April 1, 1927, the IHB was transformed into the International Health Division (IHD) as part of an internal reorganization that consolidated activities and brought together the foundation's semi-independent boards under a single roof. This change also heralded a shift in focus. Under Wickliffe Rose's direction from 1913 to 1923,[53] the IHB had implemented known public health measures in places that—it judged—could benefit from them. A nonscientist, Rose had dedicated himself to "strategy and administration," leaving trusted advisers to think through the scientific aspects of IHB programs. Though he understood "the value of research" and the need for laboratory verification of disease, the influential Rose believed that "the aim of the I.H.B. was to apply our actual knowledge which he was convinced was at least fifty years in advance of ordinary [public health] practice."[54]

But Rose's successor departed from this philosophy. Dr. Frederick Russell was a physician-bacteriologist who had enjoyed a long career in military medicine before joining the RF in 1919, initially as director of its public health laboratory service. Russell, who had helped develop a typhoid vaccine and almost singlehandedly compelled the U.S. Army to make it obligatory, pushed for the creation of a central laboratory in New York as an essential element of disease research.[55] During Russell's tenure as director, which extended from 1923 until 1935, the division's focus shifted to scientific research—including epidemiological activities and public health administration methods—under the leadership of, as he put it, "a small group of well-trained men of the best type."[56] He recalled of this period that "existing knowledge, no matter how extensive, was rarely adequate for control. Studies must be made of each disease in its own environment. [In the late 1920s] the basis of our program became simultaneous study and control in the field under natural conditions."[57] Although the IHD no longer had its own trustees, the RF's Board of Trustees agreed that the RF's international health programs needed to be evaluated for their scientific effectiveness, and in 1929 they named a Board of Scientific Directors to oversee the IHD's activities.[58] With a staff dedicated to "the spirit of inquiry and [the] desire to increase knowledge," Russell predicted, the IHD was bound to "make the greatest progress in the prevention of disease."[59]

The DSP and the IHD shared this belief in impartial scientific pursuit, but the development of local health units would remain shaped by political imperatives as much as it was by technical and scientific ones.

The First Unit

As extensive negotiations between the IHD and the DSP were underway, the first cooperative sanitary unit was established in December 1927, well before an agreement was reached. Located in a southern river valley in the state of Veracruz, the new unit was shared by the towns of Minatitlán and Puerto México, serving a combined semi-urban population of 25,000. Puerto México (today called Coatzalcoalcos) was the state's second largest seaport and served a vital purpose each time the port of Veracruz was disabled by unrest, not an infrequent occurrence in those years.

Unlike the previous yellow fever and hookworm efforts, the new unit was not based on a pact of RF–Mexico cooperation. Instead, Carr, under pressure from his superiors to begin the unit, entered uncharted waters. With the DSP reluctant to enter into a contractual arrangement for the unit, Carr temporarily bypassed it, in spite of RF principles requiring federal participation. The unit was guided by only a vague outline of financial obligations made "on a basis of friendship and voluntary desire," unlike the RF's customary binding and detailed contract. To resolve the issue of accountability for the unit's well-being, Carr convinced Veracruz Governor Heriberto Jara, a strong backer of the project, and state health officer Dr. Agustín Hernández Mejía to take responsibility for securing payment from the municipalities, warning them that the unit was certain to fail unless closely monitored.[60]

Table 3.1. Funding sources for Minatitlán–Puerto México, 1928*

	Pesos	2004 Dollars (Approximate)
Veracruz State Health Department	4,890	25,750
Municipality of Minatitlán	3,600	18,500
Municipality of Puerto México	3,600	18,500
Rockefeller Foundation	4,890	25,750
Total	16,980	88,500

*The DSP did not contribute until 1930.

Source: Carr, "Annual Report of Unidad Sanitaria Cooperativa Minatitlán–Puerto México for the Year 1928," RG 5, Series 3, Box 146, RFA.

Carr was more preoccupied by the political implications of the DSP's absence than by the question of adequate financing, since both towns "have unusually adequate incomes because refineries and oil fields of the Mexican Petroleum Company are located in the area. The situation is that the money is there, the question is to divert a part of it."[61] Senior IHD administrator Wilbur Sawyer congratulated Carr on the founding of the first unit, confident that the DSP would participate as soon as it proved stable and useful. In the meantime, Sawyer recommended that Carr lobby the state and both municipalities to assure their monthly contributions.[62]

The joint unit—which would later become two full-fledged units—opened offices in both towns, each staffed by a sanitary inspector and a nurse. To keep costs down, the two towns, separated by fifteen miles of rough terrain, shared a physician-director.[63] Operating under an annual budget of 16,980 silver pesos (the equivalent of $7300 in U.S. gold in 1927) or .70 pesos per capita ($3.00 in 2004 dollars), the unit was slated to receive 50 percent of its budget from the two municipalities, an important contribution, for "Neither Federal or State Governments would find it feasible" to fund a health unit in every municipality.[64] The first year, Puerto México and Minatitlán together financed almost 40 percent of the budget, with the balance split by the State of Veracruz and the RF (see table 3.1). For two full years the DSP remained notably absent from the list of funders.

Carr promised that the Minatitlán–Puerto México unit would adapt modern, scientific public health methods to local conditions, dealing with problems "encountered in proportion to the relative importance of the disease . . . in the locality."[65] Based on his own observations, Carr ranked the towns' principal public health priorities as malaria, hookworm, soil sanitation, smallpox, maternal and infant hygiene, child health, and regulation and instruction of midwives. These were "All the problems, in a rather exaggerated form, which would be encountered in some of the southern [U.S.] states."[66] The DSP was not satisfied with Carr's impressions, however, and commissioned its own survey of the coastal Veracruz population. The study also showed a preponderance of malaria and hookworm, the latter in part reflecting attention to hookworm in the RF-DSP campaign. Finding the crude mortality rate to be 31.5/1000, over 50 percent higher than the "accepted rate,"[67] the survey emphasized the need to combat excessive death rates rather than sickness rates (such as rates of infestation from hookworm disease), but this recommendation was ignored in the early years.

Instead, the unit's early focus was on sound administration and achievable goals. Continuity of policy, financial responsibilities shared by various levels of government, a full-time staff, and the selection of "honorable and intelligent and energetic employees" were elements that the RF deemed essential in this endeavor. Even without DSP participation, Carr claimed that the new unit met them all. Elated, he declared that the new unit "will awaken interest not only among national health authorities but also in civil leaders and the inhabitants themselves, who will cooperate with an organization directly interested in their welfare."[68]

In the first annual report of the Unidad Sanitaria Cooperativa Minatitlán-Puerto México for 1928, Carr proudly recounted that the IHD had successfully pioneered a new type of health organization in Mexico. Criticizing itinerant campaigns for failing to complete their disease control objectives, monitor recurrence of diseases, battle local health problems, and carry out effective preventive health education, Carr lauded the efforts of the joint health unit. Sized for efficient management, according to Carr, the unit had also overcome the duplication of efforts by local, state, and national entities: the unit "represents complete and effective economic and administrative cooperation," with the director receiving his instructions from a unified panel of the DSP chief, the state health officer, and the municipal president.[69]

The annual report—in Spanish and English versions—became an important tool of public relations, reflecting the unit's need to address different audiences. Carr's report to the IHD was vague about the financial contribution made by each entity because of the lingering uncertainty of regular payments, yet it outlined the annual budget in detail, proudly displaying a table of staff salaries and expenses (table 3.2). The Spanish version of the report omitted these figures, perhaps unwilling to arouse the ire of local inhabitants, most of whom earned less than one third of the lowest-paid sanitary unit employee.[70] Instead, it showered praise on the unit's state and local financiers, advertising it as a cooperative financing success, while failing to mention that the DSP's only contribution was a few pieces of equipment.

Notwithstanding Carr's vow to combat all prevalent diseases, in its first year the Minatitlán-Puerto México sanitary unit featured hookworm diagnosis and treatment, the testing of antihelminthic drugs, latrine construction, and hookworm prevention lectures. Dental hygiene, prenatal care, and routine vaccinations were later incorporated, but quarterly reports repeatedly highlighted hookworm. In

Table 3.2. Salaries and expenses for Minatitlán–Puerto México Unit, 1928

	1928 Pesos	2004 US Dollars (Approximate)
Salary of physician director	6,480	33,600
Salary of two inspectors	3,600	18,500
Salary of two nurses	3,600	18,500
Salary of secretary	1,200	6,700
Traveling expenses	420	2,200
Equipment	1,480	8,000
Contingent fund	200	1,000
Total	16,980	88,500

Source: Carr, "Annual Report of Unidad Sanitaria Cooperativa Minatitlán–Puerto México for the Year 1928," RG 5, Series 3, Box 146, RFA.

1931, for example, one report boasted that at seven each morning, dozens of people would arrive at the unit for hookworm treatment (on an empty stomach to avoid aftereffects), receiving "the same attention as in the private office of the best physician," but for free.[71] The continued emphasis on hookworm long after the establishment of the cooperative health units rested on the need to demonstrate concrete achievements. As the IHD knew intimately, hookworm's easy identification through microscopical examination of fecal samples and its straightforward treatment through oral doses of chenopodium made it far simpler to control than other ailments. Moreover, the five-year hookworm campaign in Veracruz had paved a path to popular acceptance.

In spite of his early and public optimism, Carr soon became apprehensive about the unit's ability to sustain full-time permanent personnel, and he anguished over obtaining a firm financing commitment from the federal government. Carr had promised not to break away from the work of the now DSP-based hookworm campaign until he was "sure local units will survive."[72] By mid 1929, he was having doubts about the viability of the Minatitlán–Puerto México unit. In nervous letters back to the RF home office, he advocated a return to the hookworm campaign[73] and as late as 1931, he sought to retain the last hookworm brigade in Chiapas as a mobile health unit.[74]

The stability of the first cooperative unit was not Carr's only concern: the DSP's own development of a local health unit had put him on the defensive.

The Competing Health Unit in Veracruz

While Carr was fretting over the Minatitlán–Puerto México unit, the DSP was busy launching its own model local health unit. In May 1929, the DSP inaugurated a municipal health unit in the city of Veracruz under the direction of Miguel Bustamante. The RF did not participate in the unit's founding, and Carr maintained an uncharacteristic distance from the effort.

From the beginning, the DSP and IHD units differed markedly. Serving a population of 70,000, the Veracruz unit was more comprehensive and autonomous than that of Puerto México-Minatitlán. With a budget fifteen times bigger and a large full-time staff including four doctors, a veterinarian, and a sanitary engineer, the Veracruz unit trained its own personnel, developed health education posters, films, and lectures, and collected, classified, and analyzed the city's vital statistics. At the same time, it adhered to Bustamante's vision of a federalized health service. In 1930, for example, the federal government contributed 84 percent of the Veracruz unit's budget, the city provided 12 percent, and the state contributed less than 2 percent,[75] in striking contrast to the heavily state-subsidized unit under Carr. In 1930, the Veracruz unit began to receive a symbolic contribution from the RF, ranging between 2 and 4.5 percent of the unit's budget, a share far smaller than for other units. The RF's contribution—while acknowledged in DSP reports—represented more of an afterthought than a cooperative effort.[76]

The new unit focused its attention on communicable disease control, which continued a number of existing measures in the city of Veracruz, including the tracking of typhoid, tuberculosis, and venereal disease; plague prevention and rabies vaccination; malaria and yellow fever control; and market, restaurant, and building inspections. Child hygiene was addressed through prenatal care, visiting nurse services, dental care, school physicals, and mandatory smallpox vaccinations. The diagnosis and treatment of hookworm was just one item in a comprehensive list of priorities.[77] Bustamante also marshaled change via regulatory reform. Until 1929, milk had been sold via mule-driven carts without inspection, refrigeration, or bottling. By the following year, the milk was bottled, inspected, and refrigerated in handling centers before distribution on special milk wagons, as enforced by the health unit.[78]

Bustamante admitted that the city's most pressing problems were linked to the water and sewage system, and he backed the expansion and repair of broken pipes.[79] A structural mistake, which had crossed clean water and sewage pipes, showed the need for improvements in the training of municipal sanitary engineers. Bustamante also vowed to overcome the public's refusal to allow the chlorination of water.

These activities corresponded to the city's principal causes of mortality— infectious diseases in general, infant mortality, and diarrheal diseases—unlike the Veracruz unit's Minatitlán–Puerto México counterpart, with its continued primary focus on hookworm. Bustamante strove to make his unit as wide-ranging as possible, and he sometimes employed unorthodox approaches in order to demonstrate the superiority of his unit's design.

Bustamante was quick to tie the Veracruz unit's activities to improvements in health, publicizing these successes in the United States. The 1930 crude death

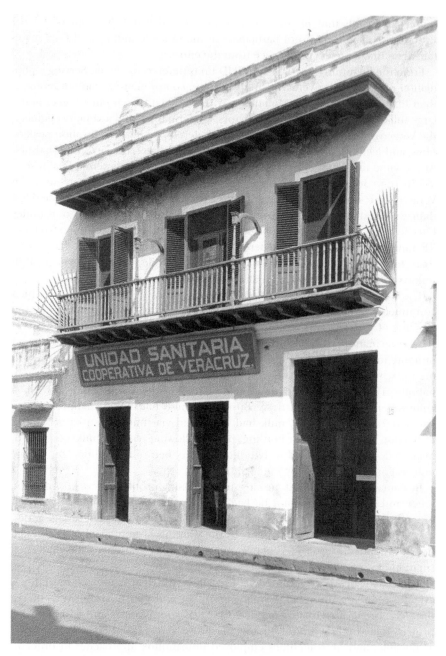

Figure 3.3. Veracruz health unit, 1929. Courtesy of the Rockefeller Archive Center.

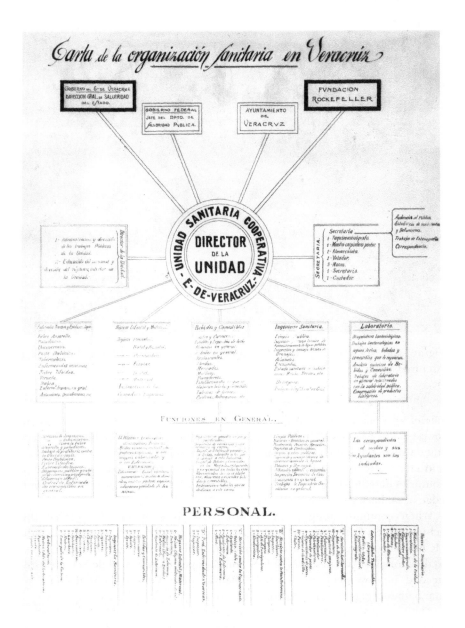

Figure 3.4. Veracruz unit organizational chart. Courtesy of the Rockefeller Archive Center.

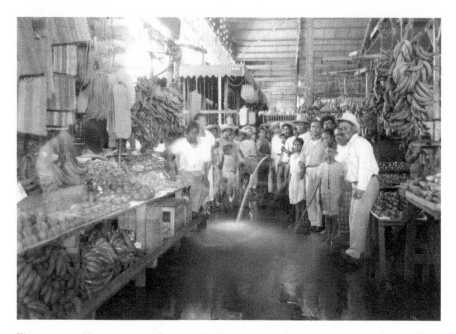

Figure 3.5. Veracruz market sanitation, 1929. Courtesy of the Rockefeller Archive Center.

rate of 25.4 per 1000, he wrote in the *American Journal of Public Health*, "was the lowest in the 40 years of our statistics." Bustamante reflected, "To be sure, we are not satisfied, but merely encouraged by present conditions. However, our desire and effort is to reduce further the rates to approximate those of the leading countries in public health work, particularly the United States, where our knowledge of sanitary science has its source."[80]

When communicating privately with Carr, Bustamante also placed the achievements of the Veracruz unit in the international context of public health. He favorably compared Veracruz's 1928–29 crude mortality rate of 28.33/1000 to the mortality level in scores of U.S. and European settings: while Veracruz still needed improvement, its mortality figures were not far behind those of Manhattan (15.3/1000) or Spain (20.7/1000).[81]

These results were especially gratifying, Bustamante reported, given the city's public health history[82] of malaria, yellow fever, tuberculosis, and gastrointestinal diseases. The Veracruz sanitary unit had been created, he argued, out of the many national and local efforts to address these problems, rather than from the IHD's yellow fever and hookworm campaigns. Bustamante's celebration of Mexican achievement did not exclude international influences, and he noted that the unit had benefited from the experiences of the League of Nations, the

American Public Health Association, and the Johns Hopkins School of Hygiene and Public Health.[83] Bustamante certainly did not object to the participation of the IHD, but his nationalistic sentiment shaped his belief that Mexico had long ago learned the lessons of modern public health and that the country had the leadership ability and technical capacity to implement them.

For DSP chief Dr. Aquilino Villanueva, the Veracruz unit was the "crowning of our efforts" to take charge of all public services related to health.[84] In 1929, on the pages of the *Boletín de la Oficina Sanitaria Panamericana*, Villanueva acknowledged the important role of the RF but failed to mention its work in Minatitlán and Puerto México. Given that he presented Mexico's principal problems and priorities as malaria, tuberculosis, and infant mortality, it is not surprising that he would overlook the hookworm-oriented IHD-sponsored initiative.

Although the Veracruz unit offered a range of services that was more comprehensive than those that were provided at Minatitlán-Puerto México, Carr repeatedly criticized it. He found the unit's reliance on the central government excessive and the low state contribution deplorable. Believing that Bustamante did not sufficiently humor state authorities, Carr complained:

> I am not sure that the Director of this unit is really convinced of the desirability of the cooperative idea or whether he would be just as satisfied to see the Unit depend straight out from the Departamento. . . . Sometimes a young man put in charge of a big organization such as the Unit, gets an exaggerated idea of his importance, especially if he has a tendency that way.[85]

Carr, himself a young man, hinted at no irony when describing his own management style: "I have complete control and can exact obedience on the part of the personnel. For that reason . . . I am able to please all the participants, Federal, State and Municipal."[86] Carr's target was also the DSP, which remained a reluctant donor to the Minatitlán–Puerto México unit.

But Carr was alone in his resentment. His supervisors in New York applauded and were encouraged by Bustamante's—and the DSP's—work in Veracruz. When IHD Associate Director Ferrell visited the Veracruz unit in 1933, he was highly impressed with the city's progress in hygiene. He sided with Carr over conflicts with Bustamante, but Ferrell could not deny the unit's achievements. He noted that since his previous trip, Veracruz's streets had become cleaner and sanitation had improved, even with continuing problems posed by malarial swamps. Despite the fact that Veracruz was "tropical and undesirable" as a major port, its health unit was a "success." Contributions from federal, state, and local governments were well coordinated, and the community as a whole enjoyed "greater health protection than ever before."[87] Though Carr and Bustamante had become rivals, the IHD was delighted to partake in the credit for the Veracruz unit's accomplishments.

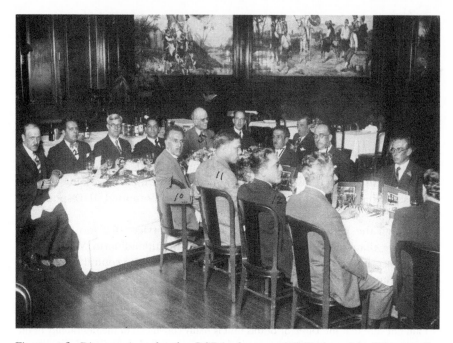

Figure 3.6. Dinner given by the DSP in honor of IHD Associate Director Dr. John Ferrell, Hotel Regis, Mexico City, 1929. Courtesy of the Rockefeller Archive Center. Photograph key (following the small numbers marked on many of the dinner guests):

 1. Dr. Francisco de P. Miranda, professor in the School of Public Health
 2. Dr. Ezequiel Padilla, secretary of Public Education
 3. Dr. John A. Ferrell, associate director of the IHD
 4. Dr. Aquilino Villanueva, director of the DSP
 5. Dr. David L. Edsall, dean of Harvard Medical School and School of Public Health
 6. Dr. Salvador Bermúdez, director of the School of Public Health
 7. Dr. Alfonso Pruneda, former secretary-general of the DSP
 8. Dr. Fernando Ocaranza, director of the General Hospital
 9. Dr. Rafael Silva, president of the Mexican Academy of Medicine
10. Dr. Gabriel Malda, former director of the DSP
11. Dr. Henry P. Carr, IHD officer in Mexico
12. Dr. Ayala González, secretary-general of the DSP

Dissemination

For the DSP, the creation of the Veracruz unit was an undeniable triumph, one that represented "a new phase in the evolving process of [Mexican] public health"[88] Thereafter, the Veracruz unit became the inspiration and the standard

Table 3.3. DSP budgets, 1922–39

Budget Year	Millions of Pesos	% of Federal Budget
1922	3.7	
1923	3.7	
1924	2,8	
1925	3.5	
1926	5.1	1.93
1927	8.4	
1928	7.5	
1929	7.1	
1930	8.9	
1931	8.6	
1932	6.4	
1933	6.5	
1934	7.5	3.4
1935	12	3.86
1936	15.6	4.2
1937	14.8	4.6
1938	13.9	5.0
1939	16.5	5.5

Sources: Public Health Department Budgets, 1932–41, RG DSP, Box 6, Folder 12/172.1/, AGN.; AGN RG DSP Box 6, 12/172.1/2; Agustín Hernández Mejía, *Dieciocho Años de Trabajos Sanitarios en México* (Mexico: D.F., 1941), 38–39; and "Report by Ferrell of his Visit to Mexico, March 14–April 13, 1941," RG 2, Series 300, Box 561, Folder 3814, RFA.

by which other local health units would be measured. If the DSP appreciated the efforts of the "noble RF," Mexico's achievements in local health were seen as homegrown. By the early 1930s, it also became clear that the DSP would not be able to provide the same level of economic support to every municipality in the country. Compared to the DSP's budget increases of the 1920s, in the early 1930s the budget stagnated and then dropped (see table 3.3) while its activities were multiplying. The DSP would have to settle for a "path more in tune with reality."[89] Other than in cash-rich and economically vital Veracruz, then, health units would initially appear slowly, with the next new DSP unit established in the city of Durango in 1931, the following in Mazatlán in 1932,[90] and statewide health services launched in Guanajuato and Querétaro in 1933.[91]

Given the DSP's limitations on expanding the number of local health units, the IHD perceived a potentially larger role for itself in this effort than had originally seemed possible. It was Carr who led the campaign for a more substantial IHD presence in the DSP's local health initiative. He had begun in mid 1930 by prodding his superiors to allow him to move his office from Veracruz back to

Mexico City. Having finally secured federal funding for the Minatitlán–Puerto México unit, Carr argued that he would have many administrative matters to attend to in the capital. First, he held, the capital was a better location from which to oversee the health units. Then, Carr cited his obligations with the ongoing hookworm campaign; he continued to serve as its chief scientific and administrative advisor even after the DSP had officially taken over the campaign.[92] It would also be advantageous, Carr maintained, to increase his personal and social relations with the "chiefs" of the DSP. Carr admitted a danger in having "field folks" travel to Mexico City, lest they "form connections which might cause them to become unduly ambitious or tend to distract them from their work," so he promised to travel to each field unit every month or two.[93]

Finally, the young doctor protested the deteriorating living conditions in Veracruz, where food prices had surged and the "American colony has almost disappeared." Carr lamented that "it is impossible for one, especially a bachelor as I am, to lead anything approaching a normal social life as one can in Mexico City where I have American and English friends." From New York, Ferrell agreed to the move, advising Carr to seek new DSP chief Rafael Silva's consent before any action was taken, to ensure that the IHD would not be viewed as too aggressive.[94]

Once in Mexico City, Carr enjoined both the RF and the DSP to fund a "Rural Hygiene Service" as the basis for ongoing cooperation. This new service would establish and administer the health units, maintain amicable relations among the various levels of government, encourage local initiatives, map the future course of the units, and secure regular state and municipal payments. Carr proposed that the IHD representative serve as subdirector, in practice functioning as the director, much as during the hookworm campaign.[95] The Rural Hygiene Service would gradually take over the RF's share of expenditures for the sanitary units, similar to the hookworm campaign arrangements.

Carr tactfully avoided the question of the DSP's budget constraints. He suggested that it was initially helpful for the RF to participate financially, proposing 40,000 pesos for 1931 ($97,000 in 2004 dollars) to be supplemented by a DSP contribution of 110,00 pesos ($270,000 in 2004 dollars). The health units still had foes, and "It is a help to the Chiefs of the Departamento if they are able to answer criticisms by saying that the Foundation supplies part of the funds for the work. It strengthens our position."[96] Moreover, Carr claimed to Ferrell, the RF's hookworm campaign had so impressed Veracruz authorities that they now supported the sanitary units, in turn making the DSP grateful to the RF. Carr's final pitch for the new Rural Hygiene Service was to show it to be "analogous to a typical situation in the [United] States where the Foundation might contribute funds and personnel to the establishment of a Bureau for County Health Work" supporting the administration—but not the operating budgets—of the units.[97]

Carr's plan, devised to help the DSP set up its administration of local health units, had further implications. With relatively minor monetary contributions,

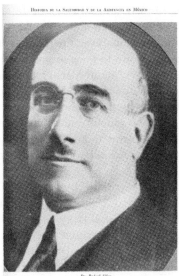

HISTORIA DE LA SALUBRIDAD Y DE LA ASISTENCIA EN MÉXICO

Dr. Rafael Silva.
Jefe del Departamento de Salubridad Pública. 7 de febrero de 1930 — 22 de enero de 1932.

Figure 3.7. Dr. Rafael Silva, director of the DSP (1930–32). From José Alvarez Amézquita, Miguel E. Bustamante, Antonio L. Picazos, and F. Fernández del Castillo, *Historia de la Salubridad y de la Asistencia en México*, vol. 2 (México, D.F.: Secretaría de Salubridad y Asistencia, 1960). Courtesy of the Secretaría de Salud, Mexico City, Mexico.

the RF sought to institutionalize its health unit model in Mexico. The home office regarded Carr's plan as an advance in the organization and stability of local health units but criticized its heavy reliance on Mexico's central government. Carr himself was troubled by the dual loyalties—between the RF and the DSP—that his position demanded. He worried that "I have to . . . satisfy the Chief of the Departamento and at the same time not to deviate from your instructions."[98]

Aware of Carr's projects and before the DSP became committed to the Rural Hygiene Service, Miguel Bustamante campaigned to credit Mexico's own laws with the growth of the local health movement. Citing the 1926 Sanitary Code as the basis for the formation of local health units, Bustamante stressed that the success of the units derived from the initiative and financial support of the country's most progressive states. Writing for a North American audience, he simultaneously praised and slighted county health work in the U.S.: even in the country that served as a model for awakening local efforts in public health, it was "necessary to insure the coöperation of the U.S. Public Health Service and the International Health Board."[99] Attempting to shape the activities of the new Rural Hygiene Service and instill confidence in his DSP superiors, Bustamante argued that Mexico's slower development of cooperative health units was based on its distinct culture, history, and health conditions. Unlike Americans, Mexican farm workers lived in towns, not on their land, sharing common water sources and trading at communal markets. Epidemics were thus much harder to control, often spreading from town to town on market days.

In addition, he noted, Mexico's "greatest general public health problem is the lack of adequate provision of pure water" and sewage disposal, a veiled attack on the RF, which refused to involve itself in water supply and sanitation. Bustamante lamented the high cost involved, which "retards the solution," maintaining that despite a knowledge of the problems and the desire to confront them, "our limitations are those of any reconstruction period, overcrowded with many pressing problems."[100]

Bustamante penned this subtle critique, but it was the DSP that faced a conundrum. Not wishing to reject needed resources and expertise, it was loath to turn down the RF's offer to establish a Rural Hygiene Service. On the other hand—as evidenced in its reluctance to sign a written agreement with the RF for the initial development of local health units—the DSP was concerned about retaining its sovereignty, both in day-to-day operations and in the design and long-term development of health services.

A few months before Bustamante had aired his views, DSP chief Silva had published his own analysis in the *American Journal of Public Health*, "The Health Problem in Mexico," based on a speech he had given to the American Public Health Association's annual meeting in Fort Worth, Texas. He laid out Mexico's commitment to sanitary improvement and its "considerable success" in addressing many challenges, making special mention of the DSP's current "promising project" of organizing cooperative sanitary units. Nonetheless, Silva stressed, Mexico's problems remained "difficult to solve." In light of this, international cooperation was "indispensable to all." Silva told his audience that he himself had come to the meeting "in search of enlightenment, which in the end will serve our people's cause."[101]

With Silva's rationale for cooperation articulated, the DSP acceded to the jointly funded Rural Hygiene Service in 1931. Now the question of *who* would head the service had to be decided, a process which took months. Notwithstanding his differences with Bustamante,[102] Carr conceded that he really was the most appropriate director because of his Johns Hopkins training, his experience heading the Veracruz unit, and his ability to survive a "shake up" in the DSP.[103] The IHD home office, concerned with Bustamante's tendency to choose his own course, tried to convince Carr to get Dr. Hernández Mejía, the Veracruz state health officer who had been supportive of both the yellow fever and hookworm campaigns, appointed to the post.[104] Ferrell began by advising Carr to make a decision based on "what will lead to efficiency in the local organization of health work and to the gradual extension of this type of service." However, he openly backed Hernández Mejía, due to his "demonstration in the State of Veracruz; the fact that he knows thoroughly the type of work that should be advocated; that he is reliable and cooperative; and that he favors the fulltime principle in public health." Ferrell went so far as to suggest that Carr make this selection himself, quickly adding that "We, of course, must not go beyond the bounds of propriety in the filling of government positions because, after all, we are a foreign, outside, private agency without and not desiring authority."[105]

Perhaps to ensure Mexican control of the service in this aggressive atmosphere, Silva named the spirited Bustamante as director of the Rural Hygiene Service—and thus Carr's new superior in the DSP. (Nevertheless, when Bustamante was appointed to a new post several years later, he was replaced by Hernández Mejía.) Bustamante was elated with his new position, for "all of Mexican hygiene has rural aspects."[106]

The question of whether or not the IHD's involvement in the creation of the Rural Hygiene Service co-opted Mexican efforts is a complicated one. Certainly Bustamante was able to stand up to Carr and develop national policies, practices, and organization of local health services. At the same time, Bustamante was an RF fellow and a strong advocate of the public health principles he had studied in the U.S. One could certainly argue, as did IHD administrator Ferrell, that the Veracruz unit represented a better-funded, more ambitious, less cautious version of the Minatitlán–Puerto México unit. But Carr and Bustamante recognized differences of substance, not only magnitude: Carr in the Veracruz unit's insufficient recognition of the cooperative principle, and Bustamante in his own unit's more preventive approach to health problems, for example, stressing provision of clean water over hookworm treatment. Still, Bustamante appeared fully committed to the technical and scientific underpinnings of public health.

As head of the Rural Hygiene Service, Bustamante saw that public health could become a tool of social empowerment even in the absence of the professional principles espoused by the RF. In his desire to be responsive to communities not served by a local health unit, Bustamante supported the use of untrained, nonmedical personnel to carry out public health activities. For example, when the director of a rural school in Huixtla, Chiapas, relayed his experiences teaching inhabitants the elements of personal hygiene and how to build and use outhouses, how to confine pigs and chickens to separate quarters, and how to pressure state authorities for better water systems, Bustamante hailed his efforts as an example of the value of popular education. Bustamante sent the school director a large packet of health education materials and encouraged him to continue his efforts.[107] Carr responded to such approaches negatively, arguing that the Rural Hygiene Service needed to accept RF principles on cooperation and public health professionalism in their entirety.

Bustamante fully backed the extension of permanent health units throughout the country. In contrast to Carr's strict advocacy of full-time professionals as purveyors of public health, Bustamante resorted to using teachers and priests in the interim before the establishment of the units. He pursued this policy even though these surrogates typically lacked formal training and the preventive, diagnostic, and treatment tools of modern medicine and public health. During his two years as head of the Rural Hygiene Service, Bustamante not only oversaw the health units, but he also set the operating principles for the rural sanitary campaigns promulgated by the DSP, effectively combining technical expertise and community leadership. Sanitary unit personnel and other Rural Hygiene Service staff worked with rural teachers and local clergy to conduct surveys of local social and economic conditions. Priests, teachers, and peasant organizations were also trained in health education and in the construction of sanitary wells and water filtering techniques.[108]

Still, the IHD managed to keep its spoon in the stew. The Rural Hygiene Service's annual reports were issued in Spanish, signed by Mexican officials, and rarely mentioned the RF or IHD, but they were written by the RF representative to Mexico, filed as routine IHD reports, and voiced an IHD perspective.[109] The DSP also used these reports in a strategic bureaucratic sense. Clearly written and illustrated, the reports demonstrated accomplishments and efficiency more than they reflected IHD control.

Bustamante's leadership of the Rural Hygiene Service complemented his practical experience in Veracruz, and in late 1933 he was chosen as founding director of the DSP's "Servicios Coordinados de Salubridad." This new national system of "Coordinated Health Services in the States" was based on a system of cooperative health units. In 1934, Bustamante outlined the policies and practices he espoused for this "Mexican sanitary institution" in a seminal article entitled "La Coordinación de los Servicios Sanitarios Federales y Locales como Factor de Progreso Higiénico en México." ("The Coordination of Federal and Local Health Services as a Factor in Public Health Progress in Mexico").[110] Published in the *Gaceta Médica de México* to mark Bustamante's acceptance into the Mexican Academy of Medicine, this manifesto called for technical centralization and administrative decentralization (to the states) of health services, an arrangement officially authorized the same year by a new sanitary code. Drawing from his organization of the Veracruz unit, Bustamante also called for physicians— together with visiting nurses, sanitary engineers, and health inspectors—to serve the "social function" of public health, incorporating geographic, economic, cultural, social, philosophical, racial, and historical factors in their efforts to realize "the progress of the nation."[111] Bustamante's ideas positioned the country for a rapid expansion in health services in the mid 1930s. His influence was not only domestic: in its day, the article had an enormous impact throughout Latin America, and it continues to be reprinted to the present.[112]

If Bustamante's ideas might be characterized as "Rockefeller with a Mexican face," they also represented a departure from the IHD's proclaimed science-based policy[113] by fusing social and technical understandings of public health. The battles between Carr and Bustamante were more than a clash of personalities; they symbolized the larger struggles taking place between a government department extending the reach of public health services to meet revolutionary demands and a private U.S. philanthropy promoting a particular structure for that effort. The

IHD was at the same time learning from the field and adapting to it—whether consenting that latrines should be built for communal rather than individual use or accepting heavy reliance on federal financing for local health units.

Bustamante publicly hoped that the foundation's "private aid will awaken the nation's sanitary conscience," and permit "the biological defense of the nation to be an element in its progress."[114] While the system of coordinated health services was in the process of being developed, he argued that the needs of the people had to be met through existing means. In effect, Bustamante wished to take pieces of his Hopkins-acquired know-how and recast it together with sovereign knowledge, population-based priorities, and local experience in the development of health units. The extent and nature of this appropriation, going back and forth between RF and DSP models of local health, would become ever more apparent in the next round of IHD units.

Expansion to Cuernavaca and Beyond

With the creation of the Rural Hygiene Service, the IHD was significantly expanding its involvement in Mexico's local health units, accepting that a U.S.-style "public health demonstration" strategy would not lead to a spontaneous generation of units. By 1931, only one municipality (Durango) had stepped up to the plate. Mexico's combination of thinly stretched resources and little experience with coordinated federalism—schools, for example, tended to be organized either as part of a state system or a federal system but not in unified systems[115]—meant that the decentralized model of financing favored by the IHD would be slow in coming.

By this time Carr had finally become satisfied with the progress of the Puerto México and Minatitlán units (now two separate units), which were beginning to include malaria control, typhoid vaccination, and two visiting nurses per unit. With the success of these measures, he noted, "one begins to see on the streets, people of the laboring class, and especially children, with some color in their faces."[116] Carr further argued that the RF was indispensable to this effort: the well functioning units "would not long survive should the Foundation withdraw" from them.[117] Mexico, Carr now realized, differed from the United States in the need for funding from the central government. State and local governments were unstable and inefficient, support could not be guaranteed to last from administration to administration, and reluctant municipalities were often bullied into making payments to the units. RF involvement provided continuity in such circumstances. In sum, Carr held that without the IHD, the cooperative sanitary units could not last; thanks to the IHD's support and supervision, the units were flourishing.

What Carr overlooked, of course, was the fact that acclaim for the units was largely based on the work of the Veracruz municipal health unit. The Minatitlán and Puerto México units began to thrive only after they went beyond hookworm to carry out much-needed activities in maternal and child health, sanitation, and other areas, emulating the broad scope of Bustamante's Veracruz unit. Though Carr failed to recognize it, the IHD had learned from the DSP that it was not hookworm control that would spark a revolution in local health but rather comprehensive public health services.

With the IHD now promoting a Veracruz-style comprehensive local health initiative, it sponsored three new units in 1931: in Tuxtepec, Oaxaca; Tierra Blanca, Veracruz; and Cuernavaca, Morelos (see table 3.4).[118] Of these, the Cuernavaca unit was the most important. The selection of Morelos became a test of the long-term viability of the sanitary units and an indicator of the continued politicized nature of their placement. In the early 1930s, Morelos, one of Mexico's smallest states, had under 150,000 inhabitants spread across 230 towns and villages, but its political importance was far greater than its size suggested. RF officials claimed to have chosen Morelos because it was located in the populous yet rural central plateau region, was less than fifty miles from Mexico City, and accessible to major roads, allowing federal officials to observe the functioning of sanitary units.[119] This description applied equally to other nearby states such as Puebla, Hidalgo, México, and Querétaro.

Tiny Morelos's disproportionate importance to Mexico's national interests derived from its status as the nearest to the capital of the country's agrarian "trouble spots." In the mid 1920s limited land reform had tempered strife; in the early 1930s, however, there was renewed agitation—and Morelos, the home state of the most popular revolutionary hero, Emiliano Zapata—was dangerously near the capital.[120] The threat was economic as well as political: unrest might disrupt the state's lucrative agricultural output which included rice, maize, bananas, tomatoes, sugar cane, and other crops. From the RF's perspective, infectious diseases were a "hindrance to the industrial, commercial, and agricultural development of a rich region." With Morelos free of malaria, one yellow fever officer had reasoned in 1924, U.S. capital could be invested in sugar cane, alcohol, and chicle cultivation, all within easy distance of Mexico City.[121] Setting up a health unit became a sound preventive strategy, on the part of Mexico and the RF alike, against agrarian mobilization.

The process of establishing a sanitary unit in Morelos began with Carr's December 1930 visit to the popular state governor, Vicente Estrada Cajigal, with a letter from DSP chief Dr. Rafael Silva in hand. Through his own negotiations, Silva had already obtained approval for a unit from the municipal president of the town of Cuautla in the Morelos highlands.[122] With Cuautla as a fallback, Carr's aim was to convince the governor to support a unit in the state capital Cuernavaca. Silva's letter promised the project would bring Morelos "transcendence for the immediate future."[123] Carr presented his position in more grounded language:

> For several years the Department of Health has been studying and testing the most appropriate and practical means of bringing the benefits of modern, scientific,

Table 3.4. Cooperative local health projects for 1932 (in 1932 pesos)

Project	Year Begun	Total	Municipality	State	DSP	IHD
Minatitlán–Puerto México Unit	1928	21,040	7,200	4,890	4,060	4,890
Veracruz Health Unit	1929	112,249	36,000	5,000	66,249	5,000
Tuxtepec Health Unit	1931	23,000	2,280	3,000	15,720	2,000
Tierra Blanca Health Unit	1931	23,000	2,400	2,400	16,200	2,000
Cuernavaca Health Unit	1931	23,000	2,400	2,700	15,600	2,000
Central office administration	1931	22,000	1931	2,700	13,010	8,990
Studies in hookworm and malaria	1931	15,000			7,500	7,500
Field Training Station	1932	24,000			12,000	12,000
Total in 1932 pesos		263,289	50,280	17,990	150,339	44,380
Approximate Total in 2004 U.S. dollars		1,152,000	219,000	81,000	657,000	195,000
% of Total (%)		100	19	7	57	17

Source: Tabular résumé (as of December 31, 1932) of Rockefeller Foundation cooperation in Mexico since termination of the hookworm campaign and establishment of first full-time health unit, RG 1.1, Series 323, Box 19, Folder 157, RFA.

efficient health and hygiene knowledge to the people of Mexico, in order to improve the public's health, improve physical welfare, protect and strengthen the race.[124]

Carr explained to the governor that the health units in Veracruz were bound by only a handful of operating principles and had met with great success. Echoing Bustamante's broad agenda, Carr assured the governor that the Morelos unit would "dedicate the majority of its attention to the region's most important problems, such as infant mortality, maternal mortality, the high incidence of gastrointestinal diseases, malaria, childhood physical defects, and hookworm, leaving problems of lesser importance for the future."[125]

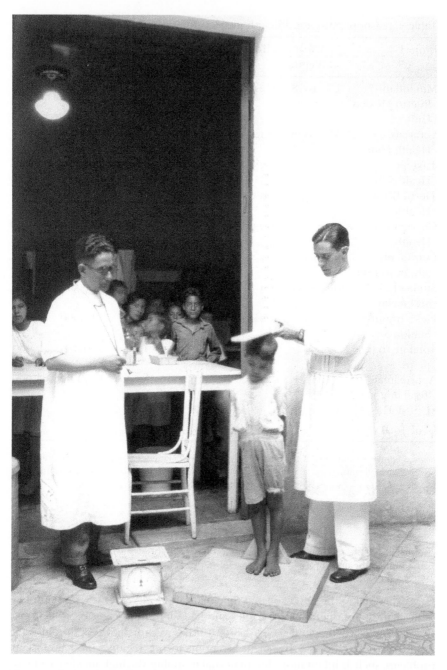

Figure 3.8. Boy being measured at a Veracruz health unit, 1929. Courtesy of the Rockefeller Archive Center.

Leaving the RF out of the equation for the moment, Carr explained that the unit would be under the joint supervision of the state, the municipality, and the DSP, with the DSP's subdirector of rural hygiene (Carr himself) responsible for the day-to-day functioning of the unit. He also advised that it was best to hire employees from the Rural Hygiene Service because, he argued, their training and experience made them the most qualified.[126] Carr's hiring scheme countered the principles of joint management—not to mention patronage practices. But Morelos Governor Estrada Cajigal agreed that a secure, centralized health service was preferable to an unstable, locally managed one. However, he was not willing to undo the Cuautla deal that DSP chief Silva had engineered.

Within a month, the governor ordered the municipal president of Cuautla to support the unit.[127] The DSP was to cover two thirds of the budget, with the state, municipality, and RF each contributing approximately 10 percent. Mexican health officials saw this as an ideal system for poorer communities; state and local governments participated only modestly in funding the units, allowing the DSP to "expand its radius of action."[128] The IHD preferred greater local funding and control, but it was the more centralized funding and management plan that Bustamante had pioneered in Veracruz that became the standard.

As soon as Cuautla's municipal president publicly approved the unit, Cuernavaca officials pressed to obtain their own unit. The Morelos capital's political pull led to a last-minute switch of the unit's locale, coinciding with Carr's intention. All along Carr had planned his visits to Morelos so that he could meet with both the governor and Cuernavaca officials; with less than two weeks to spare, he was able to prepare Cuernavaca for the unit's June 1, 1931, inauguration, pledging that a combination of patience and steady commitment would ensure the unit's success.[129]

The Cuernavaca unit operated with a budget of 23,000 pesos ($137,000 in 2004 dollars) financed in accordance with the cooperative responsibilities that had been set out for the Cuautla unit.[130] The municipality of Cuernavaca paid its monthly dues of 200 pesos ($900 in 2004 dollars) religiously, ever concerned with the possibility that the "ailing, prostrate bodies that once lined Avenida Morelos" would return.[131] Municipal President Crisóforo Albarrán recognized the "true benefit" of a sanitary unit and promised that the town would cooperate in every endeavor that bettered the community.[132]

The Cuernavaca unit's medical director, Dr. Julio Viniegra[133]—selected because of his experience in one of the Veracruz units—was quick to establish services in response to need. Local leaders pressed for attention to infant mortality, so from the start the Cuernavaca unit prioritized maternal and child health.

Within weeks of its founding, the DSP commended the Cuernavaca unit for being readily accepted by the public. In an attempt to demonstrate the unit's broad value, an early quarterly report assured that the unit served and was received by all social classes equally well. As one unit nurse recalled, not only could one attend the new units without paying a single peso, the health personnel would give away medicine and build latrines for free.[134] The surrounding rural population generated more demand than town dwellers. The local, state, and national governments were lauded, too, for their "progressive efforts to improve the nation's health."[135] Carr was more skeptical. Writing in confidence to Ferrell, he complained that the local population, "especially the lower classes," were "much more difficult to work with than" in Veracruz. Due to the "agitated" political situation, Carr warned, the work of the sanitary unit would be slower.[136]

Carr's fears were overstated: the Cuernavaca unit's activities expanded rapidly to include communicable disease control and immunizations, prenatal and postnatal clinics, instruction to midwives, preschool and school health, oral hygiene, sanitary engineering, control of food and beverage sale, vital statistics, and education.[137] As was the case with the other new units, hookworm no longer took precedence.

According to unit personnel, it was this wide array of services that drew people in. Dr. Felipe García Sánchez, an RF fellow and director of almost every IHD-sponsored unit at some time in the 1930s, recalled that so many people lined up for the units on many days that he and one nurse each saw a patient every two minutes from 7 a.m. to 7 p.m. (see figure 4.14). When he arranged to see sixty children for smallpox vaccinations in a small village one Saturday morning, two hundred people showed up, including "naked children, old people, and families who came to be cured."[138]

Employees of the Cuernavaca and other units recall that educational approaches were particularly appreciated. Prior to the establishment of the local health units, many Mexicans equated public health with coercive measures, such as quarantine of individuals with contagious diseases and fines for the violation of hygiene regulations in marketplaces.[139] The units' popularity was enhanced, a Rural Hygiene Service report stated, because "Coercion is never employed" and the work "only involves public health, not administrative matters."[140] Some health administrators seemed to lament the passing of old coercive ways. Health education was "continuously, diplomatically and tirelessly given," using a lamentably "slow though demonstrably positive method of preventive medicine, far more lasting and beneficial . . . than the application of laws, regulations and fines."[141]

Under the leadership of Viniegra, the Cuernavaca unit initiated epidemiological mapping of communicable diseases to facilitate their control. He organized a full laboratory and, thanks to the IHD, the unit received the latest professional books and journals. Thus, the unit was well equipped for modern, scientific work without being luxurious.[142]

A particular concern in Morelos was the uneven collection of death certificates, especially for infants, resulting in unreliable mortality statistics. On the advice of the IHD representative, the governor of Morelos signed a law calling on the state health director to contact the relatives of all residents who had "died without medical assistance to ascertain the cause of death and to provide a certificate of death."[143] In addition, the director of the health unit was authorized to obtain a daily summary of deaths reported to the civil registrar to ascertain agreement with the International Classification of Diseases. Birth registration, too, was improving, thanks to the "diligence of the midwives."

These activities seemed to represent an agreeable coexistence—if not fusion—of the concerns of the local population, health unit staff, DSP, and IHD. The greatest achievement may have been the "good will" of the state, acknowledged by quarterly reports for "improving the living conditions and promoting the health and happiness of its population."[144] But this story of progressive cooperation belies a more complicated interplay of perspectives, policies, and practices.

Reception

Engendering the Units

Perhaps no activities reflected this swirl of interests as much as those that took a gendered approach to health. The maternal and child health work in Cuernavaca and at the other units undoubtedly extended and even enhanced the DSP's work in this area. Since its founding in 1929, for example, the DSP's Infant Hygiene Service, together with the publicly subsidized National Association for Infant Welfare, organized free clinics for prenatal and postnatal care together with other health promotion efforts, starting in large urban settings.[145]

But the units served as more than the town and country arms of Mexico City–based services: they found women to be ideal public health conduits in rural and semi-urban settings.[146] What began as an attempt to get to hard-to-reach populations was transformed into a conscious policy to target women directly— as healers, health workers, patients, and family health intermediaries. As patients and intermediaries, women were viewed in their roles as mothers, child bearers, and teachers; their hygiene practices in the prenatal, child-rearing, and schooling phases would determine the health and productivity of the next generation of workers. As public health personnel, women carried out several functions. Working-class, and occasionally middle-class, nurses served as a gendered bridge between doctors and the sanitary units on one side and peasants and townsfolk on the other. Through home visits and their activities in the sanitary units, nurses transported the ideology of Rockefeller public health—belief in biological causes of, technical cures for, and medical authority over disease. Midwives, alternatively, were partially co-opted by the health units, which needed their labor but abhorred much of their canon. Firmly situated in their communities, midwives were brought into the units for "professional" training, and were indeed sent back with more professional—though more circumscribed—roles. Each of these gendered approaches served to generate and maintain the health units' clientele and embed public health ideas in the population.

Although neither the IHD nor the DSP set out with a deliberate "women and health" agenda for the sanitary units, women grew to play a key role as translators and targets of the RF's cooperative efforts in Mexico. From the IHD side, this orientation in part reflected growing attention to maternal and child health in the U.S. and Europe, where such concern coincided with late nineteenth-century industrialization, urbanization, fertility declines, and state-building exigencies.[147] Early on, infant mortality could be addressed principally by extending the breast-feeding period, improving the milk supply, and bettering general sanitary conditions, but by the turn of the twentieth century, a focus on mothers' childbearing and child-rearing abilities emerged, based on bacteriological advances and social reform campaigns.[148]

In the United States this growing medical and social expertise translated into fits and starts of activity in a mix of voluntary and government venues, many of which were founded by women: Josephine Baker's Bureau of Child Hygiene in New York, Jane Addams' Hull House in Chicago, the U.S. Children's Bureau, founded in 1912 by Julia Lathrop, and the short-lived Sheppard-Towner Act (1921–29), which provided federal funding for maternal and child health education in the United States.[149] In conjunction with these initiatives, many local governments hired public health nurses and a number of states sought to regulate midwives. A relatively weak national state in the early twentieth-century United States enabled social reformers—particularly feminists—to fill the social policy vacuum and become pioneers in the organization of maternal and child health services.[150] The reformers never succeeded in converting these needs into a government responsibility or a universal right. Nor were these women able to fend off the opposition of organized medicine, given the ideology of private and voluntary provision of social services that predominated in the United States. The IHD was not won over by such feminist reformers—though nursing experts Mary Beard and Mary Tennant joined the staff in the 1930s to help professionalize nursing education—but it was certainly aware of these maternalist efforts and their relevance to public health projects at home and abroad.

Mexico's longer contact with and tradition of European influences in social policy and medicine made it more attentive to continental approaches to maternal and child health. By the early twentieth century, most European countries embraced a mixture of measures to improve infants' and mothers' health and welfare, including ideological campaigns, voluntary initiatives, and large-scale state activities.[151] France—which was particularly concerned with fertility declines and infant mortality—responded with an early and extensive array of protective legislation, from the Roussel Law of 1884, which provided breast-feeding to abandoned infants to a range of maternal pensions, mandated work leaves, and child health programs in subsequent years.[152] Many of these ideas and directives drew from the field of puericulture, Adolphe Pinard's notion of the scientific cultivation of childhood and the improvement of child health and welfare through better conditions of child-rearing.[153] In contrast to the United States, France's early commitment to universally implemented state measures—which were at once medically recommended and socially oriented—were influenced more by statists, health professionals, and intellectuals than by women reformers.

A variety of factors shaped Mexico's receptivity to these modern maternal and child health efforts. Mexican—and the broader Latin American—commitment to maternal and child health had deep cultural roots in a variety of indigenous practices.[154] Pre-Columbian cultures are known for their adherence to hygienic precepts, such as bathing rituals following childbirth, testing the milk of wet nurses, and monitoring the nursing mother's diet. The Maya in particular considered children to be a sign of wealth and good fortune and paid special attention to infant health.[155] Although many of these indigenous practices were suppressed during the colonial period, in the late 1920s the DSP's Infant Hygiene Service revived interest in the *ixbut*, a lactogenous plant used by the Maya to stimulate milk production among new mothers and wet nurses. In a DSP-sponsored experiment, agricultural researchers found that a group of cows that were fed milky secretions from the *ixbut* plant experienced a threefold increase in daily milk production.[156]

Regional and national feminist movements also played an important role in maternal and child health advocacy in the early twentieth century. Movements for women's equality in Latin America—ranging from communist to liberal-elite orientations—typically did not deny femininity and motherhood, but instead embraced these roles. Mother-feminism, based in part on Catholic spirituality, protested "laws and conditions which threaten[ed women's] ability" to bear children and nurture their families, including war, drugs, prostitution, urban misery, adultery, and exclusion from suffrage and property ownership.[157] As was the case elsewhere, these movements were more influential in urban settings, where middle-class women made social issues part of public policy and mobilized to improve and regulate social conditions for poor women.

If revolution furnished hope for the advancement of women in Mexico, early achievements were ambiguous. The 1917 Constitution and related laws called for female suffrage and women's workplace protections, but these provisions translated into few changes. In some cases, laws remained unenforced for decades (women gained the right to vote only in 1953), and in others they did not pertain to women in roles outside the formal labor force, such as homemakers, small artisans and merchants, and peasants. In still other cases, the provisions were not turned into workable social policy. Revolutionary political allegiances also helped to fragment Mexico's relatively small feminist movement. The state of Yucatán was the setting for the country's most far-reaching feminist activism—including extensive civic and economic participation—but the movement was virtually eradicated after the Socialist governor was assassinated in 1924.

At a national level, a small number of women entered public life in various social policy wings of government departments (though few in the doctor-dominated DSP) and advanced a feminist agenda from their new positions. But their natural allies—middle-class and elite women of Catholic background—protested against and were isolated from the anticlerical presidencies of the 1920s. Still, some elite women, including doctors, founded their own health and social welfare agencies and worked in tandem with government initiatives. Moreover, feminists did agree on women's suffrage, and by the 1930s they were able to parlay this unity into greater political power.[158] Rural women—who were approached principally as the conduits for a male-based vision of modernizing the countryside—may also have experienced gender gains in this period thanks to the introduction of laborsaving household technologies and to their new-found relationship with the state's rural agents—women teachers and nurses.[159]

Around the same time, Mexican professionals and statesmen—as they did in other countries in Latin America— "discovered" infant mortality to be a menace to growth and modernization projects, if not a threat to population and industrial needs as in Europe.[160] Similar to France but in contrast to the United States, many Latin American physicians were supportive of the state's role in the provision of health services, and together with nurses, sociologists, policymakers, and reformers, they held leadership roles in the regional movement for maternal and child health. In 1927 the International Institute for the Protection of Childhood was founded in Montevideo, Uruguay, the first establishment of its kind in the world.[161] Prodded by its member countries, the PASB began to address the problem of infant mortality in the 1930s. Most notably, the Pan American Child Congresses—inaugurated by Latin American feminists in 1916—attracted the backing of male physicians and lawyers as well as social workers and other professionals, across the region. These groups joined forces for some four decades to craft pioneering legislation to protect children and their mothers.[162]

Another important ingredient in the region's support for maternal and child health—and a source of antagonism between North American and Latin American social policy—was the response to eugenics. Anglo-Saxon eugenics was principally informed by Mendelian genetics. Improving society's genetic stock entailed the breeding out of bad genes through sterilization and prohibitions on procreation (so-called negative eugenics). While such ideas generated tremendous divisions among researchers within the United States, the precepts of "negative eugenics" were eagerly adopted by policymakers, with thirty-one out of forty-eight states passing compulsory sterilization laws between 1907 and 1937.[163]

Eugenics in Latin American countries reflected French influences rather than Anglo-Saxon genetics. As Nancy Stepan has demonstrated for Mexico, Brazil, and Argentina, eugenics was interpreted through neo-Lamarckian ideas about the inheritance of acquired characteristics and implemented through the practices of puericulture and homiculture, the latter a Cuban-coined extension of Pinard's childhood concerns to all age groups. Latin eugenics stressed reforming the social and moral environment of prospective parents and children instead of blocking reproduction. Children raised well might not only overcome an unfavorable genetic background; they would also pass on their new traits to future generations, improving the larger society. This "positive eugenics" movement, with its emphasis on sanitation and the scientific improvement of the circumstances surrounding conception and childhood, closely overlapped with maternal and child health matters.[164]

As Alexandra Stern has shown, French-influenced Mexican eugenists dominated the Mexican medical establishment as well as a wide array of government agencies. Education and criminal justice, to mention just two arenas, joined health and medicine in making eugenic ideas central to Mexico's project of national (re)construction in the 1920s and 1930s.[165] DSP initiatives were particularly infused with eugenic thinking. The School Hygiene Service closely monitored the physical and mental development of schoolchildren and the Infant Hygiene Service—under Isidro Espinosa y de los Reyes's leadership—emphasized puericultural training, home visits, and the medical monitoring of mother and child as a means to reduce infant mortality. Though these measures were wide-ranging, they were initially implemented in Mexico City,[166] leaving activities elsewhere somewhat more open to other approaches.

At bottom, the female social agenda that emerged in these years—including regulation of wet-nursing and adoption, oversight of foundling hospitals, assessment of maternal fitness by the welfare system, organization of venereal clinics and milk stations, pregnancy surveillance and well-baby care, among other measures[167]—drew from feminist-maternalist ideas, indigenous cultural practices, nationalist concerns, physician advocacy, and eugenic puericulture. Mexican attention to maternal and child health in the 1920s and 1930s may also be framed within an understanding of state institution-building. Nineteenth-century Mexican efforts to organize health and social welfare institutions for women and children had been marred by limited government involvement.[168] Receptivity to these ideas predated the revolution, but Mexico's ability to adapt, modify, and extend maternal and child health practices grew in function with revolutionary institutional expansion.

Because the RF began working in Mexico just as this expansion was taking place and as the DSP was considering how best to reach the interior of the country, the foundation could forge a potentially larger role for itself than pervasive European medical influences might otherwise have allowed. Thus, the IHD's joint activity with the DSP in developing health units in provincial towns operated amidst competing forces but also with the possibility of considerable bearing upon public health institutionalization. How the work of the health units became gendered is an important facet of this story.

Nursing a Public Health Approach

Nurses only occasionally worked with the hookworm brigades, and for the Minatitlán–Puerto México unit, Carr did not think about nurses except as office-based assistants to the physician. Bustamante, by contrast, well aware of the pivotal role played by visiting nurses in both the United States and Mexico City, had employed visiting nurses in Veracruz beginning in 1929. The IHD's belated recognition that it was nurses—virtually all of whom were female—who could best traverse the worlds of modern public health, maternal and child welfare, and local customs was reinforced by the request by Cuernavaca and other local officials that the units address the problem of infant mortality. Once the IHD-sponsored units began using visiting nurses in 1931, they became a vital and permanent component of the full-time staff.

Visiting nurses served as a key point of outreach and contact with the local community, and they often traveled beyond the immediate radius of the units to reach women living on the outskirts of town or in rural areas. After having been trained by unit physicians, then closely supervised until approved to work independently,[169] the nurses were dispatched to the public, household by household. Though they occasionally made home visits to administer vaccines and attend to persons unwilling to undergo hookworm treatment, their main purview was maternal and infant health.

With the RF providing the framework and rationale, maternal and child health measures drew from a variety of national and international practices. Unit nurses typically devoted every afternoon to home visits to pregnant women and new mothers, showing and telling them how to care for themselves and their children. Husbands and brothers might have finished their field or town labors and returned home to rest by this time of day, but there are no records of the nurses interacting with men. During each visit, nurses surveyed the conditions of the home and assessed overall household hygiene. Pregnant women were told to bathe daily, wash their breasts, eat regularly without overindulging, defecate daily, exercise, and rest, and avoid reading "morbid literature or adventure stories."[170] The women were advised to purchase baby cribs instead of sleeping with their newborns and to stay in bed for two weeks after childbirth. Many of these recommendations challenged both the customs and the economic possibilities of many families, and suspicious mothers sometimes denied entrance to nurses, who—as retired visiting nurse Judith Castor put it—"needed to know how to talk their way in."[171]

Health unit administrators viewed home visits as principally educational and individual, not medical or social endeavors. They were simply "the most practical means of infusing the necessary personal hygiene knowledge" in the minds—and actions—of the public. "Of course," the 1931 Minatitlán–Puerto México unit report asserted, "poverty influences the development of public health problems, but poverty is not the determinant factor." Instead, "the lack of

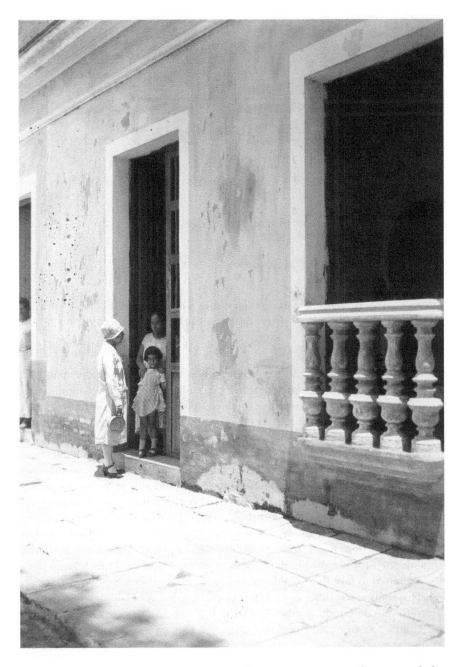

Figure 3.9. Visiting nurse on her rounds, Veracruz, 1929. Courtesy of the Rockefeller Archive Center.

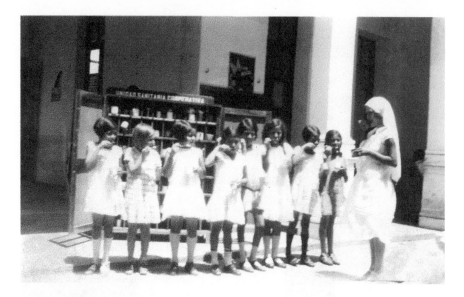

Figure 3.10. Schoolgirls brushing their teeth, with cubby holes for toothbrush storage at the health unit. Courtesy of the Rockefeller Archive Center.

knowledge of hygiene determines health, and it is precisely the poor man who needs this knowledge so that he may live healthily in spite of his economic situation."[172] Family well-being was thus reduced to maternal responsibility for good hygiene. Unlike the situation in France or even Mexico City, women were not provided with social or economic support to follow this advice.

Teachers, who were by the early 1930s far more numerous than nurses in provincial Mexico, were also engaged as mediators of modern health and hygiene.[173] As part of the Cuernavaca unit's school health program, for example, teachers were asked to organize theatrical performances demonstrating the value of health measures. In one "health play," children lined up in a row and were presented with the gift of a toothbrush. Together the members of the class would brush their teeth and carefully store the toothbrushes on a special hygienic shelf for use during daily tooth brushing exercises. The children were not permitted to take their new brushes home for fear they would be lost or dirtied. This routine was described to curious parents, many of whom could neither afford to purchase toothbrushes nor provide a sink and storage area.[174] School-age children became an important target of sanitary education because they "could be molded by the influence of their teachers" even when their families did not assimilate messages of personal hygiene.[175]

The home was the territory of the nurses, but they were also charged with attracting their subjects to the units. After a pregnant woman was examined

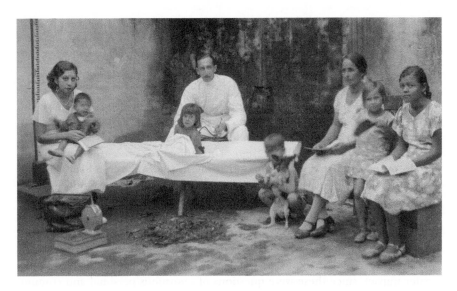

Figure 3.11. Pre-school health clinic, Puerto México health unit, 1935. Courtesy of the Rockefeller Archive Center.

by the nurse, she was given instructions for a "happy pregnancy," which entailed semi-monthly attendance at special clinics at the sanitary units. There, the women were given careful pelvic exams, urine analysis, blood pressure measurement, and treatment for syphilis, and they were also offered "the necessary medical advice to prevent difficulties and disasters." According to quarterly unit reports, these women—who often had never before visited a medical doctor—received care equivalent to "the best laboratories of the most conscientious specialists." Thus, the unit doctors assured that the "misfortunes and tragedies" resulting from poor care could be avoided. Though infant mortality rates rose in the areas surrounding IHD-sponsored health units during the 1930s,[176] the RF attributed much of the increase to better data collection and claimed success in "saving the lives of countless mothers and babies."[177]

After delivery, a visiting nurse persuaded the new mother to attend the weekly infant clinics organized by the health units for group instruction in the care of newborns. Nurses sought to convince even experienced mothers to enroll in the infant clinics so the progress of their children could be closely monitored. Visiting nurses also renewed their home visits to administer typhoid and smallpox vaccines and to continue home instruction, now covering infant bathing, regular feeding, digestion, and overall care of the baby's health.[178] Mothers were advised to boil drinking water to "kill all the little animals" so that their children would not die. As visiting nurse "La Güera" Coronel recalled:

I told the mother that boiling water was her own responsibility. I could come visit her but I did not live in her house. It was she who had to make sure that she washed her hands before eating and feeding the baby and after defecating to make sure her baby remained healthy.[179]

Given the absence of sources on women's responses to these efforts, we can reconstruct popular effects only indirectly. According to Cuernavaca unit statistics, the semi-monthly maternal and child health clinics were well attended, with twenty to forty women usually present. This number represented a small proportion of the estimated 30,000 people living in Cuernavaca and surrounding areas at the time, but it also meant that up to four hundred households (assuming that each woman attended two clinics) might have been reached each year. The effects would have been multiplied by diffusion through networks of friends, family, and neighbors.[180] Although these activities involved far smaller numbers than the many thousands of people reached annually by a single hookworm brigade, contact around maternal and child health issues had an arguably greater impact, since these were questions of enormous personal and community concern. Moreover, each health encounter was longer, and visits were repeated for up to a year or more.

As we have seen, this was also an overbearing initiative: the infant clinics occupied large amounts of the mothers' time (including travel time), and women were held responsible for their children's health based on the medical knowledge transmitted at the clinics. Grandmothers, aunts, and neighbors—a new mother's customary teachers—were systematically excluded and criticized by the nurses for their "primitive" ways. Only the advice of medical personnel was deemed valid. Even a mother's own experience was discounted by sanitary unit doctors, who admonished "Just because you have been pregnant before does not make you an expert."[181] Visiting nurses more compassionately urged their patients to heed medical recommendations but the message persisted; notwithstanding women's personal and collective experience, existing practices of motherhood needed to be medically supervised.

Why, then, might women have subjected themselves to these impositions? Certainly infant mortality was a severe problem, with some Morelos towns experiencing the death of more than one fifth of all newborns. Especially in more rural areas with few healers and a need for large families to help with agricultural work, the promise of better health outcomes might have been attractive to women and to their families. Alternatively, although birth control services were not provided by the units, some women may have sought reproductive knowledge from visiting nurses. On another front, the daily clinics of the units were filled with women and children seeking treatment for a variety of ailments. The preventive health outreach by the visiting nurses may well have generated a demand for these free services; women may have combined their attendance at the clinics with care-seeking for other family members. Visiting

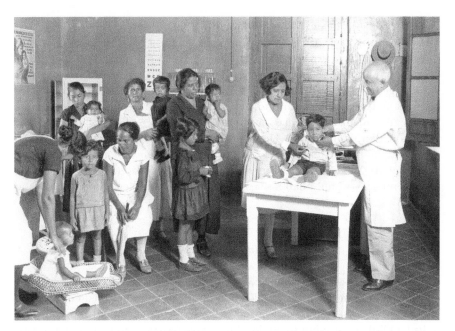

Figure 3.12. Mothers and children attending infant hygiene clinic, 1929. Courtesy of the Rockefeller Archive Center.

nurses were instrumental in this effort. They used a combination of local know-how and professional expertise to make their way into women's homes and coax and induce the women to attend the clinics, at once utilizing local systems of women's information-sharing and creating new relationships around knowledge and services.[182]

Initially, IHD officers thought that they could profitably hire middle-class nurses educated in hospital-based schools in Mexico's larger cities, for their "influence will undoubtedly gradually radiate from the urban centres as has been the history of public health nursing development in the [United] States."[183] Soon, however, it became clear that nurses would have to be trained specifically to serve in rural areas, because few middle-class city girls could be attracted to work in provincial towns. Beginning in 1932, public health nurses joined health officers and sanitary inspectors in six or eight-week courses in RF-supported field training stations. Within fifteen years almost a thousand nurses had been trained in these courses. Still, RF officers complained perennially that nurses were of "low cultural standing" and that training in Mexico was "primitive."[184] In spite of these laments, reliance on visiting nurses grew over time.

Without explicitly conceptualizing the visiting nurses as a women's initiative, the IHD-DSP health units—as did countless health departments in Europe, elsewhere in Latin America, and the U.S.[185]—engaged in cross-class and gender-specific strategies, using working-class (though preferring middle-class) nurses to bring poor, rural women into the medical fold. As guided by unit directives and their own experience, nurses employed a mixture of incentives, coercion, reprimands, and warnings. The common thread was that expert knowledge, imparted either in the health unit or in the home, should replace customs and superstition around maternal and child health. Trained nurses represented medical and class authority, and gender affinity facilitated the reception of this authority. These efforts, while challenging existing social structures in rural Mexico, were consistent with many of the goals of the revolutionary Mexican state, whereby a growing professional class—including women nurses—would enable social and economic modernization across the country.

Midwives as Midwives

Though nurses—and to some extent teachers—served as a female-friendly extension of the health units, rural communities already enjoyed an existing set of women healers—midwives. Having promised to target infant mortality, the units had little choice but to ask local midwives (*parteras*) to carry out a service that the units themselves could not fulfill—delivering babies and providing ongoing care to new mothers. While *curanderos* (traditional healers, both male and female)[186] had been swept aside as superstitious witches, the sanitary units sought to incorporate midwives through medical training and supervision. In doing this, the IHD-sponsored units—whether consciously or not—were adapting their public health model to the local reality. The units were also entering a long-standing controversy around the training of midwives in Mexico.

In addressing pregnancy, infant care, and midwifery, the health units were entering territory that had previously been the domain of women. The units justified their encroachment by linking Mexico's high infant mortality to maternal ignorance and the "erroneous practices" of midwives, who attended over 90 percent of births.[187] Infant mortality, estimated at over 200 deaths per 1000 live births, offered, according to the 1934 Annual Report of the Rural Hygiene Service, "evidence of the need for medical care and supervision for the expectant mother" and the infant. Infant mortality rates in towns with sanitary units were lower than the national average, but still high, ranging in 1934 from 88 deaths per 1000 live births in Tuxtepec, Oaxaca to 145 deaths/1000 in Puerto México.[188]

The 1934 report went on to complain that "many women, through ignorance or economy, prefer empirical midwives who charge little, creating a grave danger for both mothers and children." Because they did not restrict their activities to childbirth, midwives were also blamed for posing prenatal and postnatal dangers. It was thus necessary to identify, monitor, and train midwives in order to

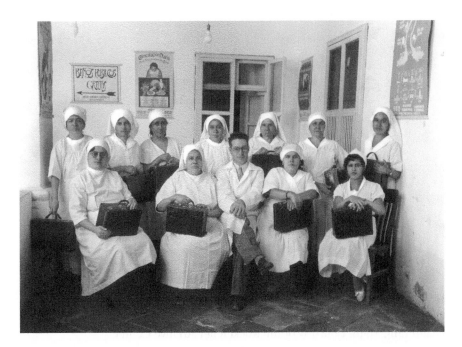

Figure 3.13. Members of the midwife club, equipped with satchels filled with scissors, soap, silver nitrate ampules, sterile tape, forceps, and other instruments, pose with the Cuernavaca health unit director, 1933. Courtesy of the Rockefeller Archive Center.

"give them a sense of responsibility and to place limits on their work so they would not threaten the lives of mothers or their children."[189]

Beginning in the early 1930s, instead of displacing them, the units sought to transform scores of "empirical"—traditional—midwives into modern childbirth attendants by paying them to attend weekly "midwife clubs." At the Cuernavaca unit, for instance, midwives were pressured to attend classes so that "the Doctor could instruct them in less dangerous birthing practices." This training in obstetrics and midwifery, as one doctor noted, consisted mainly of instruction in "what they should not do." It also allowed doctors to monitor midwives, "because for now it is impossible to get rid of them and it is worthwhile to recognize this situation and attempt to educate them in order to minimize the harm they cause."[190]

In traditional Mexican settings, the midwife—*ticitl* in Nahua—served as chief advisor, spiritual guide, and caregiver to women during pregnancy, childbirth, and the post-partum period.[191] Many midwives believed they answered a divine calling, and virtually all underwent apprenticeships to learn both ritual and clinical practices. Midwives, typically respected older women, provided continuous care through all phases of birth, earning the confidence of expectant and new

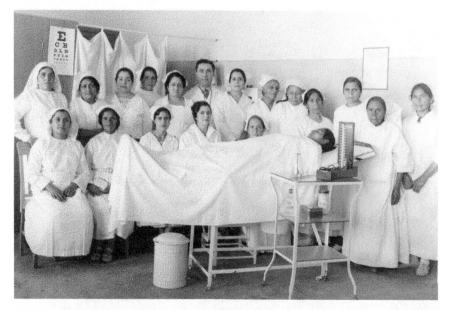

Figure 3.14. Midwives being trained in modern childbirth methods, Cuautla health unit, 1936. Courtesy of the Rockefeller Archive Center.

mothers. Although specific practices varied from culture to culture and from indigenous to mestizo communities, historians and anthropologists have documented numerous overlapping patterns. Prenatal care involved observing the color of the nipples. the shape of the womb, and the position of the fetus, and relieving physical ailments through massage and herbal remedies. Childbirth usually took place at home in the presence of the expectant mother's family. Traditionally, women gave birth in a kneeling or squatting position, aided by the forces of gravity. During difficult deliveries, midwives sometimes employed herbal medicines and gentle massage. The umbilical cord, not cut until the placenta was expelled, was normally cauterized with a candle flame or cut with a heated blade. In the weeks following the birth, the midwife aided the new mother with household chores, offering both emotional and physical support. Within a few weeks after delivery (and sometimes during pregnancy and the early stages of childbirth), the new mother took one or more *temazcalli*—therapeutic steam baths—which served to physically, ritually, and emotionally cleanse her.[192] Midwives and their patients believed the baths increased the flow of milk, prevented illness, and helped adjust the balance of hot and cold influences.[193]

Sanitary unit training sessions, on the other hand, were designed to limit the midwife's role to a medical one, discarding social and ritual functions. Doctors convinced midwives to use aseptic methods to prevent microbial infection, employ and disinfect instruments such as forceps, and deliver women in a

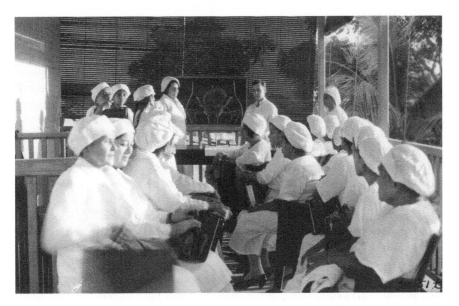

Figure 3.15. Empirical midwives being trained in reproductive physiology, Minatitlán health unit, 1935. Courtesy of the Rockefeller Archive Center.

supine position.[194] The new rules denounced the customs of herbal teas, massages, umbilical cord cauterization, and other practices, even though there was no evidence that they were harmful. The units further medicalized the child-birth process by strictly advising the midwife to recognize her limitations and to consult a physician or hospital at any sign of complication.

While it is difficult to determine the exact number of midwives trained by the units, we might estimate that with approximately ten to fifteen midwives attending each three-to-four week course, there were some 150 midwifery graduates per unit per year. With each midwife following several pregnancies at a time, thousands of women per unit may have been reached by the trained midwives. Aware of this multiplier effect of midwifery training, unit directors were unapologetic about paying them to attend. Still, gauging the extent to which the trained midwives assimilated what they had learned into their own practices requires further study.

Many of the midwives arrived at training sessions barefoot and in ragged clothes, like most of their patients; at the end of the course, midwives in starched white uniforms were awarded a bag of instruments and a Spanish translation of the Mississippi State Board of Health's *Midwife Manual.* Though few were literate, most midwives learned the new practices quickly.[195] As their medical expertise grew, their dependency on outside knowledge and products also rose.

Like midwifery training elsewhere, the health unit programs attempted to modify virtually every aspect of traditional midwifery, failing to take long-held customs into account. By replacing superstition and empirically based tradition with science, trainers made some midwives fear their own practices, warning, for example, that if the baby hit its head on the ground during delivery, it was the fault of the midwife. In training midwives, the IHD-DSP units hoped to minimize reliance on traditional medical practices and to increase the importance of the licensing and training of midwives in modern obstetrical methods. Midwives were also asked to bring their patients to prenatal and postnatal clinics at the sanitary units, both to expand the reach of these efforts and to generate further demand for trained midwives. One could argue that, although midwives were often enticed into attending the sessions, the units enhanced their skill and potentially the survival of midwifery as a profession. These strategies were similar to those followed in the South of the U.S. during the same period, when black midwives were blamed for bad outcomes and then made subject to state regulations because they served as a "vital link between poor African Americans and health departments."[196]

The cooperative health units' approach to midwifery was also consistent with— if not more welcoming than—numerous Mexican efforts beginning in the colonial period[197] and continuing to the present[198] that have culpabilized midwives for infant and maternal deaths and have called for midwifery training (and for a more circumscribed role for the midwife) and licensing, or complete replacement by nurses and doctors. Mexican midwives were not covered by licensing regulations until 1945, allowing them to practice widely but also leaving them open to often unwarranted attacks. In 1931, for example, Dr. Isidro Espinosa y de los Reyes, head of the DSP's Infant Hygiene Service, recommended to the National Commission on the Practice of Midwifery that professional training and licensing be prerequisites for any midwife wishing to practice in a town of 4,000 inhabitants or more, that midwives be required to obtain medical assistance if labor lasted more than twenty-four hours (in the case of a woman's first labor, twelve hours for a subsequent labor), and that midwives officially register all births with the DSP.[199] The measure did not pass. In 1937 Governor of Morelos José Refugio Bustamante inaugurated the state's first school of nursing and obstetrics with the declaration that empirical practices by "midwives without the least rudimentary knowledge of scientific medicine" had to be eliminated in order to "save the nation's defenseless sons and daughters from grave danger."[200]

While the experience of the IHD-DSP health units in Morelos undoubtedly informed this critique, the contention that traditional midwives in Mexico harmed more than they helped surfaced centuries before the arrival of the RF.[201] Still, the health units' articulation of this view was lasting: in 1973 the doctor heading the Health Ministry's midwife training program repeated, almost verbatim, an IHD officer's words from forty years before: "Above all, she should be instructed specifically as to what not to do."[202]

In the cooperative local health units of the 1930s, this view was translated into a small but significant effort. Because the units were closely engaged with the communities they served, they were in a position to implement midwifery train-ing. By targeting midwives, the units narrowed the understanding of both the cause and the solution to high infant mortality, at once disregarding its social and economic determinants and medicalizing midwives, childbirth, and motherhood itself. IHD personnel reinforced the ideological dimensions of this reductionist approach to health by blaming midwives and their traditional practices for high infant and maternal mortality. In addition, by severing the role of visiting nurse from that of midwife, the health units played class favorites, expanding the purview of trained, working- and middle-class public health nurses, while reduc-ing the role of empirical midwives. Yet in a sense, the units helped to rescue mid-wives through their very medicalization, in contrast to the Mexican medical profession's preference, which was to eliminate midwives outright.

One might reasonably ask how else the IHD-DSP might have dealt with mid-wives. Only a few years after the IHD left Mexico, a different approach emerged from international health circles. In 1956, Isabel Kelly, an anthropologist with the Institute of Inter-American Affairs, was asked by the WHO to develop a proposal for midwifery training in Mexico. Her plan promoted the existing skills and experience of midwives while instructing them in the medical principles of asepsis and hygiene, prenatal and postnatal care, and recognition of cases to refer to physicians. In order to maximize midwives' acceptance of the new practices, Kelly recommended integrating medical instruction with traditional beliefs surrounding pregnancy and childbirth. Thus, for example, herbal teas might be prescribed in place of water (which was believed to be detrimental to the fetus), and hospitals could be instructed to dispose of the placenta according to indigenous traditions.[203] These ideas shaped the WHO's traditional birth attendant training programs in subsequent decades but found no place in the RF's efforts in Mexico.

Of course, the RF and DSP were not the only international or national organ-izations that recognized that women—as midwives, nurses, mothers, and patients—could channel public health ideas and practices to distinct settings and be held accountable for maternal and child health outcomes. Lenore Manderson has documented a similar arrangement in colonial Malaysia starting in 1905, in which traditional midwives received basic instruction; local women were recruited to become medically trained nurses to eventually replace the midwives; and new mothers were attracted to infant health programs via home visits. The strategies of "teaching" motherhood and training women healers were modeled on British notions of maternal roles. As infant mortality-reducing policies employing the healers closest to the targeted women themselves, they were also practical and effective.[204]

The Mexican environment in which the RF cooperated bore similarities both to rural parts of the U.S. and to the tropical reaches of European empires, where the goal of modernizing health services came up against traditional practices and economic constraints. Relying on local nurses and empirical midwives, who underwent short training courses, the IHD had in essence copied at least part of Bustamante's approach to expanding public health services using available personnel. The IHD departed from its strict professional model of modern public health, fashioning together with the DSP—a set of services adapted to rural and small town settings. In Mexico, the pressure to solidify the state through public health success made these measures ever more expedient.

Displacement and Resistance

Opposition to the RF-DSP local health efforts was on a small scale and sporadic, but local resistance to the displacement of traditional medical practices and practitioners is suggestive of wider discontent. Once midwives were invited to the sanitary units, it was principally *curanderos* and *brujos* (witches) who were shunned by the local health developments.

Even before the healers began to feel threatened by their new competitors, the IHD faced the unexpected opposition of another group of practitioners— local physicians. In 1928, just a few months after the founding of the Minatitlán–Puerto México unit, Carr reported that a group of local physicians was charging that "The Unit is trying to diminish the amount of disease in the area; the physicians make their living from the disease in the locality; therefore the Unit is detrimental to the physicians." The frustrated Carr attempted to explain to them that "we have no intention of running a free treatment clinic for general diseases," and that the units were interested in preventive rather than curative medicine. He pointed out that the units would not diminish the doctors' clientele but rather boost it, for "as the people become more 'health conscious' they will be more ready to consult the physician." Further, healthy, working people would have money to visit the doctor. The units were actually encouraging these patients to visit private physicians for a range of conditions. His arguments aided little in "dealing with the Latin temperament."[205]

Carr also observed that local physicians were irritated by the modern equipment used by the sanitary units and by the physical examinations they provided to school children. According to Carr, doctors feared that their patients would begin to demand the sophisticated apparatus, requiring them to upgrade their own offices. Despite the hostility of all but a handful of local physicians, Carr optimistically noted that the controversy might "raise the standard of local medical service."[206] IHD Director Russell equated the opposition of Mexican doctors to that of U.S. doctors opposed to full-time county health departments in rural Ohio, New York, and other states. The solution was for Carr to regularly attend meetings of the local medical society, befriend its leaders, and publicly present new projects before they were initiated in order to obtain the approval of the majority of members.[207] He also recommended using the units to train a handful of local candidates for new positions, as a precursor to the creation of a formal training station.[208]

Where doctors might be convinced and midwives trained, the IHD had little interest in integrating other healers. Healers and their communities in Mexico held to a unified concept of spiritual and physical well-being as opposed to the bifurcated beliefs of the outsiders, who failed to attend to the spiritual needs of the ill: likewise, the herbal and surgical remedies of traditional Mexica, Maya, and other cultures were not separated from spiritual religious healing methods.[209] This did not make traditional and "western" medicine irreconcilable. During the colonial period, indigenous and galenic-influenced European beliefs settled in a syncretic healing system, centered on the balancing of the humors by adjusting hot and cold influences.[210] By the mid twentieth century, the empirical orientation of various regimes of indigenous medicine enabled the approval of modern medical treatment for diseases considered to be natural, as opposed to those believed to have supernatural causes.

Many in the DSP and, later, in Mexico's National Indigenous Institute also tolerated an improvised coexistence of traditional and modern medicine.[211] By contrast, IHD officers, like most North American doctors, assumed that traditional medicine was superstitious and ineffective, despite the herbalist origins of quinine and other medications.[212] IHD men were thus pleased that the units had been positively received. Yet high attendance records at the sanitary units did not necessarily indicate wholehearted acceptance of modern medicine. Many villagers may have gone out of curiosity and in response to incentives; others were brought to the clinics by their children, who had been instructed to attend by their schoolteachers.[213]

Healers themselves, though perhaps displeased at the appearance of new providers, posed few direct challenges to the sanitary units.[214] Typically only one unit was developed at a time, lessening the impact on traditional healers. In the most remote areas, traditional medicine was not joined by modern health services until at least the 1950s, when new highways facilitated the opening of rural health clinics.[215] In some places where clinics were established, traditional healers practiced alongside doctors and even adopted similar commercial practices of seeing dozens of patients per day.[216] In larger towns, the units may even have increased the demand for traditional medicine.

It was not IHD disdain but rather Mexican physician corporatism that provoked the first clash between unit doctors and traditional healers. In 1931, at the same time as the opening of the health unit in Cuernavaca, a group of hospital directors set out to regulate the practice of medicine in Morelos, proposing licensing requirements for doctors, dentists, pharmacists, veterinarians, obstetricians, and nurses. These regulations excluded *curanderos* and other so-called charlatans from practice altogether. Agricultural, mining, and industrial enterprises would be required to employ licensed practitioners. In places with no licensed physicians, the chief of the State Health Department would grant exceptions to unlicensed practitioners who had attended primary school, had a good reputation, and who, after a maximum of two chances, had passed a theoretical and practical examination (costing 25 pesos, or $150 in 2004 dollars) to prove their competence.[217] The weeding out of "unfair" competitors had long been on the agenda of medical professionals; in the early 1930s these efforts could be linked to a nation-wide unionization movement. In response to the proposed regulations, healers in seven or eight hilltop towns in Morelos staged vehement protests against doctors working for the sanitary units.[218]

Other Morelos residents—likely backed by *curanderos*—opposed specific practices promulgated by personnel of the health units and the DSP. During the same years as the healer protests, some villagers began to object to mandatory smallpox vaccination because they did not wish to take "medicine" when they were healthy. Visiting nurse-vaccinators traversed Morelos on horseback,[219] typically covering three or four towns each day. When the nurses arrived to administer the vaccines, some villagers sent dogs out to attack them. On one or two occasions, nurse-vaccinators were killed by locals unwilling to undergo vaccination. Medicalized bureaucratization became the solution: when the Morelos government began to require proof of vaccination for the registry of newborns and school attendance, objectors gradually disappeared.[220]

Still, periodic outbursts of opposition to sanitary measures persisted. In 1940, after the IHD had been working in Morelos for almost a decade, the attempt of the Cuautla unit (finally established in 1935) to impose isolation methods to control a cerebrospinal meningitis outbreak was met with fatal mob violence. The epidemic had begun at "the height of a fair . . . where there were thousands of people congregated from other parts of the state and surrounding states."[221] After that fair, six more large fairs were held around Morelos, with up to 70,000 people converging upon towns of 7,000 or 8,000 people.[222] The RF officer "did everything possible to have these fairs suppressed, by appealing to the Governor and the Federal Health Department," meeting with no success. The Cuautla health officer urged municipal authorities to close the fair, but:

> The Indians of the town remonstrated against such a closure and became rebellious and troublesome. Finally the Health Officer requested the aid of the army corps at Cuautla. A colonel and four soldiers were sent and just as they were arriving in the town, they were set upon by the mob and all five were killed. The Health Officer barely escaped hanging, although his car was almost demolished.[223]

A few people were arrested, though nobody was charged, and the fairs—highly important regional events—continued to be held. Because of the large number of carriers present and the difficulty of controlling fair crowds, seventy-four people were struck by meningitis in 1940 after three years without reported cases in Morelos. The RF home office was distressed at the situation but assured the RF officer in Mexico that, "having advised Government as to appropriate preventive measures, it seems to me that you and your associates have fulfilled your duty." Ferrell stressed that it was the Mexican government's responsibility, not the RF's, to control disease outbreaks.[224]

Through the late 1940s, RF projects met with occasional opposition, threats, and anti-"gringo" posters. During an IHD malaria survey in the state of Guerrero in 1947, for example, an armed, angry mob formed, accusing the project's physicians of sterilizing children and killing the sick. The health personnel barely survived. The same year, a large-scale cattle slaughtering effort to control hoof-and-mouth disease enraged livestock owners, who attacked visiting health authorities, including IHD men. The RF attributed this opposition to "superstitious and very suspicious . . . unlettered Indians and Mestizos" and to Communist "troublemakers" hoping to discredit the president.[225] In another instance, the spraying of DDT to control typhus in the early 1940s was linked to U.S. war-mongering; some villagers believed that DDT would increase fertility so that children could become soldiers; still others heard rumors that the chemical would assist the government in limiting the number of children in each family.[226]

The sometimes violent objections to RF-DSP initiatives might be attributed to several factors. First, in traditional cultures, healers were generally consulted in the case of illness, often considered a shameful occurrence; many people, therefore, may have been reluctant to attend health units for preventive measures. In 1952, the PASB carried out an anthropological study of the role of popular beliefs in the reception of health centers in Mexico. Many villagers felt that their time visiting a doctor was wasted due to long waits or appointments available only during the workday. Some were suspicious of health unit workers who were of a higher social class, unlike their neighbor-*curanderos*. Others felt that doctors were impolite, callous, and purposely induced fear in their patients, with nurses perceived as more humanitarian, understanding, and sincere. A large number of interviewees felt that sick children were not well treated. Health personnel told mothers to await the visits of nurses for child health problems, not explaining that these were routine, preventive visits and that signs of illness in a child merited an urgent visit to the health center.[227]

Because many Mexicans were fatalistic about their health, the report argued, many believed that their appointments at the health center were a favor to the staff rather than a benefit to themselves. A large portion of the population visited both *curanderos* and Western physicians, often to the disadvantage of the latter as they were not consulted until the *curandero* had repeatedly failed to achieve results. *Curanderos* were deemed more honest by the interviewed villagers because they recognized their limitations and occasionally referred their patients to physicians, but physicians never recommended visits to traditional healers. In allopathic medicine's defense, the PASB study also pointed out that *curanderos* treated vague symptoms that were easy to relieve, while Western medicine was based on a disease etiology that sometimes had no therapeutic component.

Given the potential for cultural conflict over public health measures, it is in some ways surprising that the IHD units did not face more opposition.[228] In part,

Table 3.5. Number of health units in Mexico by type, selected years

	1925	1929	1932	1934	1935	1936	1937	1940
Federal delegations in state capitals, ports, and border towns	34	65	62	70	77	n/a	n/a	47
IHD-DSP local health units		1	5	5	10	8	5	5
DSP local health units		1	6	10	82	138	246	427
Ejidal units					2	36	75	121

Sources: Salvador Iturbide Alvirez, "Panorama General de la Salubridad Pública en México," *Pasteur: Revista Mensual de Medicina* 10, II, no. 4 (1937): 93–102; Departamento de Salubridad Pública, *Rural Hygiene and Social Medicine Services of the Department of Public Health: Organization-Functions, Results Obtained until 1940*, (México, D.F.: Departamento de Salubridad Pública, 1941); José Siurob, *Trabajo Sanitario en los Estados Unidos Mexicanos, 1934–1940*, Departamento de Salubridad Pública, April 26, 1940; José Alvarez Amézquita, Miguel E. Bustamante, Antonio L. Picazos, and F. Fernández del Castillo, *Historia de la Salubridad y de la Asistencia en México*, 4 vols. (México, D.F.: Secretaría de Salubridad y Asistencia, 1960); "Mexico, Expenditures by Subjects and Years, July 1, 1913–December 11, 1940 (Corrected Statement as of 9/28/42)," RG 2-Stacks, Box 561, Folder 3814 RFA; Miguel E. Bustamante, "La Coordinación de los Servicios Sanitarios Federales y Locales Como Factor de Progreso Higiénico en México," *Gaceta Médica de México* 65 (1934): 207.

resistance may have been muted thanks to unit hiring practices—aside from the medical director and some other specialist posts such as those of sanitary engineers, the local population filled staff positions as secretaries, inspectors, technicians, and chauffeurs. Midwives and visiting nurses in particular served as a supportive link between populace and health unit. Just as important was the fact that most small-town and rural Mexicans had learned to patch together their health services from a variety of sources—including healers, midwives, and doctors—and thus viewed the units as an option more than as a threat. Perhaps this was not quite the revolution in rural health that the RF had in mind, but it allowed traditional and modern medicine to coexist over the long run.[229]

International Interplay

By the end of 1932, Mexico's Rural Hygiene Service was on stable footing and involved the governments of three states (Veracruz, Oaxaca, and Morelos), and five municipalities (see table 3.4). With the services running smoothly, the DSP was ready to absorb the Rural Hygiene Service into the new division of "Coordinated Health Services in the States" inaugurated under Bustamante's direction in 1933. The DSP's own health unit expansion (without IHD involvement) had thus far been limited to two extra units in the state of Veracruz, one unit each in the states of Durango and Sinaloa, and a new statewide service slated to start in Guanajuato and Querétaro in 1933. As such, there was an ambitious plan and high hopes for the "Coordinated Health Services in the States" (see table 3.5). Within just a few years, due to a big budget expansion and the power of a new Sanitary Code in 1934, which compelled state participation, more than two thirds of the states were sponsoring local health units, offering a mix of services covering sanitary engineering, nutrition, infant health, epidemiology and prevention of infectious diseases, laboratory work, health education, biostatistics, and visiting nurses.

As an international health effort, the design and implementation of the local health units involved far more national-international-local interplay than any of the parties might have expected. In part this was a question of timing: the sanitary units appeared at the confluence of several sets of interests. Perhaps more than any other area of Mexican public health, local health services constituted a revolutionary claim on the state that the new DSP was unable to meet quickly, owing to legal, financial, and infrastructural impediments. The RF expressed its support for permanent local health units in Mexico just as these obstacles were being overcome. That this ambitious initiative to design and implement a cooperative model of local health took place at a time of turmoil in Mexico, organizational changes at the RF, and difficult political relations between the two countries underscores the extent to which mutual give-and-take were required. More than in the RF's previous campaigns in Mexico, this effort was shaped by a variety of local forces and was used by Mexico to legitimize its authority domestically and to showcase its innovations to international audiences. Indeed, the local health initiative coincided with Mexico's increased participation in international health conferences and publications, giving health professionals an attractive activity to highlight.

If the political landscape of Mexico had changed since the days of the prerevolutionary dictatorship, many of the scientific and industrial goals of Porfirian liberal capitalism persisted. Elites and revolutionary politicians in the 1920s agreed that experts and scientists should guide Mexico's social and economic advancement. As open conflict subsided in much of the country, various sectors stepped up their demands for improved living and working conditions: peasants in Morelos, Veracruz, and other states mobilized around land reform and social services, and increasingly powerful labor unions fought for improved wages, working conditions, and overall welfare.[230] Public health rested at this intersection of modernization and social rights, proffering technological advancement, better living conditions, and enhanced state authority. Continuing turmoil in Mexico in the late 1920s heightened the government's need to legitimize its authority by delivering promised social services to the people, and the health units fit this bill.

The nature of the interplay between Mexico and the RF reflected the stage of the relationship as well. The yellow fever campaign served as a mutual introduction, and the mobile hookworm brigades showed each partner how the other conducted itself and what could be accomplished, but it was the founding of permanent local health units in the late 1920s that sealed the relationship. At this point the RF and DSP left politeness behind, allowing for both dynamic synergy and occasional friction.

Notwithstanding initial reluctance on the part of DSP officials, the two agencies found a way to work together, with each side proposing its own variants on the organization of local health units and each borrowing ideas and practices from the other, whether consciously or not. The IHD set a standard for full-time and exclusive employment by medical personnel and technically oriented public health services in Minatitlán-Puerto México. The Veracruz unit embedded this orientation within a broader population-based agenda for public health, which the IHD eventually recognized as feasible, effective, and attractive to the public.

Likewise, the DSP's Bustamante was applying to Mexico the knowledge and perspective that he had gained as an RF fellow, adapting this model to local circumstances, a practice the IHD had also learned over time. In the end Bustamante's much-criticized use of nonmedical personnel to extend public health coverage was imitated by the cooperative units in their ingenious use of empirical midwives. This approach, in turn, was disdained by the Mexican medical profession. Clearly this was not just a two-sided process: the gender-based maternal and child health strategies that extended the reach of the units involved a blend of feminist-maternalist, French-eugenic, U.S., colonial, and local interests and practices.

The relationship between the RF and Mexico also had its conflictive aspects. The town and semi-rural populations targeted by the units—populations that for the most part seemed to flock to the free services—occasionally erupted in opposition to particular public health measures. Likewise, the dissatisfaction of other healers was periodically visible but generally attenuated by the resilience of traditional medicine itself. Perhaps most acerbic were the struggles that took place between Carr and Bustamante, though they never reached the public eye. In this regard the RF was successful in its goal of minimizing publicity for its activities in Mexico.

Of course the RF's modesty did not extend to the DSP itself. In 1932, when the RF representative learned that DSP Director Gastón Melo was "hazy on how the RF has aided Mexico over the past 13 years," he proceeded to outline the history of RF cooperation in Mexico, including annual expenditures, salaries, and program accomplishments.[231] The DSP responded in kind: when Ferrell visited Mexico in the spring of 1933, the Mexican government treated him like a visiting dignitary.[232]

The DSP and RF's rivalry over how best to organize local health units in accordance with Mexico's needs launched an inchoate institutionalization that—after considerable negotiation and mutual borrowing—seemed amenable to all parties. As Mexico's growing demand for and capacity to deliver public health services mounted, the interplay between the entities would enter yet another phase.

Chapter Four

You Say You Want an Institution

All simple relationships are like one another, but each complicated relationship is complicated in its own way.[1] In the early 1930s, just when the DSP-IHD collaboration had settled into a comfortable pattern of give and take, Mexico began an intense period of political activism. With the waning of most regional conflict, the various parties to the Mexican Revolution vigorously reiterated their claims on the state. Peasants and industrial workers, in particular, demanded their rights, as embodied in the 1917 Constitution. Lázaro Cárdenas's election to the presidency in 1934 did not signify an end to the turbulence, instead launching an era of social rumblings, redistributive justice, and heightened nationalism—all within the context of a growing central government and continued capitalist development.

In this atmosphere, virtually every element of society—from labor to the arts, industry, and government—was undergoing a frenzy of institutionalization and bureaucratization.[2] Now that Mexico was able to channel its full energies to the building and rebuilding of the nation, the three pillars of revolutionary politics from the 1920s—education, public health, and nationalization of resources—needed to quicken their move from rhetoric to policy. In the health arena, significant expansion occurred in multiple areas, with special attention to local health services, public health research, industrial hygiene, and professional training and placement. This period of activism also framed the emergence of rural health policies that were creatively suited to Mexico's modernizing—yet still heavily agricultural—economy: growing ranks of progressive public health and medical professionals joined forces with the revived system of traditional collective farming in the provision of much-needed health care for the rural population.

How might the RF's interests fit into this agenda? At first, it was not clear if the IHD-DSP partnership would survive Mexico's political and social mobilization; the RF seemed to be pulling away despite the DSP's relentless pursuit of its cooperation. As the DSP gained momentum in implementing its own mix of social medicine and popular health, the IHD redirected its attention to the training of Mexican health professionals in both Mexico and North America.

While the IHD-DSP collaboration was facing a period of uncertainty, binational relations were on firmer ground. The United States' "Good Neighbor" policy, under President Franklin D. Roosevelt, inaugurated an era of improved U.S. behavior toward Latin America.[3] The new stance lessened Mexico's suspicion of its northern neighbor even as the oil problem festered. The "Good Neighbor" policy also meant that the RF would no longer need to play an ersatz diplomatic role. When the oil question erupted later in the decade, the RF once more found itself in a vital—if unexpected—position.

These political and social developments delineated the possibilities and the shape of IHD-DSP public health cooperation. How each party dealt with growing institutionalization and how each managed its relationship with the other demonstrate the durability and flexibility of the relationship. These interactions also show the extent to which Mexico and the RF molded one another to meet domestic and international needs.

Building a Healthy State: Cárdenas, the PNR, and the Six-Year Plan

Lázaro Cárdenas's presidency was potentially the greatest challenge to the RF since its arrival in Mexico in 1921. A mestizo and native of the state of Michoacán, Cárdenas rose from town jailer to become one of Plutarco Elias Calles's brigadier generals during the revolution, continuing his ascent to presidential advisor, governor of Michoacán from 1928 to 1932, and then head of the National Revolutionary Party (PNR).[4] As governor, Cárdenas used state-driven popular mobilization as a means to woo pro-Church constituents in the wake of the *Cristero* rebellion. He successfully organized a state confederation of workers and peasants, redistributed land, boosted educational spending, and funded technical training for rural farmers.[5] Still, as the PNR's 1934 presidential nominee, Cárdenas was Calles's man, and Calles himself showed no signs of relinquishing his stronghold over the presidency and the "maximal" influence over domestic and foreign policy he had wielded since his official presidential term ended in 1928.

But the situation was not as simple as this. Calles was under considerable pressure from agrarian and labor sectors to carry out major reforms, and he had selected Cárdenas—one of the most powerful men in the country—as a compromise candidate, whom he hoped would appease activists while maintaining the political equilibrium.[6] However, because Calles and his military and civilian cronies had created the PNR without a strong foundation of organized support, the party's left wing—which did have organizing experience at the state and local level—took charge of mobilizing the popular base in the 1934 presidential campaign. These circumstances gave Cárdenas leeway to campaign as a populist.

Cárdenas also had a new political tool at hand. In the lead-up to the campaign, Mexico's electoral cycle was modified, and a six-year, non-renewable presidential term was introduced. Accompanying this change was the institution of

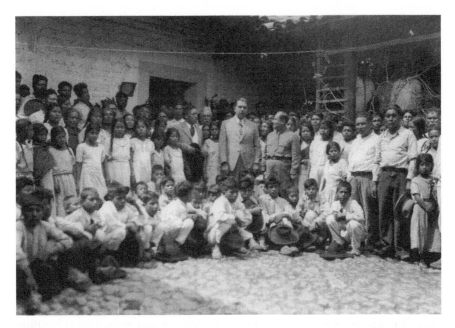

Figure 4.1. President Lázaro Cárdenas, ca. 1936. Courtesy of the Instituto Nacional de Antropología e Historia, Fototeca Nacional, Pachuca, Hidalgo, Mexico.

an officialist PNR political platform, called the Plan Sexenal—"Six-Year Plan"— a conscious echo of the Soviet "Five-Year Plans" that had begun under Joseph Stalin in 1927. Originally commissioned by Calles, the plan was radicalized by the agrarian wing of the PNR. It turned into a bold call for social and economic progress for the nation and its people, whose failure to gain the benefits pledged by the constitution was now compounded by Depression woes.[7]

The proposals outlined in the Six-Year Plan both oriented Cárdenas's campaign and informed the agenda of his presidential administration. It was Cárdenas's championing of the PNR's activist platform and, as we shall see, the support he garnered from increasingly organized sectors of workers and peasants that helped facilitate his rupture with Calles following the election. Cárdenas cut short the Maximato, but he also entrenched the *dedazo* (big finger) system, whereby each outgoing president named his party's candidate-successor, continuing—albeit in a more limited way—the connection between personal political power and state-party power that Calles had crafted.

The Six-Year Plan was the country's first systematic attempt to deliver on revolutionary promises with clear and functional objectives for national development.[8] For the rural population, the main problem identified by the plan was uneven land distribution. The corresponding goal was to provide social and economic freedom for peasants to farm their own land and enjoy the "harvest of their labor."[9] At the center of the agrarian reforms was the revival of the *ejido*—the traditional cooperative farming arrangement that was largely eroded by the end of the nineteenth century—which would be accomplished through the redistribution of large tracts of land, the improvement of agricultural methods, and the creation of public schools and medical care services on the *ejidos*.

The Six-Year Plan coupled better rural conditions with a commitment to industrialization along national needs. The government intended to renationalize subsoil rights, increase oil production, expand mining and electrical energy production, and prohibit foreign monopolies, as well as build a transportation network, essential public works, and a modern military.[10] Worker safety and welfare, wages, and the right to unionize would be protected by the government, and workers themselves would help to spur industrial development: during his campaign Cárdenas called for democratic and revolutionary action by the masses, who could "channel their enthusiasm to benefit society."[11]

Accompanying these economic and labor policies were ambitious plans for the social arena. Building upon Secretariat of Public Education founder José Vasconcelos's efforts in the 1920s, education was identified as a key element in the enhancement of social and economic conditions and in the nation-building project as a whole. Public education would be allotted a vast increase in spending, enabling the construction of 12,000 rural schools, and the training of rural teachers (who themselves would provide technical instruction in agriculture). Akin to health and medical activities, the new "socialist" education emphasized modern, science-based teaching. In promoting national identity, this approach celebrated the nation's pre-Columbian past even as it broke with indigenous and colonial Spanish legacies of superstition, ignorance, and fatalism.[12]

Public health was one of the critical building blocks of the Six-Year Plan, which declared that it was "time to pay much-needed attention to the improvement of sanitary conditions in the Republic."[13] The plan called for tripling the DSP budget, promising the additional resources to the states, given their greater needs and the fact that Mexico City had consistently received a disproportionate share of health spending. Echoing a mixture of principles advocated by Miguel Bustamante and the "Coordinated Health Services in the States" and the IHD, the plan favored decentralized services, with municipalities determining their own needs, and the states and the federal government providing moral, technical, and financial support, including loans for public works.

The plan identified the highest priorities as infant mortality and clean water and sewerage systems. Before any project was initiated, the plan cautioned, careful evaluation of economic conditions, culture, and ideals was needed. Until "current wretched conditions disappear, a restricted campaign based on medicines is worthless" for the "depressed biological condition of large groups of farmers minimizes the people's energy." The plan also promised a tropical disease research institute and national health campaigns using trained technical personnel, including a minimum of one nurse per 10,000 inhabitants. In all of these efforts, public health activities were emphasized over medical services, which was considered only "a secondary defense." In health as in other areas, the Six-Year Plan integrated technical measures with social goals.

The RF's Reaction

Cárdenas's passionate advocacy of the Six-Year Plan led the RF to pay close attention to the presidential campaign. Like other foreign interests in Mexico, RF officials studied the plan carefully, hopeful that Calles's continuing command—and several years of steady relations with the United States—would inhibit great change. Yet it remained cautious in its commitments to Mexico. Many Americans deemed Mexico "a good place to do business" through the mid 1930s, with positive relations between the countries bolstered by the "Good Neighbor" policy.[14] Still, because much of Mexico's activist ire was aimed at "imperialist gringos," U.S. political and economic radars went on alert. Given the labor militancy in the Depression-era United States, American authorities were particularly fearful of Soviet influences in Mexico. Though many of Cárdenas's supporters in intellectual and labor circles were sympathetic to Communism, the new Mexican government was no Bolshevik lackey. In 1929 the Mexican Communist Party was banned; the following year Mexico broke relations with the Soviet Union due to complaints of subversive activities, and the Cárdenas administration "refused to re-establish diplomatic relations with Moscow in the 1930s."[15] Cárdenas went so far as to give refuge to Stalin's rival Leon Trotsky in 1937. (Mexico was also a strong supporter of the Spanish Republicans, offering asylum to numerous Spanish Civil War exiles.) If the political threat to the United States was exaggerated, the Six-Year Plan did portend major economic restructuring, with potentially significant implications for foreign investors.

It was plausible that RF programs might be nested within the PNR's larger plans for a socially redistributive state, but it was not certain that the new administration would invite the RF to participate. Recognizing the importance of the Six-Year Plan to the future of public health in Mexico and to the RF's role, and just as Cárdenas's campaign was taking shape in 1934, IHD Associate Director Ferrell asked his Mexico officer to outline some ideas for a prospective program in Mexico.

By this time, IHD officer Henry Carr had been succeeded by Dr. Charles F. Bailey. A Brooklyn man, Bailey had served as a USPHS inspector at the Ellis Island Immigration Station in New York and as a quarantine officer in Canada prior to joining the RF in 1916.[16] Like other new RF officers, Bailey studied public health at Johns Hopkins University. He was then posted with RF hookworm campaigns in El Salvador and Spain and worked at the IHD's Paris office.[17] Not long after his arrival in Mexico in 1932, Bailey found that his routine administrative responsibilities overseeing local health units were taking a back seat to larger policy and political concerns.

Responding to Ferrell in a series of letters, Bailey focused on politics first, observing that "Mexico, like all Latin countries, has no united national conscience within the country. Individualism reigns supreme and politics dominates every activity."[18] Bailey worried that the likely candidate for DSP chief under a Cárdenas presidency had "radical ideas for change," which "if true would not fit in with [the RF's] policies and idea."[19] Soon after the election, Bailey voiced repeated apprehension about "this communistic movement."[20]

As for the Six-Year Plan itself, Bailey noted that infant mortality, "the causes of which are only indefinitely surmised," was not sufficiently addressed, nor was the collection of vital statistics. Bailey's main concern both before and after Cárdenas's election in July 1934 remained the viability of the IHD's local health units: 1933 was the scheduled final year of IHD participation in the Minatitlán and Puerto México units in Veracruz and their supervision was now in a holding pattern. The three other units, in Tuxtepec, Oaxaca, Tierra Blanca, Veracruz, and Cuernavaca, Morelos, had two more years of funding left. Bailey emphasized that these units operated "on a higher level than any other similar service of the Department," certain that their excellent performance would continue "just as long as the Foundation are directing their activities." "But what would happen," he wondered, "if the Foundation withdrew control of these Units?"[21]

Mexican public health officials who had worked with the IHD, particularly Bustamante, believed that the DSP could successfully run the units on its own. Bailey disagreed. Despite the RF's "relatively small" appropriation to the units, "we have practically complete autonomy in their administration and cordial cooperation with the Department." Governors and mayors changed frequently, and their payments to the units were constantly late, mostly because "The general public have little interest in civic matters."[22] Bailey—who had already employed threats and intimidation to collect the debts of the Tuxtepec unit[23]— doubted whether the DSP would be more successful than the RF in this task. In late 1934 he finally succeeded in convincing the home office to delay handing over the Veracruz units to the DSP so that much of the IHD's "considerable investment in Mexico" would not be lost.[24]

Perhaps because Bailey was so focused on day-to-day affairs, the RF was unwilling to rely exclusively on his missives to plan its next steps. RF President Max Mason was sufficiently concerned to send his own envoy, RF Vice President Selskar Gunn, to Mexico in September 1934 to evaluate the scene. After several months, Gunn reported back that "Mexico is going through a violent attack of nationalism, and it is probable that the days of foreign exploitation are ending." The PNR had "complete control of the government" and obviously intended to "eliminate the foreigner" and confiscate his property, which was "very disturbing to foreign financial interests" although "entirely reasonable to the Mexican." Gunn conceded that foreigners had occasionally "abused the Mexican hospitality," but Mexico undoubtedly "profited a great deal from this foreign contact." According to Gunn, a longtime IHD officer before becoming an RF executive, Mexico had a "rather pretentious and extensive public health program," with 3,000 employees and "magnificent buildings," modeled on a typical state health department in the United States. With the RF's continued collaboration, Gunn believed, Mexican public health had a bright future.[25] On the eve of the election, the RF's role in that future was still uncertain.

Wait and See:
The RF and the DSP in the Early Cárdenas Era

Cárdenas's campaign and election helped forge a new progressive alliance in the name of Mexico's modernization.[26] Immediately after his inauguration on December 1, 1934, Cárdenas's administration began to enact various elements of the Six-Year Plan. Within six months, his vocal support for agrarian reform and his tacit and then explicit approval of the growing number of workers' strikes led to a clash with Calles, who publicly opposed these challenges to the status quo. Cárdenas decisively neutralized Calles and his allies in the military and bureaucracy and forced Calles into exile in June 1935. Having secured the loyalty of the party, the army, and government workers—and augmented his popular support with the backing of the militant General Confederation of Mexican Workers and Peasants, and the Confederation of Mexican Peasants— Cárdenas began to promote the most far-reaching changes in Mexican society of any administration since the revolution.[27] Cárdenas was free of a powerful political bully, but he now had to contend with the challenge of aligning the often contradictory interests of workers, peasants, and the state.[28]

Having eliminated Calles's DSP chief, the Cárdenas administration created an ambitious public health, agenda under a new DSP leader, Dr. José Siurob.[29] A former general in the Revolution, member of the Constitutional Convention of 1917, and governor of various states, Siurob promised a prestigious, moral, and corruption-free administration dedicated to "convinc[ing] the masses of the necessity of health and hygiene for the preservation of life."[30] His first step was obtaining a considerable funding increase. In 1926, only 1.93 percent of the budget had gone to the DSP; beginning in 1935, the government dedicated increasing peso outlays and a larger proportion of the budget to public health, starting at 3.4 percent of the budget and reaching 5.5 percent by 1939 (see table 3.3).[31]

Under Siurob, the DSP sought to combine scientific research with social goals to shape the nation's health policies. In 1935, Bustamante formulated a set of priorities based on a nationwide survey of health conditions: (1) to promote sanitary food and water; (2) to provide clean clothes to all inhabitants; (3) to drain swamps; (4) to provide safe housing; (5) to use visiting nurses to administer smallpox vaccine and other biologics; and (6) to control syphilis.[32] Later that year, DSP chief Siurob persuaded the president to incorporate these concerns into a resolution creating sanitary services throughout the country, to address: "(1) Poor general health conditions; (2) inadequate nutrition; (3) the absence of efficient health services [particularly outside the main cities]; and (4) the public's ignorance of medicine and personal hygiene."[33]

Notwithstanding the RF's fear of the Six-Year Plan's radical rhetoric, the interests of the Cárdenas administration and the IHD coincided over Mexico's readiness to expand and solidify its public health activities. Each party recognized that Mexico had growing technical capacity and personnel, at least in the capital and leading cities, to greatly increase the purview and responsibilities of the DSP in the years ahead. Both valued the experience obtained from local health units in Veracruz, Oaxaca, and Morelos. The DSP and IHD alike understood that rural health would have to become a priority for the Cárdenas administration in order for it to meet long-standing needs and demands. In terms of the presidential resolution, the RF's interests lay principally in the area of health services, and the Cárdenas administration was intent on obtaining its support.

In February 1935, Ferrell visited Mexico to see firsthand the relationship between the Six-Year Plan's rhetoric and the reality of the early Cárdenas presidency. Praised by DSP officials for bringing the RF's "proposals of assistance in the fields of greatest human endeavor around the world,"[34] Ferrell was asked to support projects as diverse as sanitary control of the new Laredo–Mexico City highway, a circulating rural library, the founding of a Mexican public health association, and cooperation in agriculture, education, or welfare.[35] For the moment, however, the IHD was taking no action.

If the DSP was eager to retain the IHD's technical expertise, it was also under pressure to address the underlying causes of poor health. Mexican doctors working in rural areas soon chided the DSP for not making sufficient efforts to improve social conditions. The DSP, as one physician wrote, "should be the most revolutionary of all government branches . . . for those who have known the people's hunger, the hunger for liberty, the hunger for health." Calling for socialized medicine, he held that only "after doctors recognize that their knowledge belongs to the nation and not to their personal gains will the nation be able to progress politically, economically, and socially."[36]

DSP chief Siurob might have used such an opening to expand full-time salaried positions for doctors in existing sanitary units, a strategy well aligned with IHD objectives. But he had a different scale of involvement in mind. In the spring of 1935, he asked Bailey to join Bustamante in drawing up a project for extending sanitary units throughout the country, using an entire state rather than a single unit as the "demonstration." By this time, the DSP's "Coordinated Health Services" existed in fourteen states, each of which sponsored two to ten local health units or specialized clinics. In two years as director of the "Coordinated Health Services," Bustamante had engineered the integration of existing local, state, and federal services and established new services in areas where they did not exist.[37] Bailey lamented that most of these units had been created too quickly, suppressed local autonomy, operated with untrained, part-time personnel, and received low, thinly spread appropriations "instead of concentrating on a limited organization."[38]

Despite his misgivings, Bailey accepted Siurob's invitation and joined Bustamante. The pair decided on Morelos as the first demonstration state because the state's proximity to Mexico City and "fairly good means of transportation" made it "available for frequent visits and observation by Department and other Government officials." Moreover, Bailey boasted, the three years of "intensive" health work carried out by the Rural Hygiene Service in Cuernavaca under the IHD's watch had yielded "splendid results."[39] Other issues were involved in the decision as well. Morelos remained a potential setting for unrest, fueled by the 1934 election's raised expectations. Although agrarian strife surfaced only sporadically, its visibility was raising concerns for local landlords and Mexico City alike.[40] Under these circumstances, health services, whether placed in the immediate vicinity of unrest or not, served an appeasement and deterrent function.

The DSP agreed that Morelos was an excellent choice for a statewide demonstration project, but it did not stop there. The states of Tlaxcala, Hidalgo, México, and Michoacán were added to the demonstration area; the first three of these were also adjacent to Mexico City, and the last was Cárdenas's home state. Morelos itself was to have five units, one in Cuernavaca and four more in the important regional towns of Cuautla, Jonacatepec, Tetecala, and Jojutla. Representing a coordinated effort between the DSP (60 percent) and the state (40 percent), the Morelos demonstration was quickly launched under nominal supervision by Bailey's office,[41] with the four other states following apace.

Siurob soon pressed for official RF support, and Bailey in turn told Ferrell that President Cárdenas "is anxious that scientific health measures be introduced" through a cooperative project with the RF.[42] Even when Cárdenas intimated that the federal government was willing to increase its subvention to the demonstration,[43] the IHD remained reluctant to commit itself to the endeavor.

Indeed, the IHD home office appeared to have altered its modus operandi, leaving Bailey to muddle through the local scene on his own. RF officials spent much of 1935 observing Mexico from a distance, waiting to see how far the Cárdenas government would go in implementing the Six-Year Plan before deciding on any collaboration: the IHD might require flexibility in order to pull out of Mexico quickly. The tables were now turned, with the Mexican government in hot pursuit of a coy IHD.

Bailey's Crossroads

If the IHD was undecided about the future, Bailey was not. Repeating the health officer's mantra of technical and bureaucratic continuity, he beseeched his

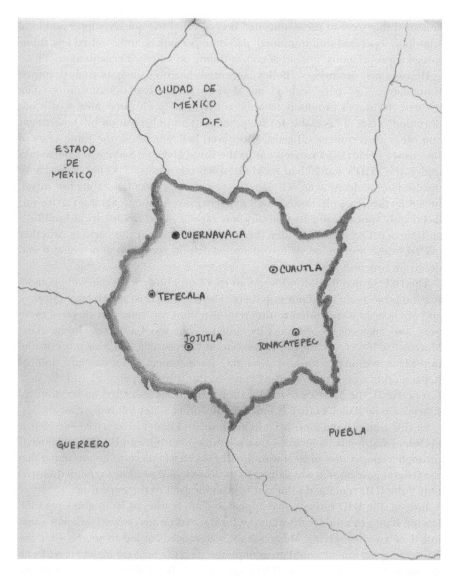

Figure 4.2. Map of Morelos Supervised District. Courtesy of Sun Wiechers de la Lama.

superiors for support. In his correspondence with the home office, Bailey expressed his displeasure with the five Morelos units in the new demonstration area, which were organized on a part-time basis with "untrained and insufficient" personnel who showed "an absolute ignorance of the principles of preventive medicine."[44] He decried these political appointees as incapable of being trained, avowing that "I would not employ a single one of the personnel of any of the five staffs."[45] At a midday visit to the Cuernavaca unit in May 1935, for example, Bailey found no one on hand to serve a room filled with prostitutes waiting for venereal treatment. His dissatisfaction was exacerbated by the new governor's refusal to make the state's stipulated contribution. Faced with the DSP's threat to rescind the Morelos agreement, Cárdenas personally appealed to the governor and the state's obligation was promptly paid.[46]

Without full IHD supervision, Bailey held, the units were not committed to fundamental RF operating principles. Not only had Bustamante's division of "Coordinated Health Services in the States" achieved "nothing" in 1935, but, Bailey feared, "three years' efforts of the Rural Hygiene Service are jeopardized." The state of affairs, he declared,

> is really pathetic and the money now being expended on these Units might better be thrown in the street, for the poor to benefit by, as compared with literally nothing new being accomplished from the point of view of health preservation or disease prevention.[47]

Bailey was convinced that the other four state health services "do not materially differ from Morelos, and how could they. They were organized in haste, with wholly untrained, underpaid, part-time personnel, merely to meet pre-election promises."[48] Bailey concluded that only the IHD's participation could rescue the situation.

Unmoved by Bailey's protestations, Ferrell urged prudence and composure. Despite the popular demand for health units, he cautioned that "We know quite well that it is futile to set up an enterprise too far in advance of public opinion and economic development. We should support only features which can be absorbed and expanded indefinitely in the near future by the governments we are trying to aid." Even in the United States, Ferrell asserted, just two states had fully developed full-time local health services, and thus, "Unless I am badly mistaken, one or two decades may be required in Mexico to reach the stage of development now to be observed in Delaware and Maryland."[49]

The IHD's shift in stance was reflected in Ferrell's diminished tolerance of the local situation. During his April 1933 visit to Mexico, he had expressed understanding of the difficulties faced by many municipalities in making regular payments to the sanitary units, comparing the Mexican situation to that experienced by numerous Mississippi counties which had had to release staff members due to budget shortfalls.[50] Two years later, Ferrell opposed funding a project "which would not stand after outside aid should be withdrawn." If one or two units could be shown to be capable of surviving without RF intervention, then the "exceptional interest in public health" displayed by the current administration would be served best by a "limited demonstration of local full-time service with trained personnel."[51]

By June 1935, desperate for home office approval, Bailey argued that Cárdenas's "sympathy with and support [for] every public health improvement" provided precisely the right "psychological moment" for the IHD to act.[52] In Veracruz, he pointed out, almost one quarter of the population was served by seven full-time health units. Four of the units "stand alone," offering "a small demonstration that the full-time principle is surviving, improving and progressing without outside aid." Bailey went so far as to praise Bustamante's organization of the "Coordinated Health Services," which, he said, met "official and public demand."

DSP chief Siurob, meanwhile, raised the stakes. Promising to quadruple the DSP's budget, he asked the RF to finance the headquarters in Cuernavaca as well as two full-time units, with state and local jurisdictions funding two part-time units. In addition, he called for the RF to subsidize a Supervised Training District in the larger Mexico City region which would oversee classroom and field activities of public health training stations.[53]

Mexico's capacity to adhere to IHD public health objectives had become secondary to larger political concerns: were conditions right for the RF to stay in Mexico?

Initial signs appeared negative. In December 1934, Ferrell had acceded to Bailey's request to postpone the transfer of the IHD's Veracruz units to the DSP, but in October 1935 Ferrell abruptly reversed the decision, after learning that the Veracruz state government was imposing a 5 percent tax on all private companies to cover public health expenditures.[54] Interpreting the tax as a challenge to the RF's cooperative principle, Ferrell ordered an immediate IHD withdrawal from the state despite his promise to Bailey that the turnover would be delayed. Hinting at the IHD's ambivalence about staying in Mexico, Ferrell remarked, "While it is complimentary to the Foundation for the government to be willing to have a member of the [IHD] staff administer important branches of the health service, it is an artificial arrangement that should not be unduly extended or prolonged."[55] As in Brazil, he argued, "In a nationalistic country we may not encounter very much opposition so long as the project is small and there is a definite, clear-cut record of transferring full responsibility to the government after a reasonable period of time." If this role were to be enlarged too much, however, "our motives will certainly be questioned and those desiring positions and unable to secure them in our Division will create opposition."[56]

In November 1935, Ferrell finally agreed to small-scale RF participation in a gradual expansion of health services in Morelos (but only in a minor supervisory role in the other four states), beginning with one or two full-time units. New units were to be added only if existing ones were operating successfully, because, as Ferrell had noted privately, "years will elapse before Mexico can finance such an intensive and extensive project. I think we had best go slow and allow time for strengthening the administrative and economic structure."[57] To Bailey, Ferrell indicated cautious optimism: "In general, I am anxious, as you know, that every phase of the enterprise [should] represent a type of thing which, if successful, can be multiplied."[58] The IHD's slow growth offer was quickly approved by the Mexican government, and Bailey assured Ferrell that the year had ended in stability: the Cárdenas transition was marked by "perfect accord, harmony, and cooperation" and a desire for continued RF participation.

As the IHD's role was being discussed, the DSP changed the name of the Rural Hygiene Service—which ran the IHD units—to the Cooperative Office of Sanitary Specialization and Rural Hygiene, reflecting both the cooperative organization and the technical nature of the initiative. In essence, this office served as the IHD's own agency within the DSP. Much as he had done since the hookworm campaign, the RF representative directed joint IHD-DSP activities while holding a DSP subdirector's title. Bailey nominated both technical and nontechnical personnel, made policy "with the advice and consent of" the DSP chief, received and disbursed funds, supervised health regulations, presented papers at conferences, and issued field reports.[59]

Though small, the Office of Sanitary Specialization's clout was considerable, most evidenced by its control of personnel decisions. A few weeks before the IHD (through this office) assumed the management of the Morelos Sanitary Services, the state health director appealed to President Cárdenas to be allowed to retain his position. Because the IHD had been promised hiring and firing privileges, however, Cárdenas denied this request and had the doctor transferred to another state.[60]

After one year of joint operation, Bailey had become satisfied with the state's administration of the revived unit in Cuernavaca, remaining adamant about the need to expand the number of units across the state to the projected total of five. A demonstration of Morelos's commitment to public health was the new State Health Department, staffed by a health officer, an epidemiologist, a sanitary engineer, and a bacteriological chemist who directed the laboratory. For the first time, the state handled all of its own bacteriological analyses and conducted epidemiological and sanitary engineering surveys. But problems with the cooperative principle persisted: in 1936 the state again suspended its payments,[61] and Siurob had to appeal to President Cárdenas once more.[62]

By this time, Cárdenas's promise to "cover [Morelos] with health activities"[63] in response to his meetings with numerous village committees had reached a new level of urgency. His administration recognized that public health measures served as a hearty appetizer to the more slow-moving main course of land redistribution. The federal government again upped its commitment so that per capita health spending in Morelos (742 pesos, or $2.80 in 2004 dollars) was almost three times the national average in 1936, with new units in Cuautla and Jojutla.[64]

Despite this increase in federal support, the health and sanitation needs of part of the state remained unmet due to shortages of personnel and poor road and rail transport, especially during the rainy season (ironically, Morelos's

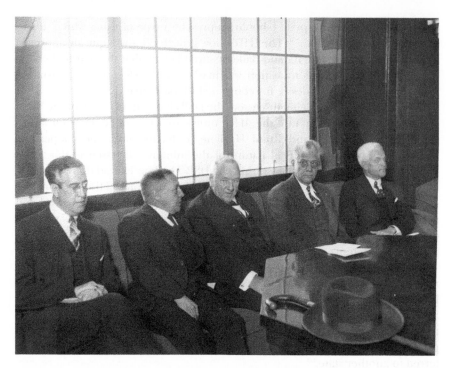

Figure 4.3. Meeting, ca. 1937, Mexico City, of DSP Director-General Dr. José Siurob; U.S. Ambassador to Mexico Hon. Josephus Daniels; RF officer Dr. Charles A. Bailey. Left to right: Lic. Octavio Reyes Espindola, DSP Chief of Protocol; Siurob; Daniels; Dr. Hernández Alvarez, director of Department of Social Assistance; and Bailey. Courtesy of the Rockefeller Archive Center.

selection had been justified by its good transport). The single contribution most villages could make to a health unit was a building, and, Bailey noted, "The economic level, in some manner, will have to be materially raised before a Municipality and the populace can, as in the United States, be expected to provide funds for preventive medicine."[65] In 1937, the state of Morelos paid only 5 percent of the total budget, and the municipalities did not contribute at all.[66] The RF had to more than double its proportion of funding, from 10 to 25 percent of the budget, to keep the demonstration afloat. With the larger federal contributions committed, Bailey remained convinced that "the country is ready for this progressive health development, the public are interested and are daily realizing the benefits and are demanding preventive measures." RF aid, he assured, "will be sufficiently repaid in permanent returns."[67]

Three years into the Cárdenas administration, Bailey praised the country's improvements in the economy, transportation, schooling for children and adults, and wages. Regretting the widespread unionization that was taking place, he remained generally optimistic about Mexico's future. He expressed confidence that IHD guidance, supervision, and incentives would continue to produce public health progress. The staff in the Morelos demonstration had expanded to ten health officers, twelve public health nurses, two dentists, twelve sanitary inspectors, one chemist, and forty-seven nontechnical personnel, including secretaries, janitors, and chauffeurs. In addition, between thirty and fifty laborers attached to two sanitary units carried out the antimalarial activities of ditching, draining, filling, and spraying.[68] Despite ongoing local funding difficulties, Bailey boasted, "The cooperation of the public has been most gratifying and their confidence has been secured in all areas, even in many districts of extreme poverty and absence of curative medicine."[69]

The RF home office's view was less rosy. Local health programs for Mexico were administered together with those for Canada and the United States, and in comparative terms, Mexico was a disappointment. Demonstration units operated for one year in the United States and Canada, while in Mexico a minimum of two years was considered necessary for the establishment of a permanent unit. Moreover, in Mexico, demonstration areas did not serve as stimuli for the development of health units in adjoining regions. As IHD administrators explained to the RF Board in 1937, little progress had been made "owing to backwardness and economic limitations in Mexico."[70] The home office complained that Cárdenas expected IHD participation at every step and had "frequently and urgently requested an extension of the full-time local health activities to reach the entire population."[71]

Another sign of the RF's mixed feelings about early Cardenismo was its unwillingness to consider new cooperative opportunities. During Ferrell's 1933 visit to Mexico, he had requested meetings with the secretaries of agriculture and education to discuss collaborative efforts with the IHD. Much to Ferrell's chagrin, the Mexican government considered these areas too sensitive for foreign participation.[72] Three years later, the new Mexican administration reversed this position, inviting RF support in both education and agriculture. Notwithstanding this keen interest—which was further augmented by the strong encouragement of U.S. Ambassador to Mexico Josephus Daniels—the foundation refused the opportunity in 1936.[73]

The Cárdenas Administration on Cárdenas Public Health

If the IHD seemed to be in a holding pattern, the DSP was moving ahead with great institutionalizing strides. Midway through his presidential term, Cárdenas showcased his administration's public health achievements at home and abroad.[74] In spite of Bailey's doubts about Mexico's ability to bring medical and public health services to the people without the RF's direct supervision, under Cárdenas the DSP became more active across the nation than it had ever been.

In two years, spending on the "Coordinated Health Services in the States" had risen by over 50 percent, totaling one third of the DSP budget. The DSP was actively enforcing the nation's 1934 sanitary code, putting into practice numerous constitutional provisions and passing new public health laws.

In the summer of 1937, a vast exhibit in Mexico City's Palace of Fine Arts (Palacio de Bellas Artes) displayed the federal government's public health accomplishments during the first half of the Six-Year Plan:[75]

(1) nutritional improvements through research, regulation, popular education, and milk pasteurization;

(2) large-scale sanitary construction, including the installation of water supply and sewage systems in 141 towns; thousands of latrines for rural villagers and septic tanks for town dwellers; 7,484 "hygienic houses" for industrial and agricultural laborers; the inspection of 129,671 buildings; the sanitary evaluation of 200 towns;

(3) infant hygiene developments, including the founding of the Department of Infant Welfare in 1937; the organization of 40 maternal and child health centers now attended by 234,000 children; study of the principal causes of infant mortality and morbidity; and cooperation with milk producers to improve the quality and distribution of milk;[76]

(4) the administration of 6.9 million smallpox vaccinations and 379,000 typhoid immunizations, and the distribution of millions more vaccine and serum units to combat pertussis, diphtheria, and tetanus;

(5) a 20 percent increase in the budget of the malaria campaign, and an increase in control measures against tuberculosis, venereal diseases, alcoholism, and other diseases;

(6) coverage of 23 of Mexico's (then) 30 states and territories by "Coordinated Health Services in the States" (by 1936).[77]

Thousands of visitors to the Palace of Fine Arts filed by the DSP's flurry of posters, brochures, and other educational materials placed alongside a grandiose display of the new technical equipment used by sanitary officers. As notable as their self-assessed epidemiological success was the national scope of these initiatives. More than 1,500 visiting nurses had been placed, with hundreds more added each year in order to fulfill the Six-Year Plan's goal of one nurse per 10,000 inhabitants.[78] The DSP had expanded into the area of occupational health, with a 1935 law resulting in the inspection of 3,200 factories and over 20,000 workers.[79]

Most far-reaching was the health education arena. In 1936, over 51 million popular health education pamphlets and books were published, up from 7 million in 1934. Hundreds of health messages had been recorded in Spanish and Maya and were heard on portable phonographs throughout the country, each shared by several villages.[80] Health education often took place in the absence of

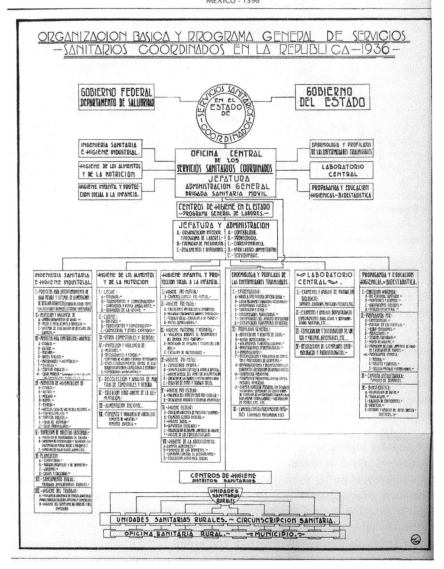

Figure 4.4. DSP organizational chart, 1936. From José Siurob, *Modern Tendencies of Public Health in the Republic of Mexico* (México, D.F.: DSP, 1936). Courtesy of the Secretaría de Salud, Mexico City, Mexico.

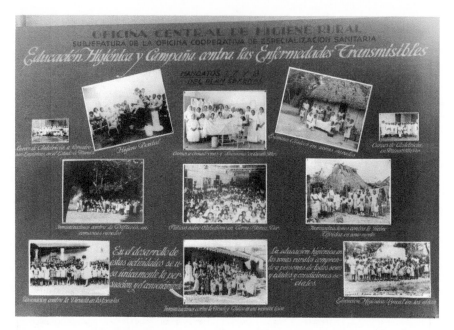

Figure 4.5. 1937 DSP exhibit in the Palacio de Bellas Artes—Communicable Diseases Display. Courtesy of the Rockefeller Archive Center.

public health infrastructure. Materials published through the Cárdenas administration's Autonomous Department of Press and Publicity (founded in 1936), such as the domestic medicine manual *¡Hermana Campesina!* (*Sister Peasant!*), assumed that its readers had little or no access to health services. The widely diffused manual celebrated women's self-sufficiency and pride, imparted basic knowledge of hygiene, child-rearing, nutrition, and first aid, and sought to dispel popular superstitions. While it emphasized schooling as a right, *¡Hermana Campesina!* called on women peasants to demand medical services from agricultural employers rather than the state.[81] This manual and other popular health education efforts suggest that the DSP's official public health modernization agenda was paired with subsidiary strategies to address the continuing obstacles to rural health coverage.[82]

The DSP's main story was of growth and progress. All told, the DSP congratulated itself for lowering infant mortality from 134 deaths/1000 live births in 1934 to 107/1000 in 1936 with the crude mortality rate dropping from 23 deaths/1000 population to 22.2/1000 over the same period according to an estimate by a Mexican RF fellow.[83] Among the "truly few" objectives that still needed to be reached to fulfill the Six-Year Plan, announced DSP chief Siurob, was the definitive fight against transmissible diseases, a goal "not even reached by the most advanced countries."[84]

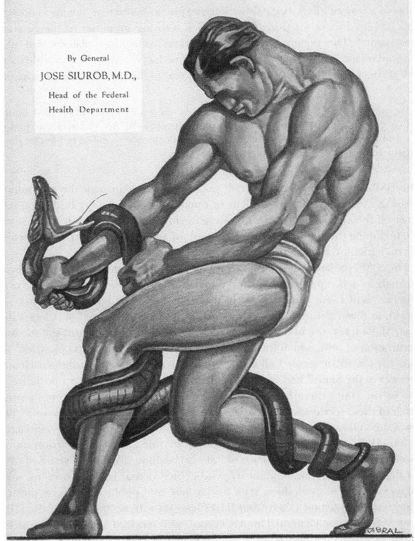

Figure 4.6. DSP pamphlet cover. From José Siurob, *Modern Tendencies of Public Health in the Republic of Mexico* (México, D.F.: DSP, 1936). Courtesy of the Secretaría de Salud, Mexico City, Mexico.

The popularity of the DSP's programs was reflected in the thousands of letters Cárdenas received from Mexican citizens, many of whom pressed him personally for the creation of health services. An entire Campeche town lamented that the newly trained local nurses were without instruments and medicines,[85] and the residents of a Sonora village begged Cárdenas to give a license to a "botanical doctor" who had lived there for thirty years and was a strong supporter of the agrarian movement.[86] The members of a gum workers' union complained that they received no medical attention, so Cárdenas immediately arranged to provide them with services.[87] Even towns with physicians turned to the President for assistance:

> We are suffering a lot from malaria and tuberculosis and the doctor paid by the Government will not see us because he is very bourgeois. We need a humanitarian doctor who behaves differently, we beg you to send a doctor who is willing to fight for these poor and forgotten agrarian communities.[88]

The DSP could further demonstrate popular support through the 2.1 million pesos ($7.62 million in 2004 dollars or one seventh of the 1937 budget) it had received through donations from state governments, oil companies, and workers, including the spontaneous contribution of 400,000 pesos by peasants working on agricultural collectives.[89]

The DSP parlayed domestic advances into international health publicity through its active participation in public health conferences in Europe, North America, and Latin America. As the DSP chief proudly recounted in a 1937 report, at these venues Mexican scientists shared their research on Chagas disease, Malta fever, the use of plant extracts to combat measles, and the vacuum sterilization of milk, which was "so important for Latin American countries."[90]

As for the RF, it seemed all but invisible. In 1936, the "Coordinated Health Services in the States" had been given heightened organizational importance as one of the DSP's three branches, and the DSP boasted of the comprehensive reach of these services to "people of all sexes, ages, and social conditions."[91] But it was the well-functioning IHD-sponsored cooperative sanitary units—packaged by the DSP—that symbolized the capacity of the Cárdenas administration's socially oriented state. The Palace of Fine Arts exhibit displayed a series of photos depicting these units' infant hygiene clinics, dental hygiene sessions, midwifery workshops, vaccination stations, latrines, and public lectures on malaria and hookworm—most taken from IHD files—yet with no mention of the IHD. Even U.S. Surgeon-General Thomas Parran, who received a report on Mexico's public health accomplishments, seemed unaware of the RF's role in developing the cooperative unit model. He was "favorably impressed" with Mexico's progress in rural hygiene and the "almost unique system of coordinating National, State and local health activities."[92]

Nonetheless, the RF did not go unappreciated. It was precisely at this time—September 1937—that the DSP organized an official ceremony to recognize

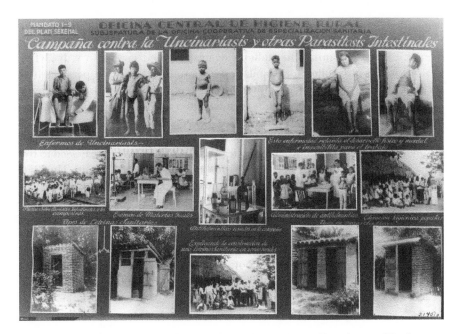

Figure 4.7. 1937 DSP exhibit in the Palacio de Bellas Artes—Hookworm Campaign Display. Courtesy of the Rockefeller Archive Center.

John D. Rockefeller's contributions to Mexico.[93] If the DSP seemed to be publicly downplaying the RF's part in institution-building, its role in promoting scientific public health was not lost on DSP personnel.

The 1937 exhibit indicated the double thrust of the Cárdenas era. The DSP remained conscious of its constituency, pledging attentiveness to the "immense proletarian and agrarian collectivity, the cradle of progress and the future." The DSP's activities also reflected its new technical orientation, based on a "vast, rational scientific and rigorous" reorganization.[94] This reorganization gave top spending priority to the Institute of Hygiene, the proposed Institute of Health and Tropical Diseases, malaria, tuberculosis, and syphilis campaigns, and the construction of rural hospitals, all of which employed largely technical approaches to public health. The more socially oriented projects—water and sewage systems, federalization of sanitation services, training visiting nurses, and increasing the minimum wage—were now nearer the bottom of the list of DSP priorities.[95]

On domestic turf, the DSP's new ranking did not go unanswered. In August 1937, the first Congress of Health Workers held in Mexico City concluded that more money needed to be spent on public health, particularly in the areas of prevention, health education, construction of rural hygiene centers, and training of personnel. Congress participants, including six former RF fellows, demanded "immediate attention to a clean water supply" as the best public health investment: over ten years it was cheaper to set up a water supply system than it was to "immunize the millions against typhoid every two years." The health workers also called for popular education efforts to teach peasants how to build latrines, septic tanks, drainage systems, and insect-free "hygienic houses."[96] In a sense, health workers seemed better able than the DSP to balance local needs and foreign approaches.

In sum, the early years of the Cárdenas administration were marked by institutional growth and commitment; public health resources were harnessed to the demands of state-building, social activism, and rural development. The RF's proven track record, its administrative capacity, experience, and interest in provincial Mexico—as well as its much hoped-for resources—were incorporated into the institution-building project, though not advertised publicly. A limited RF collaboration in Mexican public health remained useful and pursued by the DSP and President Cárdenas himself, even as the RF's interest in Mexico seemed to be waning. But a change was afoot: the RF's direct involvement in public health delivery had become subsidiary to another focus of its international health work.

The Training Touch

Whether or not the DSP or Bailey accepted it, the RF's support for local health had stagnated in the early Cárdenas period. By no means, however, had its interest in Mexico diminished. Instead, the IHD had subtly changed its emphasis from big-ticket public health projects—disease campaigns and sanitary units— to less conspicuous yet no less important backing for professional training.

The RF's activities in Mexico had included graduate fellowships in public health beginning with the yellow fever campaign. In the 1920s and early 1930s the IHD hand-picked one or two physician fellows each year to pursue advanced training in the United States. Upon their return to Mexico, the fellows were expected to commit themselves to government service, either with IHD units or in the DSP's expanding bureaucracy.

In the mid 1930s, this small educational program was turned into a major initiative. First, starting in 1932, the IHD and DSP jointly developed a set of regional training stations, typically run by returned RF fellows. Each year, scores of the nation's frontline public health workers—doctors, nurses, engineers, technicians—now underwent rigorous, advanced training in public health. The stations received added attention and resources during the Cárdenas administration.

Second, beginning in 1935, there was a marked increase in the number of Mexican RF fellows sponsored each year, and sanitary engineers and public health nurses began to be awarded fellowships alongside doctors. Third, the IHD renewed its invitation to high-level Mexican health officials to go on short-term tours of local, state, and national public health agencies and facilities in North America. The IHD hoped that having these officials witness successful public health organization firsthand would accelerate Mexico's adaptation of U.S. public health strategies. The IHD also believed the tours would induce the DSP to provide sufficient support for cooperative projects and to facilitate the work of the returned fellows. Together, these efforts constituted a multi-pronged educational strategy that complemented cooperative programs in the field and sought to bypass often thorny political considerations by appealing directly to public health personnel.

The RF Fellows

The RF's involvement in graduate public health education originated in its hookworm campaign experience in the South of the U.S. from 1910 to 1914, which revealed a dearth of trained public health personnel. Soon thereafter, it founded the United States' first schools of public health at Johns Hopkins (opened in 1918) and Harvard (1922) universities. (See chapter 1). As the RF extended its international health activities, these, and a few other schools hosted RF-funded public health fellows from around the world, many of whom came from Latin America.

The IHB's founding director, Wickliffe Rose, stressed that professional education was an essential component of public health advancement internationally. He believed that a select group of public health specialists would diffuse their acquired knowledge into their respective societies through research, administration, and teaching. Not only would this approach save money, enabling the RF to implement programs in more places, but international fellows would be in a better position than RF representatives to disseminate theory, practice, and values to researchers, government agencies, professional communities, and the public in a culturally relevant manner.[97] Having established formative ties to top universities in the United States, the returned fellows would continue their engagement with North American institutions and ideas over the course of their careers. "Incidental" advantages included the development of relationships with current and future leaders from other countries and international scientific exchange.

Rose's commitment to education was rooted in the Progressive Era's confidence in the ability of science to systematically solve society's problems: nations that failed to employ science were bound to fall behind, while those that promoted science were transforming education and "remaking . . . civilization."[98] According to Robert Kohler, this view was typical of the era's foundation officers, who believed that scientists could marshal "rational social change."[99] Because Rose held that RF public health activities should apply existing knowledge rather than engage in new research, early generations of fellows were trained primarily as public health practitioners and teachers, equipped with the knowledge and administrative skills needed by RF programs in the field. Even after the IHD's new emphasis on the "advancement of knowledge" in the late 1920s, most Latin American fellows received practice-oriented master's in public health degrees rather than research doctorates.[100]

Encouragement for the RF's international fellows program came from various quarters in the United States. In 1918, the research arm of the Council of National Defense expressed interest in helping the RF coordinate both student and faculty exchanges.[101] The same year, L. S. Rowe, assistant secretary of the Treasury and formerly an emissary to South America, recommended that the RF establish a Latin American fellows program because "there is nothing [else] that we can do at this time which will contribute so largely to the fostering of a closer understanding between the United States and the peoples of Central and South America."[102] A few years later, a U.S. general who had retired in Mexico echoed this view: fellows "think differently from their compatriots," and become "ambassadors for the U.S.," interested in peace and commerce with their "neighbor to the north."[103]

Of the 451 public health fellowships awarded to Latin America and the Caribbean between 1917 and 1949 (of a total of 2500 U.S. and international health fellows), Mexico received 68, trailing only Brazil (which received 89, but had twice the population of Mexico in the 1920s and 1930s).[104] Over three decades, the RF sponsored 32 physicians trained in public health administration, 9 physicians trained in public health laboratory methods, 6 public health nurses, 20 sanitary engineers, and 1 statistician from Mexico.[105] With the exception of the nurses, who studied at the University of Toronto and the New York City Health Department, almost all of the Mexican fellows attended either Harvard or Johns Hopkins on one- to two-year fellowships (see appendix).[106]

International fellowship applicants were typically recommended by ministries of health, approved or rejected by the IHD's country representative, and formally selected by the RF in New York. Each grant was to be made "because the individual represents the project which the I.H.D. is interested in developing."[107] The IHD officer generally knew how many grants would be available each year, and he decided on the ministry's candidates accordingly. In some settings IHD officers were concerned that few candidates were of sufficient caliber to qualify, so RF policy advised field officers to "adjust" their standards.[108] Fellowships did not always go to the best students, but often "to those needed in certain posts."[109]

Other than an instance in 1926 when a DSP official declined the RF fellowships as an infringement of national honor (see chapter 2), fellowships and the returned fellows were highly popular with the Mexican government. The DSP typically responded to the IHD's offer of free training by nominating dozens of candidates each year,[110] but the home office repeatedly emphasized that the number of fellowships awarded to any one country was limited. Ferrell reminded RF representatives to Mexico "to carefully study the organization needs of the health department and be sure that the fellowships are restricted to outstanding young men who, without doubt, will continuously hold important positions in the public health service."[111]

The most successful candidates were those who were young (and therefore not entrenched in the DSP bureaucracy) and who had already had field experience with RF programs.[112] By focusing on the elite of Mexican medical graduates, however, the RF supported primarily urban, upper-class fellows, some of whom did not wish to carry out rural campaign work. When RF representative Carr requested a fellowship for a man slated to return to Mexico as a hookworm officer in 1927, IHD director Russell sought assurances that the person would be "accustomed to rough life in tierra caliente [hot regions] and not averse to field work."[113]

Occasionally, Mexican officials came up with training plans that interfered with Rockefeller policy. In 1930, for example, returned RF fellow Dr. Alfonso Castrejón, director of the DSP's Institute of Hygiene, intended to send four fellows to Boston and Paris to learn techniques for preparing anti-typhoid vaccine, diphtheria antitoxin, and other biologicals. Carr grumbled that the four were not physicians, and "I don't see why Doctor Castrejón himself, who has had a magnificent training of more than three years in the States and abroad, can not train his own technicians to make the routine biological preparations."[114]

The fellowship period provided a combination of academic and cultural experiences. Fellows were faced with a challenging course load, and "competition with American students keeps the fellows on their toes."[115] As a U.S. newspaper reported in 1943, Latin American RF fellows constituted twenty-one out of twenty-eight international students at the Johns Hopkins School of Hygiene and Public Health, effectively forming a "Pan-American Council." The fellows interviewed expressed the belief that increased knowledge would improve relations between Latin America and the United States and that more North Americans needed to study in countries to the south. Mexican fellow J. J. Osorio suggested that Mexicans and Americans ought "to know more about each other." Others noted that the "ideal South American visitors . . . were the physicians sent south by the Rockefeller Foundation 'who settle down, study the country, learn the language—and don't write books.'"[116]

RF fellowships affected both careers and social circles. Miguel Bustamante, a 1926–28 RF fellow to Johns Hopkins (as the first Mexican to receive a doctorate in public health) kept the school closely apprised of his activities,[117] noting to a Johns Hopkins dean that in Mexico, former fellows found "a good part of our cultural activities and life tied to the School."[118]

Official expectations for RF fellows naturally focused on the practical. Even before Bustamante returned from his fellowship in Baltimore, the DSP secretary-general expressed "certainty" that he would make a "magnificent collaborator" in Mexican public health.[119] Despite keen interest from home turf, the RF sought to prevent interference with the fellows during their time abroad. When Carr

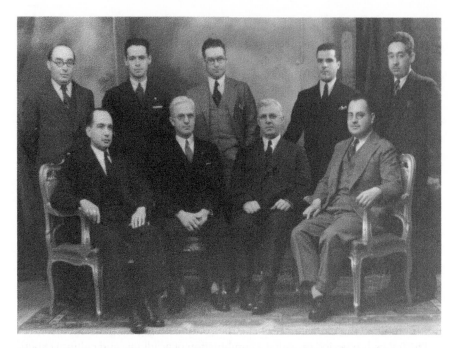

Figure 4.8. Returned RF fellows from Mexico, 1935. Standing, left to right: J. Segura, Esteban Hoyo, Dr. Pilar Hernández Lira, Dr. Ricardo Granillo, unknown. Sitting, left to right: Dr. Salvador Bermúdez, Dr. Charles Bailey, Dr. John Ferrell, and Dr. Miguel Bustamante. Courtesy of the Rockefeller Archive Center. See appendix for further details.

and the secretary-general of the DSP requested news on the Mexican fellows in 1926, Russell refused to provide it, citing violation of RF policy.[120] The RF had learned "from sad experience" that when governments maintained close contact with their fellows, they attempted to modify each fellow's curriculum as officials devised new ideas for health organization. Thus, "while a man is studying epidemiology and statistics, he might as well be getting himself trained as a pathologist, sanitary engineer, toxicologist or what have you."[121] The fellows perforce served as important information conduits, whether collecting pamphlets on maternal and child health[122] or acquiring specific expertise needed in their home countries. While the Mexican government wished to maximize the knowledge acquired by each fellow, the RF preferred to train specialized public health officers. In order to avoid "annoying" interference, the RF requested the likely return posting of each fellow before their departure to North America. Mexican fellows also favored this arrangement because it gave them independence abroad and a guaranteed position upon their return.[123]

For the individual selected, an RF fellowship was a virtual guarantee of a distinguished career; through the fellows, the RF made a lasting contribution to Mexican public health.[124] Fellow Luis Vargas, a prominent entomologist who worked with the IHD's malaria projects, believed that the RF fellowships opened Mexico to the entire field of public health; before the RF, he said, doctors were interested only in their patients and, occasionally, in hospitals.[125]

Fellows were deeply affected by their experiences in the United States, not only because of the knowledge and laboratory skills they gained, but also because they were instantly transformed into public health leaders when they returned to Mexico. Although an old guard of European and nationally trained doctors still held the DSP's directorship and remained for some time the country's most renowned researchers, the new crop of health professionals educated by the RF played a pivotal part in shaping the DSP at a critical time, building new research institutions, training the nation's health workers, and setting patterns of public health practice.[126]

Since they often headed new departments and divisions, the fellows were in a position to determine institutional orientations and priorities, reflecting—or selectively emulating[127]—some of the structures, ideas, and practices they had become familiar with in the United States.[128] In this sense the fellows, like RF officers, were transnational professionals, moving ideas and practices back and forth across borders. Dr. Alberto P. León, for example, was an assistant at Mexico's Institute of Hygiene before he received his doctorate from Harvard in 1936. He then spent a year researching typhus control methods under the eminent Harvard bacteriologist Hans Zinsser. He returned to Mexico to found and direct the DSP's Office of Epidemiology and went on to serve as secretary-general of the DSP, establish an institute for the BCG tuberculosis vaccine, and author more than ninety scientific articles.[129] León represented his country at dozens of international conferences, including the World Health Conference in 1946 and as chief of the Mexican delegation to the first World Health Assembly in 1948. For many years he was professor and department chair at Mexico's School of Public Health and the UNAM's Faculty of Medicine, and he continued in his research post at the Institute of Health and Tropical Diseases into the 1990s.[130] The direct and indirect influence of the fellows lasted for many decades; local health units, DSP divisions, and other offices were headed by returned fellows and staffed by health personnel trained under them, who in turn molded subsequent generations.

Through the fellowship program, the RF forged a heightened role for U.S. ideas and models in the development of Mexico's public health knowledge, ideologies, and practice. French textbooks continued to be used in Mexican medical schools in the 1920s and 1930s (as late as 1935, Mexican physicians deemed France the ideal locale for advanced medical training),[131] but public health was another matter. A 1936 DSP handbook for rural hygiene organization, for example, recommended that health officers stock their libraries with sixteen general public health texts, ten of which were published in the United States (beginning with Milton Rosenau's classic, *Preventive Medicine and Hygiene*), two published in France, two in the Soviet Union, and one each in Britain and Spain. The handbook's recommended journals and specialized list of holdings in epidemiology, statistics, and sanitary engineering likewise emphasized U.S. publications.[132] By 1941, Dr. Angel de la Garza Brito, the director of Mexico's School of Public Health, called for all incoming students to demonstrate English-language reading ability so they could benefit from the "excellent" American and British public health literature that had not been translated into Spanish.[133] RF fellows, for their part, formed part of the first sizeable generation of Mexican scientists to publish their own work in international journals. Starting in the 1930s they increasingly contributed to U.S. publications.[134]

The fact that most were trained in the U.S., and thanks to the RF, did not mean that the fellows simply transplanted, root to leaf, the public health curriculum and applications they had studied. Bustamante, as we have seen, selected the elements of the IHD local health model that he deemed appropriate to Mexico. As head of the Veracruz unit, for example, not only did he define public health's purview to include living and social conditions, he also refused to adhere to the IHD's hookworm preference, relegating hookworm control to a marginal role. Likewise, Alberto León modeled the DSP's new Department of Epidemiology after U.S. agencies to include divisions of research, prevention, and education, while tying epidemiological efforts directly to the social goals of the Six-Year Plan.[135]

Given the mutual importance of fellowships, both the RF and the Mexican government closely tracked the fortunes of the fellows and the fortune being spent to train them. Between 1920 and 1934, fifteen Mexican fellows were trained at a cost of $34,578.[136] By 1937, thirty-two fellowships had been furnished at a cost of over $90,000 dollars ($1.17 million in 2004 dollars).[137] This jump in the number of fellows was no clerical error: from 1920 until 1934, one or two fellows were selected each year (except in 1926, when four fellows were sponsored); in 1935 the IHD supported six fellowships and sustained four to six fellows per year through the late 1940s with increased support for engineers and nurses(see table 4.1).

Why did this change in emphasis from projects to fellows occur? Several factors were at play, all related to the Cárdenas administration. On one level, the RF was nervous about the political direction Mexico might take. Funding fellows was less risky than funding programs that might be discontinued. Even if a fellow was removed from a particular position, he would retain his expertise and might serve his country in a different venue. On another level, Mexico was already committed to local sanitary units; the extent to which the cooperative model was struggling had more to do with the politics of local and national revenues than with any technical problem the IHD might be in a position to address. On a third level, Mexico's public health expansion was so rapid and extensive that training specialists had become a more efficient way for the RF to stay involved than its

Table 4.1. Cumulative number of IHD (RF) fellows from Mexico, 1920–49

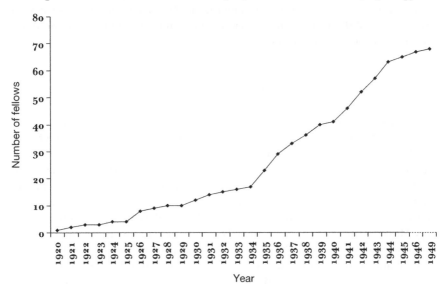

sponsorship of a small number of focused activities. Stepped up demand for trained public health professionals also stimulated the RF's participation. Advanced professional training was a propitious means of international health interchange for both sides, one which allowed a role for the donor and left ample room for local developments with selective appropriation of outside ideas.

The IHD's switch in gears seems to have yielded the desired results. As early as November 1935, Ferrell noted that "a number of changes have taken place in Mexico"[138] that would make both the president and the DSP chief "agreeable to employment of professionally trained personnel, that is, returned fellows, in all of the key positions." When Siurob reorganized the DSP that year, four hundred employees were discharged, including numerous high-ranking officials, but Bailey was relieved to report that "As yet none of the former Foundation fellows have been removed," thanks, he claimed, to his own diplomacy.[139] On the whole, Bailey sensed, the "Government realizes the benefit of trained personnel and incidentally their obligation to the Foundation."[140]

By the end of the Cárdenas administration in 1940, the RF hailed the success of the Mexican fellowship program. The IHD representative proudly reported that of thirty-nine Mexican fellows thus far, thirty-six were serving in the government. Most occupied influential positions, including secretary-general of the DSP, director of Epidemiology, chief of Biostatistics, director of the Institute of Hygiene, and director of the Cuernavaca training station.[141] The home office was elated: "If infiltration of the governmental health structure of Mexico with trained personnel continues . . . the outlook is with real optimism."[142] As evaluated in terms of prestigious job placement, the RF's perception of its successful "infiltration" of the DSP was perhaps warranted. In terms of influence, however, the story was more complicated.

Seeing is Believing

In addition to sponsoring fellowships for advanced public health study, the RF began to fund short tours for senior DSP officials to travel to the United States and Canada to observe state and local health departments, research institutes, schools of public health, and national health agencies. The IHD held that high-level officials needed to visit successful North American installations—including IHD-founded schools of public health—in order to be convinced of the cooperative model of public health work.[143] DSP chief Bernardo Gastélum was the only Mexican official to receive an IHD travel grant in the 1920s. In 1936 the program was reborn and through the mid 1940s, two or three officials per year—many of them returned fellows—were invited on public health tours.

A typical destination for Mexican visitors was Charles Chapin's famed Providence, Rhode Island Health Department. A fervent advocate of bacteriology, Chapin claimed that sanitary efforts were obsolete and that public health depended mostly on personal hygiene. He strongly favored the development of local health departments with responsibilities for disease surveillance, communicable disease control (involving vaccination, isolation, and laboratory verification), and hygiene education rather than broad social measures. Throughout his five-decade career, he maintained a position he had espoused in 1902: that it would "make no demonstrable difference in a city's mortality whether its streets are clean or not, whether the garbage is removed promptly or allowed to accumulate, or whether it has a plumbing law."[144]

The tours usually entailed extensive travel. In 1936, for example, a prominent group of officials headed by DSP chief Siurob began their journey in Washington, D.C., where they met with officials of the American Public Health Association, the USPHS, and President Roosevelt. The visitors—who included Bustamante and returned fellow Gerardo Varela—then spent a day and a half in Baltimore, visiting the campus of Johns Hopkins University and meeting with professors. They went on to visit the University of Toronto's Schools of Medicine, Nursing, and Hygiene as well as the Toronto Health Department, city laboratories, milk pasteurization facilities, and an incineration plant. After sightseeing at Niagara Falls, the group returned via New York City to meet with RF officials, the American Hospital Supplies Co. (to obtain prices), the New York Hospital, Cornell Medical School, the East Harlem Nursing and Health Service, and the New York City Department of Health. The voyage ended with stops at health departments in North Carolina and Tennessee.[145]

The Mexican press covered the trip favorably, citing dozens of "very valuable results" obtained by the health officials.[146] The officials were particularly lauded for representing Mexico's interests in spite of the limits imposed on them as observers. Upon their return, the Mexican team proposed a wide array of projects: to prepare nurses at a special training facility and equip them for home visits; to regulate the selection of health personnel and the location of health services; to train mothers to bathe, weigh, exercise, and otherwise care for their children and report to health workers; to increase collaboration between the university and the DSP for the training of health personnel; and to hold periodic conferences and an annual convention for health officers and other personnel. Above all, the team promised in an internal report to the IHD, to "Endeavor to pattern, develop, and organize Health Services as now existing in the United States."[147]

Of course, Siurob and his colleagues were telling the IHD precisely what it wanted to hear. The visitors no doubt garnered new ideas, but much of what was proposed following the trip was already well under way in Mexico. Still, this was a fine opportunity for Siurob to lobby both for greater IHD support and for an increase in government spending on health. Over the next few years a virtual "who's who" of Mexican public health went on similar trips.

Overall, between 1925 and 1950 thirty-six Mexican health officials, including each incoming director of health, received RF travel grants to visit North American public health offices and research centers.[148] RF fellows wielded the enthusiasm, institutional positions, and skills to shape Mexico's public health activities. Courting the support of DSP and government leaders—who saw for themselves the fruits of successful public health work in North America—was an effective way to keep these issues on the national political agenda.

Training Stations

The DSP had been concerned with training mid-level public health personnel since its founding in 1917. Soon after the cooperative sanitary units were established in Mexico, RF representative Carr similarly discerned a need for professional training. The RF was not inclined to grant fellowships to a large number of health workers to study in the United States, so another solution was needed. Although the DSP had intermittently operated its own educational facility starting in the early 1920s, Carr complained that "the training is entirely class room, didactic teaching and there is no opportunity to give the practical field training which is so important."[149] Equally important, large classes made it impossible to judge the ability of a student "before he is later intrusted [sic] with a position." Instead, Carr suggested that returned RF fellows, together with occasional lecturers from the United States, train the next generation of public health practitioners and administrators in Mexico.

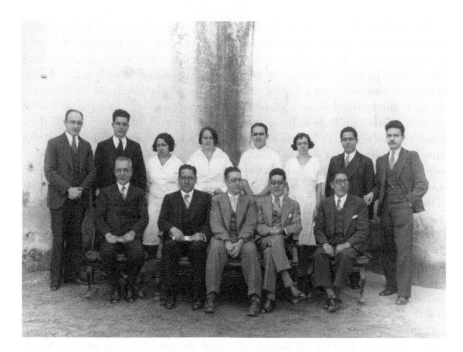

Figure 4.9. Participants in the first Cuernavaca training station course, 1932. Standing, left to right: Roberto Sánchez, Samuel Oropeza, Alicia Sosa, Julia Valladares, Dr. Félix Léceygui, Rebeca Durán, Miguel Angel Cinta, and Jesús Granados. Sitting, left to right: Dr. Agustín Hernández Mejía, Dr. Ramón Ojeda Falcón, Dr. Pilar Hernández Lira, Dr. Enrique Esparza, and Dr. Julio Viniegra. Courtesy of the Rockefeller Archive Center.

Carr called for a field training station "outside, but near" Mexico City, where the staff of an operating local health unit could teach students in the classroom and provide them with practical field training. In November 1932, the Cuernavaca health unit became the site of the first training station, fashioned after the IHD's Indianola, Mississippi station. The Cuernavaca station was headed by the health unit's physician-director and supported by the unit's sanitary engineer, nurse, sanitary inspector, and statistical clerk. The teaching staff (who themselves underwent training) provided courses in transmissible diseases, epidemiology, maternal and child health, vital statistics, school hygiene, sanitation, and health administration, with similar curricular content to North American stations. Like the sanitary unit itself, the training station was partially funded by the RF and assigned to the subdirector of the DSP's Rural Hygiene Service, IHD representative Bailey.[150]

Though meticulously planned and ably directed by RF fellow Pilar Hernández Lira, fresh from his studies at Johns Hopkins, the Cuernavaca station failed to attract sizable numbers of public health trainees, largely because of insufficient student funding. Ferrell was "favorably impressed" with the training station, which was 50 percent funded by the IHD in its first year. Yet the IHD was slow to fulfill requests to furnish stipends for students who had to pay for travel and several months of living expenses out of their own pockets.[151] Ferrell hoped that the very existence of the training station would serve as an incentive to the Mexican government to increase its financial commitment, but the station failed to thrive. Bailey claimed to "have done everything humanly possible to create interest in our training Station at Cuernavaca and to show the [training] needs of the country," but, he argued, the secretary-general was not "convinced of the need of trained personnel for Health Services."[152]

In 1934, the DSP decided to transfer the Cuernavaca training station to Xochimilco, a "crowded and insalubrious" district known for its canals and swamps, located just outside Mexico City. DSP officials believed that a location closer to the capital would draw more students and more government funding; the RF agreed to support the training station and an accompanying health unit for a five-year period. Bailey found Xochimilco to be "practically virgin soil for public health," offering opportunities for work in water supply, infant mortality, and the study of malaria, but he remained frustrated about the move.[153]

According to Bailey, the Xochimilco station's opening in January 1935 was delayed by the appointment of an unpopular communist mayor, which led to several days of mob violence.[154] The public refused to cooperate with a baseline sanitary survey, and the unit's sanitary inspectors were personally threatened. Bailey worried that health personnel were "considered part of this radical machine. The public was most suspicious of our aims, and it took weeks of cautious diplomacy to gain their confidence and cooperation."[155]

By the end of the year, however, both the local government and the training station had become "most popular." The Xochimilco station had spread "educational propaganda" around the region and had protected "practically the entire population" against smallpox, typhoid, and diphtheria.[156] This was not an easy task: the Xochimilco station covered 34,179 persons in fifteen towns, and was among the poorest districts in the nation, entirely lacking in preventive medicine services. Bailey complained that almost all of the inhabitants drank *pulque* to excess and "live in one room adobe houses or shacks with dirt floors and without beds."[157] Many lived with farm animals, and almost no one had sanitary facilities. Bailey described Xochimilco as an exceedingly unsanitary version of Venice.

Hernández Lira directed the new training station in its first year,[158] and was replaced by Bustamante in 1936. For several years Bustamante worked hard to organize training courses and outreach activities that integrated laboratory and socio-political approaches to public health. With the local population serving as

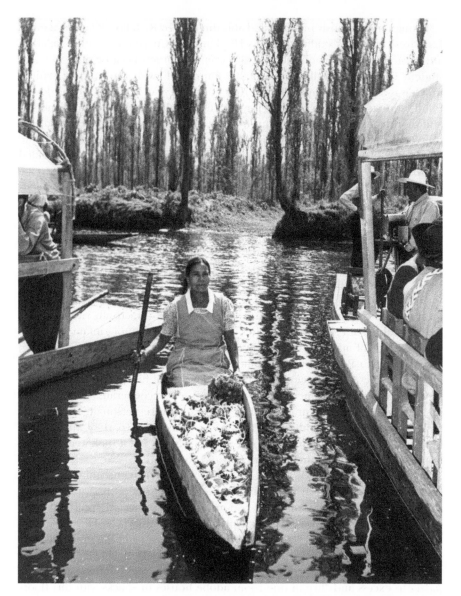

Figure 4.10. Flower-selling on Xochimilco canals. Courtesy of the Rockefeller Archive Center.

a social laboratory, physicians, nurses, and sanitary engineers spent eight weeks in the classroom, laboratory, clinic, and community. Together they studied and then implemented measures in areas of transmissible disease control, maternal and child health, social hygiene, sanitary engineering, nutrition, and health

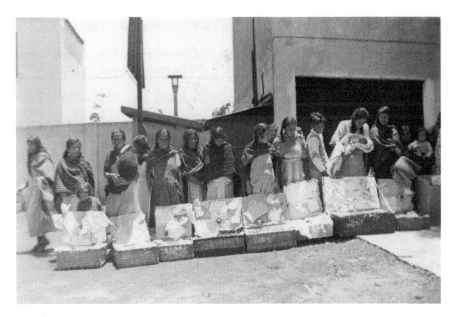

Figure 4.11. Distribution of bassinets and layettes to mothers who had attended pre-natal clinics at the Xochimilco unit, 1937. Courtesy of the Rockefeller Archive Center.

education. Trainees also learned and applied laboratory methods, assessed social conditions, and organized the collection of vital statistics. Graduates were expected to direct new sanitary units as comprehensive as the Veracruz unit that Bustamante had founded a decade earlier.

Bustamante had a second agenda as well: convincing the medical profession of the value of the training stations. In the *Gaceta Médica de México,* he argued that the training endeavor was highly beneficial to medical personnel and to the community, with both gaining from new access to clinical diagnosis, biological products, laboratory services, statistical studies of the community's disease conditions, and preventive measures.[159] Bustamante described Xochimilco's social conditions as "unfortunately fortuitous," for the "reigning ignorance, poverty, and alcoholism," made the public health training work very interesting. But, he assured his medical audience in terms that would appeal to them, "the biological and medical sciences together transcend social concerns in the age-old battle against disease and infirmity."[160]

By 1937—when Bustamante left to work at the new Department of Infant Welfare—the Xochimilco station was on solid footing. According to Bailey, the DSP—with the backing of the medical profession—had become "thoroughly aroused as to the need for trained personnel." The DSP generated an "explosive" demand for training and constantly requested new training stations and sanitary

Table 4.2. Graduates of training stations at Cuernavaca (C) and Xochimilco (X), 1932–37

	C 1932–34	X 1935	X 1936	X & C 1937	Total
Health officers (physicians)	17	40	30	71	158
Public health nurses	15	57	72	11	155
Sanitary inspectors	23	9	48	38	118
Laboratory technicians	1				1
Medical students				5	5
Total	56	106	150	125	437

Sources: Annual Reports for Xochimilco Health Unit, 1935–37, and for Cuernavaca Health Unit, 1932–34, 1937, RG 5, Series 3, Box 145, RFA.

units, especially after Siurob's trip to the United States in 1936 (see table 4.2).[161] Though the IHD was pleased at the "complete confidence and cooperation of officials and the public," it was unhappy about the effects of classroom crowding on the quality of teaching. The IHD preferred to limit admission to a few well-qualified students to keep class sizes small, while the spirit of the Cárdenas era favored expanded access to education.[162] Crowding was exacerbated by short-term attendance by medical students, military officers, and agriculture and education workers, in addition to a small number of RF fellows from other Latin American countries. To meet the long waiting list, the training period was cut from eight to five weeks; and, Bailey believed, many trainees were sent into the field with insufficient preparation.[163] Over the short term, little could be done, however, because limited RF funding (never exceeding one or two thousand dollars per year in the mid and late 1930s) placed the stations "in the hands of the Department."[164] In 1937, the backlog of students necessitated both the reopening of the Cuernavaca station and the separation of training courses into specialized sections for doctors, nurses, and sanitary inspectors.[165]

The education of nurses was of special concern to both the RF and the Cárdenas administration, and, by extension, to the training stations.[166] Not long after the founding of the Xochimilco station, Bailey complained that "not one capable nurse is available."[167] He attempted to convince the National University to raise the educational standards and salaries for nurses and create a new school of nursing because "The need for trained nurses is equal to, if not greater than for health officers." A special class was quickly organized in Xochimilco to train instructors for rural nurses. Although seven nurses qualified as instructors and the others became visiting health nurses themselves, Bailey argued that their poor training disqualified them from service entirely. Nonetheless, by the following year, the nurses proved to be highly competent instructors.

Bailey's concerns were corroborated by one of the RF's nursing experts, Mary Tennant, who in 1936 made a survey of Mexico's nursing schools. She found the level of instruction at the three schools in Mexico City to be extremely low, with virtually no preclinical training, few enrollment requirements, and little awareness of the modern nursing curriculum. The schools operated on a hospital apprenticeship model, overseen by doctors unprepared to teach the principles and practice of nursing. Tennant found only the Red Cross Hospital School to be of acceptable quality, with students who were "young women of intelligence, refinement, education, and [who] have a real interest in learning."[168] The other schools and the training station were "of inferior quality." The nurses, she lamented, "are not superior, in appearance, in dress, in intelligence, in attitude toward work or in comprehension of it. . . . The background of these nurses is so limited in education and nursing and social standards,"[169] that they required months of very basic training. Tennant also observed home visits and concluded that successful health education required nurses "from a higher social and economic level."[170]

On the heels of her visit, the RF sent five middle-class nurses on fellowships to Toronto. At the University of Toronto School of Nursing, the Mexican nurses, most of whom had trained at Mexico City's Red Cross Hospital, were highly regarded. In addition to their classroom training, they spent time working with the city of Toronto's Department of Public Health and interned with the Victorian Order of Nurses. Several of the nurses—Carmen Gómez Siegler and Bertha Heuer-Ritter—then spent a year training at the New York City Public Health Department, before returning to careers as public health nurses for the Mexico City Health Department. Unlike in Venezuela and Brazil, the RF decided against supporting a nursing school in Mexico.[171] If the training stations could do little to change the class background of nurses or improve basic nursing education, they were able to set an impressive track record in attracting nurses to public health: by the 1940s, nurses usually comprised the largest group of students (see table 4.3).

After five years of Xochimilco's operation, the IHD and Mexican officials alike were extremely pleased with the training effort.[172] Bailey applauded its accomplishments, hailing the "spirit of the staff" and "good will" of the public.[173] The IHD was ready to withdraw its support from both stations but continued to play a minor role so that it could "lend a stabilizing influence."[174] In 1941, the Xochimilco training station was moved to the Tacuba district of Mexico City, where the country's new Institute of Health and Tropical Diseases was located. Modeled on Johns Hopkins University's Eastern Health District in Baltimore,[175] Tacuba offered training, research, and practical settings for work in infectious and chronic diseases, nutrition, mental hygiene, and other areas.[176] Funded by the Mexican government, the Tacuba station received a three-year grant from the RF to carry out a survey of local nutritional patterns.[177] In the mid 1940s—even as the IHD was pulling out of Mexico—it became involved in four other training stations, financing equipment and salaries high enough to attract "first-rate" instructors.

IHD personnel judged the influence of the training programs to be "very considerable."[178] As of 1940, 587 health officers had been instructed at field training

Table 4.3. Graduates of combined training stations at Coatepec, Cuernavaca, Monterrey, Celaya, Guadalajara, and Tacuba, 1944–48

	1944	1945	1946	1947	1948	Total
Doctors	37	55	43	61	28	224
Nurses	86	11	88	160	62	407
Sanitary inspectors	77	99	79	56	62	373
Total	200	165	210	277	152	1,004

Source: Downs to Smith, February 7, 1949, RG 1.1, Series 323, Box 20, Folder 167, RFA.

stations in Mexico, including 290 health officers, 165 public health nurses, 127 sanitary inspectors, and 5 medical students.[179] By 1950, the majority of Mexico's 2,000 state and local health employees had attended one of the training stations and thousands more were trained there over the next decades. The DSP's support for and expansion of the stations indicates similar satisfaction with the endeavor.

The Mexican School of Public Health

The RF's extensive involvement in the training of Mexican public health workers both in local stations and in North American universities would seem to suggest that Mexico did not have its own school of public health. In fact, even without RF support Mexico already had one. In 1922, DSP Secretary-General Alfonso Pruneda, moved by the war-ravaged country's overall public health situation, the importance of health education, and the urgent need for trained public health personnel (including personnel for the yellow fever campaign), had started a School of Public Health directly out of the DSP.[180] Pruneda's broad vision initially mustered few resources, and in the first few years only a handful of courses were taught for existing DSP personnel.[181]

The RF's indirect role in the school grew after 1925 when the first large cohort of Mexican fellows was sent to the United States. Upon their return to Mexico, the four fellows became responsible for training "medical sanitarians."[182] Through courses in epidemiology, health administration, health legislation, demography and vital statistics, sanitary engineering, and microbiology, these instructors attempted to recreate the learning atmosphere of the North American schools where they had studied. Thereafter, each generation of RF fellows shared the latest educational innovations from Baltimore and Boston in courses organized for DSP staff members. Because Mexico's School of Public Health was a DSP dependency, it was subject to political maneuverings, often suffering due to changes in administration.[183]

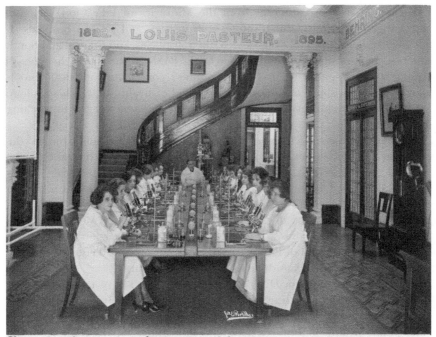

Bacteriologic Course in charge of Prof. Dr. Tomas G. Perrin, that is given in his own Laboratories. 756500

Figure 4.12. Nurses using microscopes in DSP bacteriology course. Courtesy of the Rockefeller Archive Center.

By the mid 1930s, the school faced the additional problem of competition from the Rockefeller-run training stations. As a result, aside from a few short courses in practical nursing, pharmacology, industrial hygiene, and health policy, the school was left to run correspondence courses in malariology for district health officers and in basic anatomy, physiology, and hygiene for rural schoolteachers.[184] Angel de la Garza Brito, who headed the school in the 1930s and 1940s, blamed the Cuernavaca and Xochimilco training stations for failing to work with the school.[185] Students and applicants complained that the school provided no scholarships and was too centralized and elitist, requiring long periods away from jobs.[186]

The situation improved after 1940, when government stipends began to be offered and a full-time research faculty was hired.[187] Around this time the School of Public Health and the training stations began to coordinate their efforts, with School of Public Health students required to spend several months at a practical training station, a cooperative sanitary unit, and regional health administration offices.[188] On firmer ground, the School of Public Health finally began to grow, graduating fifteen students in 1944 and over sixty per year by 1950. In the 1940s, it opened its doors to students from the Ministries of Education, Defense, and Indigenous Affairs, the Institute of Nutrition, and various hospitals. It attracted students from all over Mexico, the Caribbean, and Central and South America, many of whom were sponsored by the PASB. By the 1960s, the school's stability and independence from the country's conservative medical schools allowed the flourishing of a more social model of health, in which sociology, anthropology, psychology, history, and economics became integral to teaching and research.

Elizabeth Fee has suggested that Wickliffe Rose's desire for public health education in the United States to include both national research institutes and regional training centers was implemented on an international scale, rather than in the United States.[189] Mexico, starting in the 1940s, when its School of Public Health began to thrive and collaborate with the new Institute of Health and Tropical Diseases, was an example of this conception. Top Mexican officials envisioned training stations as the site of preliminary instruction for all health workers, with the School of Public Health providing advanced education to the "more promising individuals discovered in this program."[190]

Mexico's School of Public Health was also the beneficiary of a wartime expansion in RF fellowships. During World War II, the suspension of grant-giving in Europe opened up extra fellowships for Latin Americans. In 1939, 151 medicine, public health, natural sciences, and humanities fellows came from the United States, 141 from Europe, and 47 from Latin America. In 1943, 44 were from the United States, 4 from Europe, and 104 from Latin America, half of whom were public health fellows.[191] The increased demand for professional training stimulated the school's expansion in the mid 1940s. Following the war, European reconstruction became an urgent priority, leaving Latin American grants to plunge. Robert Lambert, associate director of the Division of Medical Sciences, explained to a concerned Mexican official that the postwar period in Europe merited "special attention. We cannot overlook the fact that during the war when practically no European could come to the U.S. for training, young men from Mexico and other countries to the south of us enjoyed an unprecedented opportunity."[192] With the reduction in RF fellowships after World War II, the Mexican government further increased the number of national fellowships it funded in public health, and starting in 1945, the School of Public Health modeled its application materials on RF fellowships, adding prestige and support to the "study at home" option.[193]

It is important to reiterate that—notwithstanding the medicalized model of public health it was promoting—the RF invested little in Mexican medical education. If public health was a field where the RF might be influential, for decades medicine was viewed as an area far too entrenched for targeted assistance to make a mark. RF medical officers Alan Gregg and Robert Lambert conducted periodic—largely denunciatory—surveys of Mexican medical education on their evaluation trips around Latin America in the 1920s and 1930s,[194] but assistance to Mexican medical schools in this period was limited to the purchase of a few laboratory instruments and a handful of graduate fellowships.[195] In part obstructed by the authority of the highly revered old guard of medical faculty, and in part resigned to Mexico's adherence to French and other European medical traditions, the RF was reluctant to commit itself to the medical arena in Mexico until the late 1940s and 1950s, when it began to furnish equipment and fellowship grants to the National University's medical school, to three regional medical schools, to the National Children's Hospital, and to the National Institute of Cardiology.[196]

In sum, central to the long-term strategies of the RF in Mexico (and elsewhere) was the creation of a breed of public health professionals who could act as scientific, administrative, and cultural translators for the IHD while it operated in situ and could substitute for it when it was gone.[197] Serving as an educational centrifugal force, the RF's extensive fellowship and training programs were vital to institutionalizing in-country cooperative efforts: only by preparing informed leaders, specialized administrators, and technically capable frontline workers could the IHD have a lasting effect on the theory and practice of public health in the many countries in which it operated.

But this was not a one-sided affair. Mexico took great advantage of the fellowship and training opportunities and called upon returned fellows to fill national needs. Though RF training stressed the biological basis of public health and disease control rather than their social dimensions, many fellows melded the technical aspects of their training with the country's social and political goals, particularly in the 1930s. Perhaps the best example of the combined forces of autochthonous developments and creative appropriation was the Cárdenas administration's new approach to rural health.

Institutionalization, Mexican Style

Health and the Ejidos

Many Cárdenas-era public health activities represented an acceleration of developments from before the revolution and tended to work in tandem with the IHD's programs and goals in Mexico. One area differed from this general pattern: the founding of rural medical services on the growing number of agricultural cooperatives or *ejidos*. Resurrection of the *ejidos*, rooted in traditional land-holding patterns of shared property that could not be sold, was the cornerstone of Cardenista politics in rural Mexico.[198] The 1917 Constitution had authorized the return of land tenure to peasant collectives, but this process was extremely slow until Cárdenas came to power: his administration redistributed over three times more land (30 million hectares) than all of his predecessors combined—doubling the beneficiaries to 1.6 million peasants—and organized extensive rural development schemes.[199]

The ground-breaking ejidal health units—which integrated medical and social services—were the brainchild of a small group of physicians based at the Universidad Michoacana de San Nicolás de Hidalgo in Cárdenas's home state of Michoacán. The *nicolaítas*—who held a range of humanist and socialist views— had discussed politics and medicine with Cárdenas when he was state governor in the early 1930s and continued to advise him and influence his health policies when he became president.[200] Most notably, Dr. Jesús Díaz Barriga guided the initiative as secretary-general of the DSP, and his disciple, Dr. Enrique Arreguín Vélez, was rector of the Universidad Michoacana where the ejidal health services were conceived.

The first ejidal clinic was founded in Zacapu, Michoacán in 1932 as a *nicolaíta* experiment to accompany agrarian reform. The unit was based on the belief that medical services were critical to and inseparable from social advancement: physicians were integral to preventive and curative services—replacing *curanderos*—and to social development. In serving this role, physicians became salaried employees of the *ejido* rather than working in private practice on a fee-for-service basis. The success of the Zacapu unit induced Bustamante to organize a similar service in Anahuac, Nuevo León in 1934, this time with federal support.[201]

These services were physically located where peasants lived, unlike the RF and DSP sanitary units, which were generally established in leading regional towns.[202] Just as important, the ejidal units were partially financed by the peasants themselves through annual contributions tagged to their earnings. In the mid 1930s, peasants typically contributed 12 pesos ($45 in 2004 dollars) per year per corn-growing family and 24 pesos per cotton, wheat, and cane-harvesting family. On one *ejido*, a health unit was founded by peasants on their own initiative, without the involvement of sanitary authorities. The community arranged to pay dues in crops instead of cash.[203] In the most densely populated areas, *ejido* dwellers contributed over 50 percent of the costs of the health services in their locale, supported by communal credit societies.

Following Mexico's first Rural Hygiene Congress held in Michoacán in 1935, the system of ejidal sanitary units was made a permanent part of the DSP, initially administered by the DSP's Office of Coordinated Health Services in the States. DSP chief Siurob personally claimed credit for the idea of "social medicine" units, established because the DSP's sanitary services were ineffectual in many rural areas.[204] At the congress, the new units were deemed "truly rural"[205] as opposed to those sponsored by the RF and the DSP through the Coordinated Health Services. The success of the ejidal units led to the creation in 1937 of a separate "Office of Social Medicine and Rural Hygiene," which borrowed the "Rural Hygiene" designation from the service that oversaw the IHD's sanitary units.

The two original units multiplied to 36 by 1936, 104 (serving 900,000 workers and their families) by 1938, and 121 by 1940 (see table 3.5).[206] Demand for the ejidal units seemed limitless. In the 1936 fiscal year, most of the DSP's 2.46

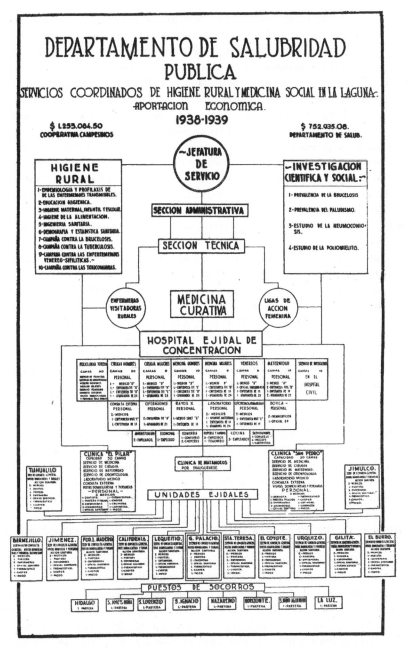

Figure 4.13. Chart of ejidal unit organization in La Laguna region, 1938–39. From José Siurob, *Social Medicine in Mexico* (México, D.F.: DSP, 1940). Courtesy of the Secretaría de Salud, Mexico City, Mexico.

million peso budget increase ($9.3 million in 2004 dollars) went to the ejidal units, which now consumed 15 percent of DSP spending.[207]

This attention was part of the Cárdenas administration's strategy of focusing on regions with the greatest social and economic needs.[208] In the mid 1930s, Mexico's federal government spent almost half of its budget on agrarian improvements including the distribution of land to *ejidos*, the development of a rural banking system, and investments in rural education, irrigation, and road construction. These efforts stemmed from the conviction that the betterment of peasant life was not separate from, but crucial to, Mexico's modernizing project.[209] Advancement required healthy and productive workers who accepted the legitimacy of the government and scientific authority. Rural medical services not only brought health care and education to the *ejidos*, they also "promote[d] progress in regions where a coordinated effort would translate into real improvement in the economic status of the peasants."[210]

Ejidal unit sites were selected on the basis of (1) the absence of medical or public health services; (2) the prohibitive cost of existing services; and (3) the location of large centers of indigenous population in need of adequate medical and sanitary services.[211] In poorer, more sparsely settled areas, the government fully funded ejidal clinics. The DSP sought to identify the special health needs of rural communities rather than merely duplicate methods and activities employed in urban areas. As part of this effort, it made use of laws and ideas from other social movements aimed at raising the lot of peasants: on many *ejidos*, social work, environmental hygiene, community organizing, and housing improvement became as valued as the treatment and prevention activities of the medical units.

What began as a modest attempt to adapt modern medicine to rural communities not served by physicians evolved into a network of integrated medical services, as engaged in social, economic, and cultural development as in health services delivery. Medical care was viewed as only the beginning of a multifaceted plan to better the lives of rural Mexicans, not as an end in itself.

While both the ejidal and IHD-sponsored sanitary units emphasized the primacy of trained health professionals, the two initiatives differed on a number of counts. The ejidal units were housed on communal lands serving populations most in need of health services, while the sanitary units were located in towns of regional and political importance where units were likely to garner public recognition and support. The ejidal units delivered a range of medical and social services, including housing assistance, construction of clean water systems, and social development activities; their sanitary unit counterparts typically limited their services to vaccination, maternal and child health care, and hookworm control. Moreover, the ejidal services were community-financed and community-controlled, unlike the sanitary units, which were government-run and funded by a combination of federal, state, and local contributions with little or no community participation.

The IHD's reaction to the ejidal medical services was decidedly muted given their importance to the Cárdenas administration and the putative competition they posed to the IHD's sanitary unit model. One explanation for the IHD's silence is that there were internal divisions in the RF over public versus private provision of medical services:[212] discussion of the ejidal model risked provoking these arguments. More likely, the IHD did not consider the ejidal units to be of particular relevance—or a threat—to the IHD sanitary units. Indeed, there is no evidence that any IHD officers ever visited an ejidal unit. In his only direct remark on the subject, RF officer Bailey called the ejidal medical units a "sound" combination of curative and preventive services, yet he held that the locations were invariably "unwisely chosen and do not actually reach those for whom they presumably were created."[213] Thus, he felt, a large quantity of low quality services was being organized, and he was skeptical of the ejidal units as "an ideal impossible to attain," because the DSP had failed to meet the basic need for trained personnel and adequate remuneration.

The ejidal project was ambitious, and the units turned to teachers in areas where trained health workers were unavailable—a large proportion of the country in the 1930s. Though this approach was a temporary stop-gap, it was the component of the DSP's rural health outreach that seemed most troubling to the RF officers. Not only did the RF disdain the use of personnel unversed in the biology of disease and its treatment, but the involvement of rural schoolteachers inspired fears about rural radicalism. Selskar Gunn, the RF's envoy to Mexico charged with assessing early Cardenista politics, had been awed at the commitment of peasants to building and maintaining "their little schools."[214] As he noted, teacher-activists served a special role in bringing the benefits of the Mexican Revolution to the rural population by increasing literacy, organizing communities, promoting cultural development, and assisting in the transformation of new communal lands for grazing and farming.[215] Beginning in the 1920s, teachers had been given rudimentary instruction in health education and were enlisted to obtain fecal cultures from students and to promote the use of outhouses.[216] Under Bustamante's guidance, teachers spearheaded demands for improving the water supply.

Yet in reality, teacher responsibility for health was carefully limited to a few activities, and most teachers remained dependent upon the closest ejidal or sanitary unit. Because the IHD supported the goal of raising public health awareness, its principal argument against the ejidal units—buried in an administrative report—was that their involvement of teachers showed that they were molded by politics more than science, providing "very questionable results and benefit to the country."[217]

If the RF was quietly critical of the ejidal units, considering them inferior to the sanitary units, the Cárdenas administration viewed the two types of units as complementary. The praise showered on the RF at the first Rural Hygiene Congress in 1935 reinforced the notion of the cohabitation of "scientific" and "social" public health. At the same time, the publication in English and distribution to the United States and elsewhere of several pamphlets describing the organization and accomplishments of the ejidal units indicates the importance the DSP attached to obtaining international recognition of this Mexican innovation.[218]

Physician Social Service

Over the long term, an even more far-reaching endeavor of the DSP under Cárdenas was its plan to redress the medical personnel shortage in rural areas through a new social service requirement for graduating medical professionals. This initiative claimed multiple fathers. Formally proposed at the first Rural Hygiene Congress, the idea also had Michoacán roots, with *nicolaítas* Díaz Barriga and Arreguín Vélez having discussed the question extensively.[219] In 1936, Cárdenas himself called for the training and placement of licensed physicians in every community as an essential investment in the nation's progress.[220] Dr. Gustavo Baz, dean of the National University's Faculty of Medicine, has also been assigned authorship of the plan,[221] and even the IHD's Bailey seems to have (wrongly) taken credit for it.[222]

At the Rural Hygiene Congress, it was RF fellow Dr. Pilar Hernández Lira who proposed a law requiring all physicians, nurses, midwives, chemists, and dentists to serve two years in a rural location before graduating. No longer would these health workers be "oblivious to the needless sacrificing of the real life and wealth of the Nation—the peasant."[223] The new rural health workers would be trained in epidemiology, maternal and infant hygiene, bacteriology, nutrition, statistics, personal hygiene, sanitary legislation, and the basics of sanitary engineering and would require "self denial, firmness of character, loyalty and benevolence for the fulfillment of their sanitary activities, which will encourage and create confidence and sympathy in the communities for which work is done." Congress participants recognized that "the great demand for properly trained personnel," had resulted from "the improvement in the installation of Municipal Sanitary Services," especially those supervised by the RF.

The proposal for rural social service was adopted first by medical schools (followed by nursing in the 1940s and other professions subsequently). In 1935, the National Autonomous University of Mexico and the University of Michoacán began requiring prospective medical graduates to train in public health and to spend six months as government-salaried doctors in rural communities, often on *ejidos*. These sixth-year medical students assumed the functions of local sanitary officers—administering immunizations and medical care free of charge, carrying out regional social and sanitary surveys, and submitting weekly reports—all the while competing against traditional healers. Faculty of Medicine Dean Baz told the entering cohort:

I have come to ask you to join patriotically one of the most singular experiments in the history of medicine. Each of you will work in a place where there is no doctor. . . . Your responsibility will be to introduce the rudimentary elements of public health, teach concepts of hygiene, and collect information about the mode of life in each locale . . . [including] its history, population characteristics, climate, alimentary patterns, economic means of survival, sanitary conditions, and the causes and levels of morbidity.[224]

Widespread satisfaction with the first 134 medical students in rural service resulted in a tripling of participants by 1936[225] and a permanent requirement in 1940. At one and the same time, the program resolved the scarcity of rural physicians; expanded the practical training of physicians; alerted medical students to the nation's medical and public health needs; encouraged doctors to practice outside the major cities; improved relations between physicians and local sanitary authorities; increased the DSP's knowledge of local health conditions (often through the theses written by medical students on social service placements);[226] and created closer ties between the universities and the people.[227] To this day, physician social service (lasting between six months and a year) remains one of the most successful legacies of the 1930s, enabling the staffing of rural health posts throughout the country.

As with the case of the ejidal units, the IHD had almost nothing to say about the social service requirement. During a 1947 visit to Mexico, IHD director George Strode noted admiringly that many physicians returned to practice in rural areas following medical school.[228] However, this comment was part of a diary entry, not for official consumption, and apart from the early remark by Bailey, who had attended the Rural Hygiene Congress, the IHD does not seem to have discussed the rural medical requirement in reports or correspondence.

Perhaps the IHD considered rural medical internships, like the ejidal units, to be medical as opposed to public health endeavors and thus beyond its purview. Maybe rural service was ignored or privately disdained because in some manner it defied the IHD's cooperative health model due to its social orientation and financing scheme, which bypassed local government authorities. Alternatively, given the involvement of RF fellows in the design of rural medical service, the IHD—as their sometime patron—may have disapproved of these efforts but felt that criticizing them was inappropriate. Possibly the IHD was divided over whether this medicalization of the countryside was a success or a failure. In the end, both the ejidal medical units and physician social service drew creatively from some RF public health precepts and diverged from others. Ironically, these efforts both involved RF fellows and disregarded some of the RF's most basic public health principles regarding cooperative financing and trained medical professionals.

If RF public health met an unexpected competitor in these rural health programs, the next challenge was from a completely different domain.

The Oil Nationalization:
Between Rockefeller and a Hard Place?

Since its arrival in Mexico in the early 1920s, the RF had carefully sidestepped the controversy over oil. Local critics of the RF raised the issue of its connections to Rockefeller-owned Standard Oil, accusing the RF of serving oil company interests, but these instances were rare.[229] Officially, Rockefeller public health and Rockefeller business interests in Mexico operated as and were considered separate entities. This was even the case when it came to the regulation of health conditions on oil company property, although DSP Chief Gastélum saw fit to notify the RF in 1925 when he discovered the appalling sanitary conditions tolerated by several oil companies.[230] For the most part, the DSP pursued these matters quietly. During the yellow fever campaign, the DSP's Antilarval Service sought to take over responsibility for mosquito control in oil worker camps, but they were not always welcomed by oil companies.[231] Inspections and sanitary efforts were stepped up in the mid 1920s, meeting with limited success, in part because there were no repercussions for oil companies that refused entry to Antilarval Service personnel.[232]

Following Cárdenas's election, the stakes with regard to the foreign ownership of Mexican oil reserves rose. The country had become more politicized, workers more organized, the effects of the Depression deeper, and expectations for improved living and working conditions higher. Cárdenas himself had had intimate experience with the oil issue as military commander of the Veracruz oil region during the mid 1920s: in the tense period before the Morrow-Calles agreement was reached in 1927, President Calles had ordered Cárdenas "to prepare to set the oil fields on fire in the event of a U.S. invasion."[233]

Amidst the mobilizations of the mid 1930s, the DSP sought to enforce various legal provisions that taxed property owners for sanitary services and street paving and required large companies to fund health services for their workers and nearby residents.[234] Despite their assurances, only a handful of oil companies instituted sanitary or antilarval measures.[235] British-Dutch-owned El Aguila, the largest oil company in Mexico, promised to work with the health units in Veracruz, but unit personnel were repeatedly refused entry to the company's walled compound.[236] After considerable aggravation, El Aguila finally agreed to pay for unit personnel to ditch and drain company property—leading to a drop in malaria incidence for 1935.[237] In 1937, El Aguila built three cooperative sanitary units near its refineries in the state of Veracruz.[238] Modeled on the DSP-RF units, these units offered preventive and treatment services, antilarval measures, dental services, and decent salaries to employees. Prospective sanitary personnel were quickly sent to Xochimilco and Cuernavaca for training.[239] By this time, the limited efforts of a single company were not enough to placate the oil workers or the Mexican government.[240]

Of course, battles over health conditions on oil company property were only part of the story. According to the Six-Year Plan, returning ownership of subsoil rights to Mexico was connected to the nation's commitment to industrial growth and social progress. Together with the president's support for unions in other industries, he backed the demands made by the Mexican Union of Oil Workers in the mid 1930s for higher wages and benefits. When the oil companies offered only 14 million pesos ($52.7 million in 2004 dollars) of the 65 million peso raise demanded by the oil workers, the workers went on strike in May 1937. Several months later, a Mexican government inquiry concluded that the companies could afford to pay workers an extra 26 million pesos per year, an amount the oil companies claimed would exceed their annual profits. The matter then went to the courts, and on March 1, 1938, the Mexican Supreme Court agreed that the companies could afford the 26 million peso raise and gave them one week to comply with the decision. After initially failing to respond, on March 16 the companies agreed to disburse the full amount, but in exchange they demanded restrictions on future union activity.

Cárdenas cited the companies' "contemptuous" behavior in choosing this as the right moment to fulfill the constitutional goal of nationalizing the oil industry: on March 18, 1938, to the surprise of Mexicans and foreigners alike, the president seized all foreign oil holdings in Mexico.[241]

Public support for the nationalization extended through most segments of Mexican society, including physicians. Within two days of the action, letters began to flood into Cárdenas's office, with letter writers volunteering financial and moral resources to help the government pay compensation to the companies. Hundreds of doctors, many working with the RF, sent telegrams to Cárdenas expressing their "faith and absolute support . . . for this act of ultimate patriotism." One doctor offered 50 percent of his salary; others begged to know how they could help increase petroleum production. Health personnel at a rural health post in the state of Aguascalientes asked to translate their approval into something concrete, for "As Mexicans we proudly accept whatever sacrifice is necessary . . . for the respect of our Nation's Sovereignty."[242] The top echelons of the San Luis Potosí state bureaucracy, including sanitary chief and returned RF fellow Felipe Malo Juvera, offered 10 percent of their paychecks to the government as long as extra revenues were needed.[243] Public health-minded mayors along the Gulf Coast thought to request permission to take over the antilarval equipment left behind by the oil companies.[244]

Not only did these responses reflect the nationalism of Mexican professionals, they had direct implications for institutional survival. Almost immediately following the nationalization, the Cárdenas government set in motion a Program for National Economic Recovery to generate savings in federal expenditures that could be applied to the payment of compensation to the oil companies whose property had been nationalized.[245] In the DSP, this program demanded an increase in productivity, punctuality, and efficiency, a strict limit on the acquisition of new equipment, and a prohibition on overtime work. While the DSP remained committed to producing vaccines and continuing disease prevention and control programs, travel and research costs were to be severely curtailed in a "patriotic" and "praiseworthy effort to support the national government."[246]

The nationalization and recovery program served as an important test of the president and his party's political transition from populism to pluralism. In the mid 1930s, Cárdenas had built his power base through populist politics. He had appealed to urban industrial workers as their ally in business-labor relations. At the same time he had reached out to peasants—the vast majority of whom remained landless and shortchanged by the promises of the revolution—through a more radical restructuring of economic relations and social conditions.

Cárdenas successfully used the state in pursuit of this dual agenda, for example, implementing both workplace protections and land reform. When his policies of protecting the petroleum industry from foreign interests escalated in 1937, however, the existing arrangement of the state as an autonomous actor began polarizing the country more than unifying it: the progressive coalition that backed Cárdenas's challenge to powerful domestic and foreign interests in Mexico had paradoxically "strengthened the opposition and increased the cohesion of these groups."[247] In December 1937, Cárdenas backed a replacement party for the PNR. The new Partido de la Revolución Mexicana (PRM) was predicated on participation of "all 'revolutionary' sectors": labor, peasant, military, and popular, crossing class and regional lines, with membership of over 4 million people. Though the new party began by advocating the nationalization of industry—starting with oil—foreseeing a longer-term goal of socializing production, this ideology was rapidly replaced with a "national unity" agenda. In embracing both progressive and conservative forces, the PRM successfully moderated left-wing forces both inside and outside the party, at once achieving "state control" over peasant and working-class organizations and neutralizing their power as the party's base in the face of capitalist interests.[248] The new party was also well suited to the nation's institutionalization project.

The IHD Response

Because of IHD officer Bailey's confidence in his good relations with the Mexican government under often trying circumstances, he was surprised and unnerved by the nationalization. Considering Cárdenas's move to be almost a personal humiliation, Bailey could not recover his faith in Mexican officials, and the remainder of his tour in Mexico was marked by cynicism and suspicion. His first comments came two weeks after the nationalization, when he explained that his knowledge of events was wildly inaccurate due to "biased" information from censored newspapers and because "Broadcasting from the [United] States

Table 4.4. Relative financial contributions to the supervised district budget—
Morelos

	1935	1936	1937	1938	1939
DSP (%)	71	64	68	67	69
State/municipality (%)	11	13	25	9	5
IHD (%)	18	23	7	24	26
Total in constant pesos	197,500	314,140	224,268	252,011	231,911
Approximate total in 2004 dollars	742,000	1,180,000	843,000	736,000	612,000
Number of employees	45	84	56	63	No data

Source: Annual Reports, 1935–39, Oficina de Especialización Sanitaria, RFA, RG 5, Series 3, Boxes 145 and 146.

is continuously purposely drowned out." With "rampant nationalism and anti-foreign sentiment" making the outcome of the situation difficult to predict, Bailey fretted about the chaotic financial situation and the scarcity of the rapidly devaluating currency.[249] Bailey was particularly worried about meeting the health units' payroll, as neither Morelos nor Cuernavaca had made paid their obligations, even though the DSP chief "spends every weekend in Cuernavaca."[250] Following several years of growing state and municipal participation in the unit budgets, the IHD ended up covering much of their share in 1938 and 1939 (see table 4.4).

Walter Earle, an IHD malariologist who was carrying out mosquito control experiments in Morelos during the year of the nationalization, held a contrasting view of events. He saw a mixture of pride and uncertainty in a "little brother when he first got up nerve to kick big brother in the pants."[251] In spite of the personal sacrifices required from Mexicans to pay for the nationalization, he observed that "The entire country seems to be united." Earle had not noticed any change in the Mexican attitude toward the RF, and, he reflected, "my own sympathies are with" Cárdenas.

Notwithstanding Bailey's fears, the nationalization did not visibly affect the IHD's commitment to Mexico. The home office spoke of the situation only in euphemistic tones. Ferrell relayed, "We have learned with deep regret of the unsettlement in Mexico which affects the public health work," and he urged Bailey to carry on courageously.[252] As Ferrell explained to U.S. Vice President Henry Wallace several years later, some Mexicans had long suspected that the RF was connected to Rockefeller business interests,[253] and this was the RF's singular opportunity to demonstrate otherwise.

Meanwhile, British, Dutch, and U.S. oil companies (including Standard Oil of New Jersey) were adamant about the $700 million ($9.3 billion in 2004 dollars) they claimed they were owed for their seized property and even more insistent about what they believed to be their rights to the subsoil.[254] The oil companies and Britain (which was much more dependent on Mexico's oil than was the U.S., and was leading an embargo of Mexico), placed mounting pressure on the State Department to exact retribution on Mexico. But at this juncture, there were larger considerations than private property. Though concerned that other oil- and mineral-rich Latin American nations might follow Mexico's example, the U.S. government did not act hastily.

From a Mexican perspective, the timing of the oil nationalization could not have been more propitious. With rising fascism in Germany and Italy in the late 1930s, any of a range of actions by countries with oil interests—economic sanctions, invading Mexico, or ousting Cárdenas—could push Mexico into the Axis camp. In the months after the nationalization, Nazi Germany became Mexico's primary petroleum customer followed by Mussolini's Italy.[255] The health sector took part in these new relationships. The DSP purchased microscopes and other medical instruments from Germany because several U.S. companies refused to do business with Mexico.[256] Most notably, in 1939 the new Institute of Health and Tropical Diseases was fully outfitted with German equipment, some of it obtained in exchange for petroleum.[257] German pharmaceutical companies had long studied disease problems in Latin America and marketed a range of drugs to the region,[258] and in 1935 Mexico had bartered rice for German medical equipment for the Military Hospital and pipes for use in the construction of water and sewage systems.[259] Now Germany was ready to step into a larger international health role. With the United States unable to afford to lose Mexico as an ally, the RF's role as health diplomat was resurrected.

Though the U.S. government initially sympathized with oil company claims, it softened its stance on the nationalization within several months. To begin, Roosevelt's "Good Neighbor" policy precluded unilateral intervention, particularly when "fair compensation" was being offered.[260] Tensions in Europe and then the outbreak of war framed Washington's soft approach in the short term. For five years, the U.S. State Department and the Mexican government haggled over the terms of compensation. In 1942, the two countries agreed that Mexico would pay slightly less than $30 million ($327 million in 2004 dollars) to U.S. oil companies for property and interest. This constituted a fraction of their value according to the oil firms, which delayed their acceptance of these terms for more than a year. Despite the acrimony of the U.S. oil sector, the settlement managed to resolve the compensation issue without jeopardizing U.S.-Mexican relations.[261]

Amidst the larger-scale politics, Bailey's world had taken on what he considered nightmarish proportions. At first blush, the problem was cognitive: if he did not understand the IHD's reservations about supporting public health upon Cárdenas's election, he was even more baffled at its staying power after the oil nationalization.

In spite of Bailey's confusion, he became the RF's eyes and ears in Mexico; the RF relied on him, while it, for the most part, maintained an official silence in the face of turmoil.

Bailey's troubles were also practical. He saw his day-to-day management difficulties soar and his power diminish. During the early Cárdenas years, Bailey was proud that not a single RF fellow had been moved from his position, even with a major reorganization of the DSP.[262] Now the situation had changed. Highly disturbed by the DSP's frequent transfers of his personnel, he asked Ferrell:

> Which of two ways should we interpret these requests and moves for our personnel? Should we consider them as a compliment in taking our trained men as the best to be had in the country, or as a means to an end in reducing our service to an unnecessary appendage? With the increasing spirit and evidence of Nationalism—Mexico for the Mexicans—socialism, and the strangle hold the syndicate now have [sic] over Government—one wonders—and I am not sure which is the correct answer.[263]

Ferrell instructed Bailey to "acquiesce cheerfully" and "undergo any inconvenience" caused by the transfer of personnel because "We are in no sense competitors of the Federal service." The IHD's role, Ferrell reminded his frustrated field officer, was to assist in the development of "sound programs and policies directed by men of training and experience." Ferrell attempted to lift Bailey's spirits by telling him of the RF's appreciation for his efficient direction of IHD activities in Mexico and for his adherence to "merit systems."[264]

Ferrell reacted coolly to the aftermath of the nationalization, noting, "When conditions become disturbed because of economic or political stress, one would not be surprised if some impairment of efficiency should arise." Encouraged by the RF's role during two decades of "consistent advances in public health" in Mexico, Ferrell recommended allowing the Mexican government "to determine the services and the conditions under which we may render aid" for existing programs without pursuing any expansion of the programs.[265] By maintaining its programs following the nationalization, the RF supported the position that its health programs were above politics. Just as important, the polarized and deteriorating international situation was no time for the RF to pull out: the IHD was needed in Mexico to promote goodwill.

To Bailey, every day brought "more demands, less work accomplished, insubordination of non-technical staff and seemingly no redress." He became a fierce critic of the union activity that he had once quietly tolerated. His request to the DSP for pay increases had been denied, leaving his office vulnerable to strikes by the "all powerful" DSP union. Bailey complained, "I have no freedom of action whatever in handling of personnel, in transferring them from one station to another, as some emergency may demand." Since the formation of the health workers' union, "The efficiency of our workers has decreased at least 25%, sick leaves and leaves demanded for syndicate and other reasons have more than doubled. Defiance and even insolence are constantly evident." Bailey resented the frequent demands that his office pay for the medical care of staff members. Bailey summarized, "In short this Service has become part of a vicious cycle and is quite remote from the principles and policies of the Foundation."[266] The institutionalization of the IHD's programs in Mexico meant that it now operated just like any other division of the DSP. To Bailey, the loss of privilege and power was an unconscionable affront.

The conflicts between unionized DSP workers and Bailey's office had come to Cárdenas's attention, but the president was careful not to take sides. DSP chief Siurob met with Cárdenas in early 1939 to try to resolve the dispute. Siurob described the RF's dedication to Mexico and defended the IHD's workplace policies as ensuring job security and program stability. According to Siurob, a problem had arisen when several workers abandoned their posts to participate in union activities. This rankled Bailey, who fired one worker from the Xochimilco unit and transferred several Morelos employees who were active in their union. Siurob argued that many of these workers had intentionally provoked the IHD by refusing to give up the right to private practice. Siurob worried that, due to the actions of these union members, the "Department's best opportunity for good health services and training would be lost together with the valuable cooperation, grants, and subsidies of the Rockefeller Foundation," and he implored the president not to jeopardize the RF's "beneficial assistance" to Mexico. Cárdenas decided that "in principle workers employed with the Rockefeller Foundation have the same rights as all other workers." "However," he added, "the DSP should resolve individual cases through monetary compensation."[267] Thanks to this loophole, the IHD would not be required to comply with union rules; individuals who were fired would be recompensed by the Mexican government.

In settling the conflict between disgruntled workers and Bailey, Cárdenas played his cards astutely. He refused to override union-protected workers' rights but allowed exceptions on a case-by-case basis, ensuring compatibility with the IHD's rules. The following year, when Nelson Rockefeller met with Cárdenas in a failed attempt to resolve the oil crisis, Rockefeller did succeed in gaining the president's approval for returned RF fellows to circumvent Mexican labor laws so that they could fill senior DSP positions.[268] Cárdenas would not violate the labor laws that he himself had championed, yet he did everything possible to appease the RF.

Bailey could not be mollified. Once optimistic, he predicted that 1940 "will be anything but a bed of roses and little will be accomplished."[269] Whereas prior to 1938 Bailey had enthusiastically presented all Mexican proposals to the IHD as his own, now he refused to back a much-favored plan to develop a training station adjacent to the School of Public Health. He warned his superiors that it was "impossible for us to engage in any cooperative project, in which we handle, supervise, and direct (or rather attempt to direct) Government personnel, unless there is a radical change" with a new president in 1941. He even lost interest in the RF fellows—nominating only one fellow in 1941—because the "Syndicate has stated they would in the future designate and control Foundation fellowships."[270] In 1940, the embattled Bailey was assigned to a new post: he left Mexico a bitter man, unable to recognize the important developments in public health that had taken place while he was there.

The Hows of Institutionalization

If the RF's field officer believed this era was a failure for international health, both the RF and the DSP smelled success. Even in a period of high nationalism, the work of the two entities had become so intertwined that the mutual appropriation of ideas went unnoticed.

The RF's New York office was undoubtedly troubled on some level by the nationalization and by rising social and political activism in Mexico during the Cárdenas years. Nonetheless it was—perhaps by nature—less excitable than its officers on the ground. Indeed, the RF had reacted to the two periods of crisis— Cárdenas's arrival in power in 1935 and the oil nationalization in 1938—in a manner completely opposite to Bailey's. The early period of the Cárdenas administration was one of wait and see: nervous at developments in Mexico, the RF wished to limit its investments, regardless of the potential consequences to its public health programs. The oil nationalization, by contrast, occurred in a context of altered world politics: in the lead-up to World War II, fending off the influence of Axis powers in Latin America was a pressing concern, and the IHD had a role to play in maintaining good relations with Mexico.

Though the RF reacted in divergent ways at these two moments, it also viewed its activities in the broader context of Mexico's ongoing institutionalization process in the 1930s. By the end of the Cárdenas presidency, the RF had become pleased with its investment in Mexico. On a 1940 trip to Mexico, Ferrell commented, "In the past there have been too frequent changes in regimes and in personnel, but in the Health Department practically all of the fellows trained by the Rockefeller Foundation grants have had continuous employment in the federal service."[271]

The Morelos health demonstration area was also entrenched. It served the state's 170,000 residents through four full-time health units and over a dozen auxiliary and branch units.[272] In 1939 alone, Morelos health personnel gave 500 conferences (to schools, midwives, personnel, and the public), treated 13,000 cases of communicable diseases, administered almost 40,000 smallpox immunizations, performed more than 10,000 laboratory tests including 4,400 Kahn reactions for syphilis, attended 2,600 expectant mothers, visited almost 4,000 infants, and examined 4,000 school and preschool children. In addition, over 5,000 stores, restaurants, hotels, markets, and dairies underwent annual

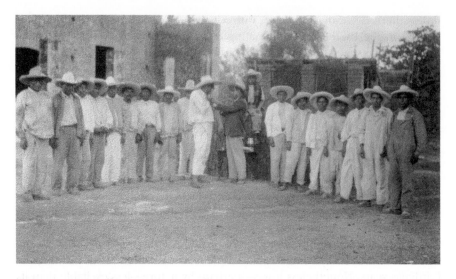

Figure 4.14. Smallpox vaccination clinic, 1935. Cuernavaca health unit. Courtesy of the Rockefeller Archive Center.

hygiene inspections, and the sanitary engineering service inspected some 2,000 schools and other public and private buildings, installing several hundred water carriage toilets, latrines, and septic tanks per year.[273] The Morelos district project reached as many people in 1939 as had the entire Rural Hygiene Service in 1935, touching, in some manner, most of the state's population. The $57,000 ($760,000 in 2004 dollars) the IHD had invested between 1936 and 1940 had helped control transmissible diseases, promote infant and child hygiene, and improve sanitation.

According to Bailey, the only flaw in the Morelos district was the apparent worsening of some health indicators, with infant mortality rates rising by 50 percent in the first two years of the supervised district before slowly falling to approximately 100 deaths per 1000 live births. Bailey claimed—probably correctly—that the rise in infant mortality could be at least partially attributed to better vital statistics collection: sanitary units personnel had convinced more inhabitants to bring the illnesses and deaths of their children to the attention of the state.[274]

The DSP agreed that the Morelos district had advanced public health and set an example for the entire country, and in 1940 returned RF fellow Alberto León, now DSP secretary-general, asked for continued IHD aid.[275] Funding was extended, but by late 1941 the home office judged the Morelos program to be "sufficiently developed . . . to permit the withdrawal of IHD support" in 1942.[276] Five years later, the RF boasted that Morelos had become "perhaps the best organized state in Mexico."[277] In 1947, the Morelos service was headed by returned RF fellow Adán Ornelas and comprised ten full-time doctors, twenty nurses, twelve sanitary inspectors, one midwife, two social workers, and two laboratory technicians. Seven health centers located around the state were coordinated by the central unit in Cuernavaca, which included both a tuberculosis dispensary and a training station that had turned out one quarter of the country's public health trainees. Based on attendance figures, the health units were "clearly appreciated by the population."[278]

After the Morelos units were handed over to the DSP, the IHD scaled back its support to Mexico, believing that—even if some individual units could not sustain full-time personnel—the DSP had learned and understood the value of the full-time model.[279] But the IHD was not ready to conclude the relationship: in 1940 it sent a new representative, Dr. George Payne, to replace Bailey in Mexico. In 1943, the DSP organized a new regional health district in the northeastern state of Nuevo León near the Texas border, an area important in agriculture, mining, industry, and petroleum. The district was wealthy enough to sponsor its own units, but the IHD insisted on paying some staff and travel costs so that it could observe the district's activities.[280]

From the DSP's perspective, there was also no question that the Cárdenas era was marked by successful institutionalization. While this was a domestic and nationalistic endeavor, the DSP recognized the part played by RF international health. Even one of the DSP's most decidedly sovereign efforts—the Institute of Health and Tropical Diseases (ISET)—bore an imprint of the RF.

Opening the institute had been a goal of the 1934 Six-Year Plan. As evidence of Mexico's scientific progress and political independence, Cárdenas inaugurated the ISET on March 18, 1939, the first anniversary of the oil nationalization. With parasitologist and public health specialist Dr. Manuel Martínez Báez as the founding director, the institute was conceived according to the principles of scientific sovereignty: studying local diseases in the context of local realities so that Mexico's health priorities could be identified and addressed by Mexican researchers.[281] Laboratory-based research on hookworm, malaria, leprosy, shigellosis, and many other diseases would now take place in Mexico—a country that suffered heavily from such ailments—rather than in Europe or the United States where these diseases were considered "exotic."[282] Most notable was the focus on onchocerciasis, which the IHD had repeatedly rejected as a cooperative project. In the late 1940s, ISET researcher Luis Mazzotti, a returned RF fellow, identified the ability of hetrazan to destroy the onchocerciasis parasite and described anaphylactoid reactions following chemotherapy; these became known worldwide as Mazzotti reactions.[283]

The illustrious Martínez Báez was the ideal leader for this undertaking. A native of Morelia, Michoacán, he—like the founders of the ejidal medical units and physician social service—was a *nicolaíta*, of the same generation as some of the country's leading medical men. After a period as head of the DSP's health education office, in the early 1930s Martínez Báez studied parasitology in Paris, Hamburg, and Rome, the latter under an RF grant. He was named Mexico's delegate to the OIHP, launching a long career in international health at the WHO, the United Nations Educational, Scientific and Cultural Organization, and other agencies.[284] A laboratory scientist, a public health man, an international player, and a medical humanist, Martínez Báez knew how to court the RF without sacrificing the ISET's independence and research integrity.

Built in Mexico City, because few "capable research workers" were willing to reside outside the capital, the modern, million-peso institute had two floors of laboratories, one floor for hospital beds for research subjects, and one for the School of Public Health.[285] Faculty members received good salaries in exchange for full-time service, but Martínez Báez knew from the first day that they lacked sufficient training and experience. Even before the ISET was founded, he implored the RF to send Johns Hopkins researchers to Mexico to help out.[286] Beginning in 1939, the RF funded short-term consultations and training sessions by Johns Hopkins faculty.[287] ISET faculty members also received RF funding to visit the Rockefeller Institute for Medical Research and the School of Tropical Medicine in Puerto Rico.[288] At the end of the ISET's first year of operation, all five divisions were headed by returned RF fellows; five years later RF fellows likewise held the ISET's directorship and occupied five out of twelve department chairships.

Back to the US(SR)?

By 1940 the RF and DSP had reached a stage in their relationship when they needed each other. In 1934, however, it was not clear that the relationship would evolve to this stage. The Cárdenas era's red politics, sovereign public health developments—particularly the ejidal medical services—and nationalization of oil each had the potential to threaten RF activities and its legacy in Mexico. In Greece, for example, political and economic instability in the interwar years prevented the RF from achieving its goals of modernizing public health.[289]

With Cárdenas in power, the RF home office feared a similarly unfavorable outcome, and it repeatedly compared Mexico to the Soviet Union in terms of such "watchwords" as socialization of land and industry, mass education and health, and reorganization and reconstruction. In the early 1940s, the RF reassured itself that despite the fact that the "anti-capitalistic and anti-church murals of Diego Rivera, Orozco, and other modernists are almost as common in Mexico as are the blatant Red posters in Moscow," the political cultures of the two countries differed markedly, with the Mexican masses interested not in ideology but in "material betterment" and not "particularly concerned over the system through which they get it." Whatever the rhetoric surrounding the oil nationalization, RF home office visitors to Mexico did not "sense any hostility whatever to the capitalistic

Yankee or any suspicion of his dollar diplomacy," reflecting, some believed, the changed attitudes resulting from the "Good Neighbor" policy.[290]

In Mexico, demonstrations of difference from the IHD's offerings—in theoretical and practical terms—did not result in the IHD's abandonment of its activities there. In large measure, this was because the IHD simultaneously permitted ample space for national developments and tried to fill this space through its own efforts.

By concentrating on a circumscribed set of health issues in a limited section of the country—turning down Mexican requests to work in a variety of areas—the RF left a wide range of public health problems open to local approaches and interests. But the IHD kept its hand in the bigger institutionalization mix by subtly shifting its emphasis in favor of educational initiatives in the mid 1930s. RF fellows, in particular, found themselves at the heart of the interplay between the RF and DSP. From the RF's viewpoint, fellows were a "select group greatly influencing medicine, education, and public health in Latin America."[291] Fellows cultivated new patterns of government service, filled important posts, and employed the latest health technologies; through the agencies and training stations they ran, the fellows diffused their knowledge and practices to Mexico's public health community and well beyond.

But the fellows did not simply learn their IHD lessons and fall into marching order. Miguel Bustamante, Pilar Hernández Lira, and other fellows played a pioneering role in developing strategies and employing resources within the country's economic possibilities and according to national ideologies. This generation of health officials certainly absorbed RF international health precepts; at the same time they were innovators themselves. They paid heed to local needs and constraints in devising rural medical student internships and socially oriented health services, ultimately creating a Mexican-style institutionalization rather than following recipes from abroad.

Still, the three-decade interaction between the IHD and DSP had results other than an apparently productive and open marriage in which each of the partners happily gave and took what they wanted. The legacy came at a price. Part of that price may have been the obstruction of national initiatives, such as ejidal units, which were ultimately overtaken by the sanitary units in the 1940s as the main model of rural health services. Much of the price was bureaucratic. For administrative and accounting ease, IHD programs were kept in separate divisions—for example, the IHD-sponsored units were housed in the Rural Hygiene Service rather than with the "Coordinated Health Services in the States"—with separate staffs and budgets, generating inefficiencies, duplication, and waste.[292] This arrangement gave the IHD more control over its investments, but it meant that its approach was never fully infused into the DSP's work. In the end, the RF's role in the institutionalization of Mexican public health under Cárdenas was ambiguous—at times controlling, at times irrelevant, at times a spark for change, at times accidentally well placed—but always locally molded.

Chapter Five

Ingredients of a Relationship

In the autumn of 1932 the Rockefeller family invited Mexican painter Diego Rivera to create a mural for the new Rockefeller Center—a distinctive urban complex of shops, offices, theaters, restaurants, and public art on Fifth Avenue in New York City. Beginning work the following spring, Rivera offered a prescient depiction of the potential directions for modern life entitled *Man at the Crossroads Looking with Hope and High Vision to the Choosing of a New and Better Future*. With a robot-like worker controlling a giant turbine at the center, the mural displayed the wonders of science. In front of the man, discoveries of biology, chemistry, and physics were represented on a luminous globe. Behind him, two diagonal lenses crisscrossed, one revealing microscopic views of germs, cells, and a developing embryo, the other showing a telescopic panorama of far-flung galaxies, stars, and planets.

The artist also portrayed contrasting scenes of human society on the left and the right of both fresco and political spectrum. *Man at the Crossroads'* right side yielded to the world of capitalism: bleak scenes of war; unemployed workers being beaten by the police; and fancy club-goers gambling, smoking, and drinking, oblivious to the world outside. To the left, conversely, were images of a socialist society: a colorful May Day Parade, a line of muscular female athletes, and a scene of African-American and white laborers joining hands with a familiar politician-philosopher. Rivera pointedly challenged the liberality of his sponsor by endowing this figure with a striking resemblance to Vladimir Lenin.

The press soon got wind of the theme of Rivera's mural, and in late April 1933 the *New York World-Telegram* headlined a story: "Rivera Paints Scenes of Communist Activity—and John D. [Rockefeller] Jr. Foots Bill."[1] The young Nelson Rockefeller—a member of the Rockefeller Center board, a trustee of the Museum of Modern Art and the second son of John D. Jr.—sought in vain to have Rivera replace Lenin's portrait with something less "offensive," such as an image of Abraham Lincoln (according to an apocryphal version of the story), but the muralist demurred. Within a few weeks, Rivera was called down from his scaffold and made to cease work while the differences were resolved. Months of public demonstrations and private negotiations proved fruitless. With neither side willing to yield, Rivera was dismissed and the mural was demolished.[2]

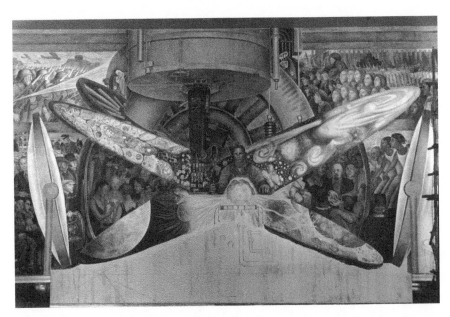

Figure 5.1. *Man at the Crossroads Looking with Hope and High Vision to the Choosing of a New and Better Future*, Rockefeller Center, 1933, by Diego Rivera. Photograph of the mural before it was destroyed, secretly taken by Lucienne Bloch, assistant to Rivera on this project. In 1934, Rivera recreated the mural for the Palacio de Bellas Artes in Mexico City, where it is on permanent display. In this subsequent rendition, Rivera balanced out the Lenin figure on the socialist side of the mural with a recognizable portrayal of John D. Rockefeller Jr. as one of the gamblers on the capitalist side. Photograph by Lucienne Bloch. Courtesy of Old Stage Studios.

Four years later, another work of public art involving the Rockefeller family and a Mexican revolutionary was unveiled—now in Mexico City. On this occasion it was Mexican President Lázaro Cárdenas who had commissioned a bronze plaque to be placed on an inner courtyard wall of the DSP headquarters in memory of the late John D. Rockefeller Sr. and in appreciation of the Rockefeller Foundation's aid in "solving many Mexican health problems."[3]

On September 18, 1937, a distinguished group of doctors, government officials, and other dignitaries gathered for a music-punctuated ceremony, with U.S. Ambassador to Mexico Josephus Daniels as the honored guest.[4] In the opening speech, Dr. Alfonso Pruneda, the first DSP official to interact with the RF, recalled that in the years since the foundation had been invited to Mexico in 1920, its officers had acted as government functionaries, facilitating cooperation, friendship, and progress among Mexican professionals and country folk

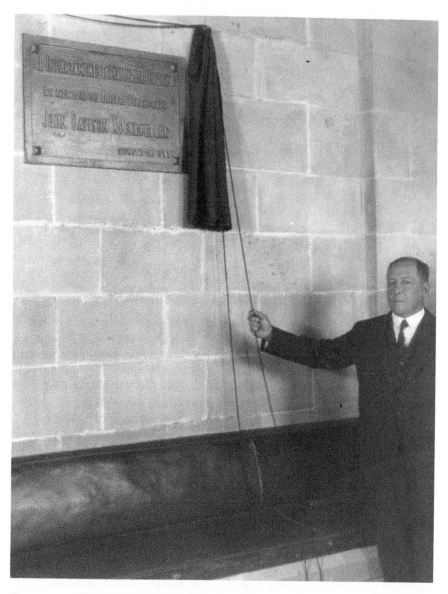

Figure 5.2. DSP chief Dr. José Siurob (1935–38 and 1939–40) unveiling DSP plaque honoring John D. Rockefeller. Courtesy of the Rockefeller Archive Center.

alike. For Pruneda, the joint programs left enduring benefits thanks to the RF's extensive training effort and its "powerful contribution to the shaping of various health activities, especially rural health services."[5]

In the keynote address, Ambassador Daniels—who as Woodrow Wilson's secretary of the navy had ordered the United States' 1914 invasion of Mexico's main port of Veracruz during the Mexican Revolution—struck an internationalist chord, stressing that "No wall has been erected so high, no barrier constructed so strong, no cordon stretched so effectively as to confine germs and bugs . . . to any one country."[6] To loud applause, he went on,

> Let us rejoice that governments and individuals are seeking . . . to provide agencies for the care of children and the protection of public health. Meeting this vision and challenge is Mr. Rockefeller's greatest claim to the gratitude of the people of the earth. Mexico honors itself in honoring a philanthropist who permitted no national boundaries to narrow his practical interest in the public weal.[7]

After unveiling the tablet, DSP chief General José Siurob declared that the philanthropic work of men like Rockefeller was the most efficient means of bringing countries closer together and was thus deserving of the highest homage.[8]

Exactly six months later on March 18, 1938, President Cárdenas nationalized the oil industry, taking over the operations of British, Dutch, and U.S. oil companies, including Rockefeller-owned Standard Oil, and raising a firestorm of controversy. Yet RF health activities in Mexico continued unabated for many more years.

Like Rivera's turbine man, Mexico was at a crossroads when it became involved with the RF. Emerging from a bloody decade-long revolution, at odds with the United States and other foreign investors over rights to the country's rich oil reserves, and needing to meet the increasingly vocal demands of its large peasant and growing working-class population, Mexico faced a challenging set of choices for the future. Although the country's ideological direction was yet to be resolved, the means were clear: Mexico would harness science to social and economic advancement. By the early 1920s, despite financial woes, human and institutional losses, and ongoing unrest, Mexico had already begun to address its ambitious agenda. Its visionary education secretary, José Vasconcelos, launched an educational plan that would one day bring a school to every hamlet, where pride in Mexico's past would unite with modern teaching methods and knowledge. In the health arena, too, the DSP sought to pick up where prerevolutionary public health had left off, drawing on European expertise, regional developments, and local resources as needed.

At the Rockefeller Center in New York, a revolutionary Mexican perspective on scientific progress tied to socialist values resulted in stalemate, while in Mexico this same commitment enabled fruitful and long-term cooperation. Ironically, Diego Rivera and the Rockefellers seemed to get along much better in Mexico than in the United States: the bronze plaque to John D. Rockefeller Sr. was located just a few feet away from a conference hall where in 1929 Rivera had painted a series of nudes depicting pre-Columbian medical traditions.

How could the RF tolerate turmoil, radicalism, and the nationalization of oil in one setting, but perceive a single figure in a large mural to be too disruptive in another? In the context of 1930s New York class conflict, art could not remain neutral. Liberal as it was in its artistic taste, the Rockefeller family was unable to reconcile the anticapitalist theme of Rivera's mural with the pressure to fill office space in the "homage to capitalism" Rockefeller Center. In Mexico, by contrast, health revolutionaries and the RF took public health to be a technical force residing at the intersection of state-building, economic growth, and material betterment.

Although unfolded on a plane of symbolic expression, these episodes are emblematic of the complexity of the relationship between the RF and revolutionary Mexico and the ability of each party to tailor cooperative public health programs to meet respective social, ideological, professional, and revolutionary goals. This dynamic rested on agreement that science was the key to human progress, regardless of political context.

The mutual belief in science is also symbolized in the strangely parallel life courses of two of the foremost personalities behind this story: John D. Rockefeller Sr. (1839–1937) and Lázaro Cárdenas (1895–1970). Both born of modest backgrounds in the nineteenth century, each was bound to shape the next. Rockefeller—the son of a snake oil salesman and himself an adherent of homeopathy—dominated and virtually single-handedly transformed the oil industry and then dedicated his colossal profits to equally groundbreaking philanthropic endeavors. His eponymous foundation hitched modern science to the mission of promoting the "well-being of mankind" by revolutionizing the fields of medicine, public health, and education. In the first half of the twentieth century, the RF was the world's leading international agency, and its experiences reverberated in countless local settings and successor organizations. Rockefeller's frugal Protestant values influenced both his business and philanthropic dealings; neither was able to escape controversy.[9]

Cárdenas—the son of an herbalist—was a little-known tax clerk and army officer on a fast track—to oil field general, minister of war, state governor, and president, all before the age of forty. Cárdenas dared to challenge both his political patron and big oil, risking foreign opprobrium and raising socialist-populism to an art form. He dedicated his presidency to the advancement of Mexico—through modern institutions, industrialization, and land reform, calling on science and technology to satisfy the social demands of revolutionaries and the economic demands of modern state-builders.[10] Minimally educated and personally austere, Cárdenas's politics resonated throughout Mexico's twentieth century and all over the developing world, where many emerging nation-states tried to follow Mexico's path of political independence and economic integration. If

Rockefeller's contradictions stemmed from his combination of exploitative and meliorative pursuits, Cárdenas's lay between his radical rhetoric and the reality of political deal-making.

The overlapping trajectories of this unlikely pair—sons of medical empirics, ambitious risk-takers, builders of institutions and industry, believers in the ability of science to better the human condition—are representative of the reasons the Mexico–RF relationship was so durable.

Conspiracy, Charity, Catalysis, Coincidence, Chaos, or All of the Above?

To assess the relationship, we return to the story itself. We begin by exploring the larger meaning of the RF and Mexico—how and why they came to one another and stayed together for so long—through a series of explanatory frameworks. Next, we examine the extended dénouement of the IHD in Mexico and the terms of disengagement. We then address the issue of public health campaigns rejected by the IHD despite persistent Mexican demands. Finally, we analyze the part played by each of the story's principals to uncover the effects of decades of this public health cooperation on the RF, on Mexico, and on international health itself.

From the 1920s to the 1940s, the RF's main involvement in Mexico was through four distinct but related public health projects: (a) a high-budget yellow fever campaign centered along the Gulf of Mexico Coast from 1921 to 1924 that inspected tens of thousands of houses, treated millions of breeding sites, and tested the (failed) Noguchi vaccine against yellow fever; (b) a lower-priced and far-reaching hookworm campaign that treated over 200,000 people and built some 15,000 latrines in dozens of villages in five central and southern Mexican states from 1924 to 1928; (c) a local health initiative that involved the founding of five cooperative health units in three states starting in 1927 and a statewide demonstration district in Morelos (five units) that lasted from 1935 until 1942, plus small-scale research and administrative activities in several other states through the 1940s; and (d) an ongoing educational effort that sent sixty-eight public health fellows to pursue graduate degrees in North American universities, trained 587 health workers in two training stations founded in Mexico by 1940 (and approximately two thousand by 1950), and sponsored study trips to North America for three dozen high-level public health officials.

How might we gauge these endeavors as a whole?

In one version of the story, the RF carried out health activities in order to protect Standard Oil and other U.S. investments in the region, boost the reputation of these companies, and generate Mexican dependency on the United States in medicine and more generally.[11] Viewed at a structural level, these efforts removed threats to the stability of the capitalist system and attenuated its flaws.

Revolutionary politicians, for their part, enlisted the RF to buy off loyalty and votes in provincial jurisdictions, and Mexican doctors used the opportunity to elevate their status and expand their reach. Or, to pose the question more pointedly, was there an international health conspiracy? That is, did the RF intentionally promote a capitalist version of public health, with the complicity of a segment of Mexican leaders, in order to implant a reductionist, biological, conservative—rather than a social, community-based, revolutionary—understanding of health and disease, staving off both anti-U.S. and pro-socialist tendencies, as well as protecting trade and enhancing the health, productivity, and consumption capacity of local employees of foreign companies?

Were this the case, how might we interpret the reciprocal belief of RF and Mexican doctors and high-level administrators on both sides in the potential of these programs to improve the health of all Mexicans and help guide a permanent government commitment to public health? What is the evidence that the various players were privy to such a plot? Was popular support for public health projects the product of "manufactured consent?"[12] The conspiracy theory of international health—with its oft-gratifying internal logic—does not begin to reflect the panoply of parties to, nor the interplay of power and interests involved in, the RF's public health programs in Mexico.

If not conspiracy, then unadorned charity? Certainly the RF's mission of advancing the "Well-Being of Mankind Throughout the World," rang pure and altruistic.[13] But the RF was established precisely as an alternative to religious charity: John D. Rockefeller Sr. and his associates sought to channel wealth systematically and to institutions, not haphazardly or to individuals.[14] From the Mexican government's perspective, the prospect of alms from its arch-adversary was variously suspect, reviling, and, at least initially, rejected. Moreover, if RF subsidies for local health campaigns, institutional development, and training were good-hearted donations, they came at a steep price that included substantial local cofinancing, outside agenda-setting and approaches, and compliance with a series of prerequisites.

Another way to consider the RF is as a catalyst for change.[15] In this understanding, RF programs helped "institutionalize" Mexico's revolution by meeting rural claims on the state and rebuilding the nation's health infrastructure. The RF's very presence in Mexico, might be viewed as the spark that ignited public health institutionalization. Not only does this interpretation overlook the older competing influence of European health and medicine in Mexico, but it disregards both the degree to which public health modernization was already occurring as part of the national agenda and Mexico's extensive refashioning of RF endeavors to serve domestic needs.[16]

In this sense, was the RF's role more coincidental than catalytic, accompanying or accelerating what was an inevitable public health model that would eventually be implemented with or without foreign participation? Or, as a variant on this notion, was the RF's interest in Mexico chiefly as a demonstration of

American scientific ingenuity to its European competitors?[17] The notion of coincidence, however, strips the players of power and intent—as though Mexico and the RF came together only incidentally and could do little about it.

With the IHD's experience in Mexico only partially explained by notions of conspiracy, charity, catalysis, and coincidence, did multiple and varied interests—philanthropy, international political relations, scientific modernization, professional advancement, diminishing the threat of disease and disorder, meeting social demands, and state-building add up to an undirected chaos? Here we return to the historical record. The priorities of Mexican leaders and RF administrators frequently overlapped and also diverged over specific policies and larger geopolitical concerns. At another level, Mexican doctors and Rockefeller public health officers in the field were trained similarly but perceived the Mexican context and the RF's role differently. Further, IHD officers and the Mexican peasants and townsfolk they targeted shared little a priori understanding of health or of one another, with each party retaining its own beliefs and preconceptions. Yet resistance and misunderstanding did not preclude partaking in the common ends of improving local health. The IHD's agenda and conditions were rigid, but they were also subject to local interpretation, contestation, and reshaping, confusing the question of who controlled whom and how success was judged. Above all, this was an interactive experience.

The answer to the question of conspiracy, charity, catalyst, coincidence, or chaos, then, is all of the above. Mexico was not simply another locale where the RF could implement its programs: IHD Director Russell closely oversaw the RF's involvement in Mexico, and in 1927 he insisted that "There is no more important country for our purposes than Mexico."[18] Attempting to understand these purposes and the unfolding Mexican positions brings to the fore the broader relevance of the RF's Mexican enterprise for the field of international health. One way of doing this is to examine the IHD's waning years in Mexico, for how things end may be as illuminating as how they begin.

The Long Goodbye

By the early 1940s, senior IHD administrators expressed satisfaction at having accomplished the agency's goals in Mexico. In early 1942, the IHD turned over responsibility for its remaining local health units to the DSP, ending more than twenty years of intensive cooperation. Instead of pulling out of Mexico, the IHD stayed on for another decade. IHD representatives to Mexico kept busy as advisors to the further extension of local health units, overseeing small malaria research projects, and consulting with the DSP on a variety of health policy matters.

Three developments—all occurring in 1943—gave new and contradictory meaning to the IHD's presence in Mexico. First, the RF invested in an enormous new venture—the Mexican Agricultural Program (MAP)—designed to increase food production through new agricultural technologies. Second, the U.S. Institute of Inter-American Affairs (IIAA) undertook a massive health and sanitation program in Mexico and fourteen other Latin American countries—the likes of which the RF would neither advocate nor afford—as part of President Roosevelt's campaign to ensure the region's support for the Allied powers in World War II. Third, the Mexican government demonstrated its institutional commitment to public health through the founding of the Mexican Institute of Social Security and the elevation of the DSP to the ministerial level. Though the IHD was partly counteracted and overshadowed by these initiatives, each was marked by the IHD's experience in Mexico.

The Mexican Agricultural Program

The near suspension of the RF's activities in wartime Europe[19] opened up significant resources for its enhanced involvement in Latin America. Perhaps the most far-reaching of these efforts was the MAP, organized by the RF's Natural Sciences Division in conjunction with the Mexican government.[20] An experiment aimed at increasing Mexico's wheat and corn output through the implementation of crop hybridization and other genetic technologies developed in the United States, the program became the first international demonstration of the Green Revolution, which would later spread to Brazil and throughout the developing world. Like IHD projects, the almost two-decade-long MAP sent U.S. advisors to Mexico and trained Mexican fellows in the United States. The $13 million program (over $130 million in 2004 dollars) also supported research at Mexico's National Agricultural University in Chapingo and funded a large supply of U.S.-made equipment. Warren Weaver, then head of the RF's Natural Sciences Division, was aware of the IHD's pattern of budget incentives and would later come to regret the large capital investment made in the MAP.[21]

The MAP relied heavily on the contacts and goodwill the IHD had generated, without engaging in the same degree of cooperation. Weaver invariably complained about Mexico's failure to pay its share of the bill, though he admitted that "this program was initially more or less stuffed down their throats" under almost complete RF control.[22] Mexican agricultural researchers at first welcomed the MAP, after some local attempts to boost the volume and efficiency of crop production had failed.[23] The program—with its full-blown transplantation of U.S. agricultural techniques—was ultimately adopted only in those areas where the assumptions and expectations of Mexican farmers resembled those of their North American counterparts, that is, in large agribusinesses rather than among small farmers.[24]

The new venture also signified a departure from the RF's normal procedures. First, the MAP was strongly advocated by U.S. Vice President Henry Wallace,[25] testing the RF's proclaimed independence from government interests. Wartime exigencies meant that standard operating principles were overridden by larger political considerations. The MAP also heralded a paradigmatic shift. With the RF's change in focus from the IHD to the MAP, public health problems were no longer viewed as the major impediment to development. Instead, the principle challenge was understood to be the pressure of feeding growing—now healthier—populations in developing countries. Of course, the two concerns were not unrelated, and the RF originally intended to integrate Mexico's agricultural advances with health projects focusing on nutrition. In anticipation, the IHD began funding community-based studies on nutritional deficiencies in 1942.[26] But the joint effort never evolved, largely because the MAP became more involved in the business than the public health side of improved agricultural output.

The MAP's approach also contrasted with the IHD's in that the agricultural experiment's technical and economic success was a more pressing goal than obtaining concomitant national contributions for long-term agenda-setting. Even so, the MAP borrowed from the IHD's style of interacting with government officials and, especially, with professionals: like the IHD—it adhered to a particular conceptualization of technology-based applied science and demonstration projects. Moreover, the MAP's overshadowing of the IHD implied a mutual Mexican-RF satisfaction: that is, the IHD was no longer needed since Mexico was fully committed to modern public health.

The Institute of Inter-American Affairs

Mexico's strong commitment to public health did not mean that all of the nation's considerable demands in this area had been met. Indeed, when the U.S. government offered to invest in the country's public health infrastructure during World War II, Mexico became an eager partner. In August 1940, as Washington's anxieties about Axis penetration into Latin America were mounting, the Roosevelt administration organized the Office of the Coordinator of Inter-American Affairs[27] to foster commercial and cultural relations and increase "solidarity" among the American republics, as well as to further hemispheric cooperation in defense.[28] Roosevelt appointed Nelson Rockefeller— who had a keen interest in Latin American business, politics, and (as we have seen) art—as the office's coordinator. Rockefeller was to formulate policy in conjunction with the State Department and report directly to the president.

Rockefeller, who was advised by RF staff in Latin America, learned that living and working conditions around proposed U.S. military bases and in areas that supplied strategic raw materials were unhealthy. A prime example was the problem of malaria in regions of the Amazon where wild rubber trees grew. In 1942 the IIAA was created as the health and sanitation subsidiary of the office Rockefeller coordinated. Beginning with Brazil, the IIAA organized an enormous campaign

Table 5.1. IHB/D expenditures in Mexico by area and year (U.S. dollars), 1920–41

Year	Yellow fever*	Hookworm	Local Health	PH Administration	Malaria	Training Stations	Total in Constant Dollars	Approximate Total in 2004 Dollars
1920	26,039**						26,039	248,300
1921	118,694						118,694	1,251,400
1922	103,485						103,485	1,167,400
1923	116,101						116,267***	1,286,000
1924	19,632	18,553					38,185	422,000
1925	32,293	21,525					53,818	578,700
1926	150	13,606					13,756	146,600
1927		6,855					6,855	73,900
1928			2,239				2,239	24,600
1929			4,402				4,402	48,100
1930			4,673				4,673	52,600
1931			9,795		1,275		11,070	137,700
1932			7,794		2,174	+	9,968	137,700
1933			7,248	1,727	1,867	+	10,842	157,800
1934			3,262	4,170		+	7,432	105,200
1935			5,836	4,074		+	9,910	136,600
1936			15,679	3,966		+	19,645	267,500
1937			11,325	4,152	3,886	+	19,363	254,100
1938			9,280	3,932	8,109	+	21,321	284,300
1939			8,006	3,320	2,670	+	13,996	190,300
1940			7,648	1,982		1,102	10,732	144,400
1941			9,968	2,760		1,580	14,308	183,600
Total								~7,300,000

IHB/D Personnel Expenses

Travel of Mexican government officials, 1927–30 (constant dollars)	1,978
IHB/D field staff salaries and expenses, 1918*–41 (constant dollars)	430,781
Fellowships (stipend, tuition, and travel), 1920–41 (constant dollars)	109,032
Total (rough estimate in 2004 dollars)	~7,000,000

* Includes small amounts for Central America.

**For provision of Noguchi vaccine.

***Includes $166 for smallpox control in Veracruz.

+ Training station expenditures not included in this résumé.

Sources: Mexico, "Expenditures by Subjects and Years, July 1, 1913–December 11, 1940 (Corrected Statement as of 9/28/42)," RG 2-Stacks, Box 561, Folder 3814, RFA. Also see "Cantidades Gastadas por la Fundación Rockefeller en su Cooperación con el Gobierno Mexicano de 1918 a 1938," RG Lázaro Cárdenas, Folder 534.1/1084, Archivo General de la Nación. Note: expenditures in 1942–51 for malaria control, nutrition studies, and health units were minor.

of public works, health programs, and propaganda designed to convince Latin Americans to support the Allies, to mobilize wartime resources, and to help prepare Latin American economies for postwar development.[29] By the late 1940s these "cooperative public health services" employed some 8,000 health workers across the region and had sponsored 600 fellows to study abroad.

The extension of Roosevelt's "Good Neighbor" policy from noninterventionist diplomacy to "no-strings attached" infrastructure-building required government-size resources—the equivalent of hundreds of millions of dollars today—unavailable to even the largest foundations. Like other philanthropies, the RF played its role in this solidarity building effort: in addition to organizing the MAP, it had stepped up cultural and educational exchanges between Latin America and the United States, which the State Department had requested in the late 1930s.[30]

In 1943, the IIAA came to Mexico, officially marking the end of the dispute over Mexican compensation to U.S. companies for the oil nationalization.[31] The IIAA's first five-year agreement with Mexico entailed U.S. government expenditures of $5 million ($48.5 million in 2004 dollars) on health, transportation, and sanitation, over five times—inflation adjusted—the amount that the IHD had spent on Mexico during the course of more than two decades (see table 5.1).[32]

Influenced by the IHD's operations in Latin America, and even though "cooperative" was part of the program's name—the U.S. government had neither the patience nor the experience to develop bona fide cooperative programs. In Mexico, the IIAA stuck to large-scale infrastructural projects including malaria dredging, water supply and drainage systems, hospital and health center construction, operating costs for tuberculosis and venereal disease clinics, equipment purchase, and road building. It relied almost exclusively on U.S. funds, materials, and technical experts, often bypassing government authorities.[33] The IIAA eschewed subtle or less visible efforts. Even its collaboration with Walt Disney on health education films, shown around the country by rural health brigades, was deemed too expensive for the results obtained.[34] The focus on public works also meant that the IIAA could pay little attention to local conditions or needs. Visiting IHD officer Hugh Smith criticized it for "undertak[ing] DDT campaigns without preliminary investigation of malaria incidence."[35] The IIAA's presence provoked IHD discomfort for further reasons.

Like the IIAA, the RF was conscious of the byproducts of its activities: generating goodwill, promoting democracy, and sharing U.S. scientific expertise. In a sense, RF sanitarians saw themselves as making up for the blunders of U.S. economic interests and foreign policy. From its inception, the RF had claimed to operate as a "scientific and humanitarian agency without connection with [the U.S.] government or with private business." Early on, according to IHD deputy John Ferrell, Mexico and other Latin American nations "did not understand this policy, but in due course they did, with the result that the Division has been welcomed by a government even at times when it might have issues with the United States or with American business corporations."[36]

The IHD was not interested in either joining or competing against the IIAA, and IHD men repeatedly criticized its operating methods. As Smith remarked,

> If we intend to go on pioneering, we have to risk failure, but often get a big return. Government agencies can hardly do this. They play safe by grafting a service operated by Americans with plenty of funds, assured of success. We build up a local group and a service the country can carry on.

When government agencies withdraw, however, "the service wilts." For the IHD, "Nothing really lives until it can reproduce itself," a goal this officer thought unattainable by the IIAA. In Latin America, "The IIAA thanks the government for their cooperation instead of vice versa. The principal objective is to better relations, not to improve and strengthen health services."[37]

If the IIAA succeeded in its mission of propaganda—leaving Mexico and other Latin American countries with U.S.-built roads, hospitals, and sanitary systems, not to mention a more positive attitude toward their northern neighbor, the IHD believed it left something on a different order. According to the RF's own assessments, it was the IHD that had played an instrumental role in solidifying Mexico's commitment to modern public health, accompanied by the necessary administrative apparatus, service delivery capacity, research institutions, and several generations of personnel who could ensure that these innovations would endure.

Nationalizing Health and Social Security in Mexico

The year 1943 was a benchmark in Mexico's commitment to public health irrespective of international cooperation. First, the DSP and the Department of Welfare merged to form the Secretariat Public of Health and Welfare (Secretaría de Salubridad y Asistencia; SSA),[38] with expanded powers, purview, and purse and "charged with the health of the entire population."[39] The DSP's elevation to the cabinet level meant that public health was further institutionalized, enabling previously tottering initiatives—such as the School of Public Health—to find firmer ground. The second development was the passage of long-awaited legislation establishing the Mexican Institute of Social Security (IMSS), which provided state health insurance, retirement, and other benefits to industrial workers.[40] The IMSS was the result of the 1917 Constitution's call for universal social security measures, and had been proposed by various legislators since the 1920s.[41] Certainly there were deficiencies: a multi-tiered, fragmented social welfare system was created with employment sector determining coverage.[42] By placing particular groups of laborers in different schemes (several smaller social security systems predated the IMSS: for the armed forces in 1926, petroleum workers in 1935, railroad workers in 1936–38, and one for civil servants founded in 1960) and

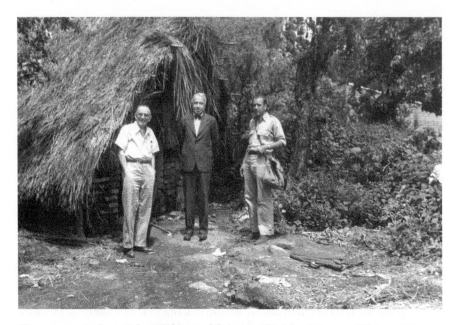

Figure 5.3. Left to right: RF Natural Sciences Division Director Warren Weaver, RF President Raymond Fosdick, and RF officer Dr. Wilbur Downs in Mexico, late 1940s. Courtesy of the Rockefeller Archive Center.

leaving agricultural, service, and informal sector workers to rely on the perennially inadequate resources of the SSA.[43] The IMSS also repeated some of the DSP's slowness in extending services beyond Mexico City.[44]

Though the decade of the 1940s was anticlimactic for the IHD-DSP relationship, this period bespoke the mutual learning that had taken place in previous decades. International health efforts had become intertwined with domestic imperatives, and both IHD and DSP personnel could take pride in the influence of their collaboration upon various agencies of the Mexican government. Under this greater stability, even Miguel Bustamante, the IHD's sometime nemesis, could be called "an old friend" by visiting IHD director George Strode in 1947.[45] In the late 1940s, RF officer Wilbur Downs thrived in his "consiglieri's" role, serving as one of seven members of the National Advisory Board for the malaria campaign,[46] one of five people reorganizing the School of Public Health,[47] and as an informal advisor on a wide range of issues. As another visiting RF official noted, Downs's studies "are being observed carefully by government officials and will no doubt have considerable influence in shaping future policies."[48]

This was also a period in which the Mexican government appeared particularly grateful to the IHD, offering accolades and honors to various IHD men. In

1943, for example, U.S. Surgeon-General Parran, a scientific director of the IHD, was awarded the Eduardo Liceaga medal—the highest public health honor in Mexico—"for service to his own country and to all American states thanks to his spirit of cooperation."[49] In 1950, the Institute of Health and Tropical Diseases dedicated an issue of its journal to RF malariologist Mark Boyd, "for his valuable original contributions, teachings, and accurate judgments concerning the control of malaria."[50] Perhaps this was simply the right time to mark several decades of joint effort, or maybe Mexico better appreciated the IHD in its smaller, informal role. In some ways, the IIAA's big-bucks, little-interaction style of foreign aid—though unsustainable over the long run—was a boon for a country that wanted infrastructure and cash without the operational interference that had characterized the IHD-DSP collaboration.

The Fading of the IHD

The IHD's waning years in Mexico were also its final years in the RF. In 1951—the year the IHD left Mexico—it was absorbed into the RF's new Division of Medicine and Public Health (headed by former Mexico hookworm campaign director Andrew Warren from 1951 to 1954, after which it was once again split into two divisions). For the next years, the RF's international health involvement was confined to scientific consulting to the United Nations (UN) and other small projects.

The IHD was disbanded for several reasons: the majority of national governments around the world had institutionalized public health activities; as African and Caribbean countries achieved independence in subsequent decades, new governments typically drew on health institution templates from the colonial period. Significantly, the WHO was founded in 1948 and—together with its expanded regional office, the PASB (from 1958, PAHO)—had taken over most of the IHD's technical cooperation functions in Latin America and around the world.[51] Many other binational and philanthropic agencies began to enter territory that had once belonged to the IHD. In addition, there were internal grounds for restructuring given that the IHD was the RF's sole field-based division.

Bearing most directly on the IHD's dissolution were geopolitical considerations relating to the Cold War and the developing world's economic and population demands.[52] The United States' Point IV Plan announced by U.S. President Harry Truman in his inauguration speech of January 1949 was designed to fend off the Soviet threat by raising the living standards of the underdeveloped world through the provision of technical skills, knowledge, and equipment. While these plans echoed the RF's development efforts, the new bilateral aid approach pursued political goals far more explicitly than had the RF. Among the justifications for the dissolution of the IHD cited by RF President Chester Barnard in 1950 was that the Point IV program would carry on public health work in "all

underdeveloped areas of the democratic world, on which we have always concentrated," and "Communism is removing great areas which were potential
fields for IHD activity." Most of all, "The U.S. can spend millions where we spend
thousands, and competition at the advisory level will breed friction."[53]

Despite the institutional soul-searching the IHD's dissolution elicited, it was,
after all, a measure of its success—indeed the self-fulfillment of its intention—
that one day it would no longer be needed.

The Diseases Less Traveled

The RF, through the administration of disease campaigns and health projects
around the world, promoted a conceptualization of public health in which the
world of sickness and health was viewed biologically more than socially; understanding of disease causation was often reduced to a single factor; solutions were
mainly technical; and public health personnel were trained medical doctors,
nurses, and engineers with a full-time commitment to public health. This model
was disseminated by RF-trained national experts and through proven, often
dramatic, techniques demonstrating the value of public health, even when the
particular ailment—initially hookworm—was not a leading local problem.
Governments were further enticed into adopting RF-style public health through
budget incentives. Each initiative received seed money from the IHD, which
gradually diminished its contribution over time while financing from local and
national governments increased.

Crucial to the RF's longevity in Mexico and elsewhere was the manner in
which it made its programs attractive to national authorities and its ability to
modify the scope and nature of its involvement as local needs and political conditions changed. While, as we have seen, Mexican counterparts molded IHD
efforts to domestic objectives, an imbalance remained between donor and coop-
erant. It was the IHD that determined the projects for cooperation; in doing so
it adhered to a principle of selecting public health activities with a known track
record, a low cost, a technical solution, the likelihood of feasibility, and the
requirement of a short time period to demonstrate accomplishment.

As important as the question of which disease campaigns the IHD would pursue, then, was which campaigns it would not pursue. Other than deciding when
and whether to work in specific settings, the IHD paid greatest attention to the
actual selection of cooperative activities. Of course, host countries sought to
influence joint projects: from early on, national officials as well as local doctors
and even IHD officers in Mexico pressed the IHD to become involved in a variety of locally determined priorities and questioned its choice of activities. The
interactions and the RF response around three diseases—tuberculosis,
onchocerciasis, and malaria—*not* selected for major collaboration are particularly illustrative of the RF's stance on disease selection.

Tuberculosis

In the 1920s, tuberculosis was a leading cause of death for adults in Mexico, as in much of the world at the time. The problem was clear to health authorities and to the population at large, who witnessed the effects of this debilitating disease among neighbors, coworkers and family members. Although bacteriological advances—beginning with Robert Koch's discovery of the tubercle bacillus in 1882—enhanced the understanding of the transmission and diagnosis of tuberculosis, definitive curative measures did not appear until the mid 1940s, with the development of the antibiotic streptomycin. During the bulk of the IHD's years in Mexico, then, tuberculosis could be addressed mainly through large-scale, collective measures: improved housing, decreased crowding, better ventilation, ample nutrition, and the isolation of patients in tuberculosis sanatoria.[54] Each of these required longtime, community-level investments, with drops in mortality and morbidity evident only after several years of activity. Tuberculosis control could hardly be a worse example for an outside agency eager to rapidly, economically, and through technical means convince officials and the public of the value of public health work.

But physicians in Veracruz had their own ideas. In the mid 1920s, with Veracruz's population having participated in the yellow fever campaign and now cooperating with the hookworm program, local doctors began to push for the RF's support in combating tuberculosis. They began by cleverly appealing to one of the RF's earliest tenets: building onto existing agencies.[55] In early 1926, RF officer Andrew Warren learned that he had been elected president of a local Antituberculosis League during a brief absence from Veracruz. He informed IHD Director Russell that he had refused the position, arguing that it ought to go to a Mexican physician, but league members insisted. When Warren presented the excuse that the RF did not work in the tuberculosis field, the well-informed physicians pointed to the case of France, where the RF had been involved in tuberculosis control during World War I.[56]

With none of the standard excuses working, Russell told Warren that it was best to "formally decline" the invitation and to offer an "explanation so simple even laymen can understand." The goal of the cooperative effort, Russell reminded Warren, was "to improve public health organizations by demonstrating what it is possible to do by coordinating intelligent government efforts." Yellow fever, hookworm, and malaria control provided effective illustrations of how to meet this goal. Tuberculosis, leprosy, and venereal diseases were never to be used, however, because "it takes too many years to show results with chronic infectious diseases, whereas with the others, particularly with hookworm, it is possible to get results in a short time." Thus, it was "improbable" that the RF would "ever finance a cooperative TB project" in Mexico.[57]

This refusal did not mean that tuberculosis would go unaddressed. In 1930, DSP authorities inaugurated a large-scale antituberculosis campaign.[58]

Ironically, by this time, health officials cited a decrease in tuberculosis morbidity and mortality even without a targeted campaign, owing in large measure, they argued, to a gradually improving standard of living.[59]

But the IHD had its own protocol and its own pocketbook to consider. Unlike the negotiated management of its programs—involving field officers, national officials, returned RF fellows, and local staff—the decisions about which disease campaigns should be pursued were made in the New York office. There, RF officials remained indifferent to local pleas and realities, including the observations and experience of their own field officers.[60]

Onchocerciasis

Over time, Mexican officials devised increasingly sophisticated pleas in favor of expanding RF efforts to other disease control efforts—still to little avail. Onchocerciasis—commonly known as river blindness, caused by a parasitic worm and transmitted via black-flies that breed in flowing waters in tropical climates—stands out as a disease that the IHD declined to support despite the Mexican government's repeated requests for assistance at the highest diplomatic levels. In 1935, U.S. Ambassador to Mexico Josephus Daniels relayed to both the U.S. State Department and the RF a conversation he had had with DSP chief José Siurob regarding onchocerciasis in the southern states of Oaxaca, Chiapas, Campeche, and the territory of Quintana Roo. Siurob had strongly praised the RF's work in Mexico and suggested that with funding from the RF or another philanthropy, the Mexican government would be able to sponsor research on the disease and a treatment.[61] IHD officer Bailey added that—though limited to a few states—onchocerciasis was spreading and was a growing economic concern for Mexico.[62] But Wilbur Sawyer, director of the IHD beginning in 1935, held that even "if Onchocerciasis is really an important public health problem in Mexico and the authorities desire assistance in working out a control program," the RF should not enter a project "in a new disease unless it is either a phase of some general rural health program or a study of great promise which would otherwise be neglected."[63]

In the meantime, the Cárdenas administration launched its own initiative, transforming the DSP's mobile onchocerciasis brigades in Oaxaca into a large project to relocate inhabitants to areas where they were less likely to be infected.[64] In three years the resettlement project "did not achieve its medical objectives,"[65] and President Cárdenas remained concerned about onchocerciasis as he was leaving office in 1940. When Bailey asked him how the IHD might render further assistance to Mexico, Cárdenas noted that he was pleased with the agency's work and "loath to ask for more aid" but would like to see onchocerciasis "scientifically studied."[66]

Again the IHD turned down this request. Until the late 1940s, the Mexican government campaigned unsuccessfully to obtain RF backing for onchocerciasis research, using more and more inventive approaches. In 1947, not long after Miguel Bustamante became its secretary-general, the PASB published a 340-page bibliography of onchocerciasis studies in Mexico and Guatemala, including a large number of articles in international journals designed to raise awareness of the disease.[67] The same year, Manuel Gamio, director of Mexico's Institute of Indigenous Affairs, advanced the case that onchocerciasis was an occupational disease. Because it was endemic in coffee-growing regions, Gamio reasoned, it was the responsibility of the United States to help control the disease, since the United States was the primary consumer and distributor of coffee.[68] Once again the RF demurred.

The IHD's inaction on onchocerciasis, even when its own officers argued in favor of collaboration, underscores the notion that the disease campaigns and locales chosen were limited to those "which were guaranteed of success."[69] It also shows how active, persistent, and creative Mexico was in seeking RF funds, expertise, and research support.

Malaria

One of the puzzles of the IHD's involvement in Mexico is why its investment in malaria control never went beyond small research projects. Beginning in the 1910s, the RF was engaged in malaria campaigns in the United States, Latin America, Europe, Asia, and elsewhere, employing antilarval strategies—such as draining and filling ditches and swamps, placing larvicidal fish in water containers, dusting Paris green, and petrolizing stagnant bodies of water—as well as administering quinine treatment to individuals.[70] Like yellow fever campaigns, malaria work typically adhered to a command-and-control approach that combined hierarchical organization with military discipline. In Mexico, however, the RF's concern with malaria remained incidental to its other activities.[71]

From before the RF's yellow fever campaign in Mexico, the DSP's yellow fever and malaria control activities had formed part of a single Antilarval Service; as we saw in chapter 2, once yellow fever was under control in 1923, DSP officials requested that the RF continue with cooperative efforts against malaria. This interest was supported by RF yellow fever officers, who repeatedly cited malaria as a major problem. The RF stalled its responses to these requests, saying that a national survey—which it did not conduct until 1936[72]—was needed before a campaign could be considered.[73]

Following the IHD's late 1920s shift in favor of scientific investigation, it began sponsoring small-scale malaria research projects at several local health units in Veracruz and Morelos. Starting in 1931, the RF sent U.S. malariologist Dr. Mark Boyd on periodic visits to advise these malaria studies, which entailed collection of climatological, entomological, and clinical information, and surveys of breeding sites and local disease prevalence.[74] Boyd worked closely with noted Mexican malariologists such as Galo Soberón y Parra,[75] but the collaboration did not induce the IHD to back a full-fledged malaria campaign.

The Cárdenas administration, unwilling to wait for the RF, made malaria a top priority. In 1935, a national malaria campaign was organized to confront this "major public health problem afflicting 1/16th of the population."[76] Financed in part by a one-cent postage stamp, the campaign also received contributions from state governors and industries in malaria-infested areas. The campaign solicited private companies to assist with sanitary engineering, while communities were invited to participate in swamp cleanups.[77]

The DSP's malaria campaign had three components—education, engineering projects, and the treatment of individuals with malaria. Like the RF's hookworm campaign, the malaria effort held that little could be accomplished unless peasants and workers were convinced of the danger that malaria presented: knowledge about the disease and the mosquito vector would enable quinine treatment and mosquito extermination to succeed. An intense educational campaign began in schools, fields, workplaces, and homes through lectures, pamphlets, films, and recordings. Scores of malariologists, technicians, and sanitary engineers were trained; the DSP sent one staff member to study methods used in Florida and Louisiana. Sanitary engineering activities included swamp drainage, canalization, and the elimination of stagnant water. Malaria dispensaries were set up in the most severely affected regions to provide free treatment to the indigenous population and agricultural laborers.[78] The Cárdenas administration claimed that these combined efforts drastically reduced malaria mortality, halving deaths to 15,000 in the first year alone.

The Mexican malaria campaign incorporated certain IHD strategies, but it also emphasized access to care, ensuring that quinine was "within the reach of the poorest classes of people."[79] At the first regional conference for the national malaria campaign, held in 1938, sixty-six conclusions were reached, including the need to cultivate rice using the English system of periodic irrigation, to develop "hygienic" houses with mosquito screens, to coordinate local antilarval services, to establish more quinine plantations, to increase research, and to mandate use of bed-netting. In addition, the conference attendees called for assistance from the IHD equivalent to that granted to Italy.[80]

Around the same time, the RF renewed its interest in malaria research, in part responding to Mexico's malaria campaign. In 1937 the IHD sent malariologist Dr. Walter Earle to Morelos for a special research program.[81] For three years he studied malaria control methods, including mosquito trapping and pesticide use.[82] He developed an experimental watering method for rice fields, which used intermittent spraying to drain excess water and prevent the proliferation of mosquito breeding sites. This method differed from the traditional method of watering rice fields: flooding them with large amounts of water, which became

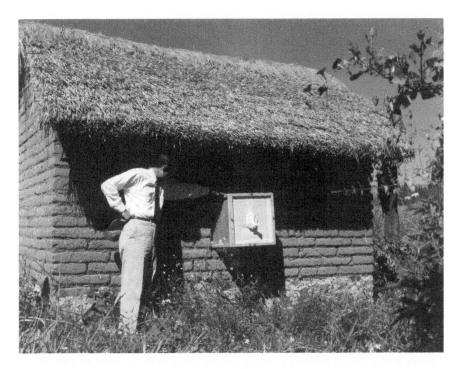

Figure 5.4. Mosquito-trapping methods in Mexico, late 1940s. Courtesy of the Rockefeller Archive Center.

stagnant over a period of weeks, attracted mosquito larvae, and exacerbated malaria.[83] In the early 1930s, the DSP and IHD had tried to limit the cultivation of rice to a distance of at least one and a half kilometers from Morelos towns in order to reduce human contact with mosquitoes but were met with strong opposition. [84] Given the sensitivity surrounding rice cultivation in Morelos—the nation's second biggest rice producer—the IHD had been forced to suspend its malaria activities. Once again, in the late 1930s, the IHD ran into problems. Earle had not sufficiently coordinated his efforts with local authorities, and his first rice paddy experiment was a technical failure because the system did not drain properly. Moreover, most local rice growers refused to participate because they feared that the new system would create more work for them and that the drained soil would quickly become impoverished, causing crop output to diminish.[85]

Ironically, in both the early and late 1930s, the IHD had set up its main malaria station in one of the states where it was least needed. With 192 malaria deaths in 1933, Morelos trailed in malaria mortality behind sixteen other states, some of which had over ten times the number (and much higher rates) of malaria deaths.[86] Nonetheless, as the center of the IHD's supervised district for local health services, Morelos was a convenient locale for malaria studies. The Mexican entomologist assigned to Earle, RF fellow Luis Vargas, believed that malaria was targeted because it was a disease that incapacitated agricultural laborers, and that Morelos was chosen due to the agrarian unrest there.[87] According to RF officer Bailey, another reason for the focus on malaria in Morelos was the state's growth as a destination for American tourists.[88]

After Earle's departure in 1939, the Mexican government took over his efforts.[89] Although it avoided a campaign, the IHD would not end its malaria story in Mexico for some time. Over the years, all of the RF's men in Mexico recognized the importance of malaria in Mexico. When Henry Carr began his tour as hookworm campaign director in 1926, he thought that malaria, not hookworm, was Mexico's biggest disease concern. Upon his departure from Mexico in 1940, Bailey called malaria the "outstanding medical problem of the country," but he considered the DSP's reported 20,000 annual malaria deaths "an exaggeration," because, he said, the majority of these cases had been attended only by lay persons and had probably been misdiagnosed.[90] At the same time, he held that the national campaign had been ineffectual because malaria's "control is politically handled." Still, "unless radical changes take place next year, I doubt if the Foundation could or should enter into this problem."[91] The RF agreed.

So the Mexican government pursued the fight against malaria alone, to considerable popular acclaim. By the mid 1940s, the campaign had a budget of 8 million pesos ($12.4 million in 2004 dollars).[92] Numerous local organizations wrote and begged the malaria campaign to work in their communities;[93] even an enlarged budget was unable to satisfy this demand.

In 1943, the RF returned to malaria, somewhat circuitously. During World War II, the RF became involved in DDT research, with the world's first field trial of DDT as a louse insecticide carried out in Morelos.[94] Previously studied in the IHD's louse-control laboratory in New York and at a conscientious objectors' camp in New Hampshire, the insecticide needed to be tested for community-wide control of louse-borne typhus "in anticipation of serious [wartime] typhus fever epidemics in Europe and elsewhere."[95] After a dubious consent process, five villages in Morelos were selected for insecticide spraying followed by deliberate louse infestation to test the insecticide's effectiveness. Only one village had actually harbored typhus prior to the experiment. A year-long effort showed that DDT was effective in controlling louse-borne typhus when sprayed inside houses and on human clothing (usually on the sash traditionally worn by Mexican men and women).

Two years later the U.S. Department of Agriculture asked the RF and the Mexican government to collaborate with experiments on the use of DDT as a residual spray for malaria. Though studies in Arkansas had proven DDT's ability to kill *Anopheles* mosquitoes for more than four months after houses were sprayed, the Department of Agriculture believed that the low incidence of malaria in the United States prevented a definitive study of DDT's effectiveness.[96] So in 1945, the ceilings and walls of most of the buildings in two Morelos villages were sprayed, and in subsequent years the population was monitored for malaria cases and, among children, enlarged spleen rates (which indicated the presence of malaria parasites in the blood). After two years, the mosquito population had been reduced by an estimated 75 percent and the cases of malaria had plunged by 90 percent. By 1947, the RF concluded that "now it is not only possible but economically practicable to free large regions, whole states and even continents, from the mosquito nuisance—and in doing so, to wipe out malaria."[97]

The results of the RF's civilian experiments in Morelos reverberated around the world, but in Mexico, full-fledged malaria campaigns were left to Mexicans. The RF limited itself to research. Until the IHD's departure from Mexico in 1951, it remained committed to malaria investigation in Baja California, Morelos, Guerrero, Nayarit, and Veracruz. In the middle and late 1940s, together with Mexican researchers, IHD representative Wilbur Downs conducted studies testing spleen rates and mosquito presence before and after DDT spraying in dozens of villages. Comparative studies of DDT's effectiveness on a variety of building materials were also conducted.[98] Downs and various colleagues published numerous articles in Mexican scientific journals on the technical control of malaria.[99] Many of these antimalaria strategies influenced and were institutionalized internationally with the creation of the WHO's Global Malaria Eradication Program in 1955.[100]

Thus, while the IHD participated in malaria campaigns in numerous settings, it used Mexico purely as a convenient locale for research—albeit with global implications—without becoming involved in actually controlling malaria. Perhaps the IHD believed that the DSP had the wherewithal and experience from the yellow fever and hookworm campaigns to run the campaign without RF collaboration, or malaria was seen as too unwieldy to combat in Mexico. The RF nevertheless had no qualms about using Mexicans as experimental subjects, taking advantage of popular goodwill generated by its long cooperation in Morelos. So, although it remained without an RF cooperative campaign, Mexico became an important testing ground for DDT, malaria's—and indeed international health's—most powerful mid-century technical weapon.

In the end, whether petitions for participation came from the local level, as in the case of tuberculosis; the presidency, as with onchocerciasis; or IHD men, Mexican doctors, and political leaders, as in the case of malaria, IHD campaign selection took place in New York. This does not mean the problems remained unaddressed— quite the contrary. Moreover, although the IHD was unmovable on disease selection, for the activities it did choose, negotiations were anything but one-sided.

¿Qué Pasó?

In Mexico, possibly more than in any other setting where the RF operated, the international health relationship endured amid contentious bilateral relations,

Table 5.2. IHB/D expenditures in Latin American countries, 1913–40 (in constant dollars)

Country	Expenditure: In-Country Activities and Fellowships	Expenditure: Fellowships, 1915–40 (and number awarded)
Argentina	108,876.79	2,417.76 (2)
Brazil	6,637,714.43	204,186.25 (77)
Colombia	518,780.37	40,745.28 (18)
Costa Rica	221,622.84	27,250.74 (15)
Cuba	143,130.83	24,434.22 (12)
Ecuador	98,616.09	2,717.92 (1)
El Salvador	80,749.44	15,105.52 (10)
Guatemala	175,361.24	24,803.92 (12)
Haiti	13,196.63	1,350.67 (1)
Honduras	23,004.08	5,660.84 (3)
Jamaica	481,236.62	34,328.52 (17)
Mexico	772,606.31	112,111.68 (54)*
Nicaragua	195,051.31	32,819.92 (14)
Panama	343,171.40	39,852.85 (21)
Paraguay	87,885.54	8,153.75 (3)
Peru	136,880.18	4,858.88 (3)
Puerto Rico	491,526.32	71,292.36 (34)
Venezuela	50,369.09	35,290.81 (16)

*Includes travel grants to government officials.
Source: International Health Division, "Appropriations for Work in Latin America, July 1, 1913 to December 11, 1940, Summary and Fellowship Tables," RG 2-Stacks 1941, Box 561, Folder 3814, RFA.

ongoing political tensions, and deep prejudices on both sides of the Rio Grande. At the same time, Mexico was the country in Latin America most attracted to U.S. precepts and in some domains beginning to resemble its northern neighbors more than its southern. But, as we have seen, Mexico forged its international ties on its own terms, holding a long record of political and professional defiance of the U.S. The French bacteriologist, Charles Nicolle, invited to Mexico in 1931 by DSP chief Rafael Silva to investigate whether European and Mexican typhus were different entities, proved an acute observer of Mexican-U.S. relations:

> Our [France's] influence is predominantly in literature, art and the pure sciences. We have but one rival in terms of cultural influence: the United States. This rival is of the most dangerous type because it represents, for many young Mexicans, a civilization better adapted to contemporary life than ours appears to be. There is no doubt that

Mexico's youth sees in this civilization above all its brilliant appearance, its economic power, and its wealth. On the other hand, no Mexican, unless he is an accomplice of these foreigners, can ignore the danger that the hand of this formidable neighbor, his money, and his intrigues poses to the independence of their country. In Mexico, Americans are admired, dreaded, and detested.[101]

Throughout the 1920s and 1930s, the RF maintained a similarly ambivalent position regarding Mexico. It was considered a "backward" country, worthy of special attention,[102] yet it was placed within the IHD's North American region, a statement and level of expectation that had more than cartographic meaning. Mexico was repeatedly compared to the American South after the Civil War, sharing "problems relating to economics, education, health, agriculture, and transportation." While Mexico's situation was deemed more extreme, Ferrell argued, "the potentialities of the Mexican masses [were] promising."[103] The RF's outlook for Mexico was far more positive than for most other developing countries,[104] and the IHD's commitment to institutionalizing public health was more sustained in Mexico than anywhere else in Latin America, notwithstanding its larger investment in Brazil (see table 5.2).[105]

Certainly, the form of the RF's programs was heavily influenced by relations between the United States and Mexico and by the preconceptions each party held of the other. Mexican political leaders initially suspected the United States—and in turn the RF—of hiding economic intentions and of interfering with national sovereignty. Many RF officers typecast the Mexican character as conniving, backward, and difficult. Mediating Mexican doctors disputed these stereotypes and contested particular RF health policies—such as the course of hookworm treatment and the design of local health services.

For the RF, the political geography of disease sparked its interest in Mexico: first, due to the potential for epidemic disease to affect commerce and the U.S. population; and second, owing to the possibility that proliferating social and health ills could further radicalize Mexico. In spite of binational hostilities, the RF's generously funded yellow fever campaign managed to overcome Mexican wariness. Lasting less than three years, the campaign served as a fruitful and extravagant mutual introduction, successfully eliminating the disease, earning popularity among politicians and the local populace alike, and sealing a long-term bond. The subsequent hookworm campaign gave a dose of reality to all: the RF discovered the challenges of working in tumultuous Mexico, and the DSP found out the scope and nature of what the RF had to offer. The two parties decided to stay together. Playing a modest yet meaningful role, the RF helped create rural health services where none existed and stimulated popular support for public health.

For Mexico, the 1928 shift from peripatetic disease campaigns to the establishment of permanent local health services was notable on several counts. Until the late 1930s, Mexico was the main setting outside North America (and Puerto

Rico) to participate in the local health units program, and the Mexican commitment survived political turmoil, philosophical battles, and funding crises. With yellow fever controlled, the hookworm campaign having increased the appetite for permanent rural health services, and other ailments requiring far too great an investment, the RF could simply have pulled out rather than contend with Mexico's challenging circumstances.

But the development of local health services presented a rare opportunity for the RF to help mold the local health services of a country that was poised to meet the public health demands of its people. In the RF's eyes, Mexico needed its guidance. Improvements in U.S.-Mexican relations resulting from a temporary resolution of the problem of foreign ownership of subsoil rights in the late 1920s framed this renewed invitation to the RF, but by no means was the DSP a supplicant. Local units became a lively venue for the continued interaction and competition between the RF and Mexico.

When Mexico's political radicalization during the Cárdenas administration made the RF reluctant to expand its in-country presence, the IHD turned to fellowships and training as a means of heightening its engagement in Mexican public health.

None of these initiatives was without conflict over public health approaches, strategies, and practices, but none was without possibility of resolution. On occasion the RF's concerns were indistinguishable from those of the DSP. Because Mexico increased its institutional commitment to public health around the same time when RF activities peaked, it is difficult to untangle who influenced whom and what derived from broader international health developments of the day.

This is not to say that the IHD-DSP relationship was uniformly effective. Health unit employees never adopted the full-time principle, instead following the longstanding practice of working for the government from 8 a.m. to 2:30 p.m. and operating a private medical practice in the afternoon, in order to supplement their salaries.[106] The IHD's desire to remove public health from the "constant interference of politicians"[107] was naïve at best, notwithstanding local assurances. IHD officers seemed to have trouble carrying out their oversight role and lobbying and bureaucratic responsibilities simultaneously, and the IHD office moved back and forth between the capital and the field in an attempt to strike the right balance. In the 1920s and 1930s, RF expectations of local financial contributions often exceeded the contents of municipal and state coffers, causing friction among the various levels of government. It is only in recent years that this "decentralized" form of health services delivery has been taken up again, and Mexico's federal government has proven slow to cede its power to subnational levels.[108] In remaining wedded to the local cofinancing model in the 1930s, the IHD misread the centralizing tendencies of Mexico's revolutionary reconstruction.

Under the expansionary Cárdenas administration, Mexican officials were also compelled to consider progressive public health ideas in crude financial terms, lamenting, for example, that it was budgetary limitations that prevented the DSP from extending the comprehensive Veracruz local health model to all of the country's municipalities. The DSP projects that were grounded in left-wing ideas—most notably rural medical internships and ejidal units—also represented a pragmatic and frugal use of scarce health resources.

Despite the IHD's inflated rhetoric of its own influence on and "infiltration" of the Mexican health establishment, its most significant achievement was its very survival in Mexico. In this sense, the IHD's patience and endurance—and the stable relationship it had developed with the DSP—were its greatest assets, for the paths that were marked during the revolutionary period set the country's public health course for many years ahead.

Would Mexico have created a comparable system and understanding of public health even without the RF? The Mexican medical elite was long tied to European medical teaching and research, and the Mexican government already favored—at least in theory—many of the modern public health interventions that had begun to emerge in the late nineteenth century. Perhaps Mexico would have heeded a stronger social medicine model had European influences persisted. On another front, given that most rural and some urban populations remained attached to traditional healers and were rarely reached by medical elites, a happier hybridization of systems might have been possible instead of the attempted displacement of indigenous healers. Certain autochthonous developments—such as the ejidal medical units—that might have formed the basis for an alternative public health system were perhaps doomed more by Mexico's conservative shift around 1940 than by RF initiatives per se, although the continued presence of the RF undoubtedly helped reinforce the hierarchical health services path over the ejidal community development approach.

Ultimately, Mexico and the RF proved dynamic partners for one another in a decidedly postcolonial relationship. While the RF shared with colonial efforts an interest in spreading Western science and values, building public health bureaucracies, improving health conditions to raise productivity and decrease the potential of local unrest, and protecting commercial routes from epidemic disease, it could not impose on Mexico. Formally invited by the national government, the IHD could not afford to be overly conflictual, coercive, or even persuasive in an unwelcome manner, for it could be uninvited at any moment (as it was from Venezuela in 1934).[109] In comparison to colonial efforts, the RF's financial outlays were small and it could remain behind the scenes as necessary. Unlike colonial or national governments, the RF was not formally accountable to political constituencies at home or abroad. This independence gave it the freedom to make decisions quickly and maintain flexibility in policies and program implementation but left it dependent on the DSP and other domestic parties for legitimacy. The marriage between the RF and Mexico was thus elastic and mutually beneficial, even as the identity of each was at times subordinate to the relationship itself.

Who, What, and How

Like all relationships, the union between the DSP and the IHD was affected by a range of dealings: assessing the years of cooperation in Mexico requires a return visit to the parties that interacted with the IHD and DSP separately and jointly. Here we look at the goals and expectations, the interplay, and the results obtained by many of these actors: Mexican physicians, mid level health workers, senior health officials, the Mexican presidency, the U.S. government, IHD officers on the ground, midwives and healers, peasants, and small-town Mexicans. Combined, these perspectives provide a sense of international health that transcends cultural imperialism, charity, or disinterested cooperation. Here we consider international health along the sometimes chaotic lines of negotiated aid from the highest diplomatic levels, through middlemen experts and administrators, to community-level health workers and peasants. It was the give-and-take between the IHD and the DSP as well as with local actors, one by one or in groups, that most marked the experience. Neither imposed from above nor innocently philanthropic, the RF's international health was shaped and reshaped by multiple parties with intersecting agendas.

We begin with Mexican politics and political leaders. Due to Mexico's long and adversarial history with the United States, an official invitation to a U.S. agency—albeit a philanthropic one—was a calculated matter. Following a bloody revolutionary decade punctuated by U.S. occupation and intervention, a joint campaign with the RF—particularly given Rockefeller oil connections— seemed at best a contradiction. Although divided on matters of land reform and labor relations, the Mexican people had become unified over the quest for economic and political sovereignty. By late 1920, President Alvaro Obregón realized that the RF's offer to help quell a frightening outbreak of yellow fever in Veracruz could turn into an opportunity, if managed astutely. Indeed the three main (post)revolutionary presidents, Obregón, Calles, and Cárdenas, all understood the value of visible public health activities (and accompanying employment opportunities) in furthering the standing and authority of the central government. Particularly in the 1920s, public health programs organized to meet at least some of the revolutionary demands of peasants and small-town dwellers appeared more feasible than large-scale land reform.

Public health lent itself to foreign participation more than did education, given the latter's national-identity-building mission. By the mid 1930s—even with Mexico well on its way to institutionalizing public health—the administration of Lázaro Cárdenas decided that the IHD offered useful resources and expertise, and his administration actively pursued the agency. IHD cooperation provided a means by which extensive—even revolutionary—Cardenista innovations could be jumpstarted domestically and showcased to the international community.

U.S. diplomatic officials said little about the specifics of RF aid, although ambassadors often served as conduits between the Mexican government and the

RF, and IHD officers served as ersatz diplomats during the 1920s when the two nations were at odds over oil rights. The State Department also encouraged philanthropic support for cultural and educational exchanges between the countries. The strongest indicator of U.S. government admiration for IHD efforts was the centrality of public health in the IIAA's wartime investments in Latin America.

Larger political concerns were also reflected in the changing interaction between the RF and the DSP. Somewhat timid in the early 1920s while political turmoil in Veracruz threatened the RF's programs, DSP leaders later courted the RF without appearing submissive. RF pressure, high expenditures in an era of scarce resources, and the birth of a new dependence upon outside models, technology, and work patterns, seemed, at least temporarily, a necessary step in Mexico's public health and social progress. Most public health leaders in Mexico agreed that the expertise of the RF could be channeled—albeit carefully—to national goals without threatening the country's sovereignty.

By the late 1920s, DSP officials began to resent the IHD's command-and-control approach and delayed further agreements until the terms became more equitable. Under Cárdenas, these dilemmas seemed to resolve themselves; RF cooperation had become so familiar that the IHD's policy differences with DSP programs—which by now had grown far larger and weightier—became marginal to the institutional relationship. Public health's "scientific basis of observation and experimentation" was fully accepted by the sanitary establishment,[110] as was the preeminence of professional training,[111] the need for technical expertise,[112] and the RF's role in these endeavors.[113]

Paradoxically, the IHD became both more and less important to Mexico over time. One indicator of its diminished importance is the coverage of IHD programs in annual DSP reports and presidential *Memorias*. In the 1925–28 *Memoria* of the DSP under Bernardo Gastélum, for example, the joint hookworm campaign was the subject of one of its twelve chapters,[114] whereas in José Siurob's 1934–40 *Memoria* the RF was mentioned only in passing in a much longer report.[115] The RF, in turn, was satisfied to remain "discretely anonymous"; so there was "no offence to local pride."[116]

From the perspective of Mexico's medical elites, the invitation to the RF demonstrated a firm belief in the power of science to improve society. Tremendous optimism had been generated by advances in medicine and technology, and Mexican professionals recognized RF cooperation as an unparalleled opportunity—certainly not one proffered by European powers—for the development of scientific public health methods and as a means of meeting the health demands of the population. RF programs presented a chance for technological progress, international interaction, graduate training, new positions, and an expanded purview for public health generally. For most Mexican physicians, professional interests overshadowed concerns of foreign interference, and many cited the dearth of trained personnel as a leading public health problem well into the 1940s. These doctors, already trained in Western medicine, stood to gain in prestige through the increased legitimacy and reach of allopathic medicine. Likewise, Mexico's small community of professional nurses recognized the advantages of advanced training and expertise, even as IHD personnel disdained Mexico's nursing profession as a whole.

Mexican doctors who worked with RF projects, RF fellows, and public health trainees—personally armed with new knowledge and skills—were the group most favorable to IHD cooperation.[117] They also understood that the public health precepts they had studied could be selectively emulated,[118] adapted to local conditions, or even ignored. And some fellows—most notably Miguel Bustamante with his Veracruz health unit and key role in developing the "Coordinated Health Services in the States"—learned to play the DSP and IHD against one another, upping the ante for public health.

Still, a small number of elite physicians intertwined scientific concerns with national pride in opposing RF strategies on grounds of medical safety, on competing visions of how best to meet the nation's health needs, and on the basis of Mexico's own traditions in the public health arena.

Predictably, IHD programs met with a less hospitable reception by other healers. Upstaged small-town doctors resented the new dependency upon and public expectations of medical technology. IHD officers deemed most traditional healers to be primitive and superstitious, and the IHD joined the Mexican medical profession's efforts to isolate them. "Empirical" midwives faced a mixed fate. Because of a shortage of physicians, the IHD sidelined its preference for physician-attended births while furthering, as much as possible, a biologically and technically oriented childbirth process. Although they were blamed by IHD units for their sanitary and extramedical practices, midwives were more co-opted than shunned. Lured to training sessions at the sanitary units, the midwives were provided with equipment and physiological and hygienic knowledge while being encouraged to abandon their social and spiritual roles. Still, decades later, many such midwives voiced appreciation for their incorporation into the country's health services formal structure, especially as midwifery might instead have been made illegal.

For the townsfolk and surrounding area peasants where the IHD and DSP operated jointly, the programs were for the most part welcomed, at least as indicated by official attendance records at hookworm clinics and health units. Purportedly asking for nothing in return, the new public health activities earned appreciation from communities whose health conditions had long been ignored by the government. Even so, we might surmise that the IHD's programs were the object of mixed sentiments. The interlopers brought relief from various health problems—not to mention mosquitoes and flies—but used alien or even dangerous methods and could upset existing structures of social authority.

Opportunistic acceptance versus outright refusal is too dichotomized an approach to understanding Mexico's interaction with the RF. Here we must return to the question of local interpretation, shaping, and appropriation. Shrewd local health unit workers developed their own explanations of the criteria the IHD used in deciding on its demonstration and research diseases. One nurse cited technical feasibility and labor productivity as the IHD's deciding factors, explaining that yellow fever's or malaria's insect vector can be interrupted, in contrast to diarrhea, whose multiple causes are more difficult to control. Moreover, "a man with fever cannot work, but a man with diarrhea can."[119] Returned RF fellow Vargas concurred, noting that "If it did not keep people from working, the IHD did not consider a disease to be important."[120]

On another front, many Veracruz peasants who refused to spend their own scant resources on latrines eventually utilized community latrines constructed by the hookworm brigades, provided they were in convenient locales—thus "accepting" latrines on their own terms. There were also many borrowings back and forth between the IHD and DSP over the use of semi-trained professionals, the scope of public health outreach, and the responsibility of federal versus local government for health services.

This dance of perspectives remains incomplete without an examination of IHD doctors in the field. Mostly hailing from rural, religious backgrounds, these men arrived at the RF convinced that science and public health could transform uneducated peoples and modernize societies. Even before they were posted overseas, officers became true believers in the IHD's rhetoric and programs. Convinced that disease campaigns and local health services could dramatically convert downtrodden people into productive members of society, IHD officers—together with returned RF fellows—became the organization's most valuable, but potentially counterproductive, tool; their daily presence, conviction, and technical and administrative capacity were instrumental in generating local enthusiasm.

The different personalities of officers made them suited to particular epochs. Andrew Warren's brash persistence made him an ideal hookworm campaign director under adverse conditions in Veracruz. Once the situation became calmer, however, his style interfered with the more delicate diplomacy required in the late 1920s. Charles Bailey was a consummate supporter of sanitary units through political thick and thin; he faithfully—and naively—shepherded the health units through the early Cárdenas administration when the IHD was on the verge of pulling out. When the IHD failed to react to the nationalization of oil in 1938, Bailey was nonplussed. Trapped between his support for the local health unit model and his abhorrence of Cárdenas's nationalization and the ongoing labor unrest, Bailey's conviction turned to despondency.

It is perhaps Henry Carr who best reveals the critical role played by IHD officers in the RF-Mexico relationship. Politically and technically adroit, Carr spent two periods in Mexico. On his first tour in 1924, he was a neophyte officer conducting a hookworm survey. His ambiguous findings on disease prevalence did not alter the IHD's decision to carry out a hookworm campaign. When Carr returned to Mexico several years later, after completing graduate public health study, he was fully convinced of the value of hookworm work. But it was his recognition of Mexico's broader needs beyond hookworm—likely prompted by the DSP's priorities—that helped marshal the IHD's interest in permanent health units to replace the hookworm campaign.

Still, Carr had not forgotten his hookworm lessons. In the late 1940s, as the IHD was deciding on its future in the postwar era, Carr was among dozens of officers who wrote to offer suggestions. He advocated the IHD's return to "fundamentals," especially hookworm control, for "there is just as much hookworm disease in countries where the climate is favorable for it, as there was in 1913 when the Foundation was established. I know because I have seen it all, and there is no public health work that benefits so many people and in such a real and vital way."[121] From the beginning, Wickliffe Rose viewed hookworm as no more than an "entering wedge," but for a true believer like Carr, thirty years in the field convinced him otherwise. This suggests that IHD officers were—and had to be— even more subject to the RF's institutional propaganda than host countries.

In sum, RF philanthropy played an influential role in Mexico's health development, but not a dominant one: it was one of numerous domestic and international tools and forces that Mexicans employed—often in creative ways—to modernize and expand the country's public health capacity. On one level, RF activities were relatively circumscribed. On another level, RF ideas and practices were pitted against other conceptions of health—European, indigenous, national, regional, revolutionary, synthetic—sometimes losing, sometimes winning, often resulting in an amalgam. On yet another level, ongoing Mexican institutional developments and larger political circumstances made the RF's impact smaller than reported in its self-assessment of success. If Mexico's reception of the RF entailed welcoming and accommodation, it was characterized just as much by resistance, negotiation, interpretive molding, and appropriation: Mexico was decidedly *not* between Rockefeller and a hard place.

Just as important, Mexico shaped the RF, and, in turn, the relationship between the two instructed international health itself. These were not lessons on how international health might best balance consent and coercion: those would have derived at least in part from the colonial health experience. Instead, the RF's programs in Mexico demonstrate a more complicated understanding of the multiple actors involved and the extent to which local and transnational actors—including both RF officers on the ground and RF fellows who studied overseas—continuously interacted in making international health cooperation serve its clients and patrons. For these reasons, the legacy of the RF's public health programs in Mexico lives on—in other settings, with other players, and other concerns.

Epilogue

International Health's Convenient Marriage

International health cooperation was an invention of the twentieth century. Not bound by colonial strictures, proselytizing mandates, or military objectives—and enabled by advancements in medicine and public health, international relations, and worldwide scholarly exchange—cooperation between specialized health agencies and willing countries offered a new form of voluntary international interaction. Part diplomacy, part development aid, part propaganda, part cultural imperialism, part economic opportunism, part humanitarianism, part scientific competition, the new international health went beyond the narrow self-interest of imperial powers or the focused agreements on nomenclature or standardization that were forged in the late nineteenth century. Unlike the health-related projects of missionaries, international health cooperation operated along strictly official terms—invited by government authorities through carefully orchestrated agreements. Though health officers may well have believed in their endeavors as much as missionaries did, they were rewarded with a paycheck and a career, not salvation. Moreover, international health agencies fostered public institutions and ideologies rather than private pieties.

By the 1930s, the Rockefeller Foundation had acquired vast experience in health cooperation in Mexico and dozens of other settings. Through its permanent field-based staff and scientific emissaries around the world, the RF had disseminated public health ideologies, implemented technological breakthroughs, and demonstrated health administration practices in cooperating countries. The RF's campaigns and activities had helped to control several diseases, promoted individual hygiene measures, and supported the development of national public health institutions. The thousands of fellows trained by the IHD had served as dynamic translators of RF public health efforts, tailoring them to local ideas and circumstances.

Mexico was just one of many venues for RF health cooperation, yet the relationship is revealing of broader patterns owing to its thirty-year duration, the variety of activities it involved, and the sometimes politically charged atmosphere in which it took place. By no means did the RF's international health work entail an outright transfer of public health ideas, methods, and technologies; nor did the various actors in Mexico or other places simply absorb the new knowledge and practices as consistent with their interests and appetite for political power. Instead, the RF joined an array of parties that included government authorities, health officials, a spectrum of healers, peasants, and labor groups, and local politicians who shaped and were shaped by their involvement with the RF and with one another.

Mexico—whose public health trajectory was marked by numerous domestic and international influences, a bold state-building imperative, popular and revolutionary demands, and pro-sovereign sensibilities—proved a formidable associate. Over and over again various interests within Mexico substantially transformed the RF's cooperative endeavors and effectively pressed the IHD to reorient its offerings to suit domestic needs.

Paradoxically, although the implementation of RF projects was inevitably subject to interaction in Mexico, as elsewhere, the IHD did not alter its operating principles to include local demands upon, responses to, and refashioning of its approach. Instead the RF's model of health cooperation was transported, largely intact, over time and place.

At the same time as the RF was involved in country-by-country cooperation, it was also influencing, directly and indirectly, the international health field writ large. Through its pioneering disease campaigns and other public health activities, the RF provided the groundwork for a new international health system featuring its own bureaucracy, legitimacy, and mode of conduct. Where other agencies, such as the PASB and the OIHP, remained for many years focused on disease surveillance and the protection of commerce,[1] the RF developed a more extensive understanding of international health cooperation. The LNHO was partially modeled after the IHD and shared many of its values, experts, and know-how in disease control, institution-building, and educational and research work. Despite the capable direction of Polish hygienist Ludwik Rajchman, the LNHO was mired in League of Nations politics, and budgetary constraints meant that it could realize only part of its ambitious agenda.[2] Rather than being supplanted by the LNHO, the IHD served as its major patron and took over some of its key activities during World War II.[3]

As the premier international health organization of its day, the RF had an overarching purview and leadership role. It was instrumental in establishing the centrality of international health activities to the realms of diplomacy, economic development, state-building, and scientific diffusion, and it institutionalized the patterns of health cooperation that remain in place to the present day. The principles that were infused both in the RF's dealings with Mexico and in the international health field as a whole are undoubtedly the RF's most important legacy: virtually all subsequent international health activities have been influenced on some dimension by these deeply-embedded principles.

The Principles

The hallmark of the RF's approach to international health derived not so much from particular successes in the field—which were molded by multiple influences and typically claimed regardless of the outcome—as from the way RF cooperation was organized. What an analysis of IHD activities in Mexico elucidates, then, is the mix of tenets, operating policies, and practices which enabled the RF to adapt to almost any political situation and to work in numerous settings simultaneously amidst a complicated swirl of local and foreign interests. Many of these ideas were developed first by colonial offices and other international agencies,[4] but it was the RF that sharpened them, made them work in concert, and applied them in a consistently effective manner.

The RF's modus operandi can be crystallized into five principles of international health cooperation, each of which is linked with a range of consequences. The principles also combine with one another in synergistic fashion, with further implications for the ideas, strategies, and practices of international health.

First is the principle that donor interests, rather than locally defined needs, determine the nature and focus of international health cooperation through direct in-country activities or the awarding of grants. The agreements between the RF and host governments—such as those governing the yellow fever campaign and local health units in Mexico—allowed the RF, through its administrators and country-based officers, an important role (albeit one subject to negotiation) in the design and implementation of cooperative activities and, indirectly, of the country's larger public health agenda. At the same time, this arrangement shielded the RF from domestic public health embroilments. The RF also furnished cooperation based on renewable grants—as was seen in targeted malaria research support in 1940s Mexico—with the RF's agenda-setting role exercised through grant application, reporting, and renewal processes.

This principle of agenda-setting from above—as practiced by virtually all donor organizations—has significant bureaucratic implications. Extensive donor involvement means that international agencies like the RF have to create their own bureaucracies to recruit and oversee officers, develop policies, approve and monitor activities, and maintain an internal infrastructure to keep themselves going. Once these systems and practices are institutionalized, international agencies are able to define and pursue high-profile global strategies, streamlining demands on the agencies and facilitating accountability.

Second is the principle that cooperative activities—while driven by donor agendas—require substantial "cooperative" financing from recipient countries. As we saw in the case of the hookworm campaign in Mexico, host countries were to provide considerable material, office, and personnel support to RF-sponsored campaigns. The host country was also expected to furnish a portion of the funding for each activity from the outset and gradually to become fully responsible

Table E.1. RF principles of international health cooperation

---

(1) Agenda-setting from above: international health activities are donor-driven, with the agenda of cooperation formulated and overseen by the international agency, whether through direct in-country activities or the awarding of grants.

(2) Budget incentives: activities are only partially funded by donor agencies; matching fund mechanisms require recipient entities to commit substantial financial, human, and material resources to the cooperative endeavor.

(3) Technobiological paradigm: activities are structured in disease control terms based upon: (a) biological and individual behavioral understandings of disease; and (b) technical tools applied to a wide range of settings.

(4) A priori parameters of success: activities are bound geographically, through time limits, by disease and intervention, and/or according to clear exit strategies in order to demonstrate efficiency and ensure visible, positive outcomes.

(5) Consensus via transnational professionals: activities depend on transnational professionals, who are trained abroad (often with donor agency staff) and involved in international networks, easing the local translation of cooperative endeavors.

---

for both financing and operations. These budget incentives were designed to encourage the sustainability of programs, while limiting the RF's financial responsibility in any one setting. Given that national matching funds were often large enough to displace other spending priorities, this arrangement served to extend the RF's agenda-setting powers well beyond the cooperative activity itself.

Accompanying the donor role in agenda-setting is the third principle, of a technobiological paradigm guiding international health projects. The RF was instrumental in furthering this enduring paradigm—that cooperative activities focus upon the control of particular diseases; that diseases are understood principally in biological and behavioral terms; and that standard technical tools be employed in the control of each disease, regardless of the setting. Typically, the RF selected one of a handful of highly visible disease campaigns—yellow fever, hookworm, or malaria—each with a specific etiology and a known technical apparatus (such as a medication, chemical prophylaxis, or method of behavior change). If the ailment was not a leading local problem or if the campaign failed to prevent the recurrence of the disease because it did not address the ailment's underlying factors (as in the case of hookworm), this approach was nevertheless retained. Even when the IHD was pushed, as in Mexico, to support local organization of health services, it continued to follow the paradigm of disease control through feasible techniques.

This narrowing of international health problems to diseases amenable to technical solutions furthers the notion that public health is a neutral force that need only be diffused to underdeveloped settings in order to spur modernization.[5] A technical orientation also has the advantage of being measurable—with each medication or liter of pesticide counted and recorded—and thus provides evidence to governing boards of quarterly or annual efficiency. It also means that a predetermined method can be applied to multiple settings at once.

The conjoined features of outside agenda-setting and the technobiological paradigm have led to the model of the "vertical" disease campaign in international health, whereby hierarchical command-and-control campaigns are organized to combat particular diseases with a single technical tool. While carefully marshaled resources and a focused target heighten the possibility that endpoints will be reached as planned, separate vertical campaign structures often lead to administrative duplication and to the neglect of broader and more permanent "horizontal" public health efforts.

The fourth principle is that a priori parameters virtually guarantee the success of cooperative international health activities. Typically projects are time-delimited (RF agreements in Mexico were usually for less than five years), place-delimited (often in locales identified by the likelihood of positive outcomes rather than health needs), and/or—particularly important for large-scale campaigns, such as that against yellow fever—include a sunset clause or exit strategy. Together with the focus on particular diseases and technically feasible interventions, these parameters of success enable cooperative activities to reach a positive outcome visibly and effectively, ensuring the donor agency's favorable reputation among local and foreign institutional interests, politicians and funders, professionals, and the public.

Coupled with the technobiological paradigm, these limits on cooperative projects enable international health agencies to show results efficiently and avoid costly, messy, underlying social investments such as those associated with tuberculosis or onchocerciasis (i.e., improvements in housing, sanitation, relocation, etc.) in revolutionary Mexico. This decidedly narrow approach to international health cooperation persists, even though many professionals and leaders in international agencies and host countries alike recognize that long-term political and social investments in combination with technical efforts will likely improve the public's health more effectively than technical measures alone.

A corollary of the limited scope of cooperative projects is the belief, pioneered by the IHD, that a demonstration activity in a defined area—as in a model health campaign—will spur local or national authorities to replicate such efforts elsewhere in the country. While this expectation yielded few results in Mexico, given that domestic agenda-making involved far more than the unfiltered imitation of international examples, the demonstration approach has resurfaced in more recent international health efforts as a subsidiary feature to the other principles.

The fifth and final principle to emerge from this analysis is the extensive involvement of transnational professionals in cooperative international health projects. As seen in the sometimes conflicting case of the RF in Mexico, transnational professionals are instrumental in building consensus around international health agendas and serve as interlocutors with regard to particular cooperative activities and approaches. Colonial agencies had begun the practice of overseas training of professionals, but the IHD perfected the fellowship system through a rigorous selection process, strict rules on the placement of returned fellows, the training of its own staff and international fellows in the same institutions, and the maintenance of ties with fellows through ongoing projects. As former head of the IHD Wilbur Sawyer noted in 1949, the training of fellows was "begun early so that leaders will be available for carrying on work later without foreign assistance."[6] Transnational professionals became part of international health networks, sharing values and understandings of international health with their donor agency counterparts. Professional training was an ideal concomitant to the other four principles; fellows educated overseas served as leaders and intermediaries for health cooperation, able to interact with both international and domestic players and to translate cooperative activities to the local scene.

As we saw in the case of Mexico, the details of these five elements of RF operations—outside agenda-setting and extensive donor involvement, budget incentives, a technobiological approach, a priori parameters of success, and transnational professional involvement—were challenged and reshaped locally and in some instances even suspended. Yet the principles took on a normative role, proving enormously useful for the bureaucratic purposes of reporting and accountability as well as for the political, economic, ideological, scientific, and humanitarian roles of health cooperation. Regardless of the extensive refashioning of particular cooperative activities on the ground, the principles have endured in the form of a common framework for international health activities.

Of course there have been numerous challenges to some of the principles, even at the RF. Just as the IHD was giving way to its heir apparent—the WHO—in the late 1940s, several internal assessments ventured toward a rather different approach to international health cooperation. In a 1947 IHD-commissioned study on international health insurance trends, its longtime China and South Africa officer John Grant called for a social medicine approach, whereby the social dimensions of human needs—ranging from universal health services to a minimum wage and to housing and nutrition needs—would be integrated with medicine and public health.[7]

Two years later, an internal report on "Efforts to Help Backward Peoples to Help Themselves" admitted that the IHD had erred in setting cooperative health agendas unilaterally, for IHD men had

a maximum sense of our own power, our own interest, our own goodness, and our own knowledge. We have very little knowledge of the parties of the second part—their social systems, their human relations situations, their resources in personnel, their philosophies and values in life. Our conceit and our desire for speed give us very little readiness to study these matters before acting. Yet, the delivery end is one of the crucial points of the whole problem.[8]

Even IHD malaria officer Paul F. Russell, who would become a key player in the WHO's global malaria campaign, acknowledged confidentially in 1950 that the IHD's long-standing practice of budget incentives was unrealistic, for "It is difficult for governments of underdeveloped countries to find money for experimental projects."[9]

By the time these critiques surfaced, the donor-driven, matching-fund-based, narrowly technical approach had become further entrenched.[10] World War II's inauguration of penicillin, and the successful use of DDT against louse-borne typhus and malaria generated renewed confidence in technical means to address public health problems, disease by disease.[11] Rather than disappearing with the demise of the IHD in 1951, the RF principles of international health cooperation found an institutional home in the WHO.

The WHO, the Cold War, and the Durability of the RF Principles

With the establishment of the WHO in 1948, international health's broadest mandate—including standard-setting, data collection, epidemiologic surveillance, training and research, emergency relief, and cooperative activities—were all located in the same agency for the first time. Thanks to its growing membership beyond the original 26 countries (especially as decolonized nations began to sign on in the 1950s) and what was planned to be an open decision-making structure through the annual World Health Assembly, the WHO enjoyed more legitimacy than its predecessors, the LNHO and the OIHP, which had been hampered by meager resources, limited mandates, and interagency jealousies.[12]

Given the broad reach and experience of the IHD, it was natural that its practices would have an important bearing on the WHO. As Lewis Hackett, who directed IHD programs in South America and Italy for over three decades, put it, "To a greater or lesser degree, all the international organizations have adopted the policies and activities in which the IHD has pioneered," through inheritance of personnel, fellows, and equipment.[13]

The RF's most direct imprint on the WHO took place through Dr. Fred Soper, who spent almost two decades at the helm of the IHD's large-scale campaigns against malaria and yellow fever in Brazil, and went on to head the PASB (as of 1949 WHO's regional office for the Americas) from 1947 to 1959.[14] According to RF President Chester Barnard, the PASB was designed to "cover most of the purposes which the IHD pursued in Latin America. Under [Soper] IHD policies and philosophies have been adopted. The PASB will eventually take over our functions."[15] The IHD model of international health cooperation found further resonance in the WHO with the election as director-general of Dr. Marcolino Candau (1953–73), who had worked with Soper in the IHD's campaigns in Brazil.

The longevity of the RF's interlocking principles of international health, however, was more than a matter of braggadocio and personal influence. Each of the five principles can be witnessed in the structure, strategies, and tenets of the WHO, and all are reflected in the current policies and practices of other leading international health agencies due to their continued ideological salience and bureaucratic convenience.

At the outset, it seemed that the WHO might defy the principle of donor-driven aid. The WHO's 1946 Constitution specified the organization's responsibilities in furnishing "appropriate technical assistance" at the request or acceptance of national governments (one of only a few specialized UN agencies with this kind of role); in strengthening health systems; in "stimulat[ing] and advanc[ing] work to eradicate epidemic, endemic, and other diseases"; and in providing direct aid during emergencies.[16] The ideas of social medicine advocates, such as Andrija Štampar and René Sand, influenced the WHO in its early planning stages,[17] and the WHO interim commission's initial activities responding to postwar epidemics in Greece, Egypt, and Turkey seemed to parallel the post–World War I Epidemic Commission, which Ludwik Rajchman had sought to use as a launching pad for a worldwide public health effort based at the League of Nations.

Hopes of a more democratized system of international health cooperation based on the WHO's idealistic definition of health "as a state of complete physical, mental, and social well-being and not merely the absence of disease" were quickly overshadowed by the ideological exigencies of the Cold War years. When the Soviet bloc pulled out of the WHO in 1949, the WHO became dominated by Anglo-American interests concerned with nesting health activities within a larger anti-Communist agenda.[18] The RF's principles and practices proved as relevant to the Cold War context as they had been to the era of waning colonial empires and waxing international economic markets.

By the early 1950s, policy decisions emanated from permanent Geneva headquarters, rather than from annual World Health Assembly deliberations or in-country negotiations. The WHO Secretariat established a set of priority disease campaigns and organized expert committees now more narrowly aimed at providing "technical assistance for disease-fighting and health-building projects wherever it is needed and requested."[19] The agenda was organized around the existence of technical weapons and the WHO's ability to provide expert advice and marshal distribution systems for the cholera vaccine, penicillin to control yaws, and BCG vaccine against tuberculosis. This technically defined approach culminated in the WHO's global DDT-based malaria campaign, which dominated the international health agenda for several decades. By the late 1950s, "extrabudgetary" funding—that is, financing that bypassed the WHO's decision-making bodies—gave even greater agenda-setting powers to large donors, most notably the United States.

The principle of international activities financed through a system of matching funds became established at the WHO in 1949, when the Expanded Program in Technical Assistance (PEAT) was created to coordinate in-country cooperative efforts by the UN's specialized agencies. Funded by voluntary donations by member countries, PEAT was to cover expert consultancies and working groups, demonstration projects, professional training and fellowships, and project materials.[20] PEAT put in place a strict system of cofinancing, similar to the system of budget incentives developed by the IHD in Mexico and other settings. Countries receiving cooperation were required to fund an increasing percentage of the project's annual costs, as well as cover the salaries of all local personnel (administrative, technical, and support staff, translators and interpreters, chauffeurs and porters, etc.); provide and maintain offices, buildings, furniture, and all materials available in the country; pay local transport, mail, and telecommunication expenses; assume health care and housing costs for local personnel carrying out the cooperative activities; and finance a considerable portion of the travel and daily expenses of foreign experts. The yaws control effort organized by the PASB in Haiti in the early 1950s, for example, was almost 50 percent funded by the Haitian government.[21]

Although the imposition of large financial burdens contradicted the declared objectives of assistance, the co-funding measures met with few internal objections. In 1951, the Regional Committee for the Americas criticized PEAT conditions for technical assistance, given the economic difficulties in many Latin American countries. The committee called on the WHO director-general to allow for more flexible terms depending on local capacity, but no such change was made either at the level of the WHO or the UN as a whole.[22]

In the end, most developing countries joined PEAT since they risked exclusion from cooperation and isolation from other international health opportunities—such as fellowships and positions within WHO—if they refused or were unable to contribute. From 1950 to 1954, voluntary payments to PEAT totaled $400 million ($2.85 billion in 2004 dollars), with developing countries contributing some 11 percent of the total. In addition to this amount, developing countries were required to allocate approximately $900 million ($6.4 billion in 2004 dollars) for in-country expenses, putting considerable strains on domestic health agendas.[23]

The synergistic effect of PEAT and central agenda-setting soon became controversial, as large donors pressured to have their own experts hired and heavily emphasized administrative over field activities. Moreover, experts tended to recommend methods and solutions employed in their home countries as generic recipes with little regard for local cultural, geo-ecological, political, and economic conditions and viability.[24]

Over time, these criticisms were attenuated, in large part thanks to the principle of building consensus via transnational professionals. With Brazilian

Candau replacing Canadian Brock Chisholm at the helm of the WHO in 1953, an increasing number of developing country nationals obtained employment at WHO's central and regional offices. By the mid 1950s, the WHO—which had started to train sanitary engineers, doctors, nurses, health administrators and other public health personnel at its founding—was offering approximately one thousand public health training fellowships each year. Within 20 years the WHO had sponsored more than 50,000 fellows.[25]

Despite these various difficulties, one might have expected developing country and central WHO agendas to overlap productively. The WHO's deliberating organs urged it to take into account socioeconomic factors as inseparable from health problems, with a special emphasis on "basic health services," prevention, and the most urgent problems of large sectors of the population, as well as public health, health education, and nutrition. But the WHO found it difficult to act on the integrated social development and health agenda advocated by its charter, because this set of activities seemed vague, costly, long-term, and hard to evaluate, all challenges inimical to the managerial objectives of the WHO bureaucracy and of demanding country donors.[26]

The WHO soon found itself mired in tensions around how broad social approaches to health might be implemented, precisely the kind of constraint that the IHD had wished to—and did—avoid. These tensions were dissipated by the launching of the WHO's flagship Global Malaria Campaign, approved by the World Health Assembly in 1955. If the principles of a technobiological paradigm and a priori parameters of success were already present by the early 1950s, they became embedded in the malaria campaign for almost a quarter century.

The Global Malaria Campaign has been analyzed as a Cold War phenomenon designed to modernize underdeveloped areas, expand biomedicine's reach, and stave off Communism,[27] but its approach can also be traced to IHD efforts in an earlier era. The initial focus of the campaign was on interrupting the transmission of the disease through the household spraying of DDT for three to four years, which meant almost total reliance on a single technical measure. Although the smallest unit of action in this military-style operation was the human dwelling, the campaign called for no familiarity with human circumstances or local context. As part of a vertical approach extolled by Fred Soper and others, specialized personnel—malariologists, educated transnationally, and sprayers, trained locally—had little contact with community health workers and paid almost no attention to other forms of malaria prevention. In most settings, national malaria eradication teams were organized in a service parallel to the Ministry of Health, duplicating activities and often monopolizing health budgets. The principle of guaranteeing success a priori was most vividly evidenced in the supposedly "global" campaign's deliberate exclusion of Africa from the campaign's purview—despite the fact that Africa had the world's worst malaria problem—due to the WHO's own recognition of numerous obstacles to the eradication of malaria in this region.[28]

When the malaria eradication campaign was abandoned in 1969, the named culprits were vector resistance and the administrative complexity of reaching out-of-the-way populations. One might even argue that the WHO's problems with malaria control stemmed from insufficient adherence to the RF model of cooperative principles. Yet more than twenty years later, at an October 1992 Ministerial Malaria Conference in Amsterdam, the failure was attributed to a set of nontechnical factors, including low education levels; low levels of community involvement; insufficient knowledge about malaria at the community level; and inadequate funding for and development of general health services.[29]

Rather than reveal publicly the limits of the technical, disease-by-disease approach to international health, the malaria fiasco only reinforced it: the WHO had simply picked the wrong disease and the wrong technique. Even before the Global Malaria Campaign was officially terminated, the WHO turned to a new disease effort—the eradication of smallpox—that would prove an easier task from a technical perspective, if one much less important in terms of annual deaths (in strange parallel to hookworm). An ancient scourge, smallpox had been subject to a range of control measures in various cultures—variolation, inoculation, inhalation of desiccated smallpox scabs, and the less toxic vaccination. By 1950, mandatory vaccination had successfully protected the populations of most developed and many developing countries. Even in the most affected countries, by this time annual smallpox deaths rarely exceeded a few thousand (outside of India there were typically no more than a few hundred deaths per year),[30] and smallpox ranked far below the leading fifteen or twenty causes of death. Still, when the Soviet Union rejoined the WHO in 1956, its delegates pushed for a WHO smallpox campaign as a measure of both domestic and international concern: students and other travelers to Russia from the developing world were importing the disease at troublesome rates.[31]

According to D. A. Henderson, the U.S. Center for Disease Control (now Centers for Disease Control and Prevention) epidemiologist who directed the campaign, the smallpox campaign was a "Cold War victory," involving both East-West and North-South collaboration.[32] For the World Health Assembly to endorse a new high-profile campaign while the malaria effort was ailing demanded an assurance of success that only a non-zoonotic disease (one without an animal host) and an effective vaccine could provide. But vaccines required infrastructure: because of the dearth of health services, trained personnel, and electricity, particularly in South Asia and Africa, the smallpox campaign required a delivery mechanism that could overcome these social and economic barriers. The development of an easy-to-use bifurcated needle, a rapid fire jet injector, and a vaccine compound that required no cold storage meant that virtually anyone could administer the vaccine virtually anywhere.

If the $1 billion spent on the global smallpox campaign from 1966 to 1980 resulted in eradication this time, the price of adherence to the RF's five principles was even higher than before. Enormous national resources—developing countries funded two-thirds of the cost of the smallpox campaign—had been marshaled to achieve the international goal of eradication at the expense of more pressing health needs in sanitation, housing, poverty, basic health infrastructure, and access to primary care services. Moreover, coercive vaccination practices in some areas jeopardized the ability of public health efforts to reach certain populations with subsequent endeavors.[33]

Challenging the Principles

Although by the mid 1950s the "W.H.O. vs. Disease" approach—reflecting the RF's five principles of health cooperation—was well-entrenched, proponents of social and infrastructural approaches to health problems persisted both within and outside the WHO. The culmination of these efforts in international terms was the 1978 WHO/UNICEF Alma-Ata (USSR) Declaration, signed by 175 countries, which called for the promotion of "Health for All" by the year 2000 through an international, national, and local commitment to primary health care within the context of social change.[34] The Alma-Ata conference and declaration entailed complex political negotiations at all levels. Using China's experience with barefoot doctors as an example, Alma-Ata was an effort to replace the WHO's disease campaigns with a broader public health perspective. The declaration reflected health activists' and developing countries' demands for a combined social and medical approach to health needs. It also emerged from internal WHO struggles—in part mirroring Cold War rivalries—over the public health ideologies the agency would pursue.

At last, it seemed, the donor-driven, technical, circumscribed, disease-based model of international health might be at least supplemented by a more integrative approach. But if the conference was a "coup" for the Soviets, Western interests responded by reshuffling their deck. The heart of the Alma-Ata strategy—the commitment to address the leading health problems of each locality, including food supply, basic sanitation, and disease prevention, from a community-based, primary-care approach—generated enormous discursive currency, but in practice it was quickly fragmented.[35] In the wake of Alma-Ata, the RF sponsored a conference from which a focus on "*selective* primary health care" emerged to replace the broad view of primary health care, which was deemed insufficiently cost-effective because it required longterm and infra-structural efforts.[36] This renewed technical approach led UNICEF, the WHO, and various bilateral agencies to work for several decades on a far narrower agenda—of children's vaccines, growth monitoring, oral rehydration, and breast-feeding (and later contraception and micronutrient supplement)—than that set out by Alma-Ata.[37]

The Alma-Ata Declaration was the first large-scale challenge to the RF model of international health principles: it defied the technobiological paradigm of health cooperation and the institutional demands that health activities be measurable and efficient (parameters of success), focused on local, rather than transnational, health personnel and derived from local and national agendas rather than those of donor agencies. This "medicine of liberation," as it was referred to in Mozambique, challenged both the ideological and bureaucratic underpinnings of international health cooperation's "business as usual." But the comprehensive primary health care approach was never fully embraced by the WHO's largest donors, and the initiative was poorly implemented, and—stripped down to its technical elements—ultimately unrealizable according to the original vision.

The Alma-Ata conference and its aftermath coincided with a movement of international health authority away from the WHO into the hands of the World Bank, the International Monetary Fund, bilateral agencies, and private entities.[38] By no means did this lead to an abandonment of the RF principles. Several key agencies turned their attention to health services and the social context of health, but with a focus on "maximizing efficiency" through health system privatization reforms and basic packages of technical interventions. The World Bank's seminal 1993 report, *Investing in Health*,[39] for example, cited poverty and lack of education as important determinants of health, yet called for a larger private sector role and investment in curative and diagnostic technologies as the best means of improving health in developing countries.[40] The principles of measurable success, agenda-setting from above, and budget incentives have likewise been built into these programs.

While it would be an oversimplification to attribute the sidelining of the WHO purely to its deviation from the RF principles of cooperation, the organization's loss of leadership is undeniable: today the WHO is just one among numerous agencies involved in international health.[41] The WHO has sought to remake itself as a central actor in global health following sustained critiques and defunding in the 1980s and 1990s.[42] It has regained prominence by partnering with the private sector and returning to technical, circumscribed approaches based upon donor-driven agendas. These include initiatives such as distributing antiretroviral drugs (the "3 x 5" initiative), directly observed therapy to "stop tuberculosis," insecticides and drug treatment to "roll back malaria," as well as global infectious disease surveillance (harking back to international health's earliest concerns).

Enshrining the RF Model

In recent decades, international health has become a far more complex field involving many thousands of players: bilateral development agencies, small and large nongovernmental organizations, private and religious charitable groups, local companies and multinational corporations, multiple UN agencies, private and development banks, philanthropic foundations, individuals, and community groups involved in direct assistance.[43]

Today, multilateral agencies spend several billion dollars per year on international health activities, and bilateral development agencies from industrialized countries spend at least double this amount. Particularly since 1980, literally thousands of small and large nonprofit aid organizations and foundations have become extensively involved in emergency assistance and local-level cooperation. Major private firms—pharmaceutical companies, banks, and insurance companies—which are now players in the business of international health, generate untold billions of dollars in loans, sales, and contracts.

For the most part, donors continue to set the international health agenda, satisfying bureaucratic needs more than those of local populations.[44] Like the RF, these agencies do not simply contribute money, equipment, and personnel—they expect their cooperative efforts to be evaluated in order to demonstrate effectiveness: a technical, disease-by-disease approach is most amenable to such ends. Although Alma-Ata temporarily derailed the vertical disease eradication approach, eradication has returned with even more vitality than before. In the mid 1980s a vaccine-based polio eradication campaign, spearheaded by Rotary International, emerged on the global health agenda and has now become the most expensive disease campaign ever.[45] Measles eradication and other technically-oriented childhood disease campaigns are high on the international cooperation agenda. The Global Fund to Fight AIDS, Tuberculosis, and Malaria, established in 2001 by UN Secretary-General Kofi Annan to increase public-private partnerships to combat three of the world's leading killers, is designed to respond to the most pressing health problems in many settings. In bringing corporate interests to the international health table, the Global Fund follows an a priori parameters of success model, requiring applicant countries to propose narrow technical approaches to each disease rather than addressing the underlying determinants of all three.[46] The mantra of evaluating cost-effectiveness as the only "credible basis" for foreign assistance, even by organizations that claim to take an integrated approach to improving global health means that social, political, and redistributive efforts—proven global health successes from Sri Lanka to Sweden—are delegitimized by the international health establishment.[47] The extensive involvement of transnational professionals in cooperative activities further inhibits the pursuit of alternate approaches to those set by donor agencies.[48] In most developing countries today, less than 20 percent of health spending comes from foreign aid,[49] but budget incentives continue to influence spending priorities.

Discovering the RF's organizational fingerprints all over international health agencies does not constitute a triumph of detective work—on the contrary, it would be surprising if the prints could not be identified. The resilience of the RF's model of international health cooperation through decades of mixed experience with outside agenda-setting, disease-based campaigns, and budget incentives suggests far more than the influence of a powerful player: the RF principles are ideally suited to supragovernmental institutions seeking to justify their own growing bureaucracies. As carried out by the IHD, disease campaigns incorporated all the elements of managerial accountability: clear objectives, guarantees of success, favorable reports to stakeholders, and ready scapegoats—faulty technical tools (which needed further development or better implementation)—for failures.

This is not to say that the RF principles of international health cooperation are universal, all-encompassing, or immutable. As we have seen in the case of the RF and Mexico, international health activities are shaped by the political, social, and public health agendas of a variety of players, all of whom interact around questions of public health models, administrative arrangements, funding policies, institutional commitments, priority-setting, and personnel decisions. Moreover, numerous nongovernmental organizations, relief agencies, medical, religious, educational or humanitarian groups, individual donors, and other entities involved in international health cooperation operate according to different principles from those developed by the RF. Doctors for Global Health, for example, is engaged only in community-oriented initiatives where the agenda is set locally.[50] The much larger Oxfam, indirectly an international health agency, focuses on economic and social justice campaigns without requiring matching funds. The People's Health Movement challenges the role of transnational professionals as a bridge to international health cooperation, instead advocating the notion that locally based (often democratically elected) health workers in conjunction with the voices of the marginalized offer more appropriate, valid, and useful channels for setting health agendas.[51]

At the same time, however, the bureaucratic model of international health crafted by the RF has proven remarkably durable, with the five principles evident in the policies and practices of the most powerful international health players, be they bilateral aid agencies, United Nations organizations, international financial institutions, or philanthropies.[52] Of course bureaucratic expedience only partially explains why the RF principles continue to govern the terms of most international health cooperation. The ideological and political relevance of the principles is equally—if not more—important. Health cooperation remains a force of international relations and statecraft,[53] having survived—in much the same guise—several reconfigurations of the world order from early twentieth-century imperialism, through the Cold War, to the contemporary context of borderless corporate capitalism.

International health is necessarily shaped by global politics. This was perhaps most evident from the end of World War II until the early 1990s when the Cold War defined international health's reach and orientation.[54] As the Western and Eastern blocs competed for power and influence throughout the developing world, international health became a pawn, used variously as outright propaganda, to promote particular variants of public health, to show off technological superiority, and, in the case especially of the United States, to defuse population pressures.[55]

Today the stakes have shifted, but many of the same motivations—now defined in terms of global security, human rights, and economic profitability—have persisted. For example, a 2001 Council on Foreign Relations document entitled *Why*

Health Is Important to US Foreign Policy[56] cites narrow self-interest, enlightened self-interest, and human rights leadership as the principal justifications for international health, harking back to concerns over the global spread of disease and the risks of economic, social, and military disruption if health needs remain unmet. But the document also presents a diplomatic benefits argument whereby U.S. involvement in international health demonstrates its altruistic leadership. Similarly, the imperative driving development along globalized market economy lines has brought international financial agencies—such as the World Bank—to the forefront of public health lending and investment "cooperation."

Most importantly, despite the demise of the ideological competition between "East" and "West" and the growing evidence of the importance of socially integrated approaches to public health, the end of the Cold War seems to have only further ingrained the RF's legacy. Part of the technical temptation in public health has, of course, derived from the postwar development, diffusion, and reception of wonder-measures, such as antibiotics, DDT, and a variety of vaccines. These innovations have increased public health's capacity but also further reinforced a medicalized approach to disease that gives short shrift to social factors.

Addressing the underlying causes of illness and early death—most notably societal inequalities in economic, political, social, and cultural conditions[57]—has been recognized by researchers and advocates as a vital means of improving global health. Although this approach may be more politically charged and less bureaucratically convenient than attacking diseases one by one, in 2005 the WHO responded to a crescendo of voices and created a Commission on Social Determinants of Health. Alas, most leading international health agencies have yet to heed this call: they remain focused on efficiency arguments to divide up responsibility for combating different diseases with various technical tools rather than integrating technical and social approaches.[58]

Inside the Gates

In an ironic parallel, almost a century after the RF's international health efforts began, a new health philanthropy is in its nascent stages. Unlike the RF, the Bill and Melinda Gates Foundation, launched in 2000 and now with a $29 billion endowment from Microsoft profits, has not spread itself thin through multiple initiatives across the globe, instead focusing on a few disease-control efforts as a grant-making agency (rather than through its own officers on the ground). As did the RF, it relies on a technical, disease-based approach, with a priori parameters of success and agenda-setting from above, using transnational professionals to legitimize its efforts. In its recent "Grand Challenges in Global Health" initiative, for example, developing-country professionals served on the board that designed the initiative and evaluated projects, and ideas for grand challenges were solicited from both developed and developing-country health researchers.[59]

As with Rockefeller, although Gates himself is an outsider to international health, his ideas have become emblematic of the entire field. In May 2005, the WHO extended an unprecedented invitation to Gates (not a member country representative) as the keynote speaker at the 58th World Health Assembly. He used his address to defend the technical, disease-based, donor-driven paradigm of international health and was unapologetic in response to charges that his foundation ignores poverty:

> Some point to the better health in the developed world and say we can only improve health when we eliminate poverty. And eliminating poverty is an important goal. But we have a different view. The world didn't have to eliminate poverty in order to eliminate smallpox—and we don't have to eliminate poverty before we reduce malaria.[60]

In a biting response to Gates's controversial appearance at the WHO, the People's Health Movement demanded that the Microsoft Corporation be declared an honorary member of the WHO, which would both justify Gates's presence at the World Health Assembly and explicitly recognize corporate influences on the international public health policies.

In the end, international health's bureaucratic and ideological imperatives continue to keep the five RF principles in play, seemingly extending the RF's legacy into the next century. The marriage of these principles and international health has indeed proven convenient, but as the People's Health Movement satire portends, international health may yet find a new partner.

Postscript: Remaking International Health

In the last several years, an international health movement called "Barrio Adentro" ("Inside the Neighborhood") started in an unlikely corner: some of the poorest neighborhoods of Caracas, Venezuela. Tired of incessantly delayed implementation of government promises of health care and Venezuelan doctors' refusal to serve them, local activists and politicians turned the principles of international health cooperation upside down. Rather than the international agency selecting the activity, funding it via budget incentives, and setting the terms of cooperation, community-level committees—now formed throughout the country—are hosting 13,000 Cuban doctors who come to live in their neighborhoods and serve as their primary care practitioners, following a principle of solidarity (at a popular level) and exchange (at the level of the state— Cuban medicine for Venezuelan oil) rather than aid. These doctors are not privileged short-term consultants, but rather eat and sleep in the same shantytown dwellings where they practice. The bona fide "bottom-up" approach of Barrio Adentro emphasizes participatory democracy and management and covers a wide range of areas, including housing, education, employment, and neighborhood improvement. Thus far, barrio-dwellers have evaluated the open-ended health program as a great success by the simplest of measures: before this program was implemented they had no primary care services, and now they do.[61]

For the moment, the Barrio Adentro movement is a unique refashioning of international health cooperation. But the experience also suggests that local social movements may serve as the boldest challenge to the RF model of principles. What if the Barrio Adentro mode of international health solidarity were to spread? What might be the implications for the participants, ideologies, and practices of international health cooperation? As in the case of the RF-Revolutionary Mexico relationship, international health would continue to be marked by interaction among players, but the terms of the game would change.

For example, the locale and population for cooperation would be self-defined, based on community initiative. The agenda and approach of joint activity would not be imposed from outside, but developed at a local level with priorities and methods deriving from truly democratic decision-making. Likewise, the criteria for evaluation would come from local determination of satisfaction of needs rather than international agency accountability systems. The time frame of the cooperation would not be set a priori but would remain open-ended, based on local needs and developments. The balance of interests of the donor, the host country, and the local arena of activity would tip in favor of the last named, with transnational consensus-building processes minimized. Where available and involved, local health workers, healers, and other community health "experts" would be incorporated into the agenda-setting and cooperative process, so that their knowledge and role would not be automatically superseded by a cooperative agenda. Training efforts would take into account local health needs and approaches, rather than imparting "value-free" scientific expertise in a social or political vacuum.

Undoubtedly, the financing—indeed, the financial viability—of such a system of democratic cooperation seems an insurmountable obstacle. With or without matching budget mechanisms, what funder, one might rightfully ask, would subject itself to such rigorous terms? Plainly it would be a "donor" that is not interested in aid per se but one whose aims are to achieve health through solidarity and universally shared rights—concepts present in the mission of many international health agencies.

Which of the range of players we have witnessed might support or withstand such a transformation? Here the answer might be broader than expected, including, potentially, not only community-level interests and local health workers, but also progressive-minded national politicians and doctors—and their institutions—keen on setting the basis for health cooperation closer to population needs. Similarly, the growing number of scientists interested in the relationship between technical interventions and community, social, and political determinants of health might jump at the chance of circumventing the standard research funding parameters. Even, or especially, staff within international health institutions might welcome an "inside the neighborhood" paradigm of cooperation, enabling the integrated goals of collective health—which may have motivated their own entry to the international health field—to transcend bureaucratic and funder interests.

This exercise leaves us with the major funding and institutional interests in international health as almost certain opponents to such a challenge to their modus operandi. Might the principles of these lead players also be reshaped through such a locally driven, needs-based, integrated, and politically grounded model in the interest of maintaining relevance? Or will parties to international health turn to new ways of financing cooperative activities—for example, through barter and exchange rather than strings-attached aid—or even a politics of radical redistribution that addresses the social and political determinants of health? That will be for the next generation of international health players—at all levels—to act upon and decide.

Acknowledgments

The fresh pages of a new book hide the countless fingerprints of the colleagues, mentors, archivists, students, and friends who have helped bring it to life.

I am grateful to the archivists and librarians at the several dozen organizations listed in the bibliography. The archivists at the two most important institutions for this story stand out for their extraordinary generosity and support. At the Archivo Histórico de la Secretaría de Salud in Mexico City, former director José Alonso Felix Gutiérrez and current director Irma Betanzos Cervantes and their staff, particularly Rogelio Vargas and Margarito Crispín, welcomed me warmly on many trips and found the time to share sweets from the Pastelería Ideal in between advising me on sources and hunting down documents. The staff at the Rockefeller Archive Center in Sleepy Hollow, New York, were likewise enormously helpful before, during, and between visits. My greatest appreciation goes to the recently retired Thomas Rosenbaum, who will be missed by several generations of historians. I am grateful to the center's director, Darwin Stapleton, for his support in reproducing many of the photos in this volume, to Michele Hiltzik for scanning the photos, and to Ken Rose for his ongoing assistance and for an archival pizza party many moons ago. My thanks go also to Omar Echegoyen of the History of Medicine Division, U.S. National Library of Medicine in Bethesda, MD, and Tonatiuh Herrera Gutiérrez at the Fototeca Nacional in Pachuca, Hidalgo, for their help in procuring photos. Dr. Juan Bustamante has been a tireless correspondent and generously shared many of his brother's papers from the Fundacíon Cívico–Cultural Bustamante Vasconcelos in Oaxaca.

My research was supported by grants from the Rockefeller Archive Center, the Indiana University Center on Philanthropy, and the Canada Research Chairs program. Passages and arguments from chapters 2 and 3 were presented at various talks in Brazil, Mexico, France, the U.S., Canada, El Salvador, Colombia, Hungary, and Spain and published in several of my articles listed in the bibliography.

Three people were instrumental in having inspired this book and shaped my thinking on the history of international health, revolution, and Latin America: Elizabeth Fee, Vicente Navarro, and Marcos Cueto. Over the years, my work has also been greatly enriched by discussions with mentors, friends, colleagues, students, and fellow travelers in the worlds of history of medicine and public health, including Ana Cecilia Rodríguez de Romo, Guadalupe Serrano Cruz, José Ronzón, Irma Gutiérrez, René Leyva, Julia Rodriguez, Armando Solórzano, Elisabeth Benjamin, Alberto Pellegrini, Chris Abel, Patrick Zylberman, Adriana Alvarez, Steven Palmer, Gilberto Hochman, Paulo Gadelha, Diego Armus, Paul Weindling, Mary Kay Vaughan, Seth Fein, Claudia Agostoni, Paul Gootenberg, Julyan Peard, Alex Stern, Emilio Quevedo, Juliana Martínez, Gerard Fergerson, Ilana Löwy, Nancy Krieger, Ana María Kapelusz-Poppi, Alex Schwartz, Carmen Concepción, and María Isabel Rodríguez. Howard Berliner, Marcos Cueto, M. Elizabeth Madigan, Charles Rosenberg, and Susan Solomon have read all or part of the manuscript at crucial moments and offered most useful feedback. Héctor Gómez-Dantés (who is but two degrees of separation from any source of consequence), Octavio Gómez-Dantés, and their entire extended family—including Josefina González Rivera—have made my times in Mexico both intellectually stimulating and enjoyable. *Gracias por todo.*

Ana María Carrillo and Nikolai Krementsov have served as this book's *parteras*. In the fine tradition of no good deed going unpunished, they have coaxed, coached, and graciously critiqued me through several manuscript drafts. *Gracias* and *Spasibo*.

I am grateful to Theodore Brown, Suzanne E. Guiod, and the University of Rochester Press staff (especially Katie Hurley and Sue Smith) for supporting the book and shepherding it—and me—through the publishing process. At the University of Toronto, my students Klaudia Dmitrienko and, especially, René Guerra Salazar provided invaluable assistance with bibliography, notes, and photographs, as well as critical reflections on the contemporary relevance of this story.

Richard and Jacqueline Mendels Birn have supplied me with never-ending encouragement, language advice, and editorial assistance, and it is to them that I dedicate this book.

In the time that it took to complete this book, Esperanza Francesca learned to chew, crawl, walk, talk, count, read and write. To her repeated question, "Are you done with your book yet?" I can finally say, "Oui, mon amour." And that goes for her papa too.

Appendix

Rockefeller Foundation Public Health Fellowships Awarded to Mexico, 1920–49

Name	Place of Training	Period of Fellowship	Position before Fellowship	Latest Known Position
Ricardo Granillo	Harvard	1920–21		Chief, Biostatistics Section, DSP
Salvador Bermúdez	Johns Hopkins	1922–23	Sub-Prof. Hygiene, DSP	Dir., School of Public Health, DSP
J. Zozaya	Harvard	1924–25	Student	Director, Institute of Hygiene, DSP
X. Hernández	Harvard	1926–27	Doctor, TB Dispensary	Unknown, not governmental
Miguel E. Bustamante	Johns Hopkins	1926–28	Ch. Vacc. Off., DSP	Chief, Division of Statistics, Inst. of Tropical Diseases, DSP
Maximiliano Ruiz Castañeda	Johns Hopkins	1926–27	Bacteriologist, DSP	Chief, Typhus Lab., General Hospital
Gerardo Varela	Harvard	1926–27	Bacteriologist, DSP	Chief Bacteriologist, Inst. of Hygiene, DSP, and Prof. of Bacteriology, Polytechnic Inst.

Appendix (*continued*)

Name	Place of Training	Period of Fellowship	Position before Fellowship	Latest Known Position
Alfonso Castrejón	Harvard	1927–28	Bacteriology Student	Hydraulic Resources
Roberto Del Valle	Harvard	1928–29	DSP, Baja California	Medical Delegate, DSP, Nuevo Laredo
E. Uribe Guerola	Johns Hopkins	1930–31	Bacteriologist, DSP	Lecturer, Mexican Red Cross
Joaquín Segura	Harvard	1930–31	Sanitary Engineer, DSP	Sanitary Engineer, Morelos Project
Fernando Tejeda	Harvard	1931–32	Sanitary Engineer, San Cristóbal	Federal Dept. of Irrigation
Pilar Hernández Lira	Johns Hopkins	1931–32	Dir., Health Unit	State Epid. Morelos and Dir. Cuernavaca Unit
Esteban Hoyo	UNC-Chapel Hill	1932–33	Assistant Engineer, Gov. Road Dept	Sanitary Engineer, Oficina de Especialización Sanitaria, DSP
Roberto Velasco	Harvard	1933–34	Chief, San. Brigades, DSP	Inst. of Hygiene, DSP
Alberto P. León	Harvard	1934–36	Assistant, Inst. of Hygiene	Chief, Div. of Bacteriology, Inst. Tropical Diseases, DSP
Luis Mazzotti	Johns Hopkins	1935–36	Chief, Coordinated Services, DSP	Chief, Div. of Helminthology, Inst. Tropical Diseases, DSP
Antonio Candano	Johns Hopkins	1935–36	Med. Insp., Child Hygiene Bureau, DSP	Epidemiologist, Federal District Health Department, DSP
Alberto Jacqueminot	Johns Hopkins	1935–36	Dir., Health Unit	Unit Dir., Oficina de Especialización Sanitaria, DSP
Luis Vargas García	Johns Hopkins	1935–36	Assistant Parasitologist	Chief, Div. of Entomology, Inst. Tropical Diseases, DSP
Andrés Lazaga Sepúlveda	Harvard	1935–36	Engineer	International Water and Sewage Commission
Rutilio Torres Saravia	Harvard	1935–36	Engineer	Unknown
Gustavo Rovirosa	Johns Hopkins	1936–37	Chief Veracruz, H. Service	Chief, Bureau of Epidemiology, DSP

Name	University	Years		
Felipe García Sánchez	Johns Hopkins	1936–37	Assistant Director, Xochimilco Health Unit	State Health Officer, Morelos
Manuel Calderón	Harvard	1936–38	Engineer, DSP	Div. San. Eng., Hydraulic Resources
Bertha Heuer-Ritter	Toronto-NY	1936–38	Head Nurse, Infant Hygiene Service, DSP	Public Health Nurse, Mexico City Health Dept.
Matilde Prida	Toronto	1936–37	Visiting Nurse, Xochimilco Unit	Field Supervisor Nurse, DSP
Carmen Gómez Siegler	Toronto-NY	1936–38	Division of Nursing, DSP	Public Health Nurse, Mexico City Health Dept.
Adán Ornelas Hernández	Johns Hopkins	1937–38	Director, Health Unit Cuernavaca	State Health Officer, Jalisco
Silvestre López Portillo	Harvard	1937–38	Public Health Officer	Physician, Hospital of Inst. of Tropical Diseases, DSP
Mercedes Miranda	Toronto	1937–38	Luis E. Ruiz Health Center	Public Health Nurse, Mexico City Health Dept.
Ma. Luisa Salgado	Toronto	1937–38	Visiting Public Health Nurse, Xochimilco	Visiting Public Health Nurse, Xochimilco
José Bustos	Harvard	1938–39	Chief, Health Services, Veracruz	State Health Officer, Jalapa, Veracruz
Felipe Malo Juvera	Harvard	1938–39	State Health Officer, San Luis Potosí	State Health Officer, Tlaxcala
Manuel Márquez-Escobedo	Johns Hopkins	1938–39	Health Officer, City of Cuernavaca	Health Officer, City of Cuernavaca
Jesús Villalpando	Johns Hopkins	1939–40	Assistant Health Officer, Cuernavaca	Assistant Medical Dir., Cuernavaca
Pedro Daniel Martínez	Johns Hopkins	1939–40	State Health Officer, Michoacán	State Health Officer, Michoacán, DSP
Victor Ocampo	Johns Hopkins	1939–40	Health Officer, Nogales	State Health Officer, Sonora, DSP

Appendix (*continued*)

Name	Place of Training	Period of Fellowship	Position before Fellowship	Latest Known Position
Guillermo Román y Carrillo	Johns Hopkins	1939–40	Health Officer, Durango	State Health Officer, Durango, DSP
Carlos Ortiz Mariotte	Johns Hopkins	1940–41	Senior Technician, DSP	Epidemiologist, DSP
José Calvo y de la Torre	Johns Hopkins	1941–42	Chief, Health Unit, Jojutla	Dir., Inst. of Nutrition
Ramón Pintado-Pérez	Johns Hopkins	1941–42	Epidemiologist, DSP	Epidemiologist, DSP
Carlos López-Fuentes	Harvard	1941–42	Sanitary Engineer, DSP	PASB officer
Antonio Sierra-Salinas	Harvard	1941–42	Sanitary Engineer, DSP	Construction Chief, Hydraulic Resources
Mario Solano-González	Harvard	1941–42	Sanitary Engineer, DSP	
A. Aldama-Contreras	Johns Hopkins	1942–43	Statistician, DSP	Biostatistics professor, School of Public Health
L. Molina-Johnson	Johns Hopkins	1942–43	Assistant Director, Tacuba Health Unit	Epidemiologist with IIAA
C. Cabrera-Moreno	Harvard	1942–43	Sanitary Engineer	
José Garza-Larumbe	Harvard	1942–43	Engineer	Chief Engineer, State Health Service, Cuernavaca
C. Rendón-Anaya	Harvard	1942–43	Engineer	
J. J. Osorio-Aguilar	Johns Hopkins	1942–43	Chief, Sanitary Unit, Guadalajara	Dir., Training Station, Guadalajara
Candelario Cárdenas	Harvard	1943–44	Sanitary Engineer, DSP	Hydraulic Resources, SSA
J. Lamberto González Hernández	Harvard	1943–44	Engineer	Hydraulic Resources, SSA
Raúl Enrique Ochoa Elizondo	Harvard	1943–44	Sanitary Engineer, DSP	Hydraulic Resources, SSA

Carlos Plancarte Haro	Harvard	1943–44	Engineer, DSP	
Joaquín de Araoz	Harvard	1943–44	Sanitary Engineer, DSP	
Carlos Calero Elorduy	Johns Hopkins	1944–45	Chief, Health Unit Orizaba, Veracruz	
Roberto Acosta Vallardo	Johns Hopkins	1944–45	Epidemiologist, Nayarit	Health Officer, Nayarit
Juan Alanís-Perea	Johns Hopkins	1944–45	Epidemiologist, Morelia, Michoacán	
Heliodoro Celis Salazar	Johns Hopkins	1944–45	Health Officer, Cuernavaca	State Health Officer, Morelos
Salvador Leal	Michigan	1944–45	Sanitary Engineer, SSA	Hydraulic Resources, SSA
Salvador Gallo Sarlat	Harvard	1944–45	Sanitary Engineer, SSA	
Juan Alcocer Campero	Johns Hopkins	1945–46	Epidemiologist, Mexicali	
Carlos Campillo Sainz	Berkeley	1945–46	ISET	Professor Tropical Diseases
Eduardo Joublanc	Harvard	1945–46	Sanitary Engineer, SSA	
Miguel Silva Martínez	Johns Hopkins	1946–47	Director, Training Station, Coatepec, Veracruz	Coordinated Health Services in the States, SSA
Roberto Silva Goytia	USPHS-Montana	1949	Clinic Director, Mexico City	IMSS

Sources: International Health Division, "Fellowships to Mexico 1920–1944"; and *The Rockefeller Foundation Directory of Fellowship Awards, 1917–1950,* RG 1.2, Series 100, Box 32, Folder 239, RFA.

Charles Bailey, "List of IHD Fellowships to Mexico, Indicating Duration, School Attended, Assignments and Estimated Cost, 1935," RG 1.1, Series 323, Box 20, Folder 161, RFA.

List of Rockefeller Foundation Fellowships Awarded to Mexico, RG2, Series 323, Box 199 Folder 1409, RFA.

Abbreviations

AGN   Archivo General de la Nación (National Archives of Mexico)
AHEM Archivo Histórico del Estado de Morelos (Historical Archives of the State of Morelos)
AHSSA Archivo Histórico de la Secretaría de Salud (Historical Archives of the Secretariat of Health)
CROM Confederación Regional de Obreros Mexicanos (Regional Confederation of Mexican Workers)
DSP   Departamento de Salubridad Pública (Department of Public Health)
FCCBV Fundación Cívico-Cultural Bustamante Vasconcelos (Bustamante Vasconcelos Civic and Cultural Foundation)
IHB   International Health Board
IHD   International Health Division
IIAA Institute of Inter-American Affairs
IMSS Instituto Mexicano del Seguro Social (Mexican Institute of Social Security)
INI   Instituto Nacional Indigenista (National Indigenous Institute)
INAH Instituto Nacional de Antropología e Historia (National Institute of Anthropology and History)
ISET Instituto de Salubridad y Enfermedades Tropicales (Institute of Health and Tropical Diseases)
LNHO League of Nations Health Organization
MAP   Mexican Agricultural Program
NARA National Archives and Record Administration (U.S.)
OIHP Office International d'Hygiène Publique (International Office of Public Hygiene)
OPS   Organización Panamericana de la Salud
PAHO Pan American Health Organization
PASB Pan American Sanitary Bureau
PEAT Expanded Program in Technical Assistance
PNR   Partido Nacional Revolucionario (National Revolutionary Party)
PRM   Partido de la Revolución Mexicana (Party of the Mexican Revolution)
RF   Rockefeller Foundation

RFA   Rockefeller Foundation Archives

SSA   Secretaría de Salubridad y Asistencia (Secretariat of Health and Welfare)

UN   United Nations

UNAM   Universidad Nacional Autónoma de México (National Autonomous University of Mexico)

USPHS   United States Public Health Service

WHO   World Health Organization

Notes

Introduction

NB. All translations made by Anne-Emanuelle Birn unless otherwise indicated.

1. Miguel E. Bustamante to William Howell, January 19, 1929, Alan Mason Chesney Medical Archives of the Johns Hopkins Medical Institutions, Baltimore, MD, RG JHU SHPH, Office of the Dean—Correspondence, Series 3A, Box 20, Folder Bru. For more on the Rockefeller Foundation (RF) and Johns Hopkins, see Elizabeth Fee, *Disease and Discovery: A History of the Johns Hopkins School of Hygiene and Public Health, 1916–1939* (Baltimore: Johns Hopkins University Press, 1987).

2. Among the many works discussing these efforts are Marcos Cueto, ed. *Missionaries of Science: The Rockefeller Foundation and Latin America* (Bloomington: Indiana University Press, 1994); Ilana Löwy, *Virus, moustiques et modernité: La fièvre jaune au Brésil entre science et politique*, Series histoire des sciences, des techniques et de la médecine (Paris: Editions des Archives Contemporaines, 2001); Luiz A. de Castro Santos, "Power, Ideology, and Public Health in Brazil, 1889–1930" (PhD diss., Harvard University, 1987); and John Farley, *To Cast Out Disease: A History of the International Health Division of the Rockefeller Foundation, 1913–1951* (New York: Oxford University Press, 2004).

3. See, for example, Lewis Pyenson, "In Partibus Infidelium: Imperialist Rivalries and Exact Sciences in Early Twentieth Century Argentina," *Quipu* 1 (1984): 253–303.

4. Alan Knight, "Popular Culture and the Revolutionary State in Mexico, 1910–1940," *Hispanic American Historical Review* 74, no. 3 (1994): 394–95.

5. Ilona Kickbusch, "From Charity to Rights: Proposal for Five Action Areas of Global Health," *Journal of Epidemiology and Community Health* 58, no. 8 (August 2004): 630–31.

6. José Saralegui, *Historia de la Sanidad Internacional* (Montevideo: Imprenta Nacional, 1958); José Ronzón, *Sanidad y Modernización en los Puertos del Alto Caribe 1870–1915* (México, DF: Universidad Autónoma Metropolitana, Unidad Azcapotzalco/Grupo Editorial Miguel Angel Porrúa, 2004); and Alexandra M. Stern and Howard Markel, "International Efforts to Control Infectious Diseases, 1851 to the Present," *JAMA* 292 (2004): 1474–79.

7. David Arnold, *Colonizing the Body: State Medicine and Epidemic Disease in Nineteenth-Century India* (Berkeley: University of California Press, 1993); Heather Bell, *Frontiers of Medicine in the Anglo-Egyptian Sudan, 1899–1940* (Oxford: Oxford University Press, 1999); Philip D. Curtin, *Disease and Empire: The Health of European Troops in the Conquest of Africa* (Cambridge: Cambridge University Press, 1998); Megan Vaughan, *Curing their Ills: Colonial Power and African Illness* (Oxford: Polity Press, 1991); David Arnold, *Imperial Medicine and Indigenous Societies* (Manchester, UK: Manchester University Press, 1988); Mark Harrison, *Climates and Consitutions: Health, Race, Environment and British Imperialism in India, 1600–1850* (Oxford: Oxford University Press, 1999); Maryinez Lyons, *The Colonial Disease: A Social History of Sleeping Sickness in Northern Zaire, 1900–1940* (Cambridge: Cambridge University Press, 1992); Warwick Anderson, "Immunities of Empire: Race,

Disease, and the New Tropical Medicine, 1900–1920," *Bulletin of the History of Medicine* 70, no. 1 (Spring 1996): 94–118; Margaret Jones, *Health Policy in Britain's Model Colony: Ceylon, 1900–1948* (New Delhi: Orient Longman, 2004); and Roy MacLeod and Milton Lewis, eds., *Disease, Medicine, and Empire: Perspectives on Western Medicine and the Experience of European Expansion* (London: Routledge, 1988).

8. Simon Szreter, "Economic Growth, Disruption, Deprivation, Disease and Death: On the Importance of the Politics of Public Health for Development," *Population Development Review* 23 (1997): 693–728.

9. Max von Pettenkofer, *The Value of Health to a City: Two Popular Lectures*, trans. Henry E. Sigerist (Baltimore: Johns Hopkins University Press, 1941), 15–52.

10. Peter Baldwin, *Contagion and the State in Europe, 1830–1930* (Cambridge University Press, 1999); and Dorothy Porter, ed., *The History of Public Health and the Modern State*, Wellcome Institute for the History of Medicine (Amsterdam: Rodopi, 1994).

11. Richard Evans, *Death in Hamburg: Society and Politics in the Cholera Years 1830–1910* (Oxford: Oxford University Press, 1987); and Paul Weindling, "Public Health in Germany," in *The History of Public Health and the Modern State*, Wellcome Institute for the History of Medicine, ed. Dorothy Porter (Amsterdam: Rodopi, 1994), 119–31.

12. Susan G. Solomon and John F. Hutchinson, eds., *Health and Society in Revolutionary Russia* (Bloomington: Indiana University Press, 1990).

13. Krista Maglen, "The First Line of Defence: British Quarantine and the Port Sanitary Authorities in the Nineteenth Century," *Social History of Medicine* 15, no. 3 (December 2002): 413–28; Anne Hardy, "Cholera, Quarantine and the English Preventive System, 1850–1895," *Medical History* 37 (1993): 250–69; and Dorothy Porter, *Health, Civilization, and the State: A History of Public Health from Ancient to Modern Times* (London: Routledge, 1999).

14. Ka-che Yip, *Health and National Reconstruction in Nationalist China: The Development of Modern Health Services, 1928–1937* (Ann Arbor, MI: Association for Asian Studies, Inc., 1995).

15. Gilberto Hochman and Diego Armus, eds., *Cuídar, Controlar, Curar: Ensaios Históricos. Sobre Saúde e Doença na América Latina e Caribe* (Rio de Janeiro: Editora Fiocruz, 2004); Diego Armus, ed., *Disease in the History of Modern Latin America: From Malaria to AIDS* (Durham, NC: Duke University Press, 2003); Diego Armus, ed., *Entre Médicos y Curanderos: Cultura, Historia y Enfermedad en la América Latina Moderna* (Buenos Aires: Grupo Editorial Norma, 2002); Marcos Cueto, ed., *Salud Cultura y Sociedad en América Latina: Nuevas Perspectivas Históricas* (Lima: IEP y OPS, 1996); Marcos Cueto, *El Regreso de las Epidemias: Salud y Sociedad en el Perú del Siglo XX* (Lima: IEP, 1997); Emilio Quevedo et al., *Café y Gusanos, Mosquitos y Petróleo: El Tránsito desde la Higiene hacia la Medicina Tropical y la Salud Pública en Colombia, 1873–1953* (Bogotá: Universidad Nacional de Colombia, Facultad de Medicina, Instituto de Salud Pública, 2004); Adriana Alvarez, "Resignificando los Conceptos de la Higiene. El Surgimiento de una Autoridad de las Primeras Instituciones Públicas de Salud. Buenos Aires 1880–1920," *História, Ciências, Saúde—Manguinhos* 6, no. 2 (1999): 293–314; and Steven Palmer, *From Popular Medicine to Medical Populism, Doctors, Healers, and Public Power in Costa Rica 1800–1940* (Durham, NC: Duke University Press, 2003).

16. Elizabeth Fee, "The Origins and Development of Public Health in the United States," in *Oxford Textbook of Public Health*, 3rd edition, ed. Roger Detels, Walter Holland, James McEwen, and Gilbert S. Omenn (Oxford: Oxford University Press, 1997), 35–54; Elizabeth Fee, "Public Health and the State: The United States," in *The History of Public Health and the Modern State*, 224–75; and Fitzhugh Mullan, *Plagues and Politics: The Story of the United States Public Health Service* (New York: Basic Books, 1989).

17. The U.S. Social Security Act of 1935 provided grants to the states for the health care of the indigent, as well as supporting various regional activities, such as the Tennessee Valley Authority's malaria eradication effort and the Farm Security Administration's health units. See Margaret Humphreys, "Kicking a Dying Dog: DDT and the Demise of

Malaria in the American South, 1942–1950," *Isis* 87, no.1 (March 1996): 1–17; and Michael Grey, *New Deal Medicine: The Rural Health Programs of the Farm Security Administration* (Baltimore: Johns Hopkins University Press, February 1999). To this day, national public health efforts are focused on research and surveillance through the National Institutes of Health and other research and demonstration agencies such as the Centers for Disease Control and Prevention; regulation via the Food and Drug Administration; vital statistics compilation, and analysis; and grant-making to individuals, local health departments, universities, and other institutions, rather than the direct delivery of public health services. The Indian Health Service, mandated by treaty to provide health services to Native Americans, is the main exception.

18. Neville Goodman, *International Health Organisations and their Work* (Edinburgh: Churchill Livingstone, 1971); Norman Howard-Jones, *The Scientific Background of the International Sanitary Conferences, 1851–1938* (Geneva: World Health Organization, 1975); David Fidler, "The Globalization of Public Health: The First 100 Years of International Health Diplomacy," *Bulletin of the World Health Organization* 79 (2001): 842–49; William Bynum, "Policing Hearts of Darkness: Aspects of the International Sanitary Conferences," *History and Philosophy of the Life Sciences* 15 (1993): 421–34; Paul Weindling, ed., *International Health Organisations and Movements, 1918–1939* (Cambridge: Cambridge University Press, 1995). The International Classification of Diseases devised by Parisian statistician-bureaucrat Jacques Bertillon in 1893 and adopted by dozens of countries (first revision 1900) was an exception to this pattern of international cooperation failure.

19. Marcos Cueto, *El Valor de la Salud: Una Historia de la OPS* (Washington DC: OPS, 2004); Miguel E. Bustamante, "Los Primeros Cincuenta Años de la Oficina Sanitaria Panamericana," *Boletín de la Oficina Sanitaria Panamericana* 33, no. 6 (1952): 471–531; and Aristides Moll, "The Pan American Sanitary Bureau: Its Origin, Development and Achievements: A Review of Inter-American Cooperation in Public Health, Medicine, and Allied Fields," *Boletín de la Oficina Sanitaria Panamericana* 19 (1940): 1219–34. Also see Anne-Emanuelle Birn, "No More Surprising than a Broken Pitcher? Maternal and Child Health in the Early Years of the Pan American Health Organization," *Canadian Bulletin of Medical History* 19, no. 1 (2002): 17–46.

20. Farley, *To Cast Out Disease*; and Raymond B. Fosdick, *The Story of the Rockefeller Foundation*, 2nd edition (New Brunswick, NJ: Transaction Publishers, 1989).

21. John Boli and George M. Thomas, eds., *World Polity Formation since 1875: World Culture and International Non-Governmental Organizations* (Stanford, CA: Stanford University Press, 1999); and John W. Meyer, John Boli, and George M. Thomas, "World Society and the Nation- State," *American Journal of Sociology* 103, no. 1 (1997): 144–81.

22. Greer Williams, *The Plague Killers* (New York: Charles Scribner's Sons, 1969); and Lewis Hackett, "Once upon a Time," *American Journal of Tropical Medicine and Hygiene* 9 (1960): 105–15. The American Public Health Association noted in 1950 that the International Health Division (IHD) "has for about a third of a century been a pioneer, a leader, and a catalyst in the development of measures for the improvement of health throughout the world." Quoted in Paul F. Russell, "Some Comments Regarding the IHD—Past and Future," November 3, 1950 (a confidential memo written at the invitation of the director), pp. 2–3, RG 3.1, Series 908, Box 14, Folder 148, Rockefeller Foundation Archives, Rockefeller Archive Center, Sleepy Hollow, NY, hereafter RFA.

23. Luiz A. de Castro Santos, "A Fundacaõ Rockefeller e o Estado Nacional: História e Política de uma Missão Médica e Sanitária no Brasil," *Revista Brasileira de Estudos de Populacão* 6, no. 1 (1989): 105–10.

24. E. Richard Brown, "Public Health in Imperialism: Early Rockefeller Programs at Home and Abroad," *American Journal of Public Health* 66, no. 9 (1976): 879–903; Saúl Franco Agudelo, "The Rockefeller Foundation's Antimalarial Program in Latin America: Donating or Dominating?" *International Journal of Health Services* 13, no. 1 (1983): 51–67; Soma Hewa, *Colonialism, Tropical Disease and Imperial Medicine: Rockefeller Philanthropy in Sri Lanka* (Lanham, MD: University Press of America, 1995); Armando Solórzano, "The

Rockefeller Foundation in Mexico: Nationalism, Public Health, and Yellow Fever, 1911–1924" (PhD diss., University of Wisconsin–Madison, 1990); and Annette B. Ramírez de Arellano, "The Politics of Public Health in Puerto Rico: 1926–1940," *Revista de Salud Pública de Puerto Rico* 3 (1981): 35–58.

25. See, for example, Marcos Cueto, "The Cycles of Eradication: the Rockefeller Foundation and Latin American Public Health, 1918–1940," in *International Health Organisations and Movements, 1918–1939*, 222–43; Ilana Löwy, "What/Who Should Be Controlled: Opposition to Yellow Fever Campaigns in Brazil, 1900–1939," in *Contested Knowledge: Reactions to Western Medicine in the Modern Period*, ed. Andrew Cunningham and Bridie Andrews (Manchester, UK: Manchester University Press, 1997), 124–46; Anne-Emanuelle Birn, "A Revolution in Rural Health?: The Struggle over Local Health Units in Mexico, 1928–1940," *Journal of the History of Medicine and Allied Sciences* 53, no. 1 (1998): 43–76; Steven Palmer, "Central American Encounters with Rockefeller Public Health, 1914–1921," in *Close Encounters of Empire: Writing the Cultural History of U.S.-Latin American Relations*, ed. Gilbert Joseph, Catherine LeGrand, and Ricardo Salvatore (Durham, NC: Duke University Press, 1998), 311–32; Shirish Kavadi, *The Rockefeller Foundation and Public Health in Colonial India, 1916–1945: A Narrative History* (Pune/Mumbai, India: Foundation for Research in Community Health, 1999); Paulo Gadelha, "Conforming Strategies of Public Health Campaigns to Disease Specificity and National Contexts: The Rockefeller Foundation's Early Campaigns against Hookworm and Malaria in Brazil," *Parassitologia* 40, nos. 1 and 2 (June 1998): 159–75; Lion Murard and Patrick Zylberman, "Les fondations indestructibles: La santé publique en France et la Fondation Rockefeller," *Médicine/Sciences* 18, no. 5 (2002): 625–32; and Susan Solomon, "Knowing the Local: Rockefeller Foundation Officers' Site Visits to Russia in the 1920s," *Slavic Review* 62, no. 4 (Winter 2003), 710–32.

26. See, for example, William H. Schneider, ed., *Rockefeller Philanthropy and Modern Biomedicine: International Initiatives from World War I to the Cold War* (Bloomington and Indianapolis: Indiana University Press, 2002); special issue of *Studies in History and Philosophy of Science, Part C: Studies in History and Philosophy of Biological and Biomedical Sciences* 31, no. 3 (September 2000) on the RF as promulgator of medical research and public health; Peter J. Brown, "Failure-as-Success: Multiple Meanings of Eradication in the Rockefeller Foundation Sardinia Project, 1946–1951," *Parassitologia* 40 (June 1998): 117–30; Pnina G. Abir-Am, "The Rockefeller Foundation and the Rise of Molecular Biology," *Nature Reviews* 3 (January 2002): 5–10; Theodore M. Brown, "Alan Gregg and the Rockefeller Foundation's Support of Franz Alexander's Psychosomatic Research," *Bulletin of the History of Medicine* 61, no. 2 (Summer 1987): 155–82; Lily E. Kay, *The Molecular Vision of Life: Caltech, the Rockefeller Foundation, and the Rise of the New Biology* (New York: Oxford University Press, 1993); Robert E. Kohler, *Partners in Science: Foundations and Natural Scientists, 1900–1945* (Chicago: University of Chicago Press, 1991); Lily E. Kay, "Rethinking Institutions: Philanthropy as a Historiographic Problem of Knowledge and Power," in "Philanthropy and Institution-Building in the Twentieth Century," a special issue of *Minerva* 35, no. 3 (Autumn 1997): 283–93; Paul Weindling, "Philanthropy and World Health: The Rockefeller Foundation and the League of Nations Health Organization," in "Philanthropy and Institution-Building in the Twentieth Century," a special issue of *Minerva* 35, no. 3 (Autumn 1997): 269–81; Susan G. Solomon and Nikolai Krementsov, "Giving and Taking across Borders: The Rockefeller Foundation and Soviet Russia, 1919–1928," *Minerva* 3 (2001): 265–98; and Jack Pressman, "Human Understanding: Psychosomatic Medicine and the Mission of the Rockefeller Foundation," in *Greater than the Parts: Holism in Biomedicine, 1920–1950*, ed. Christopher Lawrence and George Weisz (New York: Oxford University Press, 1998), 189–208.

27. Some of the older and newer "classics" on the revolutionary period, its causes, and consequences are: Daniel Cosío Villegas, ed., *Historia Moderna de México*, 8 vols. (México, D.F.: Hermes, 1955–1974); Jean Meyer, *La Revolution Mexicaine, 1910–1940* (Paris: Calmann-Levy, 1973); Jesús Silva Herzog, *Breve Historia de la Revolución Mexicana* (México,

D.F.: Fondo de Cultura Económica, 1960); Friedrich Katz, *The Secret War in Mexico* (Chicago: University of Chicago Press, 1981); Alan Knight, *The Mexican Revolution*, 2 vols. (Cambridge: Cambridge University Press, 1986); James Cockroft, *Precursores Intelectuales de la Revolución Mexicana* (México, D.F.: Siglo Veintiuno Editores, 1971); Michael J. Gonzalez, *The Mexican Revolution, 1910–1940* (Albuquerque: University of New Mexico Press, 2002); and Hans Werner Tobler, *La Revolución Mexicana: Transformación Social y Cambio Político, 1876–1940* (México, D.F.: Alianza Editorial, 1994). A sampling of studies of the revolution in particular settings includes the following: Marcel Morales, *Morelos Agrario: La Construcción de una Alternativa* (México, D.F.: Plaza y Valdés, 1994); Friedrich Katz, ed., *Riot, Rebellion, and Revolution: Rural Social Conflict in Mexico* (Princeton, NJ: Princeton University Press, 1988); Mary Kay Vaughan, *Cultural Politics in Revolution: Teachers, Peasants, and Schools in Mexico, 1930–1940* (Tucson: University of Arizona Press, 1997); Andrew Wood, *Revolution in the Street: Women, Workers, and Urban Protest in Veracruz, 1870–1920* (Wilmington, DE: Scholarly Resources, 2001); and Patience A. Schell, *Church and State Education in Revolutionary Mexico City* (Tucson: University of Arizona Press, 2003).

28. For just a small sampling, see Claudia Agostoni, *Monuments of Progress. Modernization and Public Health in Mexico City, 1876–1910* (Calgary: University of Calgary Press; Denver: University Press of Colorado; México, D.F.: Instituto de Investigaciones Históricas, UNAM [Universidad Nacional Autónoma de México], 2003); Ann S. Blum, "Children without Parents: Law, Charity, and Social Practice, Mexico City, 1870–1940" (PhD diss., University of California, Berkeley, 1997); Katherine Elaine Bliss, *Compromised Positions: Prostitution, Public Health and Gender Politics in Revolutionary Mexico City* (University Park, PA: Penn State University Press, 2001); Ronzón, *Sanidad y Modernización*; Ana Cecilia Rodríguez de Romo and Xóchitl Martínez Barbosa, eds., *Estudios de Historia de la Medicina: Abordajes e Interpretaciones*. (México, D.F.: UNAM, 2001); Ana María Carrillo, "Economía, Política y Salud Pública en el México Porfiriano, 1876–1910," *História, Ciências, Saúde—Manguinhos* 9 (Supplement 2002): 67–87; Fernanda Núñez Becerra, *La Prostitución y su Represión en la Ciudad de México (Siglo XIX): Prácticas y Representaciones* (Barcelona: Biblioteca Latinoamericana de Pensamiento, 2002); Lilia Oliver, "El Cólera en los Barrios de Guadalajara," in *Salud, Cultura y Sociedad en América Latina: Nuevas Perspectivas Históricas*, ed. Marcos Cueto (Lima: IEP y OPS, 1996), 87–109; Ana Maria Kapelusz-Poppi, "Physician Activists and the Development of Rural Health in Postrevolutionary Mexico," *Radical History Review* 80 (Spring 2001): 35–50; and Ernesto Aréchiga Córdoba, "Dictadura Sanitaria, Educación y Propaganda Higiénica en el México Revolucionario, 1917–1932," *Dynamis* 25 (2005): 117–44.

29. Even in Brazil, where the development of basic rural health outposts had accompanied a hookworm campaign in the late 1910s, these posts were soon folded into a new National Department of Health, leaving the RF to concentrate on large-scale disease efforts. See Gilberto Hochman, *A Era do Saneámento: As Bases da Política de Saúde Pública no Brasil* (São Paulo: Editora Hucitec Anpocs, 1998); Nilson do Rosario Costa, *Lutas Urbanas e Controle Sanitário: Origens das Políticas de Saúde no Brasil* (Petropolis, Brasil: Vozes & Abrasco, 1985); and de Castro-Santos, "Fundacão Rockefeller," 105–10.

Chapter One

1. Valuable studies of the Progressive Era include Richard Hofstadter, *The Age of Reform* (New York: Alfred A. Knopf, 1955); and Robert Wiebe, *The Search for Order, 1877–1920* (New York: Hill & Wang, 1967). More recent works include Lewis L. Gould, *America in the Progressive Era, 1890–1914* (New York: Longman, 2001); Alice O'Connor, *Poverty Knowledge: Social Science, Social Policy, and the Poor in Twentieth-Century U.S. History* (Princeton, NJ: Princeton University Press, 2001); and Sidney M. Milkis and Jerome M.

Mileur, eds., *Progressivism and the New Democracy* (Amherst: University of Massachusetts Press, 1999).

2. Andrew Carnegie, "The Gospel of Wealth," *North American Review* 148 (1889): 653–64, and 149 (1889): 682–98.

3. The classic biography of Carnegie is Burton J. Hendrick, *The Life of Andrew Carnegie* (London: William Heinemann, Ltd., 1933). Related works include Ellen C. Lagemann, *Private Power for the Public Good: A History of the Carnegie Foundation for the Advancement of Teaching* (Middletown, CO: Wesleyan University Press; Scranton, PA: Harper & Row, 1983); and Joseph Frazier Wall, *Andrew Carnegie* (New York: Oxford University Press, 1970).

4. The most recent and comprehensive biography of John D. Rockefeller is Ron Chernow, *Titan: The Life of John D. Rockefeller, Sr.* (New York: Random House, 1998). Also see Fosdick, *Story of the Rockefeller Foundation*, 4–6; chapter 3 in John Ettling, *The Germ of Laziness: Rockefeller Philanthropy and Public Health in the New South* (Cambridge, MA: Harvard University Press, 1981); and Judith Sealander, *Private Wealth and Public Life: Foundation Philanthropy and the Reshaping of American Social Policy from the Progressive Era to the New Deal* (Baltimore: Johns Hopkins University Press, 1997).

5. Chernow, *Titan*; and Ettling, *Germ of Laziness*, both discuss Gates's key role in Rockefeller philanthropy.

6. Real dollar conversions have been calculated using the Composite Consumer Price Index from John J. McCusker, *How Much Is That in Real Money? A Historical Price Index for Use as a Deflator of Money Values in the Economy of the United States* (Worcester, MA: American Antiquarian Society, 1992), table A-2, 323–32; and the Consumer Price Index Home Page inflation calculator of the US Department of Labor, Bureau of Labor Statistics, http://www.bls.gov/cpi/home.htm. Peso to dollar conversions were made using Banking and Monetary Statistics tables, "Foreign Exchange Rates by Countries," published in Board of Governors of the Federal Reserve System, *Banking and Monetary Statistics* (Washington, DC: Board of Governors of the Federal Reserve System, 1943), 674.

7. Raymond Fosdick, *Adventure in Giving: The Story of the General Education Board* (New York: Harper and Row, 1962); and Eric Anderson and Alfred A. Moss, Jr., *Dangerous Donations: Northern Philanthropy and Southern Black Education, 1902–1930* (Columbia: University of Missouri Press, 1999). The General Education Board later became involved in higher education, especially the reform of medical education. See E. Richard Brown, *Rockefeller Medicine Men* (Berkeley: University of California Press, 1979); Howard Berliner, *A System of Scientific Medicine: Philanthropic Foundations in the Flexner Era* (New York: Tavistock, 1985); Kenneth M. Ludmerer, *Learning to Heal: The Development of American Medical Education* (New York: Basic Books, 1985); and Steven C. Wheatley, *The Politics of Philanthropy: Abraham Flexner and Medical Education* (Madison: University of Wisconsin Press, 1989).

8. In 1838, Italian physician Angelo Dubini was probably the first to discover the presence of hookworms in humans. It was Brazilian physicians who were among the earliest to debate the etiology of hookworm, with old-school Rio de Janeiro-based Dr. José Martins de Cruz Jobim holding that climatic and meteorological conditions combined with bad hygienic habits were the cause of hookworm disease and upstart Dr. Otto Wucherer of the Bahian Tropicalista School averring that hookworm parasites, together with secondary factors relating to diet and hygiene, caused the ailment. See Julyan Peard, "Tropical Disorders and the Forging of a Brazilian Medical Identity," *Hispanic American Historical Review* 77, no. 1 (1997): 1–45. Helminthological and entomological references from the early twentieth century include Robert Hegner and William Taliaferro, *Human Protozoology* (New York: MacMillan Company, 1924); Millard Langfeld, *Introduction to Infectious and Parasitic Diseases including their Cause and Manner of Transmission* (Philadelphia: P. Blakiston, 1907); and Ernest Carroll Faust, *Human Helminthology: A Manual for Clinicians, Sanitarians, and Medical Zoologists* (Philadelphia: Lea and Febiger, 1929). A current medical school text that discusses hookworm is Dickson D. Despommier et al., *Parasitic Diseases*, 4th ed. (New York: Apple Tree, 2000).

9. On Ashford's campaign in Puerto Rico, see Ramirez de Arellano, "Politics of Public Health in Puerto Rico," 35–58. For more on the competition between Stiles and Ashford, see Ettling, *Germ of Laziness*, 29–32 and 124–27.

10. Palmer, "Central American Encounters,"316.

11. For a thorough account of the Rockefeller Sanitary Commission, see Ettling, *Germ of Laziness*. Also see Stephen J. Kunitz's "Hookworm and Pellagra: Exemplary Diseases in the New South," *Journal of Health and Social Behavior* 29 (1988): 139–48; Mary Boccaccio, "Ground Itch and Dew Poison: The Rockefeller Sanitary Commission: 1909–1914," *Journal of the History of Medicine and Allied Sciences* 27 (1972): 30–53; James H. Cassedy, "The 'Germ of Laziness' in the South, 1900–1915: Charles Wardell Stiles and the Progressive Paradox," *Bulletin of the History of Medicine* 45 (1971): 159–69; and William Link, "Privies, Progressivism, and Public Schools: Health Reform and Education in the Rural South, 1909–1920," *Journal of Southern History* 54 (1988): 623–42. For an economic perspective, see Garland L. Brinkley, "The Economic Impact of Disease in the American South, 1860–1940," *Journal of Economic History* 55, no. 2 (June 1995): 371–73.

12. See Ettling, *Germ of Laziness*; and Warwick Anderson, "Going through the Motions: American Public Health and Colonial 'Mimicry,'" *American Literary History* 14 (Winter 2002): 686–719.

13. These trials and tribulations can be followed through the very different perspectives of Fosdick, *Story of the Rockefeller Foundation*; and Brown, *Rockefeller Medicine Men*.

14. Fosdick, *Story of the Rockefeller Foundation*, 24.

15. The story of the International Health Board/International Health Division (IHB/IHD) has been told by Hackett, "Once Upon a Time," 105–15; Williams, *Plague Killers*; Fosdick, *Story of the Rockefeller Foundation*; and, most recently, Farley, *To Cast Out Disease*. For a brief but excellent introduction to the IHB's work in Latin America, see Marcos Cueto, "Visions of Science and Development: The Rockefeller Foundation's Latin American Surveys of the 1920s," in *Missionaries of Science: The Rockefeller Foundation and Latin America*, ed. Marcos Cueto (Bloomington: Indiana University Press, 1994), 1–22. There are numerous memoirs and biographies of physicians who worked with the International Health Board: M. E. M. Walker, *Pioneers of Public Health: The Story of Some Benefactors of the Human Race* (Edinburgh: Oliver & Boyd, 1930); Wilder Penfield, *The Difficult Art of Giving: The Epic of Alan Gregg* (Boston: Little, Brown and Company, 1967); Benjamin E. Washburn, *As I Recall* (New York: Rockefeller Foundation, 1960); Hugh H. Smith, *Life's a Pleasant Institution: The Peregrinations of a Rockefeller Doctor* (Tucson, AZ: self-published, 1978); Victor Heiser, *An American Doctor's Odyssey: Adventures in Forty-Five Countries* (New York: W. W. Norton and Company, Inc., 1936); and Fred Soper, *Ventures in World Health: The Memoirs of Fred Lowe Soper*, ed. John Duffy (Washington, DC: Pan American Health Organization [PAHO], 1977).

16. See Robert Shaplen, *Toward the Well-Being of Mankind: Fifty Years of the Rockefeller Foundation* (New York: Doubleday and Company, Inc., 1964).

17. "Committee on Appraisal and Plan," 1934, as cited in "Report of the Inter-Divisional Committee on Latin America to RBF [Raymond B. Fosdick]," ca. 1944, RG 1.2, Series 300, Box 1, Folder 7, 1–2, RFA. Also see Fosdick to Douglas Freeman, October 31, 1938, RG 2, Series 300, Box 160, Folder 1177, RFA.

18. See Fosdick, *Story of the Rockefeller Foundation*; Ettling, *Germ of Laziness*; Chernow, *Titan*; and Martin Morse Wooster, *The Foundation Builders: Brief Biographies of Twelve Great Philanthropists* (Washington D.: The Philanthropy Roundtable, 2001).

19. Kohler, *Partners in Science*.

20. Farley, *To Cast Out Disease*, 6–12.

21. Merle Curti, "Philanthropy," in *Dictionary of the History of Ideas*, ed. Philip P. Wiener (New York: Scribner, 1973–74), 486–93.

22. Robert Arnove, ed., *Philanthropy and Cultural Imperialism: The Foundations at Home and Abroad* (Boston: G. K. Hall and Co., 1980).

23. A more recent text that takes up these questions is Ellen C. Lagemann, *Philanthropic Foundation: New Scholarship, New Possibilities* (Bloomington: Indiana University Press, 1999).

24. Barry Karl and Stanley Katz, "Foundations and Ruling Class Elites," *Daedalus* 116, no. 1 (1987): 14.

25. John D. Rockefeller Jr. to John D. Rockefeller Sr., April 17, 1917, Rockefeller Family Archives, Rockefeller Archive Center, Box 26, as quoted in Karl and Katz on p. 13.

26. Franklin McVaugh to Secretary of State Knox, March 28, 1911; Department of State General Instruction, Consular No. 20, April 3, 1911 (File 102.15/3), "Hookworm Infection," and responses from American consuls and vice consuls throughout the world. For example, Lewis Haskell, American Consul in Salina Cruz, Mexico, to Secretary of State Knox, June 1, 1911, RG 59, Decimal File 1910–29, Box 460, National Archives and Record Administration, College Park, MD, hereafter NARA.

27. Fosdick, *Story of the Rockefeller Foundation*, 33; Shaplen, *Toward the Well-Being*, 30; and Farley, *To Cast Out Disease*, 62–74.

28. Memorandum from George Vincent to Wickliffe Rose, April 23, 1919, RG 5, Series 2, Subseries 323, Box 33, Folder 197, RFA.

29. Rose, "Memorandum on the Principles of Administration of the IHB," 1922, RG 3.1, Series 908, Box 12, Folder 128, RFA.

30. Fosdick, *Story of the Rockefeller Foundation*, 34.

31. Cueto, "Visions of Science and Development," 2–3.

32. Rose, "Memorandum on the Principles of Administration of the IHB," 1922, RG 3.1, Series 908, Box 12, Folder 128, RFA.

33. As one IHD officer to Mexico put it: because over the years the RF remained "discretely [*sic*] anonymous," seeking no public recognition, there was "no offence to local pride." George Payne, interviewed by Lewis Hackett, ca. 1950, and Notes, Vol. 1, RG 3.1, Series 908, Box 3, Folder 19, RFA.

34. Rose to Jerome Greene, September 30, 1915, RG 1.2, Series 300, Box 2, Folder 16, RFA.

35. Fee, *Disease and Discovery*, 26.

36. Minutes of the Rockefeller Foundation, June 27, 1913, p. 1027 as cited in Fosdick, *Story of the Rockefeller Foundation*, 24.

37. Rose to Greene, September 30, 1915, RG 1.2, Series 300, Box 2, Folder 16, RFA. Also see Cueto, "Cycles of Eradication"; and John Farley, "The International Health Division of the Rockefeller Foundation: The Russell Years, 1920–1934," in *International Health Organisations and Movements, 1918–1939*, ed. Paul Weindling (Cambridge: Cambridge University Press, 1995), 203–21; and Roy Acheson, *Wickliffe Rose of the Rockefeller Foundation: 1862–1914* (Cambridge, UK: Killycarn Press, 1992).

38. International Health Board, Summary of Policies in Force, Public Health Work, May 25, 1927, RG 3.1, Series 908, Box 11, Folder 123, RFA.

39. The IHB's tuberculosis program in France was an exception to this rule. See Lion Murard and Patrick Zylberman, "La Mission Rockefeller en France et la creation du Comité National de Defense contre la Tuberculose, 1917–1923," *Revue d'histoire moderne et contemporaine* 34 (April–June 1987): 257–81; and Lion Murard and Patrick Zylberman, "Seeds for French Health Care: Did the Rockefeller Foundation Plant the Seeds between the Two World Wars?" *Studies in the History and Philosophy of Biological and Medical Sciences* 31, no. 3 (2000): 463–75.

40. Rose, memorandum, 1920, RG 1.2, Series 300, Box 2, File 14, RFA.

41. Rose to Greene, September 30, 1915, RG 1.2, Series 300, Box 2, Folder 16, RFA.

42. Darwin H. Stapleton, "Lessons of History? Anti-Malaria Strategies of the International Health Board and the Rockefeller Foundation from the 1920s to the Era of DDT," *Public Health Reports* 119 (March–April 2004): 206–15.

43. International Health Board, Summary of Policies in Force, Public Health Work, May 25, 1927, RG 3.1, Series 908, Box 11, Folder 123, RFA.

44. Darwin H. Stapleton, "A Success for Science or Technology? The Rockefeller Foundation's Role in Malaria Eradication in Italy, 1924–1935," *Medicina nei Secoli* 6, no.1 (1994): 213–28.

45. Brown, "Failure-as-Success"; Giovanni Berlinguer, "Parasitoses and Development: Malaria and Echinococcosis," *Parassitologia* 33, no. 1 (1991): 1–10.

46. Randall M. Packard and Paulo A. Gadelha, "A Land Filled with Mosquitoes: Fred L. Soper, the Rockefeller Foundation, and the *Anopheles gambiae* Invasion of Brazil," *Parassitologia* 36, nos. 1–2 (1994): 197–213.

47. Stapleton, "Lessons of History?"

48. Yellow fever intermittently plagued the Americas from the seventeenth to the early twentieth centuries. See Donald C. Cooper, "Brazil's Long Fight against Epidemic Disease, 1849–1917, with Special Emphasis on Yellow Fever," *Bulletin of the New York Academy of Medicine* 51 (1975): 672–96; François Delaporte, *The History of Yellow Fever: An Essay on the Birth of Tropical Medicine* (Cambridge, MA: MIT Press, 1991); William Coleman, *Yellow Fever in the North: The Methods of Early Epidemiology* (Madison: University of Wisconsin Press, 1987); John Duffy, "Yellow Fever in the Continental United States during the Nineteenth Century," *Bulletin of the New York Academy of Medicine* 54 (1968): 687–701; John Duffy, *Sword of Pestilence: The New Orleans Yellow Fever Epidemic of 1853* (Baton Rouge: Louisiana State University Press, 1966); Martin S. Pernick, "Politics, Parties, and Pestilence: Epidemic Yellow Fever in Philadelphia and the Rise of the First Party System," in *Sickness and Health in America: Readings in the History of Medicine and Public Health,* ed. Judith Walzer Leavitt and Ronald Numbers (Madison: University of Wisconsin Press, 1985), 356–71; Margaret Humphreys, *Yellow Fever and the South* (New Brunswick, NJ: Rutgers University Press, 1992); John H. Ellis, *Yellow Fever and Public Health in the New South* (Lexington: University Press of Kentucky, 1992); Nancy Stepan, "The Interplay between Socio-Economic Factors and Medical Science: Yellow Fever Research, Cuba and the United States," *Social Studies of Science* 8 (1978): 397–423; Henry Hanson, *The Pied Piper of Peru: Dr. Henry Hanson's Fight against "Yellow Jack" and Bubonic Plague in South America, 1919–1922,* ed. Doris Hurnie (Jacksonville, FL: Convention Press, 1961); Henry Rose Carter, *Yellow Fever: An Epidemiological and Historical Study of Its Place of Origin* (Baltimore: Williams and Wilkins, 1931); and Wilbur Downs, "History of Epidemiological Aspects of Yellow Fever," *Yale Journal of Biology and Medicine* 55 (1982): 179–85.

49. José López Sánchez, *Finlay: El Hombre y la Verdad Científica* (La Habana, Cuba: Editorial Científico-Técnica, 1986); and William B. Bean, *Walter Reed: A Biography* (Charlottesville: University Press of Virginia, 1982).

50. Vincent J. Cirillo, *Bullets and Bacilli: The Spanish-American War and Military Medicine* (New Brunswick, NJ: Rutgers University Press, 2004); William Crawford Gorgas, *Sanitation in Panama* (New York, Appleton, 1915); and J. Ewing Mears, *The Triumph of American Medicine in the Construction of the Panama Canal,* 3rd ed. (Philadelphia: William J. Dornan, 1913).

51. See George Vincent, "The Work of the Rockefeller Foundation. Health as an International Bond," speech given at the Empire Club, Toronto, March 9, 1920, *The Empire Club of Canada Speeches 1920* (Toronto, Canada: Empire Club of Canada, 1921), 126–45.

52. Herbert Joseph Spinden, "Yellow Fever—First and Last," *World's Work* 41 (December 1922): 31–43. Found in RG 5, Series 2, Subseries 323, Box 33, Folder 198, p. 181, RFA.

53. Joseph H. White, "The Method of Dissemination and the Possibility of Elimination of Yellow Fever," March 5, 1915, RG 5, Series 2, Special Reports, Box 22, File 135, RFA.

54. Quevedo, et al., *Café y Gusanos,* 157–58, Benchimol, *Febre Amarela.*

55. See Lois Parks and Gustave Nuremberger, "The Sanitation of Guayaquil," *Hispanic American Historical Review* 23 (1943): 197–221; Marcos Cueto, "Sanitation from Above: Yellow Fever and Foreign Intervention in Peru, 1919–1922," Hispanic American Historical Review 72, no. 1 (1992): 1–22; and Farley, *To Cast Out Disease.*

56. Löwy, "What/Who Should Be Controlled"; Steven C. Williams, "Nationalism and Public Health: The Convergence of Rockefeller Foundation Technique and Brazilian

Federal Authority during the Time of Yellow Fever, 1925–1930," in *Missionaries of Science: The Rockefeller Foundation and Latin America*, ed. Marcos Cueto (Bloomington: Indiana University Press, 1994); Löwy, *Virus, moustiques, et modernité;* Jaime L. Benchimol, *Dos Micróbios aos Mosquitos: Febre Amarela e a Revolução Pasteuriana no Brasil* (Rio de Janiero: Editora Fiocruz and Editora Universidade Federal de Rio de Janeiro, 1999); and Benchimol, *Febre Amarela*. For a firsthand account of the yellow fever control program in Brazil, see Fred Soper et al., *The Organization of Permanent Nation-Wide Anti-Aedes Aegypti Measures in Brazil* (New York: Rockefeller Foundation, 1943).

57. See Abraham Flexner, *Medical Education in the United States and Canada* (New York: Carnegie Foundation for the Advancement of Teaching, Bulletin no. 4, 1910). There is a large literature on Flexner and the "Flexner Report." For Flexner's views on preventive medicine, see Brown, *Rockefeller Medicine Men;* Berliner, *System of Scientific Medicine;* Paul Starr, *The Social Transformation of American Medicine* (New York: Basic Books, 1982); and Gert H. Brieger, "The Flexner Report: Revised or Revisited?" *Medical Heritage* 1 (1985): 24–34. For Flexner's role in promoting a medical model of public health, see Fee, *Disease and Discovery*. For Flexner's relationship with foundations and philanthropists, see Wheatley, *Politics of Philanthropy*. For a view from the 1920s see Hans Zinsser, "The Perils of Magnanimity: A Problem in American Medical Education," *Atlantic Monthly* 139, no. 2 (1927): 246–50.

58. Fee, *Disease and Discovery;* and Elizabeth Fee and Roy Acheson, eds., *A History of Education in Public Health: Health that Mocks the Doctors' Rules* (Oxford: Oxford University Press, 1991).

59. The succession of name and organizational changes reveals the conceptual and factional shifts within and between these fields and at the RF. In 1955, the Division of Medicine and Public Health once again split into the Division of Medical Education and Public Health and the Division of Biological and Medical Research. In 1959, the two joined again to become the Division of Medical and Natural Sciences and then the Division of Biomedical Sciences in 1970. In 1974, the Division of Health Sciences superseded its predecessor, and in 1978, the Division of Population Sciences was added to the RF. See William H. Schneider, "The Men who Followed Flexner: Richard Pearce, Alan Gregg, and the Rockefeller Foundation Medical Division, 1919–1951," in *Rockefeller Philanthropy and Modern Biomedicine: International Initiatives from World War I to the Cold War*, ed. William H. Schneider (Bloomington and Indianapolis: Indiana University Press, 2002), 7–60.

60. As Robert Lambert pointed out, occasionally a first-rate scientific researcher emerged out of deplorable Latin American medical schools, just as Simon Flexner had graduated from one of the worst proprietary medical schools of his day. Lambert, "Visit to Mexico," March 1–14, 1941, RG 1.1, Series 323, Box 13, Folder 95, RFA.

61. Fosdick, *Story of the Rockefeller Foundation,* 114.

62. Cueto, "Visions of Science and Development."

63. Fosdick, *Story of the Rockefeller Foundation,* 114; Maria G. S. M. C. Marinho, *Norte-Americanos no Brasil: Uma História da Fundação Rockefeller na Universidade de São Paulo, 1934–1952* (Campinas: Editora Autores Associados, 2001); and Amy Kemp, "The Rockefeller Foundation and the Faculdade de Medicina de São Paulo: A Case Study in Philanthropy as Policy" (PhD diss., Indiana University, 2004). Kemp and Coelho Edler argue that Flexner's influence in Brazil was limited. Amy Kemp and Flavio Coelho Edler, "Medical Reform in Brazil and the U.S.: A Comparison of Two Rhetorics," *História, Ciências, Saúde—Manguinhos* 11, no. 3 (September/December 2004): 569–85. For more on the Brazilian medical profession, see Jaime L. Benchimol, *Manguinhos do Sonho à Vida: A Ciência na Belle Epoque* (Rio de Janeiro: Casa de Oswaldo Cruz/Editora Fiocruz, 1990); and Nancy Stepan, *Beginnings of Brazilian Science: Oswaldo Cruz, Medical Research and Policy, 1890–1920* (New York: Science History Publications, 1981).

64. Lambert to Fosdick, July 14, 1943, RG 2, Series 300, Box 252, Folder 1738, RFA.

65. Lambert to Fosdick, July 14, 1943, RG 2, Series 300, Box 252, Folder 1738, RFA. The Peking Union Medical College received by far the RF's largest single overseas investment;

the $45 million it received from 1915 to 1949, compared to less than one million in constant dollars for all public health activities in Mexico over a similar period. Standard accounts include Mary Bullock, *An American Transplant: The Rockefeller Foundation and Peking Union Medical College* (Berkeley: University of California Press, 1980); Mary Ferguson, *China Medical Board and Peking Union Medical College: A Chronicle of Fruitful Collaboration, 1914–1951* (New York: The China Medical Board of New York, 1970); and John Bowers, *Western Medicine in a Chinese Palace: Peking Union Medical College* (New York: Josiah Macy Jr. Foundation, 1972). More critical perspectives include Frank Ninkovich, "The Rockefeller Foundation, China, and Cultural Change," *Journal of American History* 70, no. 4 (1984): 799–820; E. Richard Brown, "Rockefeller Medicine in China: Professionalism and Imperialism," in *Philanthropy and Cultural Imperialism: The Foundations at Home and Abroad*, ed. Robert Arnove (Boston: G. K. Hall and Co., 1980), 123–46; and Qiusha Ma, "The Rockefeller Foundation and Modern Medical Education in China, 1915–1951" (PhD diss., Case Western Reserve University, 1995). See also George Basalla, "The Spread of Western Science," *Science* 156 (1967): 611–22; and Ralph Croizier, *Traditional Medicine in Modern China: Science, Nationalism, and the Tensions of Cultural Change* (Cambridge, MA: Harvard University Press, 1968).

66. See Hebe Vessuri, "Enfermería de Salud Pública, Modernización y Cooperación Internacional: El Proyecto de la Escuela Nacional de Enfermeras, 1936–1950," *História, Ciências, Saúde—Manguinhos* 8, no. 3 (September–December 2001): 507–39; and Martha C. Nunes Moreira, "A Fundação Rockefeller e a Construção da Identidade Profissional de Enfermagem no Brasil na Primeira República," *História, Ciências, Saúde—Manguinhos* 5 (November 1998–February 1999): 621–45.

67. The Liverpool and London schools of tropical medicine founded in 1899 initially focused on health and disease research in tropical climates, overlapping with, but not identical to, public health and training concerns. In 1922, the RF endowed the London school, which was to become the London School of Hygiene and Tropical Medicine. It finally opened in 1929. See Lise Wilkinson and Anne Hardy, *Prevention and Cure: The London School of Hygiene and Tropical Medicine* (London: Kegan Paul, 2001).

68. Fosdick, *Story of the Rockefeller Foundation*, 42; Lina Rodrigues de Faria, "A Fundação Rockefeller e os Serviços de Saúde em São Paulo, 1920–1930: Perspectivas Históricas," *História, Ciências, Saúde—Manguinhos* 9, no. 3 (September–December 2002): 561–90; Luiz A. de Castro Santos, "Os Primeiros Centros de Saúde nos Estados Unidos e no Brasil: Um Estudo Comparativo," *Teoria e Pesquisa* 40/41 (January–July 2002): 137–81; and Heloísa H. Pimenta Rocha, *A Higienização dos Costumes: Educação Escolar e Saúde no Projeto do Instituto de Higiene de São Paulo, 1918–1925* (Campinas, Brasil: Mercado das Letras, 2003).

69. Cueto, "Visions of Science and Development," 1–22. De Castro Santos, "Power, Ideology, and Public Health in Brazil," argues that Brazil's strong tradition in preventive medicine, the acceptance of sanitary reform ideas among elites, and a "growing wave of federal intervention in the states" made it a favorable setting for public health activities.

70. According to Lambert, "That is not Latin American either but just human nature." Lambert to Fosdick, July 14, 1943, RG 2, Series 300, Box 252, Folder 1738, RFA.

71. Table IIa, Public Health Fellowships and Nursing Fellowships for the Years 1917–1950, *The Rockefeller Foundation Directory of Fellowship Awards, 1917–1950*, RG 12, Series 100, Box 32, Folder 239, RFA.

72. See, for example, Wilson G. Smillie, "La Salubridad en Latino América," *Boletín de la Oficina Sanitaria Panamericana* 29, no. 2 (1950): 171–80; interview with Augusto Fujigaki Lechuga, May 31, 1991, Cuernavaca, Morelos; and interview with Luis Vargas, March 5, 1991, Mexico City.

73. Löwy, *Virus, moustiques et modernité*, 14–15; Miguel E. Bustamante, *La Fiebre Amarilla en México y su Origen en América* (México, D.F.: Secretaría de Salubridad y Asistencia [SSA], 1958); Helen J. Power, *Tropical Medicine in the Twentieth Century* (London: Kegan Paul International, 1999); and Anne Marie Moulin, "Patriarchal Science: The Network of

Overseas Pasteur Institutes," in *Science and Empires*, eds. Patrick Petitjean et al. (Dordrecht, Netherlands: Kluwer Academic Press, 1992), 307–320.

74. Office International d'Hygiène Publique, *Vingt-cinq ans d'activité de l'Office International d'Hygiène Publique, 1909–1933* (Paris: Office International d'Hygiène Publique [OIHP], 1933). See also Paul F. Basch, "A Historical Perspective on International Health," *Infectious Disease Clinics of North America* 5 (1991): 183–96.

75. During the Cold War, U.S. philanthropy was again accused of being a willing partner to U.S. hegemony. Robert Arnove has argued that foundations promote the dominance of American cultural values overseas, enhancing the United States' economic power. Other researchers have come to similar conclusions: see Edward H. Berman, *The Influence of the Carnegie, Ford, and Rockefeller Foundations on American Foreign Policy* (Albany: State University of New York Press, 1983); and Emily Rosenberg, *Spreading the American Dream: American Economic and Cultural Expansion, 1890–1945* (New York: Hill and Wang, 1982).

76. The IHD was self-reflective on this point. See, for example, "Draft of Notes on Backward Areas Discussion," March 5, 1949, RG 3.2, Series 900, Box 60, Folder 332, RFA. Graham Hancock, *Lords of Poverty: The Power, Prestige and Corruption of the International Aid Business* (New York: Atlantic Monthly Press, 1989), offers a sinister analysis of the overlapping work of bilateral foreign aid agencies, international financial institutions, and foundations.

77. Warwick Anderson, "Colonial Pathologies: American Medicine in the Philippines, 1898–1921" (PhD diss., University of Pennsylvania, 1992).

78. Cirillo, *Bullets and Bacilli.*

79. Birn, "No More Surprising than a Broken Pitcher?" 17–46; and Cueto, *El Valor de la Salud.*

80. See David McBride, *Missions for Science: U.S. Technology and Medicine in America's Africa World* (New Brunswick, NJ: Rutgers University Press, 2002).

81. Charles Morrow Wilson, *Ambassadors in White: The Story of American Tropical Medicine* (New York: Henry Holt and Company, 1942), 279 and chapter 12, "Banana Medicine."

82. In 1916, the United Fruit Company's agents in Cartagena, Colombia sought to influence the Colombian government to invite the U.S. Public Health Service (USPHS) to station quarantine officers in Colombia in order to "be freed from quarantine restrictions in the U.S." In this instance the attempt was unsuccessful, but in many others, USPHS officers worked closely with U.S. business interests overseas. See Leonard Blake Modeta to Secretary of State, July 7, 1916, RG 59, Department of State Decimal File, 1910–29, Box 461, NARA.

83. Wilson, *Ambassadors in White*, chapter 7, "Deeks of Canada," 156–83; and Aviva Chomsky, *West Indian Workers and the United Fruit Company in Costa Rica, 1870–940* (Baton Rouge: Louisiana State University Press, 1996), 110–43.

84. See, for example, William E. Deeks, *A Review of the Digestive Functions and Food Requirements for the Maintenance of Health with Particular Reference to the Tropics* (Boston: United Fruit Company, 1925). Deeks also pioneered a powder-based infant formula that would not spoil, promoting consumption of a product to be bought in the marketplace rather than addressing maternal nutrition to improve breast-feeding.

85. Russell to Deeks, September 11, 1923, RG 5, Series 1.1, Box 72, Folder 1026, RFA.

86. Deeks to Russell, April 6, 1923, RG 5, Series 1.1, Box 72, Folder 1026, RFA. Deeks published his own hookworm pamphlet in 1925: *The Cause of Hookworm Disease and Its Prevention.*

87. See Stabler's hand-written notes on Rose to Jordan Stabler, July 19, 1918, RG 59, Decimal File 1910–29, Box 7295, NARA.

88. J. A. Ryan to George Vincent, December 1, 1922, RG 1.1, Series 323, Box 13, File 93, RFA.

89. James R. Sheffield to Vincent, April 7, 1925, RG 1.1, Series 323, Box 13, File 93, RFA.

90. Vincent to Sheffield, May 5, 1925, RG 1.1, Series 323, Box 13, File 93, RFA.

91. Sheffield to Vincent, May 13, 1925, and Vincent to Sheffield, May 21, 1925, RG 1.1, Series 323, Box 13, File 93, RFA.

92. Sydnor Walker, interview with Laurence Duggan, Division of Latin American Affairs, Department of State, October 23, 1936, Washington, DC, RG 2, Series 300, Box 133, Folder 997, RFA.

93. See memorandum of John A. Ferrell of conference: Vice President Wallace, Raymond B. Fosdick and John A. Ferrell, regarding "Mexico—Its Problems and Remedies," February 3, 1941, Senate Office Building, Washington, DC. RG 1.1, Series 323, Box 1, Folder 2, RFA.

94. Pyenson, "In Partibus Infidelium."

95. J. D. Long, "Memorandum to U.S. Surgeon General re Contemplated Conference between Surgeon General. Cumming and Dr. Alfonso Pruneda, Secretary General, Department of Health, Mexico," March 1, 1923, RG 90, Central File, 1897–1923, Box 177, Yellow Fever, Category 1876, Year 1923, NARA.

96. Miguel E. Bustamante, "La Situación Epidemiológica de México en el Siglo XIX," in *Ensayos Sobre la Historia de las Epidemias en México,* ed. Enrique Florescano and Elsa Malvido, vol. 1 (México, D.F.: Instituto Mexicano del Seguro Social [IMSS], 1982), 37–66.

97. A standard introductory treatment of modern Mexico is Leslie Bethell, ed., *Mexico since Independence* (Cambridge: Cambridge University Press, 1991).

98. John Mason Hart, *Empire and Revolution: The Americans in Mexico since the Civil War* (Berkeley: University of California Press, 2002).

99. Recent accounts of the Porfiriato include Paul Garner, *Porfirio Díaz: Del Héroe al Dictador: Una Biografía Política* (Mexico City: Editorial Planeta, 2003); and Claudia Agostoni and Elisa Speckman, eds., *Modernidad, Tradición y Alteridad: La Ciudad de México en el Cambio de Siglo XIX–XX* (México, D.F.: Universidad Nacional Autónoma de México [UNAM], 2001).

100. For a detailed discussion of the Mexican economy in this period, see Jeffrey L. Bortz and Stephen Haber, *The Mexican Economy, 1879–1930: Essays on the Economic History of Institutions, Revolutions, and Growth* (Stanford, CA: Stanford University Press, 2002).

101. Britain's investments were 29.1 percent and France's were 26.7 percent of the total foreign investment. In 1911, 41.3 percent of U.S. investment was in railroads, 38.6 percent was in mines and metallurgy, and the remainder was in real estate, oil, public debt, banks, and industry. These numbers come from Roger D. Hansen's calculations in *The Politics of Mexican Development* (Baltimore: Johns Hopkins University Press, 1971), tables 2-2 and 2-3, 16–17.

102. Fernando Rosenzweig, "El Comercio Exterior," in *Historia Moderna de México,* vol. 7, ed. Daniel Cosío Villegas (México, D.F.: Hermes, 1965), 635–729.

103. See Hansen, *Politics of Mexican Development,* tables 2-1 and 2-4, 15 and 22; Rosenzweig, "Comercio Exterior"; and Meyer, "Mexico in the 1920s."

104. Leopoldo Solís Manjarrez, *La Realidad Económica Mexicana: Retrovisión y Perspectivas* (México, D.F.: Siglo XXI Editores, 1970); and Enrique Cárdenas, ed., *Historia Económica de México, Lecturas,* vol. 3 (México, D.F.: Fondo de Cultura Económica, 1992).

105. For a discussion of Mexican positivism, see Leopoldo Zea, *El Positivismo en México* (México, D.F.: Biblioteca del Instituto Nacional de Estudios Históricos de la Revolución Mexicana, 1953); Moisés González Navarro, *Sociedad y Cultura en el Porfiriato* (México, D.F.: Cien de México, 1994); Charles A. Hale, *The Transformation of Liberalism in Late Nineteenth Century Mexico* (Princeton, NJ: Princeton University Press, 1989); and Alexandra M. Stern, "Eugenics beyond Borders: Science and Medicalization in Mexico and the U.S. West, 1900–1950" (PhD diss., University of Chicago, 1999).

106. Much of this discussion derives from Friedrich Katz's seminal article, "Labor Conditions on Haciendas in Porfirian Mexico: Some Trends and Tendencies," *Hispanic American Historical Review* 54, no. 1 (1974): 1–47. Prior analyses offer a level of certainty and generalization that Katz masterfully disputes.

107. See B. R. Mitchell, *International Historical Statistics: The Americas 1750–1993,* 4th ed., New York: Stockton Press, 1998); and, for example, Anne-Emanuelle Birn, Raquel Pollero, and Wanda Cabella, "No Hay que Llorar sobre Leche Derramada: El

Pensamiento Epidemiológico y la Mortalidad Infantil en Uruguay, 1900–1940," *Estudios Interdisciplinarios de América Latina* 14 (2003): 35–65.

108. Rodolfo Flores Talavera and Miguel E. Bustamante, "Salud Pública y Desarrollo Económico y Social," *Salud Pública de México* 5 (1963): 777–91.

109. Pedro Daniel Martínez, "Planeación de la Salud Pública como Factor de Desarrollo Nacional" *Salud Pública de México* 5 (1963): 621–26.

110. Alberto Pani, *Hygiene in Mexico: A Study of Sanitary and Educational Problems*, trans. Ernest L. de Gogorza (New York and London: Knickerbocker Press, 1917), table I, 4–5. Table II shows that Mexico City has the highest mortality rate of all the American capitals. Pani undertook his study of hygiene at the request of President Venustiano Carranza. Pani argued that with far more physicians and engineers practicing "scientific hygiene," over one third of Mexico City's deaths could be prevented (37–39). He believed that the only solution to Mexico's health problems was to federalize public health services with implementation authority instead of mere advisory status, and he lobbied for the creation of a Department of Health in the 1917 Constitution. For more on Pani, see Keith Allen Haynes, "Orden y Progreso: The Revolutionary Ideology of Alberto J. Pani," in *Los Intelectuales y el Poder en México*, ed. Roderic Camp, Charles Hale, and Josefina Zoraida Vásquez (México, D.F.: El Colegio de México, 1981).

111. Pani, *Hygiene in Mexico*, table IV, 10–11.

112. Claudia Agostoni, "Sanitation and Public Works in Late Nineteenth Century Mexico City," *Quipu* 12, no. 2 (1999): 187–201; and Agostoni, *Monuments of Progress*.

113. Literary depictions of disease in Mexico City appear in novels by Emilio Rabasa and Fernando Gamboa as well as in virtually all travelers' accounts of the period. See Agostoni, *Monuments of Progress*.

114. Pani, *Hygiene in Mexico*, 7. Anthony Mazzaferri, "Public Health and Social Revolution in Mexico: 1870–1930" (PhD diss., Kent State University, 1968) cites a number of further sources describing Mexico's social conditions on the eve of the revolution.

115. There is a vast literature on the Mexican Revolution. See, for example, Adolfo Gilly, *La Revolución Interrumpida; México, 1910–1920: Una Guerra Campesina por la Tierra y el Poder* (México, D.F.: Ediciones El Caballito, 1971, repr. 1994); Meyer, *Revolution Mexicaine*; Jorge Vera Estañol, *La Revolución Mexicana: Orígenes y Resultados* (México, D.F.: Editorial Porrúa, S.A., 1957); Silva Herzog, *Breve Historia*; Knight, *Mexican Revolution*; John Mason Hart, *Revolutionary Mexico: The Coming and Process of the Mexican Revolution* (Berkeley: University of California Press, 1987); Katz, *Secret War*; Cockroft, *Precursores Intelectuales*; John Lear, *Workers, Neighbors, and Citizens: The Revolution in Mexico City* (Lincoln: University of Nebraska Press, 2001); Gonzalez, *Mexican Revolution*; Tobler, *Revolución Mexicana*; and Friedrich Katz, *The Life and Times of Pancho Villa* (Stanford, CA: Stanford University Press, 1998).

116. See John Womack, "The Mexican Revolution, 1910–1920," in *Mexico since Independence*, ed. Leslie Bethell (Cambridge: Cambridge University Press, 1991); and Alan Knight, "The Mexican Revolution: Bourgeois? Nationalist? Or Just a 'Great Rebellion'?" *Bulletin of Latin American Research* 4, no. 2 (1985): 1–37.

117. See Katz, *Secret War*, 3–27.

118. For a broader discussion of these issues, see, for example, Alan Knight, *U.S. Mexican Relations, 1910–1940: An Interpretation* (San Diego: University of California, Center for U.S.-Mexican Studies, 1987).

119. John Skirius, "Railroad, Oil and Other Foreign Interests in the Mexican Revolution, 1911–1914," *Journal of Latin American Studies* 35 (2003): 25–51.

120. Sandra Kuntz Ficker, "The Export Boom of the Mexican Revolution: Characteristics and Contributing Factors," *Journal of Latin American Studies* 36 (2004): 267–96.

121. Katz, *Life and Times*; and James Cockroft, *Mexico's Hope: An Encounter with Politics and History* (New York: Monthly Review Press, 1998).

122. Hart, *Empire and Revolution*.

123. John Womack, *Zapata and the Mexican Revolution* (New York: Knopf, 1969).

124. *Constitución Política de los Estados Unidos Mexicanos* (México, D.F.: Dirección General de Educación Pública, 1917); and Mazzaferri, "Public Health."

125. Jonathan C. Brown, *Oil and Revolution in Mexico* (Berkeley: University of California Press, 1993).

126. See James Angus McLeod, "Public Health, Social Assistance, and the Consolidation of the Mexican State: 1877–1940" (PhD diss., Tulane University, 1990).

127. Robert McCaa, "Spanish and Nahuatl Views on Smallpox and Demographic Catastrophe in the Conquest of Mexico," *Journal of Interdisciplinary History* 25, no. 3 (Winter 1995): 397–431; and Noble David Cook, *Born to Die: Disease and New World Conquest, 1492–1650* (Cambridge: Cambridge University Press, 1998).

128. Suzanne Austin Alchon, *A Pest in the Land: New World Epidemics in a Global Perspective* (Albuquerque: University of New Mexico Press, 2003).

129. Jacques Soustelle, *Daily Life of the Aztecs on the Eve of the Spanish Conquest* (Stanford, CA: Stanford University Press, 1970); and Bernard Ortiz de Montellano, *Aztec Medicine, Health and Nutrition* (New Brunswick, NJ: Rutgers University Press, 1990). On Mexica medicine, see Carlos Viesca Treviño, *Medicina Prehispánica de México: El Conocimiento Médico de los Nahuas* (México, D.F.: Panorama Editorial, 1986).

130. Donald B. Cooper, *Epidemic Disease in Mexico City, 1716–1813: An Administrative, Social, and Medical Study* (Austin: Institute of Latin American Studies, University of Texas Press, 1965).

131. The history of medicine in the colonial period has been studied in such classic works as Josefina Muriel, *Hospitales de la Nueva España*, 2 vols. (México, D.F.: UNAM/Cruz Roja Mexicana, 1991); Francisco A. Flores, *Historia de la Medicina en México desde la Epoca de los Indios hasta el Presente* (México, D.F. Oficina de la Secretaría de Fomento, 1886–88); Fernando Ocaranza, *Historia de la Medicina en México* (México, D.F.: Laboratorios Midy, 1934); Ignacio Chávez, *México en la Cultura Médica* (México, D.F.: El Colegio Nacional, 1947); German Somolinos d'Ardois, *Capítulos de Historia Médica Mexicana* (México, D.F.: Sociedad Mexicana de Historia y Filosofía de la Medicina, 1978); Francisco Fernández del Castillo, *Antología de los Escritos Histórico-Médicos del Doctor F. Fernández del Castillo* (México, D.F.: Facultad de Medicina, UNAM, 1982); and Gordon Schendel, *Medicine in Mexico: From Aztec Herbs to Betatrons* (Austin: University of Texas Press, 1968). More up-to-date studies include Luz María Hernández Sáenz, *Learning to Heal: The Medical Profession in Colonial Mexico, 1767–1831* (New York: Peter Lang, 1997); Martha Eugenia Rodríguez, "Las Juntas de Sanidad en la Nueva España, Siglos XVIII y XIX," *Revista de Investigación Clínica* (México) 53, no. 3 (May–June 2001): 276–80; Carlos Viesca Treviño, "La Medicina Novohispana," in *Un Siglo de Ciencias de la Salud en México*, ed. Hugo Aréchiga and Luis Benitez-Bribiesca (México, D.F.: Fondo de Estudios e Investigaciones Ricardo J. Zevada: Consejo Nacional para la Cultura y las Artes: Fondo de Cultura Económica, 2000), 56–99; and Rodríguez de Romo and Martínez Barbosa, *Estudios de Historia*.

132. George M. Foster, "On the Origin of Humoral Medicine in Latin America." *Medical Anthropology Quarterly* 1 (1987): 355–99; Alfred W. Crosby Jr., *The Columbian Exchange: Biological and Cultural Consequences of 1492* (Westport, CT: Greenwood Press, 1972); and Gonzalo Aguirre Beltrán, *Medicina y Magia: El Proceso de Aculturación en la Estructura Colonial* (México, D.F.: Instituto Nacional Indigenista/Secretaría de Educación Pública [INI/SEP], 1980).

133. John Tate Lanning, *The Royal Protomedicato: The Regulation of the Medical Profession in the Spanish Empire* (Durham, NC: Duke University Press, 1985); Hernández Sáenz, *Learning to Heal*; and Cooper, *Epidemic Disease*.

134. Andrew L. Knaut, "Yellow Fever and the Late Colonial Public Health Response in the Port of Veracruz," *Hispanic American Historical Review* 77 (1997): 619–44; and Martha Eugenia Rodríguez and Ana Cecilia Rodríguez de Romo, "Asistencia Médica e Higiene Ambiental en la Ciudad de México, Siglos XVI–XVIII," *Gaceta Médica de México* 135, no. 2 (1999): 189–98.

135. Claudia Agostoni, "Médicos Científicos y Médicos Ilícitos en la Ciudad de México Durante el Porfiriato," *Estudios de Historia Moderna y Contemporánea de México* 19 (2000): 13–31.

136. Luz Fernanda Azuela, "Médicos y Farmacéuticos en las Sociedades Científicas Mexicanas del Siglo XIX," *Boletín Mexicana de Historia y Filosofía de Medicina* 5, no. 2 (2002): 15–20.

137. Important medical texts by Mexicans were often published in French. See, for example, Manuel Carmona y Valle, *Leçons sur l'étiologie et la prophylaxie de la fièvre jaune, données à la fin de l'année 1884 aux élèves de clinique interne* (México, D.F.: Imp. du Ministère des Travaux Publiques, 1885). On the French influence on Mexican medicine, see Jaime Mendiola Gómez, "Historical Synthesis of Medical Education in Mexico," in *Aspects of the History of Medicine in Latin America, Report of a Conference*, ed. John Z. Bowers and Elizabeth Purcell (New York: Josiah Macy Jr. Foundation, 1979), 88–96; Pedro Ramos et al., *Proyección Social del Médico* (México, D.F.: Manuel Casas, 1965); Moisés González Navarro, *Historia Moderna de México: El Porfiriato, la Vida Social* (México, D.F.: Editorial Hermes, 1957), 102–34; and José Alvarez Amézquita et al., *Historia de la Salubridad y de la Asistencia en México* (México, D.F.: Secretaría de Salubridad y Asistencia, 1960), for example, vol. 1, 430–44 and vol. 2, 113–15.

138. Ana María Carrillo, "La Patología del Siglo XIX y los Institutos Nacionales de Investigación Médica en México," *LABORAT-acta* 13, no. 1 (2001): 23–31; Alejandro Cervera Andrade, "El Doctor Harald Seidelin," *Boletín Informativo de la Facultad de Medicina, Universidad de Yucatán* 1, no. 4 (1966): 34–36; and Hugo Aréchiga, "La Medicina en México," in *Un Siglo de Ciencias de la Salud en México*, ed. Hugo Aréchiga and Luis Benitez-Bribiesca (México, D.F.: Fondo de Estudios e Investigaciones Ricardo J. Zevada: Consejo Nacional para la Cultura y las Artes: Fondo de Cultura Económica, 2000), 204–43. A few Mexican scientists began to venture even further afield; one example was a famed government-sponsored trip by a group of astronomers to Japan in 1874. See Marco Arturo Moreno Corral, *Odisea 1874 o el Primer Viaje Internacional de Científicos Mexicanos* (México, D.F.: Fondo de Cultura Económica, 1986).

139. J. J. Izquierdo, "Al Terminar los Estudios Médicos a Principios del Siglo," *Gaceta Médico de México* 95, no. 1 (1965): 91–96; and Adrián Torres Muñoz, "Los Cursos de Perfeccionamiento en París," *Pasteur: Revista Mensual de Medicina* 8, II, no. 2 (1935): 38–41. Manuel Martínez Báez, for example, studied in Paris, Hamburg, and Rome in the early 1930s. See Rodríguez de Romo, Factores Determinantes. On the field of microbiology, see Manuel Servín Massieu, *Microbiología, Vacunas y el Rezago Científico de México a Partir del Siglo XIX* (México, D.F.: Plaza y Valdés Editores, 2000).

140. Alfredo Saavedra, "Historia del Movimiento Eugenésico en México," *Pasteur: Revista Mensual de Medicina* 8, I, no. 1 (1935): 19–26; Alexandra M. Stern, "Responsible Mothers and Normal Children: Eugenics, Nationalism, and Welfare in Post-Revolutionary Mexico, 1920–1940," *Journal of Historical Sociology* 12, no. 4 (1999): 369–97; Alberto del Castillo Troncoso, "La Visión de los Médicos y el Reconocimiento de la Niñez en el Cambio del Siglo XIX al XX," *Boletín Mexicana de Historia y Filosofía de Medicina* 6, no. 2 (2003): 10–16; and Birn, "No More Surprising than a Broken Pitcher?" 17–46.

141. "Grandes Sabios Franceses que nos Visitan," *Pasteur: Revista Mensual de Medicina* 3, II, no. 2 (1930): 67.

142. Hernández Sáenz, *Learning to Heal*. On the nineteenth century, see Ana María Carrillo, "Médicos del México Decimonónico: Entre el Control Estatal y la Autonomía Profesional," *Dynamis* 22 (2002): 351–75. For a regional perspective on this matter, see Ana María Dolores Huerta Jaramillo, *Salus et Solatium: El Desarrollo de las Ciencias Médicas en Puebla durante el Siglo XIX* (Puebla, México: Benemérita Universidad Autónoma de Puebla, Cuadernos del Archivo Histórico Universitario, 2000), 91–111.

143. Ana María Carrillo, "Profesiones Sanitarias y Lucha de Poderes en el México del Siglo XIX," *Asclepio, Revista de Historia de la Medicina y de la Ciencia* 50, no. 2 (1998): 149–68; and Claudia Agostoni, "Médicos y Parteras en la Ciudad de México Durante el

Porfiriato," in *México en el Siglo XIX: Cuatro Estudios de Género*, ed. Gabriela Cano and Georgette José Valenzuela, 71–95 (México, D.F.: UNAM, 2001).

144. Ana Cecilia Rodríguez de Romo, "Los Médicos como Gremio de Poder en el Porfiriato," *Boletín Mexicana de Historia y Filosofía de Medicina* 5, no. 2 (2002): 4–9; and Ana María Carrillo, "Epidemias, Saber Médico y Salud Pública en el Porfiriato" (PhD diss., UNAM, forthcoming).

145. Ramos et al., *Proyección Social.*

146. The important role of traditional medicine in Mexico both historically and contemporarily is discussed in a wide variety of studies. See, for example, Xavier Lozoya and Carlos Zolla, eds., *La Medicina Invisible: Introducción al Estudio de la Medicina Tradicional de México* (México, D.F.: Folios Ediciones, 1983); María del Carmen Anzures y Bolaños, *La Medicina Tradicional en México: Proceso Histórico, Sincretismos y Conflictos* (México, D.F.: UNAM, 1983); and Brad R. Huber and Alan R. Sandstrom, eds., *Mesoamerican Healers* (Austin: University of Texas Press, 2001). On the state regulation of herbalists, see Martha Eugenia Rodríguez, "Legislación Sanitaria y Boticas Novohispanas," *Estudios Historicos Novohispanos* 17 (1997): 151–69. Further discussion of these questions can be found in chapter 3.

147. Lilia Oliver, "La Pandemia de Cólera Morbus. El Caso de Guadalajara," in *Ensayos sobre la Historia de las Epidemias en México*, ed. Enrique Florescano and Elsa Malvido, vol. 2 (México, D.F.: Instituto Mexicano del Seguro Social, 1982), 565–81; Elsa Malvido and Miguel Ángel Cuenya, "La Pandemia de Cólera de 1833 en la Ciudad de Puebla," in *El Cólera de 1833: Una Nueva Patología en México. Causas y Efectos*, ed. Miguel Ángel Cuenya et al. (México, D.F.: Instituto Nacional de Antropología e Historia [INAH], 1992), 11–45; and Lourdes Márquez Morfin, *La Desigualdad ante la Muerte en la Ciudad de México* (México, D.F. Siglo XXI, 1994).

148. Rosalina Estrada Urroz, "Control Sanitario o Control Social: La Reglamentación Prostibularia en el Porfiriato," *Boletín Mexicana de Historia y Filosofía de Medicina* 5, no. 2 (2002): 21–25.

149. See Ann S. Blum, "Conspicuous Benevolence: Liberalism, Public Welfare, and Private Charity in Porfirian, Mexico City, 1877–1910," *The Americas* 58, no. 1 (2001), 7–38; Bliss, *Compromised Positions*; Alvarez Amézquita et al, *Historia de la Salubridad*; and Christina Jiménez, "Popular Organizing for Public Services: Residents Modernize Morelia Mexico, 1880–1920," *Journal of Urban History* 30, no. 4 (2004): 495–518.

150. On the role of public health authorities in Veracruz starting in the late nineteenth century, see Ronzón, *Sanidad y Modernización*. On the popular protests surrounding housing destruction and evictions, see Wood, *Revolution in the Street.*

151. Ana María Carrillo, "Los Dificiles Caminos de la Campaña Antivariolosa en México," *Ciencias* 55–56 (July–December 1999): 18–25.

152. A variety of sources discuss the history of public health and welfare in Mexico. See, for example, Alvarez Amézquita et al., *Historia de la Salubridad*; Miguel E. Bustamante and Fernano Martínez Cortés, "Nota sobre los Trabajos Iniciales de Investigación en Salud Pública en México," *Salud Pública de México* 28, no. 2 (1986): 191–97; Enrique Moreno Cueto et al., *Sociología Histórica de las Instituciones de Salud en México* (México, D.F.: Instituto Mexicano del Seguro Social, 1982); Miguel E. Bustamante, "Hechos Sobresalientes en la Historia de la Secretaría de Salubridad y Asistencia," *Salud Pública de México* 25, no. 5 (1983): 465–82; Fernando Martínez Cortés, "La Historia de la Salubridad en México," *Médico Moderno* 38, no. 2 (1999): 7–95; and Guillermo Fajardo Ortiz, Ana María Carrillo, and Rolando Neri Vela, *Perspectiva Histórica de Atención a la Salud en México, 1902–2002* (México, D.F.: Organización Panamericana de la Salud, 2002).

153. See Mazzaferri, "Public Health"; Ana Cecilia Rodríguez de Romo and Martha Eugenia Rodríguez Pérez, "Historia de la Salud Pública en México: Siglos XIX y XX," *Historia, Ciencias, Saude—Manguinhos* 5, no. 2 (1998): 293–310; and Arturo Erosa Barbachana, "El Gobierno de Juárez y la Salud Pública de México," *Salud Pública de México* 19, no. 3 (1977): 375–81.

154. Carrillo, "Economía".

155. González Navarro, *Historia Moderna de México*, 105–7.

156. Eduardo Liceaga, "Algunas Consideraciones acerca de la Higiene Social en México," (paper presented in the name of the Sociedad Médica "Pedro Escobedo," México, D.F., 1911); and Miguel E. Bustamante, "El Doctor Liceaga, Higienista," *Gaceta Médica de México* 70 (1940): 79–91. His posthumous autobiography is Eduardo Liceaga, *Mis Recuerdos de Otros Tiempos* (México, D.F.: 1949).

157. Carrillo, "Economía."

158. Ana Cecilia Rodríguez de Romo, "La Ciencia *Pasteuriana* a través de la Vacuna Antirrábica," *Dynamis* 16 (1996): 291–316; and González Navarro, *Historia Moderna de México*, 105–7.

159. Ana María Carrillo, "Los Médicos ante la Primera Campaña Antituberculosa en México," *Gaceta Médica de México* 137, no. 4 (2001): 361–69.

160. Ana María Carrillo, "Estado de Peste o Estado de Sitio: Sinaloa y Baja California, 1902–1903," *Historia Mexicana* 54 (2005): 1049–1103.

161. Eduardo Liceaga, *Memoria Leida en la Reunión de la Asociación Americana de Salubridad Pública Verificada en Boston, Mss., E.U.A., del 25 al 29 de septiembre de 1905* (México, D.F.: A. Carranza y Compañía, Impresores, 1905). See, for example, *Transactions of the Fourth International Sanitary Conference of the American Republics, held in San José, Costa Rica, December 25, 1909 to January 3, 1910* (Washington, DC: Pan American Union, 1910).

162. "Peril in the Germs that Infect Mexico" *New York Times*, April 26, 1914, p. 4.

163. Eduardo Liceaga's autobiography, *Mis Recuerdos de Otros Tiempos*, dedicates a chapter to his involvement in the American Public Health Association and two to his role in the International (Pan American) Sanitary Congresses. Liceaga's involvement was part of a flurry of cross-border public health exchange in the late Porfiriato. Irving Watson, secretary of the American Public Health Association, compiled a pamphlet in 1894, *Sanitary Authorities of the United States of America, the Dominion of Canada, and the Republic of Mexico* (American Public Health Association, 1894). A few years later, I. Prieto published *The Supreme Board of Health of Mexico: Its History* (México, D.F.: Consejo Superior de Salubridad, 1903) and a companion piece that explained the board's organization. These English-language documents were sent to various U.S. health authorities. Also see Ana María Carrillo, "National and Imperial Interests in the American Public Health Association" (paper presented at the Latin American Perspectives on International Health symposium, University of Toronto, Toronto, Canada, May 5–7, 2005); and Alfonso Pruneda, "El Papel de México en la Cooperación Sanitaria Interamericana," *Boletín de la Oficina Sanitaria Panamericana* 23, no. 9 (September 1944): 780–85.

164. See correspondence between Eduardo Liceaga and Walter Wyman in the years 1905–1910, RG 90, Public Health Service, General Records, Correspondence of the International Sanitary Bureau, 1903–7, vol. 1, NARA; and Carlos Viesca Treviño, "Eduardo Liceaga y la Participación Mexicana en la Fundación de la Organización Panamericana de la Salud," *Revista Cubana de Salud Pública* 24, no. 1 (1998): 11–18.

165. Ana María Carrillo, "Surgimiento y Desarrollo de la Participación Federal en los Servicios de Salud," in *Perspectiva Histórica de Atención a la Salud en México, 1902–2002*, ed. Guillermo Fajardo Ortiz, Ana María Carrillo, and Rolando Neri Vela (México, D.F.: Organización Panamericana de la Salud, 2002), 17–64.

166. Julio Sesto, *A través de América: El México de Porfirio Díaz*, 2nd ed. (México D.F.: F. Sempere y Cia, Editores, 1910).

167. Miguel A. González-Block, "Génesis y Articulación de los Principios Rectores de la Salud Pública de México," *Salud Pública de México* 32 (1990): 337–51, argues that the creation of two health agencies initially fragmented power, although forces favoring centralized health authority won out by 1925 with the abolition of the Council of Health. Likewise, the ambiguous division of responsibility for social security between the states and the federal governments caused a delay in implementation until 1943 despite

repeated attempts to pass social security legislation beginning in 1921. Also see Moreno Cueto et al., *Sociología Histórica*, 38–40.

168. See his biography in Miguel E. Bustamante, *Cinco Personajes de la Salud en México* (Mexico, D.F.: Miguel Angel Porrúa, 1986), 63–96.

169. José María Rodríguez, "Informe que el Jefe del Departamento de Salubridad Pública rinde al C. Presidente de la República sobre las labores ejecutadas por dicho Departamento durante el periodo comprendido del 10 de mayo de 1917 al 10 de agosto del mismo año," History of Medicine Division, National Library of Medicine, Bethesda, MD. Rodríguez's influenza instructions reached the state of Tlaxcala, for example, but, as elsewhere, public health measures had a limited effect and the population resorted to traditional medicine and religious alternatives. See Marciano Netzhualcoyotzi Méndez, "La Influenza de 1918 en Tlaxcala: Mortadad y Efectos Sociales," *Boletín Mexicana de Historia y Filosofía de Medicina* 6, no. 1 (2003): 23–31.

170. Alvarez Amézquita et al., *Historia de la Salubridad*, 53–161; and Miguel E. Bustamante, "Hechos Sobresalientes en la Historia de la Secretaría de Salubridad y Asistencia," April 19, 1983, RG Dr. Miguel E. Bustamante V, Archives of the Fundacion Civico Cultural Bustamante Vasconcelos, Oaxaca, Mexico (hereafter refered to as FCCBV).

171. Aréchiga Córdoba, "Dictadura Sanitaria."

172. See Carrillo's chapter in Fajardo Ortiz et al., *Perspectiva Histórica*.

173. A British engineer who visited Mexico in the mid 1920s noted medical and health conditions quite similar to those of prior decades. Frances E. Smith, "Medicine in Mexico," *The Lancet* 208, no. 5373 (1926): 413.

174. From the late nineteenth century, U.S. newspapers published records of confirmed and suspected typhus, yellow fever, and other outbreaks in northern and coastal Mexico. See, for example, "A Possible Path for Cholera," *New York Times*, February 28, 1887, 4; and "Yellow Fever in Mexico: Washington Takes Quarantine Measures against Puerto Mexico," *New York Times*, November 29, 1913, 2. For the medical community's discussion of the threat to the United States from disease in Latin America, see, for example, "Epidemics in Mexico," *The Lancet* 140, no. 3616 (1892): 1404; *Proceedings of the International Conference on Health Problems in Tropical America, Held at Kingston, Jamaica July 22 to August 1, 1924* (Boston: United Fruit Company, 1924); and F. W. O'Connor, "Concern of the United States with Tropical Diseases," *American Journal of Public Health and The Nation's Health* 25, no. 1 (1935): 1–10.

175. Marine Hospital Service, Weekly Abstracts of Sanitary Reports. These bulletins, later called the *Public Health Reports*, published warnings about yellow fever, plague, cholera, and other disease outbreaks from U.S. informants and local authorities in ports and border towns around the world.

176. Anne-Emanuelle Birn, "Six Seconds Per Eyelid: The Medical Inspection of Immigrants at Ellis Island, 1892–1914," *Dynamis* 17 (1997): 281–316.

177. Famed U.S. Marine Hospital Service Officer Joseph Goldberger, for example, was sent on two semi-confidential reconnaissance trips to the port of Tampico in 1902 and 1904 in relation to yellow fever and to Mexico City in 1909 to enforce a typhus quarantine. Alan Kraut, *Goldberger's War: The Life and Work of a Public Health Crusader* (New York: Hill and Wang, 2003), 48–54, 75–77.

178. See Wickliffe Rose to Jordan Stabler, July 19, 1918, RG 59, Decimal File 1910–29, Box 7295, NARA.

179. Capt Jen Bugge, "Sanitary Statistics of Certain Cities of Mexico, Compiled from Geographia Medico-Militar, 1907," Army War College, March 26, 1911, History of Medicine Division, National Library of Medicine, Bethesda, MD, MS F 72.

180. Wood, *Revolution in the Street*, 12–19.

181. Although the USPHS acknowledged that smallpox had been less prevalent in Veracruz than in Texas before the invasion, its contempt of Mexican public hygiene persisted: "Considering the fact that Vera Cruz is a tropical town with a mixed Spanish and

Indian population, its sanitary condition at the time of the American occupation was better than one might have expected." G. M. Guiteras, "Sanitary Work in Vera Cruz during the First Three Weeks of the American Occupation," *Public Health Reports* 29 (1914): 1619.

182. William Phillips to Eliseo Arredondo, December 22, 1915, RG 59, Decimal File 1910–29, Box 2688, NARA.

183. Jerome Greene to Secretary of State, January 6, 1916, RG 59, Decimal File 1910–29, Box 2688, NARA.

184. Victor Heiser, "Memorandum with Regard to Typhus in Mexico," January 15, 1916, RG 5, Series 2, Subseries 323, Box 33, Folder 196, RFA.

185. Memorandum from Vincent to Rose, April 23, 1919, and memorandum from W. D. Garvey to Victor Heiser, June 24, 1919, RG 5, Series 2, Subseries 323, Box 33, Folder 197, RFA.

186. Joseph H. White, "The Method of Dissemination and the Possibility of Elimination of Yellow Fever," March 5, 1915, RG 5, Series 2, Special Reports, Box 22, File 135, RFA.

187. See Rose to Stabler, July 19, 1918, RG 59, Decimal File 1910–29, Box 7295, NARA.

188. Rose, "Memorandum of Dr. Rose's Interviews in Washington, September 22–23, 1919," p. 2, Wickliffe Rose Diaries, RG 12, RFA.

189. Theodore Lyster Diaries, December 5, 1919, p. 70, RG 12, RFA.

190. Ramón Ojeda Falcón, "Apuntes sobre el Ultimo Brote de Fiebre Amarilla Ocurrido en el Puerto de Veracruz, 1920–1921," *Boletín Epidemiológico* 19, no. 1 (1955): 71–77.

191. Pruneda to Heiser, November 8, 1920, RG 5, Series 1.2, Subseries 323, Box 96, Folder 1329, RFA.

192. Francisco Castillo Nájera, "Acta de la Tercera Sesión Plena, Octubre 18 de 1921," in *Memoria de la Primera Convención de Fiebre Amarilla, Octubre 15–20 de 1921* (México, D.F.: Departamento de Salubridad Pública [DSP], 1921), 148.

193. Theodore C. Lyster, "Plan de Campaña, 12 de diciembre de 1920," reprinted in *Memoria de la Primera Convención de Fiebre Amarilla, Octubre 15–20 de 1921* (México, D.F.: DSP, 1921), 13–16.

194. Obregón also approved free telegraph, telephone, mail, and rail service for the commission members. Alvaro Obregón, "Acuerdo del C. Presidente de los Estados Unidos Mexicanos, por el que se Crea 'La Comisión Especial para la Campaña contra la Fiebre Amarilla,'" in *Historia de la Salubridad y de la Asistencia en México*, ed. José Alvarez Amézquita et al. (México, D.F.: Secretaría de Salubridad y Asistencia, 1960), 154.

195. More details of the IHB's yellow fever campaign may be found in the provocative work of Armando Solórzano Ramos, *¿Fiebre Dorada o Fiebre Amarilla? La Fundación Rockefeller en México, 1911–1924* (Guadalajara: Universidad de Guadalajara, 1997).

196. See Bustamante, *Fiebre Amarilla*; Alvarez Amézquita et al., *Historia de la Salubridad*, 21–23; *Memoria de la Primera Convención de Fiebre Amarilla, Octubre 15–20 de 1921*; and Salvador Novo, *Breve Historia y Antología sobre la Fiebre Amarilla* (México, D.F.: La Prensa Médica Mexicana, 1964).

197. Recognition of Obregón's government also hinged on Mexico's international debt, in default since 1913, and payment of property damages to foreigners incurred during the revolution. See Knight, *U.S. Mexican Relations*, 131.

198. Various U.S. oil and business interests—including Rockefeller—were accused of interfering with Mexico, especially influencing the U.S. invasion of Veracruz. See Skirius, "Railroad."

199. Solomon and Krementsov, "Giving and Taking": 265–98.

200. See Romana Falcón and Soledad García Morales, *La Semilla en el Surco: Adalberto Tejeda y el Radicalismo en Veracruz, 1883–1960* (México, D.F.: El Colegio de México, 1986); Wood, *Revolution in the Street*; Benedikt Behrens, *Ein Laboratorium der Revolution: Städtische Soziale Bewegungen und Radikale Reformpolitik im Mexikanischen Bundesstaat Veracruz, 1918–1932* (Frankfurt: Peter Lang AG, 2002); Aurora Gómez-Galvarriato Freer, "The Impact of Revolution: Business and Labor in the Mexican Textile Industry, Orizaba, Veracruz, 1900–1930" (PhD diss., Harvard University, 1999); and Heather Fowler-Salamini,

"Women Coffee Sorters Confront the Mill Owners and the Veracruz Revolutionary State, 1915–1918," *Journal of Women's History* 14 (Spring 2002): 34–63.

201. Secretaría de la Economía Nacional, *El Café. Aspectos Económicos de su Producción y Distribución en México y en el Extranjero* (México, D.F.: Secretaría de la Economía Nacional, 1933).

202. Brown, *Oil and Revolution*.

203. Hans Werner Tobler, "Peasants and the Revolutionary State, 1910–1940," in *Riot, Rebellion, and Revolution: Rural Social Conflict in Mexico*, ed. F. Katz (Princeton, NJ: Princeton University Press, 1988), 487–518.

204. Robert Freeman Smith, *The United States and Revolutionary Nationalism in Mexico, 1916–1932* (Chicago: University of Chicago Press, 1972).

205. See Armando Solórzano, "Sowing the Seeds of Neo-imperialism: The Rockefeller Foundation's Yellow Fever Campaign in Mexico," *International Journal of Health Services* 22 (1992): 529–54; and Solórzano Ramos, *¿Fiebre Dorada o Fiebre Amarilla?*

206. Later reported as 580 cases and 353 deaths: see Miguel E. Bustamante, "Distribución Geográfica de la Fiebre Amarilla en México de 1800 a 1923," *Revista del Instituto de Salubridad y Enfermedades Tropicales* 3, no. 2 (June 1942): 93–105; and Bustamante, *Fiebre Amarilla*.

207. Bustamante, *Cinco Personajes*, 146; and Carrillo, "Surgimiento y Desarrollo," 32.

208. M.E. Connor, "Informe Preliminar sobre la Campaña contra la Fiebre Amarilla, en Mérida, Yuc," and Theodore C. Lyster, "Informe del Director de la Comisión Especial Contra la Fiebre Amarilla," in *Memoria de la Primera Convención de Fiebre Amarilla, Octubre 15–20 de 1921* (México, D.F., DSP, 1921), 2126 and 11–20.

209. Lyster, "Informe del Director."

210. H. R. Carter to W. Rose, RG 5, Series 2, Special Reports, Box 2, File 135, RFA.

211. M. E. Connor, "Acta de la Primera Sesión Plena, Octubre 15 de 1921," in *Memoria de la Primera Convención de Fiebre Amarilla, Octubre 15–20 de 1921* (México, D.F.: DSP, 1921), 78.

212. Bustamante, *Fiebre Amarilla*, 164–90.
Amarilla, Octubre 15–20 de 1921 (México, D.F., DSP, 1921), 2126 and 11–20.

213. M. E. Connor, "Reporte Final de la Campaña Contra la Fiebre Amarilla en la Zona No. 1," RG 5, Series 2, Box 33, Special Reports, 323 Mexico File 194, RFA.

214. Genaro Angeles, "Informe Rendido por el Delegado en la Ciudad de Córdoba, Ver," in *Memoria de la Primera Convención de Fiebre Amarilla, Octubre 15–20 de 1921* (México, D.F., DSP, 1921), 31.

215. Liceaga, *Memoria Leida*; and Bustamante, *Fiebre Amarilla*, 139–45. Similar sanitary approaches had successfully controlled yellow fever outbreaks in Veracruz during the colonial period. Knaut, "Yellow Fever."

216. Hugh S. Cumming to F. F. Russell, July 12, 1923, RG 90, Central File, 1897–1923, Box 177, Yellow Fever, Category 1876, Year 1923, NARA.

217. Lyster, "Annual Report for the Year of 1921 to the IHB by the Director of Yellow Fever Control for Mexico and Central America," RG 5, Series 2, Subseries 323, Box 33, File 195. RFA.

218. See for example, A. Gutiérrez, "Informe de la Campaña contra la Fiebre Amarilla que se ha Desarrollado en Papantla, Ver. desde el Mes de Noviembre de 1920 a la Fecha," in *Memoria de la Primera Convención de Fiebre Amarilla, Octubre 15–20 de 1921* (México, D.F.: DSP, 1921), 111.

219. Lyster to Alfonso Pruneda, February 26, 1921, RG DSP, Epidemiology Series, Box 17, Folder 12, Archivo Histórico de la Secretaría de Salud, Mexico, D.F., hereafter AHSSA.

220. This oral discussion is captured in "Acta de la Sesión Celebrada por la Comisión Especial para la Campaña contra la Fiebre Amarilla, Octubre 19 de 1921, Presidencia del Sr. Dr. T. C. Lyster," in *Memoria de la Primera Convención de Fiebre Amarilla, Octubre 15–20 de 1921* (México, D.F.: DSP, 1921), 155–63.

221. Angel Brioso Vasconcelos, quoted in "Acta de la Sesión Celebrada por la Comisión Especial," 161.

222. Mauro Loyo, "Informe de los Trabajos Efectuados en el Puerto de Veracruz, con el Objeto de Dominar el Brote de Fiebre Amarilla que Comenzó en Junio de 1920," and Victoriano Montalvo, "Informe Presentado por el Delegado Sanitario en Puerto México, Ver," in *Memoria de la Primera Convención de Fiebre Amarilla, Octubre 15–20 de 1921* (México, D.F.: DSP, 1921), 128–31 and 132–35.

223. "Narrative Report of Yellow Fever Control Measures—Tampico," p. 3, RG 5, Series 2, Subseries 323, Box 33, Folder 196, RFA; Bert Caldwell to Henry Carter, August 29, 1924, Philip S. Hench Walter Reed Yellow Fever Collection, Historical Collections and Services of the Health Sciences Library, University of Virginia, accessed online, (hereafter Hench collection).

224. Enrique Osornio, "Nota presentada por el Jefe del Cuerpo Médico Militar," and Castillo Nájera, "Acta de la Tercera Sesión Plena," 105–7 and 147–48.

225. See for example, Bert W. Caldwell, "Informe de los Trabajos Efectuados en e Mes de Septiembre de 1921 contra la Fiebre Amarilla en la Zona de Tampico-Túxpam," in *Memoria de la Primera Convención de Fiebre Amarilla, Octubre 15–20 de 1921* (México, D.F.: DSP, 1921), 85–92.

226. Lyster, "Informe del Director," 17; and Joseph H. White, "Epidemiologia y Profilaxis de la Fiebre Amarilla," *Boletín de la Oficina Sanitaria Panamericana* 3 (1924): 5–9.

227. The doubts of commission member Dr. Pérez Grovas were mentioned (and deemed unjustified) by Brioso Vasconcelos and repeated by Gabriel Malda. Connor spoke for himself. See Connor, "Informe Preliminar," 23; and Brioso Vasconcelos in "Acta de la Segunda Sesión Plena," and Gabriel Malda, "Sesión Plena del 20 de Octubre de 1921, Alocución de Clausura," in *Memoria de la Primera Convención de Fiebre Amarilla, Octubre 15–20 de 1921* (México, D.F.: DSP, 1921), 120 and 168. Also see Aristides Agramonte, "Some Observations upon Yellow Fever Profilaxis," and "Discussion" in *Proceedings of the International Conference on Health Problems in Tropical America, Held at Kingston, Jamaica July 22 to August 1, 1924*, ed. United Fruit Company (Boston: United Fruit Company, 1924), 201–227; and Tomás Perrín, "¿Virus, o Leptospiras?" *Pasteur: Revista Mensual de Medicina* 3, II, no. 1 (1930): 11–13.

228. Noguchi's vaccine and continued research, though questioned by Latin American researchers starting in the early 1920s, was strongly supported by the Rockefeller Institute, and the vaccine was widely distributed for use in IHB campaigns in Peru, Central America, and Mexico. Noguchi continued testing his vaccine in West Africa, where he died of yellow fever in 1928. After more than a decade of use, Hideyo Noguchi's yellow fever vaccine was discovered to be erroneously based on the spirochetal agent *leptospira icteroides*; researchers in an RF laboratory in West Africa uncovered the viral origins of the disease. See Isabel R. Plesset, *Noguchi and His Patrons* (Rutherford, NJ: Fairleigh Dickinson University Press, 1980); George Strode, ed., *Yellow Fever* (New York: McGraw Hill, 1951); Cueto, "Sanitation from Above"; and Soper, "*Ventures in World Health*," 82–89.

229. M. E. Connor, "Reporte Final de la Campaña Contra la Fiebre Amarilla en la Zona No. 1," p. 24, RG 5, Series 2, Box 33, Special Reports, 323 Mexico, File 194, RFA.

230. A. M. Walcott to Angel Brioso Vasconcelos, June 4, 1923, RG Public Health, Section Epidemiology, Box 39, Folder 7, AHSSA. On fears that unstable conditions in Mexico might interrupt the campaign, see Michael Connor to Henry Rose Carter, October 11, 1922, Hench Collection.

231. Connor to Carter, February 4, 1923; and Caldwell to Carter, October 6, 1921, Hench Collection.

232. Bert Caldwell to Alfonso Pruneda, "Report on the Campaign in Veracruz and the Second Yellow Fever Zone," December 23, 1922, RG 5, Series 2, Box 33, Special Reports, 323 Mexico, File 195, RFA.

233. "Informes de los trabajos contra la fiebre amarilla en la segunda zona y reportes de vigilancia epidemiológica," 1922, RG Public Health, Epidemiology Series, Box 26, Folder 16, AHSSA; "Petición de un grupo de hoteleros de Veracruz para retardar la clausura de la Oficina Especial contra la Fiebre Amarilla." "Implementación de la campaña en

Cosamaloapan," 1921, RG Public Health, Epidemiology Series, Box 20, Folder 15, AHSSA; "Informe de los trabajos realizados en la segunda zona, con sede en Veracruz. Envío de brigadas volantes a Tabasco. Súplicas para evitar el retiro de la campaña en Veracruz," 1923, RG Public Health, Epidemiology Series, Box 35, Folder 9, AHSSA, as cited in Carrillo "Surgimiento y Desarrollo," 33.

234. Solórzano, "Sowing the Seeds"; and Armando Solórzano, "The Rockefeller Foundation in Revolutionary Mexico: Yellow Fever in Yucatán and Veracruz," in *Missionaries of Science: The Rockefeller Foundation and Latin America,* ed. Marcos Cueto (Bloomington: Indiana University Press, 1994), 52–71, table 2, 58. See also Bert W. Caldwell, "The Conduct of the Yellow Fever Campaign in Vera Cruz and the Second Yellow Fever Zone, 1921–1922," July 30, 1922, Hench Collection.

235. Caldwell to Carter, October 6, 1921; and Connor to Carter August 23, 1923, Hench Collection.

236. M. E. Connor, "Log of Yellow Fever Inspection Trip to Mexico," September 1924, p. 18, RG 5, Series 2, Subseries 323, Box 33, Folder 194, RFA.

237. Bustamante, *Fiebre Amarilla,* 181; "Dr. H. B. Cross Dies, Martyr to Science," *New York Times,* December 28, 1921, 13; and Alvarez Amézquita et al., *Historia de la Salubridad,* 184.

238. Angel Brioso Vasconcelos, "El Vocal del Consejo, Casos Registrados de Junio 8 a Diciembre 28 de 1920, 11 de octubre de 1921," in *Memoria de la Primera Convención de Fiebre Amarilla, Octubre 15–20 de 1921* (México, D.F.: DSP, 1921), 18.

239. L. Guadarrama, "Informe de la Campaña Sanitaria contra la Fiebre Amarilla, en Túxpam, Ver. y Algunas Consideraciones sobre la Enfermedad," in *Memoria de la Primera Convención de Fiebre Amarilla, Octubre 15–20 de 1921* (México, D.F.: DSP, 1921), 40–61.

240. Túxpam later became known as Tuxpan. E. Vaughn to W. Rose, September 24, 1921, RG 5, Series 2, Box 33, Special Reports, 323 Mexico, File 197, RFA.

241. Falcón and García Morales, *Semilla en el Surco,* 124–28.

242. Angel Brioso Vasconcelos, "Ultima Palabra sobre los Peces Larvicidas," June 1, 1923, RG Public Health, Section Epidemiology, Box 39, Folder 7, AHSSA.

243. Gil Rojas Aguilar, "Informe del Delegado Sanitario en Yucatán," in *Memoria de la Primera Convención de Fiebre Amarilla, Octubre 15–20 de 1921* (México, D.F.: DSP, 1921), 143–46.

244. Although the convention included talks by two dozen IHB and DSP officers, Graham Casasús had to speak from the floor. "Acta de la Primera Sesión Plena," 79.

245. M. E. Connor, "Log of Yellow Fever Inspection Trip to Mexico," September 21, 1924, p. 23, RG 5, Series 2, Subseries 323, Box 33, Folder 194, RFA.

246. See Loyo, "Informe de los Trabajos Efectuados," 128–31; and Montalvo, "Informe Presentado," 132–35.

247. See, for example, Gutiérrez, "Informe de la Campaña," 111.

248. Alfredo Cuarón, "Informe Presentado por el Delegado Sanitario Especial en Tampico," in *Memoria de la Primera Convención de Fiebre Amarilla, Octubre 15–20 de 1921* (México, D.F.: DSP, 1921), 93–96.

249. Cuarón to Brioso Vasconcelos, October 8, 1922, RG Public Health, Epidemiology Series, Folder 17, AHSSA. As cited in Solórzano, "The Rockefeller Foundation in Revolutionary Mexico."

250. Brioso Vasconcelos to Secretary General of the Department of Public Health, July 9, 1923, RG Public Health, Presidency Series, Box 8, Folder 11, AHSSA.

251. Servicio Antilarvario, Departamento de Salubridad Pública, "Sumario sobre el Informe de los Trabajos Realizados en 1924 en Vera Cruz, México," *Boletín de la Oficina Sanitaria Panamericana* 4 (1925): 168–73.

252. See, for example, Cuarón to F. Echevarria, Sub-director Comisión Especial contra F.A., January 18, 1924, RG Public Health Epidemiology Series, Box 40, Folder 1, AHSSA.

253. Hugh S. Cumming to Medical Officers in Charge, July 12, 1923, RG 90, Central File, 1897–1923, Box 177, Yellow Fever, Category 1876, Year 1923; Alexander Weddell,

Consul General to Mexico, "Excerpts from Political and Economic Conditions in Mexico during July 1926," July 3, 1926, p. 9, RG 90, General Records, General Subject File, 1924–35, Foreign Governments—Mexico, File 1850, Box 831, NARA.

254. Andrew Wood, "Close Encounters of Empire? The Rockefeller Foundation and the Battle against Yellow Fever in Veracruz, Mexico," unpublished manuscript, 2000.

255. Solórzano, "Sowing the Seeds," 529 (abstract); Connor to Carter, July 20, 1923, Hench Collection.

256. M. E. Connor, "Log of Yellow Fever Inspection Trip to Mexico," September 21, 1924, p. 23, RG 5, Series 2, Subseries 323, Box 33, Folder 194, RFA.

Chapter Two

1. "Extracto del Mensaje del General Alvaro Obregón, Presidente de los Estados Unidos de México," *Boletín de la Oficina Sanitaria Panamericana* 2 (1923): 301–4.

2. Frederick Russell to Brioso Vasconcelos, May 5, 1923, RG 5, Series 1.2, Box 163, File 2116, RFA.

3. M. E. Connor, "Log of Yellow Fever Inspection Trip to Mexico," 1924, RG 5, Series 2, Special Reports, Subseries 323, Mexico, Box 33, File 194, p. 9, RFA; and Russell to Vasconcelos, May 5, 1923, RG 5, Series 1.2, Box 163, File 2116, RFA.

4. Brioso Vasconcelos to Pruneda, July 9, 1923, RG Public Health, Presidency Series, Box 8, Folder 11, AHSSA.

5. Connor to Florence Read, March 16, 1924, RG 5, Series 1.2, Box 193, File 2469.

6. Russell to Brioso Vasconcelos, May 5, 1923, RG 5, Series 1.2, Box 163, File 2116, RFA.

7. Brioso Vasconcelos to Pruneda, July 9, 1923, RG Public Health, Presidency Series, Box 8, Folder 11, AHSSA.

8. Hewa, *Colonialism*; Rita Pemberton, "A Different Intervention: The International Health Commission/Board, Health, Sanitation in the British Caribbean, 1914–1930," *Caribbean Quarterly* 49, no. 4 (2003): 87–103; Palmer, "Central American Encounters," 311–32; de Castro Santos, "Power"; Gadelha, "Conforming Strategies"; Christian Brannstrom, "Polluted Soil, Polluted Souls: The Rockefeller Hookworm Eradication Campaign in São Paulo, Brazil, 1917–1926," *Historical Geography* 25 (1997): 25–45; Ka-che Yip, "Health and Society in China: Public Health Education for the Community, 1912–1937," *Social Science and Medicine* 16 (1982): 1197–1205; James Gillespie, "The Rockefeller Foundation, the Hookworm Campaign and a National Health Policy in Australia, 1911–1930," in *Health and Healing in Tropical Australia and Papua New Guinea*, ed. Roy MacLeod and Donald Denoon (Townsville, Australia: James Cook University, 1991), 64–87; Esteban Rodriguez Ocaña, "Foreign Expertise, Political Pragmatism, and Professional Elite: The Rockefeller Foundation in Spain, 1919–39," *Studies in History and Philosophy of Biological and Biomedical Sciences* 31, no. 3 (2000): 447–61; Lise Wilkinson, "Burgeoning Visions of Global Public Health: The Rockefeller Foundation, the London School of Hygiene and Tropical Medicine, and the 'Hookworm Connection,'" *Studies in History and Philosophy of Biological and Biomedical Sciences* 31, no. 3 (2000): 397–407; William A. Link, "'The Harvest Is Ripe, but the Laborers Are Few': The Hookworm Crusade in North Carolina, 1909–1915," *North Carolina Historical Review* 67 (January 1990): 1–27; and Shirish Kavadi, "'Wolves Come to Take Care of the Lamb': The Rockefeller Foundation's Hookworm Campaign in the Madras Presidency, 1920–1928," in *The Politics of the Healthy Life. An International Perspective*, ed. Esteban Rodríguez-Ocaña (Sheffield, UK: European Association for the History of Medicine and Health [EAHMH] Publications, 2002), 89–111.

9. The countries composing the West Indian colonies were Antigua, British Guiana, Dutch Guiana, Grenada, St. Lucia, Saint Vincent, and Trinidad. The control of the disease

was carried out through the "intensive method," which consisted of identifying all infected persons within an area, providing them with a treatment, and applying microscopic examination at the end of the procedure to show that a cure had been effected. See H. H. Howard, *The Control of Hookworm Disease by the Intensive Method* (New York: Rockefeller Foundation, International Health Board, Publication no. 8, 1919).

10. Heiser, *American Doctor's Odyssey*, 369.

11. B. E. Washburn, "The Economic Value of a Hookworm Campaign," in *Proceedings of the International Conference on Health Problems in Tropical America, Held at Kingston, Jamaica July 22 to August 1, 1924*, ed. United Fruit Company (Boston: United Fruit Company, 1924), 619.

12. See Farley, *To Cast Out Disease*.

13. Christopher Abel, "External Philanthropy and Domestic Change in Colombian Health Care: The Role of the Rockefeller Foundation, ca. 1920–1950," *Hispanic American Historical Review* 75, no. 3 (1995): 339–75, 343.

14. Rose to Pruneda, December 4, 1922, RG 5, Series 1.2, Box 137, File 1820, RFA.

15. Pruneda to Rose, February 19, 1923; and Alfonso Pruneda to Frederick Russell, March 20, 1923, RG 5, Series 1.2, Box 162, File 2110, RFA.

16. Russell to Pruneda, April 2, 1923, RG 5, Series 1.2, Box 162, File 2110, RFA.

17. "International Health Board, Summary of Policies in Force, Public Health Work," May 25, 1927, RG 3.1, Series 908, Box 11, Folder 123, RFA.

18. Vincent to Sheffield, May 21, 1925, RG 1.1, Series 323, Box 13, File 93, RFA.

19. "Report by John A. Ferrell on Visit to Mexico," March 14–April 13, 1941, Statement Corrected September 28, 1942, RG 2—Stacks, Box 561, Folder 3814, RFA.

20. While yellow fever spending—mostly for Central American efforts—continued to be counted in the Mexican budget in 1924 and 1925, by 1926 the budget had dropped to $13,756 ($149,000 in 2004 dollars), in 1927 to $6,855.39 ($73,000 in 2004 dollars), and in 1928 to $2,239.15 ($25,000 in 2004 dollars). See table 5.1.

21. Read to Warren, July 3, 1924, RG 1.1, Series 323, Box 17, File 139, RFA.

22. "Proyecto para el plan en participación que deberá seguirse por un período de cinco años entre el Gobierno de México y la International Health Board para dominar la Uncinariasis," November 12, 1923, RG Public Health, Presidency Series, Box 8, Folder 17, AHSSA.

23. Ibid.

24. Andrew J. Warren, interviewed by Greer Williams, July 31, 1963, RG 3, Series 908, Box 71, Folder 86.122, RFA.

25. Bustamante, *Cinco Personajes*, 129–56; and "Pruneda, Alfonso," in *Who's Who in Latin America: A Biographical Dictionary of the Outstanding Living Men and Women of Spanish America and Brazil*, ed. Percy Alvin Martin (Palo Alto, CA: Stanford University Press, 1935), 320–21.

26. Knight, *U.S. Mexican Relations*, Ficker, "Export Boom," and Rosenzweig, "Comercio Exterior."

27. See Thomas Benjamin and Mark Wasserman, eds., *Provinces of the Revolution: Essays on Regional Mexican History, 1910–1929* (Albuquerque: University of New Mexico Press, 1990); and Tobler, "Peasants,"

28. Heather Fowler-Salamini, *Agrarian Radicalism in Veracruz, 1920–1938* (Lincoln: University of Nebraska Press, 1978), 25–47; and Helga Baitenmann, "Rural Agency and State Formation in Postrevolutionary Mexico: The Agrarian Reform in Central Veracruz, 1915–1992" (PhD diss., New School for Social Research, 1997), 81–91.

29. See Daniela Spenser, "Mexico Seen as a Link in the Chain of World History" (paper presented at the Latin American Studies Association 22nd International Congress, Miami, March, 2000); Daniela Spenser, *Impossible Triangle: Mexico, Soviet Russia, and the United States in the 1920s* (Durham, NC: Duke University Press, 1998); and Nora Hamilton, *The Limits of State Autonomy: Post-Revolutionary Mexico* (Princeton, NJ: Princeton University Press, 1982), 90–94.

30. Baitenmann, "Rural Agency," 246–52.

31. Falcón and García Morales, *Semilla en el Surco*, 209-13.

32. Wood, *Revolution in the Street*, 71-154; and Elizabeth Jean Norvell, "Syndicalism and Citizenship: Postrevolutionary Worker Mobilizations in Veracruz," in *Border Crossings: Mexican and Mexican-American Workers*, ed. John Mason Hart (Wilmington, DE: Scholarly Resources, 1998), 93-116.

33. Fowler-Salamini, *Agrarian Radicalism*, 100-103; and Falcón and García Morales, *Semilla en el Surco*.

34. Mary Kay Vaughan, *The State, Education, and Social Class in Mexico, 1880-1928* (DeKalb: Northern Illinois University Press, 1982), discusses the ideology, politics, and impact of the Vasconcelos reform. On the reforms in Veracruz, see 150-58 and 278-79.

35. See Emmett Vaughn to A. J. Warren, 7 January 1924, RG 5, Series 1.2, Box 193, Folder 2475, RFA. The need to protect Rockefeller-owned Standard Oil Company of New Jersey has been cited by Solórzano as the reason for the IHB's selection of Veracruz. This argument is overly simplistic, however: the RF's interests might be better understood as a means of ensuring the overall stability of U.S. interests than of protecting particular business concerns of the Rockefeller family. See Cueto, *Missionaries of Science*, xi.

36. Vaughn to Warren, 7 January 1924, RG 5, Series 1.2, Box 193, Folder 2475, RFA.

37. Pruneda to Vaughn, March 14, 1924, RG 5, Series 1.2, Box 193, File 2475, RFA.

38. de la Garza Brito to Russell, February 26, 1924, RG 5, Series 1.2, Box 192, File 2468, RFA.

39. Vaughn to Russell, March 15, 1924, RG 5, Series 1.2, Box 193, File 2474, RFA.

40. Russell to Vaughn, March 25, 1924, RG 5, Series 1.2, Box 193, File 2475, RFA.

41. The most belabored point in the survey was that the microscopic examination of fecal specimens for the presence of ova was a faulty measure because not all persons with positive stools had the disease, a discovery previously made by Samuel Darling, William Smillie, and William Cort. Warren and Carr, "The Incidence of Hookworm Disease in Mexico, Technical Report to the IHB," 1925, RG 5, Series 2, Subseries 323, Box 33, Folder 199, RFA.

42. Carr to Vaughn, April 19, 1924, RG 5, Series 1.2, Box 193, File 2470, RFA.

43. Vaughn to Carr, April 16, 1924, RG 5, Series 1.2, Box 193, File 2470, RFA.

44. Russell to Carr, September 15, 1924, RG 5, Series 1.2, Box 193, File 2470, RFA.

45. Carr to Russell, October 18, 1924, RG 5, Series 1.2, Box 193, File 2470, RFA; and Henry P. Carr, "Observations upon Hookworm Disease in Mexico," *American Journal of Hygiene* 6 (July supplement 1926): 42-61.

46. Russell to Vaughn, March 25, 1924, RG 5, Series 1.2, Box 193, File 2470, RFA.

47. Wilson G. Smillie, "The Results of Hookworm Disease Prophylaxis in Brazil," *American Journal of Hygiene* 2, no. 1 (1922): 77-94. Smillie's finding may have resulted from the difference in the reliability of quantitative measuring tools as compared with their qualitative counterparts. A 1929 text recommended that the selection of a survey population should include both clinical symptoms of the disease, as measured by the hemoglobin index, and the average intelligence of each race, as "determined through a few leading questions from a person speaking the native language fluently, and acquainted with the psychology of the population." Faust, *Human Helminthology*, 374.

48. N. R. Stoll, "Investigations on the Control of Hookworm Disease. XV. An Effective Method of Counting Hookworm Eggs in Feces," *American Journal of Hygiene* 3, no. 1 (1923): 59-70; N. R. Stoll, "Investigations on the Control of Hookworm Disease. XVIII: On the Relation between the Number of Eggs Found in Human Feces and the Number of Hookworms in the Host," *American Journal of Hygiene* 3, no. 2 (1923): 156-79; and Warren, "Hookworm Study of a Small Town (Alvarado) in the State of Veracruz," 1925, RG 5, Series 3, Box 144, RFA.

49. Carr, "Observations," 52.

50. Ibid., 56.

51. Carr to Russell, October 18, 1924, RG 5, Series 1.2, Box 193, File 2470, RFA; and Carr, "Observations".

52. Carr to Russell, July 24, 1926, RG 5, Series 1.2, Box 257, File 3274, RFA.

53. See Farley, To *Cast Out Disease*, Kavadi, "'Wolves'"; and Soma Hewa, "The Hookworm Epidemic on the Plantations in Colonial Sri Lanka," *Medical History* 38 (1994): 73–90.

54. Washburn, "Economic Value," 631–632. For earlier reports of hookworm rates in Mexico, see Lewis Haskell, American Consul in Salina Cruz, Mexico to Secretary of State Knox, June 1, 1911, William Edwards, American Consul in Veracruz to Secretary of State Knox, November 4, 1911, Richard Stadden, Vice Consul in Manzanillo to Secretary of State Knox, June 23, 1911, among other letters citing similar findings, RG 59, Decimal File 1910–29, Box 460, NARA.

55. The DSP chief under the next president reiterated that hookworm was limited to a very defined zone. Bernardo Gastélum, *Memoria de los Trabajos Realizados por el Departamento de Salubridad Pública 1925–1928*, vol I (México, D.F.: Ediciones del DSP, 1928), 102. Steven Palmer echoes this finding for Central America, where Guatemalan and Salvadoran physicians argued that hookworm was not a public health priority, but the RF was "unimpressed" with this opinion and persisted with a hookworm campaign. Palmer, "Central American Encounters," 316.

56. Carr to Warren, October 23, 1924, RG 1.1, Series 323, Box 17, File 139, RFA.

57. See Anne-Emanuelle Birn and Armando Solórzano, "Public Health Policy Paradoxes: Science and Politics in the Rockefeller Foundation's Hookworm Campaign in Mexico in the 1920s," *Social Science and Medicine* 49 (1999): 1197–1213.

58. See Soledad García Morales, *La Rebelión Delahuertista en Veracruz* (Jalapa, México: Universidad Veracruzana, 1986); Fowler-Salamini, *Agrarian Radicalism*, 41–45; and Smith, *United States*.

59. Government Printing Office, *Foreign Relations of the United States 1924*, vol. 1 (Washington, D.C.: Government Printing Office, 1939).

60. Read to Vaughn, January 10, 1924, RG 5, Series 1.2, Box 193, File 2475, RFA.

61. Vaughn to Warren, January 7, 1924, RG 5, Series 1.2, Box 193, Folder 2475, RFA. Meanwhile, departing yellow fever officer Connor complained of continuing problems in Yucatán with de la Huertistas: "'Leninists' and 'non-thinkers' destroying everything in sight."

62. Vaughn to Warren, January 7, 1924, RG 5, Series 1.2, Box 193, Folder 2475, RFA.

63. Vaughn to Russell, January 21, 1924 and March 4, 1924, RG 5, Series 1.2, Box 193, Folder 2475, RFA.

64. Brioso Vasconcelos to Russell, February 22, 1924, RG 5, Series 1.2, Box 193, File 2469, RFA.

65. Alvarez Amézquita et al., *Historia de la Salubridad*, 201.

66. "Necrología," *Gaceta Médica de México* 58 (1927): 632.

67. Vaughn to Russell, March 17, 1924, RG 5, Series 1.2, Box 193, File 2475, RFA.

68. See Salvador Bermúdez to Clifford Wells, September 14, 1924, RG 5, Series 1.2, Box 192, File 2468, RFA.

69. Warren to Russell, September 24, 1923, RG 5, Series 2, Subseries 323, Box 33, Folder 198, RFA.

70. Carr, "Observations." While the article was not published until 1926, Carr's colleagues at the IHB had received news of his findings before this date.

71. Vaughn, "Narrative Report of Work Done in the State of Tlaxcala," 1924, RG 3, Series 3, Box 143, RFA.

72. In 1932, Tlaxcala had a crude mortality rate of 31.2 per 1000, the fourth highest in Mexico. See Miguel E. Bustamante, "La Coordinación de los Servicios Sanitarios Federales y Locales como Factor de Progreso Higiénico en México," *Gaceta Médica de México* 65 (1934): 181–228.

73. Vaughn, "Narrative Report of Work Done in the Mining District of Pachuca," 1924, RG 3, Series 3, Box 143, RFA.

74. Warren to Read, June 17, 1924, RG 5, Series 1.2, Box 193, Folder 2473, RFA.

75. Warren, "Narrative Report of the Work of the Lucha contra la Uncinariasis for the Córdoba Area," 1925, RG 5, Series 3, Box 144, RFA.

76. Florence Read to Warren, July 3, 1924, RG 1.1, Series 323, Box 17, File 139, RFA.

77. Carr, "Observations," 59.

78. Warren to IHB, August 28, 1924, RG 1.1, Series 323, Box 17, Folder 139, RFA.

79. Samuel Darling et al., *Hookworm and Malaria Research in Malaya, Java and the Fiji Islands, Report of the Uncinariasis Commission to the Orient* (New York: Rockefeller Foundation, International Health Board Publication no. 9, 1920).

80. Smillie, "Results"; and Faust, *Human Helminthology,* 378–79.

81. Warren to IHB, August 28, 1924, RG 1.1, Series 323, Box 17, Folder 139, RFA.

82. Florence Read to Warren, June 7, and July 3, 1924, RG 1.1, Series 323, Box 17, File 139, RFA.

83. Warren, "Narrative Report of the Work of the Lucha contra la Uncinariasis for the Córdoba Area," 1925, RG 5, Series 3, Box 144, RFA.

84. Warren to Read, July 26, 1924, RG 1.1, Series 323, Box 17, File 139, RFA.

85. Warren, "First Annual Report of the Activities of the Hookworm Campaign for Mexico during the Year 1924," RG 5, Series 3, Box 143, RFA.

86. Warren, "Narrative Report of the Hookworm Work in Mexico for the Year 1925," RG 5, Series 3, Box 144, RFA.

87. Warren, "Narrative Report of the Work of the Lucha contra la Uncinariasis for the Córdoba Area," 1925, RG 5, Series 3, Box 144, RFA.

88. Warren, "Report on Hookworm," 1925, RG 5, Series 3, Box 644, RFA.

89. See Heather Fowler-Salamini, "Gender, Work, and Coffee in Córdoba, Veracruz, 1850–1910," in *Women of the Mexican Countryside, 1850–1990: Creating Spaces, Shaping Transitions,* ed. Heather Fowler-Salamini and Mary Kay Vaughan (Tucson: University of Arizona Press, 1994), 51–73; and Heather Fowler-Salamini, "Gender, Work, and Working-Class Women's Culture in the Veracruz Coffee Export Industry, 1920–1945," *International Labor and Working-Class History* 63 (Spring 2003): 102–21.

90. Tzvi Medin, *El Minimato Presidencial: Historia Política del Maximato, 1928–1935* (México D.F.: Ediciones Era, 1982); Tzvi Medin, *Ideología y Praxis Política de Lázaro Cárdenas* (México, D.F.: Siglo XXI, 1982), 16–17; and Hamilton, *Limits of State Autonomy,* 90–95.

91. Fowler-Salamini, *Agrarian Radicalism,*18–59.

92. Ettling, *Germ of Laziness.*

93. There is a large literature on traditional medicine among various Mexican cultures, including anthropological literature that spans the twentieth century. See, for example, William Robert Holland, *Medicina Maya en los Altos de Chiapas: Un Estudio del Cambio Socio-Cultural,* trans. Daniel Cazes (México, D.F.: Instituto Nacional Indigenista, 1963); and Anzures y Bolaños, *Medicina Tradicional.* On healing practices in southern Veracruz and eastern Oaxaca, see Leova Espinosa Yunis, *Tradiciones y Costumbre del Sur de Veracruz: Recopilación y Rescate de las Raíces de Nuestra Identidad* (Guadalajara: Editorial Pandora, 2000); Guido Munch Galindo, *Etnología del Istmo Veracruzano* (México, D.F.: UNAM, 1983), 187–242; and Frank J. Lipp, *The Mixe of Oaxaca: Religion, Ritual, and Healing* (Austin: University of Texas Press, 1991), 147–94. On the Mexico City area, see Claudia Madsen, *A Study of Change in Mexican Folk Medicine* (New Orleans: Tulane University Middle American Research Institute, 1965). On Morelos, see Bernardo Baytelman, *De Enfermos y Curanderos: Medicina Tradicional en Morelos* (México, D.F.: Instituto Nacional de Antropología e Historia, 1986). On rural Morelos in the 1940s, see Oscar Lewis, *Life in a Mexican Village: Tepoztlán Restudied* (Urbana: University of Illinois Press, 1963), 280–83. In a population of 3,230 people, Lewis counted twenty-eight *curanderos* and midwives, even though there was a local doctor present.

94. Eduardo Menéndez, *Poder, Estratificación Social y Salud: Análisis de las Condiciones Sociales y Económicas de la Enfermedad en Yucatán* (México, D.F.: La Casa Chata, 1981).

95. Munch Galindo, *Etnología,* 212–13.

96. See photographs in RG 5, Series 3, Box 144, pp. 8–9, RFA, and in Series 323I, 323J, and 323K, RFA.

97. Lewis, *Life in a Mexican Village*, 175–76.
98. Warren, "Final Narrative Report of the Hookworm Campaign in Tlacotalpan, Veracruz," 1925. RG 5, Series 3, Box 144, RFA.
99. Carr, "Annual Report of the Lucha contra la Uncinariasis, Section for Tropical Diseases of the Departamento de Salubridad Pública, for the year 1927," p. 3, RG 5, Series 3, Box 144, RFA.
100. Interview with Alberto P. León, former RF fellow, Health Department official, and Institute of Health and Tropical Diseases professor, Mexico City, April 10, 1991.
101. See, for example, Elsa Malvido and Maria Elena Morales, eds., *Historia de la Salud en México* (Mexico City: Instituto Nacional de Antropología e Historia, 1996); Kaja Finkler, *Spiritualist Healers in Mexico: Successes and Failures of Alternative Therapeutics* (New York: Praeger Publishers, 1985); and Lozoya and Zolla, *Medicina Invisible*.
102. For an analysis of the effects of foreign enterprise upon local belief systems, see Michael Taussig, *The Devil and Commodity Fetishism* (Chapel Hill: University of North Carolina Press, 1980).
103. See, for example, Holland, *Medicina Maya*; and Munch Galindo, *Etnología*.
104. Warren, "Report of the Lucha contra la Uncinariasis for the Quarter ending March 31, 1925," RG 5, Series 3, Box 144, RFA.
105. Warren to Read, July 26, 1924, RG 1.1, Series 323, Box 17, File 139, RFA.
106. Russell to Warren, August 25, 1924, RG 1.1, Series 323, Box 17, File 139, RFA.
107. Russell to Warren, September 13, 1924, RG 1.1, Series 323, Box 17, File 139, RFA.
108. Warren to Russell, October 3, 1924, RG 1.1, Series 323, Box 17, File 139, RFA.
109. Warren to IHB, August 28, 1924, RG 1.1, Series 323, Box 17, Folder 139, RFA.
110. Russell to Warren, September 23, 1924, RG 1.1, Series 323, Box 17, File 139, RFA.
111. Juan Solórzano Morfín, "Tratamiento de la Uncinariasis," *Gaceta Médica de México* 58, no. 6 (1927): 363.
112. Carr to Russell, September 3, 1926, RG 5, Series 1.2, Box 257, File 3275, RFA.
113. Andrew Warren, "Report of Case of Poisoning by Antihelminthic," March 29, 1926, RG 5, Series 2, Subseries 323, Box 33, File 196, RFA.
114. Ibid.
115. Solórzano Morfín, "Tratamiento," 336.
116. Warren, "Narrative Report of the Hookworm Work in Mexico for the Year 1925," RG 5, Series 3, Box 144, RFA.
117. Warren to Russell, May 17, 1926, RG 5, Series 1.2, Box 258, File 3281, RFA.
118. Warren to Russell, July 15, 1926, RG 5, Series 1.2, Box 258, File 3282, RFA.
119. Warren to Russell, July 9, 1925, RG 5, Series 1.2, Box 226, Folder 2875, RFA.
120. Russell to Warren, July 1, 1925, RG 5, Series 1.2, Box 226, Folder 2875, RFA.
121. Warren to Russell, July 9, 1925, RG 5, Series 1.2, Box 226, Folder 2875, RFA.
122. Ibid.
123. After seeing the Aztec calendar, RF yellow fever officer M. E. Connor declared, "at least some of the ancients possessed culture." Connor to Read, March 16, 1924, RG 5, Series 1.2, Box 192, File 2468, RFA.
124. In the 1930s, for example, RF officer Charles Bailey was said to rely excessively on translators. Marrón to Ferrell, February 11, 1936, RG 2, Series 323, Box 134, Folder 1004, RFA.
125. Vaughn, "Narrative Report of Work Done in the Mining District of Pachuca," 1924, RG 3, Series 3, Box 143, RFA.
126. Warren, "Narrative Report of the Hookworm Work in Mexico for the Year 1925," RG 5, Series 3, Box 144, RFA.
127. Charles Bailey, "Medical Assistance in Rural Populations of the Country," presented to the First National Congress of Rural Hygiene, Morelia, Michoacán, October 1935, RG 2, Series 323, Box 119, Folder 907, RFA.
128. Warren to Russell, July 9, 1925, RG 5, Series 1.2, Box 226, Folder 2875, RFA.
129. Russell to Warren, July 18, 1925, RG 5, Series 1.2, Box 226, Folder 2875, RFA.

130. Russell to Warren, March 19, 1925, RG 5, Series 1.2, Box 226, Folder 2875, RFA.

131. Warren, "Severe Hookworm Infestation in Alvarado, Mexico, An Urban Community; The Epidemiology of Which Was Not Influenced by Agricultural Occupations," July 20, 1925, RG 5, Series 2, Subseries 323, Box 33, File 198, RFA.

132. See Solórzano Morfín, "Tratamiento"; and Smillie, "Results." On the nineteenth-century Brazilian variant of this debate, see Julyan Peard, *Race, Place, and Medicine: The Idea of the Tropics in Nineteenth-Century Brazil* (Durham, NC: Duke University Press, 1999).

133. Warren to Russell, May 28, 1925, RG 5, Series 1.2, Box 226, Folder 2875, RFA.

134. Vaughn to Russell, March 4, 1924, RG 5, Series 1.2, Box 193, File 2472, RFA.

135. Warren to Russell, May 28, 1925, RG 5, Series 1.2, Box 226, Folder 2875, RFA.

136. Warren to Russell, December 12, 1924, RG 1.1, Series 323, Box 17, File 139, RFA.

137. Warren, "Routine Report," November 7, 1925, RG 5, Series 3, RFA.

138. Pruneda to Russell, December 3, 1924, RG 5, Series 1.2, Box 193, File 2472, RFA.

139. See Medin, *Ideología*, 16–17; and Fowler-Salamini, *Agrarian Radicalism*, 18–59.

140. Warren to Russell, May 28, 1925, RG 5, Series 1.2, Box 226, Folder 2875, RFA.

141. Russell to Vaughn, March 31, 1924, RG 5, Series 1.2, Box 193, File 2475, RFA.

142. Vaughn to Warren, June 4, 1924, RG 5, Series 1.2, Box 193, File 2475, RFA.

143. Juan López to Read, September 12, 1924, RG 5, Series 1.2, Box 193, File 2473, RFA.

144. The physician, Gabriel Garzón Cossa, went to work for a petroleum company at a higher salary, a considerable loss for the campaign.

145. Carr to Russell, March 24, 1927, RG 5, Series 1.2, Box 296, File 3753, RFA.

146. Warren to Russell, October 12, 1925, RG 5, Series 1.2, Box 226, Folder 2876, RFA. A letter written by Warren on December 12, 1925, described continuing chaos, with squatters occupying newly built houses, the buildings ransacked, and unpaid teachers on strike. As a result, Oaxaca was also going bankrupt. Warren remained surprisingly calm, noting, "conditions barely affect [our] immediate work."

147. Fowler-Salamini, *Agrarian Radicalism*, 55–58; and Wood, *Revolution in the Street*.

148. Russell to Read, September 18, 1925, RG 5, Series 1.2, Box 226, Folder 2872, RFA.

149. Warren to Russell, October 12, 1925, RG 5, Series 1.2, Box 226, Folder 2876, RFA.

150. Russell to Warren, December 31, 1925, RG 5, Series 1.2, Box 226, File 2876, RFA.

151. Russell to Read, September 18, 1925, RG 5, Series 1.2, Box 226, Folder 2872, RFA.

152. Russell to Warren, December 31, 1925, RG 5, Series 1.2, Box 226, File 2876, RFA.

153. Warren to Russell, December 31, 1925, RG 5, Series 3, Box 144, RFA.

154. Carr, "Annual Report of the Lucha contra la Uncinariasis, Section for Tropical Diseases of the Departamento de Salubridad Pública, for the Year 1926," RG 5, Series 3, Box 144, RFA.

155. Warren to Russell, May 17, 1926, RG 5, Series 1.2, Box 258, File 3281, RFA.

156. Carr, "Narrative Report of the Lucha contra la Uncinariasis for the 4th Quarter of 1926," RG 5, Series 3, Box 144, RFA.

157. Fowler-Salamini, *Agrarian Radicalism*, 159.

158. Warren, "Narrative Report of the Hookworm Work in Mexico for the 2nd Quarter of 1926," RG 5, Series 3, Box 144, RFA.

159. Warren to Russell, May 27, 1926, RG 5, Series 1.2, Box 258, File 3281, RFA.

160. He subsequently praised the preventive work of the campaign. See Solórzano Morfín, "Tratamiento," 331.

161. The IHB representative continued to write hookworm campaign reports for several years after the campaign had been turned over to the Mexican government. See Henry P. Carr, "Lucha contra la Uncinariasis," *Salubridad* 1, no. 1 (1930): 175–82; and Henry P. Carr, "Trabajos Desarrollados en la Lucha contra la Uncinariasis," *Salubridad* 1, no. 3 (1930): 784–88.

162. Warren to Russell, May 27, 1926, RG 5, Series 1.2, Box 258, File 3281, RFA.

163. *Enciclopedia de México*, vol. 5 (México, D.F.: Enciclopedia de México, 1978), 240; Bustamante, *Cinco Personajes*; "Gastélum, Bernardo," in *Who's Who in Latin America: A*

Biographical Dictionary of the Outstanding Living Men and Women of Spanish America and Brazil, ed. Percy Alvin Martin (Palo Alto, CA: Stanford University Press, 1935), 167.

164. Bernardo Gastélum, "Report of the Lucha contra la Uncinariasis," May 1925, RG 5, Series 3, Box 144, RFA. Carr subsequently published a gender-based description of defecation patterns, but he attributed differential rates to cleaner habits among girls and women rather than to occupational differences. Carr, "Observations," 57.

165. Warren, "Severe Hookworm Infestation in Alvarado, Mexico, An Urban Community; The Epidemiology of Which Was Not Influenced by Agricultural Occupations," July 20, 1925, RG 5, Series 2, Subseries 323, Box 33, File 198, RFA.

166. Bernardo Gastélum, "Report of the Lucha contra la Uncinariasis," May 1925, RG 5, Series 3, Box 144, RFA.

167. Carrillo, "Surgimiento y Desarrollo."

168. Carr to Russell, August 19, 1928, RG 1.1, Series 323, Box 19, Folder 156, RFA.

169. See Solórzano Morfín, "Tratamiento"; F. Bulman et al., "Dictamen Presentado a la Academia Nacional de Medicina, por la Comisión Encargada de Estudiar el Trabajo de Concurso Titulado: Tratamiento de la Uncinariasis, y Emparado por el Problema: Pro Aris et Focis Certare," *Gaceta Médica de México* 58, no. 6 (1927): 372–81; Juan Solórzano Morfín, "Algunos Datos para el Estudio de las Parasitosis Intestinales de México," *Gaceta Médica de México* 58, no. 12 (1927): 742–59; and E. Cervera, "Contestación al Trabajo del Nuevo Académico, Dr. Juan Solórzano Morfín," *Gaceta Médica de México* 58, no. 12 (1927): 760–64.

170. Solórzano Morfín, "Tratamiento," 329.

171. Ibid., 329–33.

172. Ibid., 329–71.

173. Bulman et al., "Dictamen Presentado."

174. Solórzano Morfín, "Algunos Datos."

175. Cervera, "Contestación."

176. "Necrología."

177. "Las Parasitósis Intestinales de México," *Boletín de la Oficina Sanitaria Panamericana* 7 (1928): 575–79.

178. Russell to Brioso Vasconcelos, January 17, 1924, RG 5, Series 1.2, Box 193, Folder 2469, RFA.

179. De la Garza Brito to Russell, November 1, 1925, RG 3, Series 1.2, Box 226, Folder 2872, RFA.

180. Russell to Read, September 18, 1925, RG 5, Series 1.2, Box 226, Folder 2872, RFA.

181. Warren to Russell, April 12, 1926, RG 5, Series 1.2, Box 257, File 3272, RFA.

182. Gastélum, *Memoria,* 57.

183. Russell to Read, September 18, 1925, RG 5, Series 1.2, Box 226, Folder 2872, RFA.

184. Alvarez Amézquita et al., *Historia de la Salubridad,* 283.

185. Gastélum, *Memoria,* vii–viii.

186. Warren to Russell, April 12, 1926, RG 5, Series 1.2, Box 257, File 3272, RFA.

187. Russell to Warren, July 27, 1926, RG 5, Series 1.2, Box 258, File 3282, RFA.

188. Warren to Russell, January 25, 1926, RG 5, Series 1.2, Box 258, File 3281, RFA.

189. Warren to Russell, April 24, 1926, RG 5, Series 1.2, Box 257, File 3272, RFA.

190. Warren to Russell, July 15, 1926, RG 5, Series 1.2, Box 258, File 3282, RFA.

191. Warren to Russell, April 24, 1926, RG 5, Series 1.2, Box 257, File 3272, RFA.

192. Carr to Russell, July 24, 1926, RG 5, Series 1.2, Box 257, File 3274, RFA.

193. Henry P. Carr, "Conferencia sobre la Uncinariasis Sustentada por el Doctor Henry Carr en el Departamento de Salubridad," *Salubridad* 3 (1932): 463–72.

194. Carr, "Narrative Report of the Lucha contra la Uncinariasis for the 4th Quarter of 1926," RG 5, Series 3, Box 144, RFA.

195. Russell to Carr, March 24, 1927, RG 5, Series 1.2, Box 296, File 3753, RFA.

196. Russell to Carr, April 19, 1927, RG 5, Series 1.2, Box 296, File 3753, RFA.

197. Carr to Russell, November 23, 1928, RG 1.1, Series 323, Box 17, File 140, RFA.

198. Carr to Ferrell, April 5, 1930, RG 2, Series 323, Box 41, Folder 337, RFA.

199. Vanderbilt University pharmacologist Paul Lamson's work proposed that sodium sulphate could be used as a purge for carbon tetrachloride. Russell wanted to see if Lamson's work would hold up in the field, but magnesium sulphate was difficult to replace because it was cheap, universally familiar, and more soluble. See Russell to Carr, July 11, 1927, RG 5, Series 1.2, Box 296, File 3754, RFA.

200. Carr to Ferrell, April 20, 1931, RG 1.1, Series 323, Box 19, File 157, RFA.

201. Russell to Warren, August 25, 1924, RG 1.1, Series 323, Box 17, File 139, RFA. A low "worm burden" would signal infection without clinical manifestation of the disease.

202. In the IHB's campaign in Sri Lanka there was also tension over the matter of reinfection. There, IHB staff members supported prevention via latrine construction, but they ultimately succumbed to pressure from plantation owners and the government to administer large numbers of hookworm treatments instead. Treatment quickly and dramatically demonstrated the effectiveness of curative medicine by reducing absenteeism. See Hewa, "Hookworm Epidemic."

203. Russell to Carr, October 2, 1928, RG 1.1, Series 323, Box 17, File 140, RFA.

204. Solórzano Morfín, "Tratamiento."

205. Carr to Ferrell, April 5, 1930, RG 2, Series 323, Box 41, Folder 337, RFA.

206. Carr to Russell, November 17, 1928, RG 1.1, Series 323, Box 17, File 140, RFA.

207. Ferrell to Carr, February 3, 1930, RG 1.1, Series 323, Box 17, File 141, RFA.

208. Carr to Ferrell, February 11, 1930, RG 1.1, Series 323, Box 17, File 141, RFA.

209. Carr to Ferrell, telegram, June 6, 1930, RG 1.1, Series 323, Box 17, File 141, RFA.

210. Warren to Carr, June 9, 1930, RG 1.1, Series 323, Box 17, File 141, RFA.

211. Pilar Hernández Lira, "Distribución Geográfica y Patología de la Uncinariasis en la República Mexicana," Boletín Epidemiológico 8, no. 4 (1949): 111.

212. All citations in this paragraph are from "Report of the Hookworm Campaign, the Minatitlán-Puerto México Cooperative Sanitary Unit, and the Puerto México Antilarval Service for the Fourth Quarter, 1930." Communicable Diseases Section, DSP, México, D.F. Section II/021/241, Box 39, Folder 83, Archivo Histórico del Estado de Morelos, Cuernavaca, Morelos, hereafter referred to as AHEM.

213. Anne-Emanuelle Birn, "Eradication, Control or Neither? Hookworm vs. Malaria Strategies and Rockefeller Public Health in Mexico," Parassitologia 40, nos. 1–2 (1998): 137–47.

214. Carr, "Lucha contra la Uncinariasis of the Departamento de Salubridad Pública for the 3rd Quarter of 1926," RG 5, Series 3, Box 144, RFA.

215. Warren, "The First Annual Report of the Activities of the Hookworm Campaign for Mexico during the Year 1924," RG 5, Series 3, Box 143, RFA.

216. Russell to Carr, March 24, 1927, RG 5, Series 1.2, Box 296, File 3753, RFA. Russell to Carr, May 19, 1927, RG 5, Series 1.2, Box 296, File 3753, RFA.

217. "La Historia de un Niño," Health Education and Propaganda Section, Lucha contra la Uncinariasis, DSP, Mexico, 1930, Section II/021/241, Box 39, Folder 83, AHEM. Also see Anne-Emanuelle Birn and Armando Solórzano, "The Hook of Hookworm: Public Health and the Politics of Eradication in Mexico," in Western Medicine as Contested Knowledge, ed. Andrew Cunningham and Bridie Andrews (Manchester, UK: Manchester University Press, 1997), 147–71.

218. El Istmo, June 4, 1927, RG 5, Series 1.2, Box 296, File 3753, RFA.

219. Carr to Russell, July 5, 1927, RG 5, Series 1.2, Box 296, File 3753, RFA.

220. See, for example, Thomas Perrín to George Vincent, April 6, 1926, RG 5, Series 1.2, Box 257, File 3272, RFA.

221. Ferrell to Carr, October 8, 1929, RG 1.1, Series 323, Box 17, File 140, RFA.

222. Carr, "Métodos Modernos para el Dominio de la Uncinariasis Ejemplificado en el Trabajo del Departamento de Salubridad Pública de México. Informe del Progreso de la Campaña contra la Uncinariasis, 1927," RG 5, Series 2, Subseries 323, Box 33, File 195, RFA.

223. Carr to Russell, December 11, 1928, RG 1.1, Series 323, Box 21, File 169, RFA.
224. Warren, "Brief Narrative Report on the Work of the Hookworm Campaign in Mexico for the Second Quarter of 1925," RG 5, Series 3, Box 144, RFA.
225. Carr, "Annual Report of the Lucha contra la Uncinariasis, Section for Tropical Diseases of the Departamento de Salubridad Pública, for the Year 1927," p. 3, RG 5, Series 3, Box 144, RFA.
226. See Cueto, *Missionaries of Science*; and John Farley, "Species Eradication: The Sardinia Anopheles Eradication Project, 1945–1950" (paper presented at the Conference on Disease and Society in the Developing World: Exploring New Perspectives, Philadelphia, September, 1992).
227. Manuel Martínez Báez, "El Instituto de Salubridad y Enfermedades Tropicales," *Anales de la Sociedad Mexicana de Historia de la Ciencia y de la Tecnología* 1 (1969): 146; see, for example, A.R. Ochoa to Chief of Health Ministry in Russia, January 29, 1924, RG A482 (Narkomzdrav), Inventory 35, File 57, p. 21, GARF (State Archive of the Russian Federation, Moscow).

Chapter Three

1. Francisco de P. Miranda, "Evolución de la Sanidad en México," *Boletín de la Oficina Sanitaria Panamericana* 9 (1930): 233–40.
2. Ibid., 233.
3. Ibid., 240.
4. See chapter 1; and Miguel Bustamante, "Hechos Sobresalientes en la Historia de la Secretaría de Salubridad y Asistencia," April 19, 1983, RG Dr. Miguel E. Bustamante V, FCCBV.
5. José Alvarez Amézquita et al., "Servicios Médicos Rurales Cooperativos en la Historia de la Salubridad y de la Asistencia en México," in *La Atención Médica en el Medio Rural Mexicano, 1930–1980*, ed. Héctor Hernández Llamas (México, D.F.: IMSS, 1984), 93–107.
6. *Transactions of the Seventh Pan American Sanitary Conference of the American Republics, held in Havana, Cuba, November 5 to 15, 1924* (Washington, DC: Pan American Sanitary Bureau [PASB], 1924).
7. "Código Sanitario de los Estados Unidos de México," *Boletín de la Oficina Sanitaria Panamericana* 5 (1926): 367–456.
8. Bustamante, "Hechos Sobresalientes."
9. Carrillo, "Surgimiento y Desarrollo."
10. Alvarez Amézquita et al., *Historia de la Salubridad*, 275–85.
11. Ibid., 306; and Bustamante, "Coordinación de," 209.
12. Francisco Vásquez Pérez, cited in Alvarez Amézquita et al., *Historia de la Salubridad*, 278–79.
13. Henry P. Carr, "Lucha contra la Uncinariasis del Departamento de Salubridad Pública para el Tercer Trimester de 1926," RG 5, Series 3, Box 144, RFA.
14. Carr to Ferrell, July 18, 1930, RG 1.1, Series 323, Box 19, Folder 156, RFA.
15. See Bustamante, "Coordinación," 179–228; Weindling, *International Health Organisations and Movements, 1918–1939*.
16. See Charles V. Chapin, "State Health Organization," *Journal of the American Medical Association* 66, no. 10 (March 4, 1916): 699–703. In Chapin's view, the functions of a local health department included the gathering of vital statistics, control of communicable diseases, infant hygiene, supervision of water and sewerage, public health education, and the regulation of food handling. Success depended on having a "man on the spot," especially in rural areas, and on the cooperation of the state health department when necessary. Chapin's ideas were put into practice in countless North American municipalities, and in the 1920s and 1930s, Chapin's Rhode Island Health Department was a routine stop on the IHD's North American tours for health officials from all over the world. See James

Cassedy, *Charles V. Chapin and the Public Health Movement* (Cambridge, MA: Harvard University Press, 1962).

17. See Rodríguez Ocaña, "Foreign Expertise"; Esteban Rodríguez Ocaña, "La Salud Pública en la España de la Primera Mitad del Siglo XX," in *El Centro Secundario de Higiene Rural de Talavera de la Reina y la Sanidad Española de su Tiempo,* ed. Juan Atenza y José Martínez (Toledo, España: Junta de Comunidades de Castilla la Mancha, 2001), 21–42.

18. During the first years following the Russian Revolution, the Soviet regime sought to replace *feldshers* (physician's assistants or paramedics), who played an important role in providing free rural health care under the *zemstvo* tradition, with full-fledged physicians partially funded by local authorities. See Samuel C. Ramer, "Feldshers and Rural Health Care in the Early Soviet Period," in *Health and Society in Revolutionary Russia,* ed. Susan Gross Solomon and John F. Hutchinson (Bloomington: Indiana University Press, 1990), 121–45.

19. Farley, *To Cast Out Disease,* 31–43, 82–84. The RF carried the county health unit structure to Puerto Rico in 1926, under the direction of officer George C. Payne, who was the RF representative in Mexico in the early 1940s. Because of Puerto Rico's status as a U.S. territory, the politics of organizing public health programs differed both from the southern U.S. states and from foreign countries. A useful article on the role of the RF and the U.S. government in Puerto Rican public health is Ramírez de Arellano, "Politics of Public Health in Puerto Rico."

20. "Principles and Policies of International Health Division of the Rockefeller Foundation for Cooperating with Official Health Agencies in Developing County Health Work in the United States," March 5, 1926, RG 3.1, Series 908, Box 4, Folder 23, RFA.

21. "Dr. John Ferrell, Public Health Pioneer, Dies at Rex Hospital Today," *Raleigh Times,* February 18, 1965.

22. "Memorandum Concerning John A. Ferrell's Trip to Mexico April 21st–May 2nd, 1927," Diary Excerpt, May 19, 1927, RG 12.1, Box 19, RFA.

23. "Address by John A. Ferrell at Dinner Given to Him by the Federal Department of Health of Mexico, Mexico City April 26, 1927," Exhibit "A," Diary Excerpt, May 19, 1927, RG 12.1, Box 19, RFA.

24. Russell to Carr, November 16, 1928, RG 1.1, Series 323, Box 19, File 156, RFA.

25. Russell to Carr, December 29, 1928, RG 1.1, Series 323, Box 19, File 156, RFA.

26. Russell to Carr, December 24, 1928, RG 1.1, Series 323, Box 21, File 169, RFA.

27. Carr to Russell, December 19, 1928, RG 1.1, Series 323, Box 19, File 156, RFA.

28. See Alvarez Amézquita et al., *Historia de la Salubridad,* 275–85; Rafael Silva, "Memorandum to the President," May 2, 1930; "Organización de Unidades Sanitarias," Minutes from a Meeting between Doctors Francisco Bulman, Miguel Bustamante, Juan Graham Casasús, Francisco Valenzuela, José Díaz Iturbide, and Angel de la Garza Brito, January 20, 1931; and Francisco Valenzuela, memorandum, March 5, 1931, RG Public Health, Juridical Section, Box 13, Folder 1, AHSSA.

29. Personal correspondence from Juan I. Bustamante, dated September 25, 1992.

30. Anne-Emanuelle Birn, "Dr. Miguel Bustamante," in *Doctors, Nurses, and Practitioners,* ed. Lois Magner (Westwood, CT: Greenwood Press, 1997), 30–36; and Ana Maria Carrillo, "Miguel E. Bustamante," in *Ciencia y Tecnología en México en el Siglo XX. Biografías de Personajes Ilustres,* vol. 3 (México, D.F.: Secretaría de Educación Pública/Academia Mexicana de Ciencias/Consejo Consultivo de Ciencias de la Presidencia de la República/Consejo Nacional de Ciencia y Tecnología, 2003), 143–58.

31. The influence of Johns Hopkins University on international health and the symbiotic relationship between Hopkins and the Rockefeller Foundation are discussed by Fee *Disease and Discovery.*

32. Miguel E. Bustamante, "Proyecto para la Organización Económica de las Unidades Sanitarias Cooperativas que se Establezcan en la República," May 1930, DSP; Rafael Silva, "Unidades Sanitarias Memorandum," December 21, 1931, DSP; and Departamento de

Salubridad Pública, "Circular a los Delegados Sanitarios," 1931, RG Public Health, Juridical Section, Box 13, Folder 1, AHSSA. Also see Miguel E. Bustamante and Luis Mazzotti, "Programa Mínimo de Trabajo e Instructivos para los Médicos Encargados de Oficinas Sanitarias en Lugares Pequeños," DSP, 1931, RG Dr. Miguel E. Bustamante V., FCCBV; and Miguel E. Bustamante, "Higiene Municipal," *Revista Médica Veracruzana* 11 (1930): 81.

33. Charles A. Bailey to John Ferrell, 12 May 1935, RG 2, Series 323, Box 119, Folder 907, RFA.

34. Wickliffe Rose, "Memorandum on the Principles of Administration of the International Health Board," 1922, RG 3.1, Series 908, Box 12, Folder 128, RFA.

35. See table 3.5.

36. The first official support for the creation of sanitary units was Circular Number 512, dated April 30, 1927, from the DSP chief (with presidential approval) to the state governors. See Miguel E. Bustamante and Luis Mazzotti, "Programa Mínimo de Trabajo e Instructivos para los Médicos Encargados de Oficinas Sanitarias en Lugares Pequeños," 1931, DSP, RG Dr. Miguel E. Bustamante V, FCCBV.

37. Héctor Aguilar Camín and Lorenzo Meyer, *In the Shadow of the Mexican Revolution: Contemporary Mexican History*, trans. Luis Alberto Fierro (Austin: University of Texas Press, 1993), 95–96; and Knight, *U.S. Mexican Relations*, 137–44.

38. Jean A. Meyer, "Mexico in the 1920s," in *Mexico since Independence*, ed. Leslie Bethell (Cambridge: Cambridge University Press, 1991), 218–27.

39. See David C. Bailey, *¡Viva Cristo Rey! The Cristero Rebellion and the Church-State Conflict in Mexico* (Austin: University of Texas Press, 1974); Jennie Purnell, *Popular Movements and State Formation in Revolutionary Mexico: The Agraristas and Cristeros of Michoacán* (Durham, NC: Duke University Press, 1999); and Jean A. Meyer, *The Cristero Rebellion: The Mexican People between Church and State, 1926–1929* (Cambridge: Cambridge University Press, 1976), 178–80.

40. Medin, *Ideología*, 18–20; and Arnaldo Córdova, *La Ideología de la Revolución Mexicana* (México, D.F.: Ediciones Era, 1973), 307–67.

41. See table 3.3.

42. Luis Javier Garrido, *El Partido de la Revolución Institucionalizada: Medio Siglo de Poder Político en México: La Formación del Nuevo Estado, 1928–1945* (México, D.F.: Siglo Veintiuno Editores, 1982).

43. A sardonic play on words with regard to the assassination goes as follows: "¿Quién asesinó al Presidente Obregón? Shhh. . . . que se *Calle!*" Translation: Who assassinated President Obregón? Shh—be quiet!" (Also meaning "It was Calles.").

44. Garrido, *Partido*, 63.

45. Predecessor to what in the 1940s would become the Partido Revolucionario Institucional (PRI), which would dominate Mexico for the rest of the twentieth century.

46. Hamilton, *Limits of State Autonomy*, 76–77.

47. Medin, *Minimato Presidencial.*

48. Sergio Aguayo, *Myths and [Mis] Perceptions: Changing U.S. Elite Visions of Mexico*, trans. Julián Brody (San Diego: Center for U.S.-Mexican Studies, University of California, 1998).

49. Lewis Hackett, an IHD officer who researched and wrote a detailed manuscript on the history of the IHD, argues that the RF expected the stock market crash and took measures to protect itself, such as only committing program funds that could be covered by money in the bank. Lewis Hackett, vol. 1, RG 3.1, Series 908, Box 3, Folder 19, RFA.

50. Ferrell to Carr, September 18, 1930, RG 1.1, Series 323, Box 19, Folder 156, RFA.

51. Local Health Departments Program for 1932, RG 5, Series 3, Box 19, Folder 154, RFA. Also see Carr to Ferrell, August 4, 1928, RG 1.1, Series 323, Box 19, Folder 157, RFA.

52. Ferrell to Carr, September 18, 1930, RG 1.1, Series 323, Box 19, Folder 156, RFA.

53. On March 1, 1923, Rose became president of the RF's General Education Board and International Education Board.

54. Wilbur Sawyer, interviewed by Lewis Hackett, August 29, 1950 and Notes, vol. 1, RG 3.1, Series 908, Box 3, Folder 19, RFA.

55. Farley, "International Health Division."

56. Russell to First Board of Scientific Directors, "The Program for Future Work of the International Health Division," ca. October 1929, RG 3.1, Series 908, Box 3, Folder 19, RFA.

57. Frederick Russell, "Talk on Policy in Response to Presentation of the Marcellus Hartley Medal by the National Academy of Sciences," 1936, RG 3.1, Series 908, Box 3, Folder 19, RFA.

58. "Report and Recommendations as to the Future Status of the International Health Division," presented at the Rockefeller Foundation trustees' meeting November 9, 1928, by a Special Divisional Committee of the IHD with Simon Flexner, Chairman, RG 3.1, Series 908, Box 4, Folder 20, RFA.

59. Frederick Russell, "Memorandum Concerning Future Developments in the International Health Division of the Rockefeller Foundation," 1928, RG 3.1, Series 908, Box 11, Folder 124, RFA.

60. Carr to Russell, December 5, 1927, RG 5, Series 1.2, Box 296, Folder 3754, RFA.

61. Ibid.

62. Sawyer to Carr, December 15, 1927, RG 5, Series 1.2, Box 296, Folder 3754, RFA.

63. Carr to Russell, December 5, 1927, RG 5, Series 1.2, Box 296, Folder 3754, RFA.

64. Carr, "Annual Report of Unidad Sanitaria Cooperativa Minatitlán-Puerto México for the Year 1928," RG 5, Series 3, Box 146, RFA.

65. Carr to Russell, December 5, 1927, RG 5, Series 1.2, Box 296, Folder 3754, RFA.

66. Ibid.

67. Carr, "Unidad Sanitaria Cooperativa Minatitlán-Puerto México—Informe trimestral de labores del 10 de Abril al 30 de Junio de 1928," RG 5, Series 3, Box 146, RFA.

68. Ibid.

69. Carr, "Annual Report of Unidad Sanitaria Cooperativa Minatitlán-Puerto México for the Year 1928," RG 5, Series 3, Box 146, RFA.

70. Interview with Dr. Felipe García Sánchez, June 5, 1991, Mexico City. Also see table 3, Summary View of Comparable Conditions in the Regions, appendix I, Howard F. Cline, The United States and Mexico (New York: Atheneum, 1966), 435; México Salario Mínimo Medio, Dirección General de Estadística, Cincuenta Años de Revolución Mexicana en Cifras, Nacional Financiera, S.A. (México, D.F.: Subgerencia de Investigaciones Económicas, 1963); and Hansen, Politics of Mexican Development, 20–95.

71. "Report of the Hookworm Campaign, the Minatitlán-Puerto México Cooperative Sanitary Unit, and the Puerto México Antilarval Service for the Second Quarter, 1931," Communicable Diseases Section, DSP, México, D.F. Section II/021/242, Box 39, Folder 84, AHEM.

72. Carr to Ferrell, September 30, 1929, RG 1.1, Series 323, Box 19, File 156, RFA.

73. Carr to Ferrell, October 14, 1929, RG 1.1, Series 323, Box 19, File 156, RFA.

74. Carr to Ferrell, January 3, 1931, RG 1.1, Series 323, Box 19, File 157, RFA.

75. Departamento de Salubridad Pública, "Campaña Pro-Mejoría del Aprovisionamiento de Agua," ca. 1935, RG SSA, Section Subsecretariat, Box 28, Folder 9, AHSSA.

76. Alvarez Amézquita et al., Historia de la Salubridad, 310.

77. Miguel E. Bustamante, "Local Public Health Work in Mexico," American Journal of Public Health 21 (1931): 725–36.

78. Departamento de Salubridad Pública, "Campaña Pro-Mejoría del Aprovisionamiento de Agua," ca. 1935, RG SSA, Section Subsecretariat, Box 28, Folder 9, AHSSA.

79. Bustamante, "Informe Trimestral de Labores de la Unidad Sanitaria de Veracruz," October–December 31, 1930, RG 5, Series 3, Box 147, RFA. Also see H. E. Gimler, Acting Assistant Surgeon, U.S. Public Health Service, Veracruz, to Surgeon General of the U.S.

Public Health Service, May 16, 1929, RG 90, General Records, General Subject File, 1924–35, Foreign Governments, Box 830, File Mexico 0123-0415, NARA.

80. Bustamante, "Local Public Health Work," 733.

81. Bustamante to Carr, January 1930, "Notes on the General Mortality of the Port of Veracruz," RG 2, Series 300, Box 553, Folder 3736, RFA.

82. Bustamante believed that an understanding of history was a necessary precursor to public health work. After his retirement, Bustamante became a prolific historian of public health in Mexico. See Carrillo, "Miguel Bustamante."

83. Bustamante, "Local Public Health Work," 729.

84. Aquilino Villanueva, "Los Problemas Fundamentales en México en Materia de Salubridad," *Boletín de la Oficina Sanitaria Panamericana* 8 (1929): 1194–96.

85. Carr to Ferrell, April 5, 1930, RG 2, Series 323, Box 41, Folder 337, RFA.

86. Ibid.

87. "Notes on Dr. Ferrell's Trip to Mexico, March 15–April 21, 1933," RG 2, Series 300, Box 553, Folder 3736, RFA.

88. Alvarez Amézquita et al., *Historia de la Salubridad*, 306.

89. Ibid., 313.

90. See Bernardo J. Gastélum, *Dos Años Seis Meses de Higiene en Sinaloa* (México, D.F.: DSP, 1934).

91. Bustamante, "Coordinación," 207.

92. Indeed, Carr continued to write the hookworm campaign reports several years after the campaign had been turned over to the Mexican government. See Carr, "Trabajos Desarrollados," 784–88; and Carr, "Lucha contra la Uncinariasis," 175–82.

93. Carr to Ferrell, July 10, 1930, RG 1.1, Series 323, Box 17, File 141, RFA.

94. Ferrell to Carr, July 22, 1930, RG 1.1, Series 323, Box 17, File 141, RFA.

95. More than a dozen high-ranking public health officials interviewed recalled no objection to having an RF representative serve in a DSP position.

96. Carr to Ferrell, July 18, 1930, RG 1.1, Series 323, Box 19, Folder 156, RFA.

97. Ibid.

98. Carr to Ferrell, April 5, 1930, RG 2, Series 323, Box 41, Folder 337, RFA.

99. Bustamante, "Local Public Health Work," 725.

100. Ibid., 726–27.

101. Rafael Silva, "The Health Problem in Mexico," *American Journal of Public Health* 21, no. 1 (1931): 31–36.

102. Carr did not miss a chance to remark upon Bustamante's "not ideal" characteristics, but he conceded that Bustamante was likely to carry out the work successfully. Carr to Ferrell, May 18, 1932, RG 2, Series 323, Box 71, Folder 582, RFA.

103. Carr to Ferrell, May 18, 1932, RG 2, Series 323, Box 71, Folder 582, RFA.

104. Such views and interchanges on Bustamante on the part of the RF home office and IHD officers in Mexico continued through the 1930s. See, for example, Bailey to Ferrell, May 12, 1935, RG 2, Series 323, Box 119, Folder 907, RFA.

105. Ferrell to Carr, July 5, 1932, RG 2, Series 323, Box 71, Folder 582, RFA.

106. Bustamante, "Coordinación," 198.

107. Sr. Professor Cesar Reyes to Bustamante, ca. 1932, RG Public Health, Health in Territories Section, Parts and Borders, Box 16, Folder 2, AHSSA.

108. Departamento de Salubridad Pública, "Campaña Pro-Mejoría del Aprovisionamiento de Agua," ca. 1935, RG SSA, Section Subsecretariat, Box 28, Folder 9, AHSSA; and Alfonso Pruneda, "La Secretaría de Educación Pública de México y la Difusión de la Higiene," *Pasteur: Revista Mensual de Medicina* 2, I, no. 42 (1929): 52–54. Also see Vaughan, *State, Education, and Social Class*; and Vaughan, *Cultural Politics in Revolution*.

109. See "Informe Anual del Servicio de Higiene," 1933 through 1939, RG 5, Series 3, Box 145, RFA.

110. Bustamante, "Coordinación," 179–228.

111. Ibid., 180.

112. For example, it is the first article in the Pan American Health Organization's *Health Services Research: An Anthology* (Washington, DC: PAHO, 1992).

113. See Birn and Solórzano, "Public Health Policy Paradoxes" 1197-1213.

114. Bustamante, "Coordinación," 194.

115. See, for example, Vaughan, *State, Education, and Social Class*; Alec Gershberg, "Fiscal Decentralization and Intergovernmental Relations: An Analysis of Federal versus State Education Finance in Mexico," *Review of Urban and Regional Development Studies* 7, 2 (1995): 119-42; and Carlos Ornelas, *La Descentralización de la Educación en México* (Santiago, Chile: Comisión Económica para la América Latina y el Caribe, 1997).

116. Carr to Ferrell, April 5, 1930, RG 2, Series 323, Box 41, Folder 337, RFA.

117. Carr to Ferrell, July 18, 1930, RG 1.1, Series 323, Box 19, Folder 156, RFA.

118. Henry P. Carr, "Trabajos Especiales del Servicio de Higiene Rural, a Cargo del Señor Dr. Henry P. Carr," *Salubridad* 3, no. 2 (1932): 443-45.

119. Carr to Vicente Estrada Cajigal, December 18, 1930, Section II/021/241, Box 39, Folder 83, AHEM.

120. See Roberto Melville, *Crecimiento y Rebelión: El Desarrollo Económico de las Haciendas Azucareras en Morelos, 1880-1910* (México, D.F.: Editorial Nueva Imagen, 1979); Patricia Arias and Lucia Bazán, *Demandas y Conflicto: El Poder Político en un Pueblo de Morelos* (México, D.F.: Editorial Nueva Imagen, 1979); Everardo Escárcega López and Saúl Escobar Toledo, *Historia de la Cuestión Agraria Mexicana, 5. El Cardenismo: Un Parteaguas Histórico en el Proceso Nacional, 1934-1940* (México, D.F.: Siglo Ventiuno Editores, 1990); Womack, *Zapata*; Arturo Warman, *We Come to Object: The Peasants of Morelos and the National State*, trans. Stephen K. Ault. (Baltimore: Johns Hopkins University Press, 1980); Morales, *Morelos Agrario*; and Guillermo de la Peña, *A Legacy of Promises: Agriculture, Politics and Ritual in the Morelos Highlands of Mexico* (Austin: University of Texas Press, 1981).

121. Connor to Read, March 16, 1924, RG 5, Series 1.2, Box 193, File 2469, RFA.

122. On the surrounding region, see de la Peña, *A Legacy of Promises*.

123. Silva to Estrada Cajigal, December 15, 1930, Section II/021/241, Box 39, Folder 83, AHEM.

124. Carr to Estrada Cajigal, December 18, 1930, Section II/021/241, Box 39, Folder 83, AHEM.

125. Ibid.

126. Ibid.

127. Estrada Cajigal to President of Cuautla Municipality, January 17, 1930, Section II/021/241, Box 39, Folder 83, AHEM.

128. Budget No. 3, Rural Hygiene Service, Projected Cooperative Sanitary Unit of Cuautla, Morelos, December 1 to 31, 1931, Section II/021/241, Box 39, Folder 83, AHEM.

129. Carr to Cajigal, May 22, 1931, Section II/021/242, Box 39, Folder 84, AHEM.

130. Carr, "Tabular Résumé (as of December 31, 1932) of Rockefeller Foundation Cooperation in Mexico since Termination of the Hookworm Campaign and Establishment of First Full Time Health Unit," RG 1.1, Series 323, Box 19, Folder 157, RFA.

131. Interview with Hermillo Espinoza Canales, retired sanitary unit chauffeur, April 15, 1991, Cuernavaca, Morelos.

132. Crisóforo Albarrán to Secretary General of the Government, April 29, 1931, Section II/021/242, Box 39, Folder 84, AHEM.

133. A few years later, Viniegra was transferred to a clinical setting because the IHD found him "too curative," and they could not convince him to change to a more preventive orientation. Bailey to Ferrell, March 4, 1933, RG 1.1, Series 323, Box 19, Folder 158, RFA.

134. Interview with Esther "La Güera" Coronel, April 15, 1991, Cuernavaca, Morelos. The units were so popular that some people recall them giving away free bread, milk, and breakfasts for school children, programs that had actually been run by the Ministry of Education since the early 1920s well before the RF became involved in the health units. See Vaughan, *Cultural Politics in Revolution*, 27; and Vaughan, *State, Education, and Social Class.*

135. "Report of the Hookworm Campaign, the Minatitlán-Puerto México Cooperative Sanitary Unit, and the Puerto México Antilarval Service for the Second Quarter, 1931," Communicable Diseases Section, DSP, México, D.F. Section II/021/242, Box 39, Folder 84, AHEM.

136. Carr to Ferrell, June 13, 1931, RG 5, Series 3, Box 19, Folder 157, RFA.

137. "Annual Report," 1934, Rural Hygiene Service, DSP, RG 5, Series 3, Box 145, RFA.

138. Interview with Dr. Felipe García Sánchez, June 5, 1991, Mexico City.

139. The yellow fever campaign, for example, threatened fines of 5 to 500 pesos for disobeying rules. Alfonso Pruneda, "Disposiciones Relativas a la Campaña Contra la Fiebre Amarilla," Diario Oficial, March, 30 1921, RG Public Health, Juridical Section, Box 34, Folder 6, AHSSA. Interviews with Hermillo Espinoza Canales, retired sanitary unit chauffeur, April 15, 1991, Cuernavaca, Morelos, and with Joel Rogelio Sandoval, retired administrator, April 12, 1991, Cuernavaca, Morelos.

140. "Annual Report," 1932, Rural Hygiene Service, DSP, RG 5, Series 3, Box 145, RFA.

141. "Annual Report," 1934, Rural Hygiene Service, DSP, RG 5, Series 3, Box 145, RFA.

142. "Report of the Hookworm Campaign, the Minatitlán-Puerto México Cooperative Sanitary Unit, and the Puerto México Antilarval Service for the Second Quarter, 1931," Communicable Diseases Section, DSP, México, D.F., Section II/021/242, Box 39, Folder 84, AHEM.

143. Bailey to Ferrell, November 1, 1933, RG 1.1, Series 323, Box 19, Folder 158, RFA.

144. "Report of the Hookworm Campaign, the Minatitlán-Puerto México Cooperative Sanitary Unit, and the Puerto México Antilarval Service for the Second Quarter, 1931," Communicable Diseases Section, DSP, México, D.F. Section II/021/242, Box 39, Folder 84, AHEM.

145. Silva, "Health Problem," 34.

146. On nurses playing this role in the South of the U.S., see Susan M. Reverby, "Rethinking the Tuskegee Syphilis Study: Nurse Rivers, Silence, and the Meaning of Treatment," reprinted in *Tuskegee's Truths: Rethinking the Tuskegee Syphilis Study*, ed. Susan M. Reverby (Chapel Hill: University of North Carolina Press, 2000), 365–85; and Darlene Clark Hine, "Reflections on Nurse Rivers," reprinted in *Tuskegee's Truths: Rethinking the Tuskegee Syphilis Study*, ed. Susan M. Reverby (Chapel Hill: University of North Carolina Press, 2000), 386–95.

147. See Deborah Dwork, *War Is Good for Babies and Other Children: A History of the Infant and Child Welfare Movement in England, 1898–1918* (London: Tavistock, 1987); Valerie Fildes, Lara Marks, and Hilary Marland, eds., *Women and Children First: International Maternal and Infant Welfare, 1870–1945* (London: Routledge,1992); and Seth Koven and Sonya Michel, eds., *Mothers of a New World: Maternalist Politics and the Origins of Welfare States* (New York: Routledge, 1993).

148. Richard A. Meckel, *Save the Babies: American Public Health Reform and the Prevention of Infant Mortality, 1850–1929* (Baltimore: Johns Hopkins University Press, 1990), 5–6. Also Charles R. King, *Children's Health in America: A History* (New York: Twayne Publishers, 1993); Rima D. Apple, *Mothers and Medicine: A Social History of Infant Feeding, 1890–1950* (Madison, University of Wisconsin Press, 1987); Janet Golden, *A Social History of Wet-Nursing in America: From Breast to Bottle* (Cambridge: Cambridge University Press, 1996); and Samuel H. Preston and Michael R. Haines, *Fatal Years: Child Mortality in Late Nineteenth-Century America* (Princeton, NJ: Princeton University Press, 1991), 3–48.

149. See Molly Ladd-Taylor, ed., *Raising a Baby the Government Way: Mothers' Letters to the Children's Bureau, 1915-1932* (New Brunswick, NJ: Rutgers University Press, 1986), and Molly Ladd-Taylor, "'Why Does Congress Wish Women and Children to Die?': The Rise and Fall of Public Maternal and Infant Health Care in the United States, 1921-1929," in *Women and Children First: International Maternal and Infant Welfare, 1870-1945*, ed. Valerie Fildes, Lara Marks, and Hilary Marland (London: Routledge,1992), 121-32. The rise and fall of Sheppard-Towner typifies the ambivalent backing for these services in the U.S. cultural context. The Sheppard-Towner law was passed the year after women obtained the right to vote, in a highly politicized bid by the U.S. Congress to meet women's claims on the state. But right-wing hysteria about growing socialism, buoyed by the jealousy of private-practice doctors, led to bitter polemics about the appropriate role of government in the provision of health services. By the late 1920s, organized medicine's promise that doctors would meet maternal and child health needs through routine and charity care—coupled with the now diminished menace of the "women's vote"—doomed Sheppard-Towner, and the legislation was not renewed.

150. Kathryn Kish Sklar "The Historical Foundations of Women's Power in the Creation of the American Welfare State, 1830-1930," in *Mothers of a New World: Maternalist Politics and the Origins of Welfare States*, ed. Seth Koven and Sonya Michel (New York: Routledge, 1993), 43-93. Also see Theda Skocpol, *Protecting Soldiers and Mothers: The Political Origins of Social Policy in the United States* (Cambridge, MA: Belknap Press of Harvard University Press, 1992), especially 311-539, for a discussion of how means-tested New Deal programs displaced the maternalist social policies of the "woman movement."

151. Studies of the history of maternal and child health and welfare movements in Latin America include the following: Donna J. Guy, "The Pan American Child Congresses, 1916 to 1942: Pan Americanism, Child Reform, and the Welfare State in Latin America," *Journal of Family History* 23, no. 3 (July 1998): 272-91; Victoria Lynn Black, "Taking Care of Baby: Chilean State-Making, International Relations and the Gendered Body Politic, 1912-1970" (PhD diss., University of Arizona, 2002); Christine Ehrick, "Affectionate Mothers and the Colossal Machine: Feminism, Social Assistance and the State in Uruguay, 1910-1932," *The Americas* 58 (2001): 121-39; and María Soledad Zárate Campos, "De Partera a Matrona. Los Inicios de la Profesionalización del Cuidado de la Madre y de los Hijos en Chile, 1870-1920," *Revista Colegio de Matronas* 7, no. 2 (1999): 13-18. For European comparisons, see Koven and Michel, eds., *Mothers of a New World*; Fildes et al., eds., *Women and Children First*; Gisela Bock and Pat Thane, eds., *Maternity and Gender Policies: Women and the Rise of the European Welfare States 1880s-1950s* (New York and London: Routledge, 1991); and Diane Sainsbury, *Gender Equality and Welfare States* (Cambridge: Cambridge University Press, 1996).

152. On the pre-welfare state period, see: Christine Adams, "Maternal Societies in France: Private Charity before the Welfare State," *Journal of Women's History* 17, no.1 (2005): 87-111. See Lion Murard and Patrick Zylberman, *L'hygiene dans la république: La santé publique en France, ou l'utopie contrariée, 1870-1918* (Paris: Fayard, 1996); Catherine Rollet, "La lutte contre la mortalite internationale infantile dans le passé: Essai de comparaison internationale," *Santé publique* 2 (1993): 4-20; Alisa Klaus has argued that "making maternity compatible with wage labor was a primary focus of many French maternal-and infant-health programs." In the French case, concern about babies dying when mothers gave up breast-feeding to return to work and low fertility because working class women did not want to undergo the physical and financial suffering of pregnancy and motherhood led to protective maternalist legislation. Such legislation served multiple interests—nationalism, women's rights, and the quelling of working class strife. See Alisa Klaus, "Depopulation and Race Suicide: Maternalism and Pronatalist Ideologies in France and the United States," in *Mothers of a New World: Maternalist Politics and the Origins of Welfare States*, ed. Seth Koven and Sonya Michel, 195 (New York: Routledge, 1993); and Alisa Klaus, *Every Child a Lion* (Ithaca, NY: Cornell University Press, 1993).

153. Nadine Lefaucheur, "La puériculture d'Adolphe Pinard," in *Darwinisme et societé*, ed. Patrick Tort (Paris: Presses Universitaires de France, 1992); and William H. Schneider, "Puericulture and the Style of French Eugenics," *History and Philosophy of the Life Sciences* 8 (1986): 265–77.

154. Birn, "No More Surprising than a Broken Pitcher?": 17–46.

155. Max Shein, *El Niño Precolombino* (Mexico, D.F.: Editorial Villicaña, S.A., 1986).

156. G. Gándara, "La Hierba de Leche o Ixbut, para la sesión del 7 de octubre de 1929 de la sociedad científica Antonio Alzate," RG Public Health, Infant Hygiene Section, Box 7, Folder 10, AHSSA.

157. Francesca Miller, *Latin American Women and the Search for Social Justice* (Hanover, NH: University Press of New England, 1991). See especially chapter 4, "Feminism and Social Motherhood, 1890–1938," 68–109; Christine Ehrick, "Madrinas and Missionaries: Uruguay and the Pan-American Women's Movement," *Gender and History* 10 (1998): 406–24. Also, on some of the divisions within the Latin American feminist movement, see Asunción Lavrin, *Women, Feminism, and Social Change in Argentina, Chile, and Uruguay* (Lincoln and London: University of Nebraska Press, 1995). On women's movements and state-building, see Ehrick, "Affectionate Mothers"; Barbara Potthast and Eugenia Scarzanella, eds., *Mujeres y Naciones en América Latina: Problemas de Inclusión y Exclusión* (Frankfurt: Iberoamericana/Vervuert, 2001); and Maxine Molyneux, *Women's Movements in International Perspective: Latin America and Beyond* (Basingstoke, UK, and New York: Palgrave, 2001); María Soledad Zárate Campos, "Proteger a las Madres: Origen de un Debate Público, 1870–1920," *Revista Nomadías—Serie Monográfica* 1 (1999): 163–82.

158. See, for example, Anna Macías, *Against All Odds: The Feminist Movement in Mexico to 1940* (Westport, CT: Greenwood Press, 1982); Shirlene Ann Soto, *Emergence of the Mexican Woman: Her Participation in Revolution and Struggle for Equality, 1910–1940* (Denver, CO: Arden Press, Inc., 1990), especially chapter 3 on Elvia Carrillo Puerto and the feminist movement in Yucatán; and Julia Tuñon, *Mujeres en México: Una Historia Olvidada* (México, D.F.: Editorial Planeta, 1987).

159. Mary Kay Vaughan, "Modernizing Patriarchy: State Policies, Rural Households and Women in Mexico 1930–1940," in *Hidden Histories of Gender and the State in Latin America*, ed. Elizabeth Dore and Maxine Molyneux (Durham, NC, and London: Duke University Press, 2000), 194–214.

160. See, for example, Pani, *Hygiene in Mexico*.

161. Anne-Emanuelle Birn, "Uruguay on the World Stage: How Child Health Became an International Priority," *American Journal of Public Health* 95 no.9 (2005): 1506–17.

162. Guy, "Pan American Child Congresses." Latin American feminists were also active in the League of Nations' efforts to protect women and children in the 1920s. See Eugenia Scarzanella, "Proteger a las Mujeres y los Niños. El Internacionalismo Humanitario de la Sociedad de las Naciones y las Delegadas Sudamericanas," in *Mujeres y Naciones en América Latina: Problemas de Inclusión y Exclusión*, ed. Barbara Potthast and Eugenia Scarzanella (Frankfurt: Iberoamericana/ Vervuert, 2001).

163. *Eugenic News*, 22 (1937): 94.

164. Nancy Leys Stepan, *"The Hour of Eugenics": Race, Gender, and Nation in Latin America* (Ithaca, NY: Cornell University Press, 1991).

165. Alexandra M. Stern, "From Mestizophilia to Biotypology: Racialization and Science in Mexico, 1920–1960," in *Race and Nation in Modern Latin America*, ed. Nancy Appelbaum, Anne S. Macpherson, and Karin Alejandra Rosemblatt (Chapel Hill: University of North Carolina Press, 2003), 187–210; and Alexandra M. Stern, "Unraveling the History of Eugenics in Mexico," *The Mendel Newsletter* (August 1999): 1–10. Also see Saavedra, "Historia del Movimiento Eugenésico."

166. Francisco de P. Miranda, "The Public Health Department in Mexico City," *American Journal of Public Health* 20, no. 10 (1930): 1125–28.

167. See Bliss, *Compromised Positions*; Ann S. Blum, "Public Welfare and Child Circulation, Mexico City, 1877 to 1925," *Journal of Family History* 23, no. 3 (July 1998): 240–71; and Stern, "Responsible Mothers."

168. See, for example, Margarito Crispín Castellanos, "Hospital de Maternidad e Infancia. Una Perspectiva Histórica de un Centro de Beneficencia Pública de Fines del Siglo XIX," in *La Atención Materno Infantil: Apuntes para su Historia*, ed. México, Secretaría de Salud, Dirección General de Atención Materno Infantil (México, D.F.: Secretaría de Salud, 1993), 95–115.

169. "Report of the Hookworm Campaign, the Minatitlán-Puerto México Cooperative Sanitary Unit, and the Puerto México Antilarval Service for the First Quarter, 1931," Communicable Diseases Section, DSP, México, D.F. Section II/021/241, Box 39, Folder 83, AHEM.

170. Examples of forms giving advice to pregnant women. Included with Bailey to DSP chief, January 23, 1934, RG 1.1, Series 323, Box 19, Folder 159, RFA.

171. Interview with retired nurse Judith Castor, April 12, 1991, Cuernavaca, Morelos.

172. "Report of the Hookworm Campaign, the Minatitlán-Puerto México Cooperative Sanitary Unit, and the Puerto México Antilarval Service for the Second Quarter, 1931," Communicable Diseases Section, DSP, México, D.F. Section II/021/242, Box 39, Folder 84, AHEM.

173. Vaughan, "Modernizing Patriarchy," 202.

174. "Report of the Hookworm Campaign, the Minatitlán-Puerto México Cooperative Sanitary Unit, and the Puerto México Antilarval Service for the Second Quarter, 1931," Communicable Diseases Section, DSP, México, D.F. Section II/021/242, Box 39, Folder 84, AHEM.

175. "Annual Report," 1935, Rural Hygiene Service, DSP, RG 5, Series 3, Box 145, RFA. For the history of school health in Mexico in the Porfiriato and revolutionary Mexico, see Ana María Carrillo, "El Inicio de la Higiene Escolar en México: Congreso Higiénico Pedagógico de 1882," *Revista Mexicana de Pediatría* 66, no. 2 (March–April 1999): 71–74; and Patience A. Schell, "Nationalizing Children through Schools and Hygiene: Porfirian and Revolutionary Mexico City," *The Americas* 60, no. 4 (April 2004): 558–87.

176. Miguel E. Bustamante, "Mortalidad de Menores de un Año por Entidades Federales, México, 1923–1941," *Revista del Instituto de Salubridad y Enfermedades Tropicales* 5, no. 2 (1944): 101–15.

177. "Report of the Hookworm Campaign, the Minatitlán-Puerto México Cooperative Sanitary Unit, and the Puerto México Antilarval Service for the Second Quarter, 1931," Communicable Diseases Section, DSP, México, D.F. Section II/021/242, Box 39, Folder 84, AHEM. Also interview with Judith Castor, April 12, 1991, Cuernavaca, Morelos.

178. "Report of the Hookworm Campaign, the Minatitlán-Puerto México Cooperative Sanitary Unit, and the Puerto México Antilarval Service for the Second Quarter, 1931," Communicable Diseases Section, DSP, México, D.F. Section II/021/242, Box 39, Folder 84, AHEM. Also interview with Judith Castor, April 12, 1991, Cuernavaca, Morelos.

179. Interview with Esther "La Güera" Coronel, April 15, 1991, Cuernavaca, Morelos. She recalled that, after much convincing, they succeeded in saving many children's lives.

180. See, for example, Susan Cotts Watkins, "Social Networks and Social Science History," *Social Science History* 19, no. 3 (Fall 1995): 295–311.

181. Examples of forms giving advice to pregnant women. Included with Bailey to DSP chief, January 23, 1934, RG 1.1, Series 323, Box 19, Folder 159, RFA.

182. This notion is inspired by the ideas of Mary Kay Vaughan in "Modernizing Patriarchy," 26 and 30.

183. Carr to Ferrell, October 14, 1929, RG 1.1, Series 323, Box 19, Folder 156, RFA.

184. Bailey to Ferrell, April 23, 1935, RG 1.1, Series 323, Box 19, Folder 160, RFA. For more on nursing education see chapter 4.

185. For example, Barbara Melosh, *"The Physician's Hand": Work, Culture and Conflict in American Nursing* (Philadelphia: Temple University Press, 1982); Susan Reverby, *Ordered to*

Care: The Dilemma of American Nursing, 1850–1945 (Cambridge: Cambridge University Press, 1987); and Karen Buhler-Wilkerson, "Bringing Care to the People: Lillian Wald's Legacy to Public Health Nursing," *American Journal of Public Health* 83 (1993): 1778–86.

186. Holland, *Medicina Maya*, argues that Tzotzil healers of Chiapas are often older men: 171.

187. "Annual Report," 1934, Rural Hygiene Service, DSP, RG 5, Series 3, Box 145, RFA.

188. Ibid.

189. In the United States, too, midwives were blamed for high maternal and infant mortality. See Frances E. Kobrin, "The American Midwife Controversy: A Crisis of Professionalization," *Bulletin of the History of Medicine* 40 (1966): 350–63.

190. "Report of the Hookworm Campaign, the Minatitlán-Puerto México Cooperative Sanitary Unit, and the Puerto México Antilarval Service for the Second Quarter, 1931," Communicable Diseases Section, DSP, México, D.F. Section II/021/242, Box 39, Folder 84, AHEM.

191. Although historical evidence of midwifery in the 1930s is incomplete, anthropological studies conducted from the 1920s through the 1970s offer a consistent portrayal of the practice. Among the first foreign anthropological studies of this kind was Robert Redfield's *Tepoztlán: A Mexican Village* (Chicago: University of Chicago Press, 1930). Oscar Lewis returned to the same Morelos village in the mid 1940s. His massive study, *Life in a Mexican Village*, includes a comprehensive chapter on pregnancy and birth. In the mid 1950s, the WHO commissioned Isabel Kelly to write "An Anthropological Approach to Midwifery Training in Mexico," *The Journal of Tropical Pediatrics* 1 (1956): 200–205. Nicolas León's *La Obstetricia en México* (México, D.F., 1910) provides a good introduction to pregnancy and childbirth practices in early twentieth-century Mexico. More recent practices are documented in Donato Ramos Pioquinto, ed., *Salud y Tradiciones Reproductivas en la Sierra Norte de Oaxaca: Un Estudio de Caso* (Oaxaca, México: Secretaría Académica, 1998), 102–42. Also see Judith Friedlander, "Doña Zeferina Barreto: Biographical Sketch of an Indian Woman from the State of Morelos," in *Women of the Mexican Countryside, 1850–1990*, ed. Heather Fowler-Salamini and Mary Kay Vaughan (Tucson: University of Arizona Press, 1994), 125–39.

192. José Alcina Franch, *Temazcalli: Higiene, Terapéutica, Obstetricia y Ritual en el Nuevo Mundo* (Sevilla, España: CSIC, 2000), has documented evidence of archaelogical and other physical evidence of the temazcal among numerous meso-American cultures, including Huastecas, Mixtecas, Zapotecas, Nahuas, Tzotziles, and many others. See 57–131. See also Enrique Eroza Solana and Miguel Ángel Marmolejo, *El Agua en la Cosmovisión y Terapéutica de los Pueblos Indígenas de México* (México, D.F.: INI, 1999).

193. See Prudencio Moscoso Pastrana, *La Medicina Tradicional de los Altos de Chiapas* (San Cristóbal de las Casas, México: Editorial Tradición, 1982), 194–95; Guadalupe Trueba, "Birth in Pre-Hispanic Mexico," *International Midwife* (Winter 1997): 45–47; Madsen, "*Study of Change*"; Munch Galindo, *Etnología*; Lipp, *Mixe of Oaxaca*, 117–23; Sheila Cosminsky, "Midwifery and Medical Anthropology," in *Modern Medicine and Medical Anthropology in the United States–Mexico Border Population*, ed. Boris Velimirovic (Washington, DC: Pan American Health Organization, Scientific Publication no. 359, 1978).

194. Interview with Judith Castor, April 12, 1991, Cuernavaca, Morelos.

195. Interview with Esther "La Güera" Coronel, April 15, 1991, Cuernavaca, Morelos.

196. Susan L. Smith, *Sick and Tired of Being Sick and Tired: Black Women's Health Activism in America, 1890–1950* (Philadelphia: University of Pennsylvania Press, 1995), 119. Also Margaret Charles Smith and Linda Janet Holmes, *Listen to Me Good: The Life Story of an Alabama Midwife* (Columbus: Ohio State University Press, 1996).

197. Hernández Sáenz, *Learning to Heal*.

198. Circa 1990 an estimated 40 percent of all births in Mexico were attended by one of 26,000 registered and unknown numbers of unregistered midwives. See Ulises Mercado, "The Traditional Midwife in Mexico," *Scalpel and Tongs* (January–February 1994): 11. For a profile of training, practices, and characteristics of traditional midwives

in the state of Morelos, see Xóchitl Castañeda Camey et al., "Una Alternativa para la Atención Perinatal: Las Parteras Tradicionales en el Estado de Morelos," *Ginecología y Obstetricia de México* 55 (December 1991): 353–57.

199. Isidro Espinosa y de los Reyes to Lic. Francisco Vásquez Pérez, July 4, 1931, "Sugestiones que Presenta el Suscrito a la Comisión del Comité Organizador del Congreso Nacional de la Ley Reglamentaria sobre el Ejercicio de la Profesión de Partera," RG Public Health, Infant Hygiene Section, Box 8, Folder 4, AHSSA.

200. José Refugio Bustamante, "Declaration for the Foundation of the School of Nursing and Obstetrics," January 30, 1937, Section II/021/241, Box 40, Folder 62, AHEM. According to Governor Bustamante, this ignorance stemmed from the "economic and cultural backwardness of the majority of the population, a situation incompatible with the country's growing economy and its cultural improvement, deriving from the revitalizing action of the Revolution."

201. See Ana María Carrillo, "Nacimiento y Muerte de una Profesión: Las Parteras Tituladas en México," *Dynamis* 19 (1999): 167–90. Carrillo argues that the movement to license midwives that began in 1833 was crushed by the growing power of specialist gynecologists. See also Claudia Agostoni, "Médicos y Parteras."

202. J. Arias Huerta, "El Papel de la Empírica como Promotora de Salud Materno-Infantil" (paper presented at the National Conference on Health, Mexico City, 1973), as quoted in Cosminsky, "Midwifery and Medical Anthropology." More recently, various scholars and health programs have called for greater sensitivity to traditional midwifery practices, leading to a more harmonious blend of popular midwifery and modern medicine. See, for example, Pilar Alicia Parra, "Midwives in the Mexican Health System," *Social Science and Medicine* 37, no. 11 (1993): 1321–29; and Ana María Carrillo, "Physicians 'Who Know' and Midwives who 'Need to Learn,'" in *Midwives in Mexico: Controversy and Change*, ed. Robbie Davys-Floyd, Marcia Good-Maust, and Miguel Guernez (Austin: University of Texas Press, forthcoming).

203. Kelly, "Anthropological Approach," 201–5.

204. See Lenore Manderson, *Sickness and the State: Health and Illness in Colonial Malaysia, 1870–1940* (Cambridge: Cambridge University Press, 1996), 206–29; and Margaret Jones, "Infant and Maternal Health Services in Ceylon, 1900–1948: Imperialism or Welfare?" *Social History of Medicine* 15, no. 2 (2002): 263–89.

205. Carr to Russell, August 19, 1928, RG 1.1, Series 323, Box 19, Folder 156, RFA.

206. Ibid.

207. Russell to Carr, August 31, 1928, RG 1.1, Series 323, Box 19, Folder 156, RFA.

208. Russell to Carr, September 18, 1928, RG 1.1, Series 323, Box 19, Folder 156, RFA.

209. Henryk Karol Kocyba, "La Medicina y la Religión entre los Mayas Prehispánicos," in *Historia de la Salud en México*, ed. Elsa Malvido and Maria Elena Morales (México, D.F.: Instituto Nacional de Antropología e Historia, 1996), 13–26. See also Elois Ann Berlin and Brent Berlin, *Medical Ethnobiology of the Highland Mayas of Chiapas, Mexico: The Gastrointestinal Diseases* (Princeton, NJ: Princeton University Press, 1996), especially 52–60.

210. See Finkler, *Spiritualist Healers*; Francisco Guerra, "Pre-Columbian Medicine: Its Influence on Medicine Today," in *Aspects of the History of Medicine in Latin America*, ed. John Z. Bowers and Elizabeth F. Purcell (New York: Josiah Macy Jr. Foundation, 1979), 1–15; Lozoya and Zolla, *La Medicina Invisible*; Carlos Zolla and Viginia Mellado, *La Medicina Tradicional de los Pueblos Indígenas de México* (México, D.F.: INI, 1994); Arthur J. Rubel et al., *Susto, A Folk Illness* (Berkeley, CA: University of California Press, 1984); Noemí Quezada, *Enfermedad y Maleficio: El Curandero en el México Colonial* (México, D.F.: UNAM, 1989); and James Clay Young, *Medical Choice in a Mexican Village* (New Brunswick, NJ: Rutgers University Press, 1981). Also see Libbet Crandon-Malamud, *From the Fat of Our Souls: Social Change, Political Process, and Medical Pluralism in Bolivia* (Berkeley, CA: University of California Press, 1991); and Foster, "On the Origin."

211. See Holland, *Medicina Maya*, chapter 9; Lipp, *Mixe of Oaxaca*, chapter 8; Munch Galindo, *Etnología*, 214–16; Gonzalo Aguirre Beltrán, a physician-anthropologist who directed the INI's first medical clinics in San Cristóbal, Chiapas, beginning in 1951 reflected on these issues some thirty years later in *Programas de Salud en la Situación Intercultural* (México, D.F.: IMSS, 1980). A study of tensions between "cosmopolitan" and local medicine is Steffan Igor Ayora-Díaz, "Globalization, Rationality and Medicine: Local Medicine's Struggle for Recognition in Highland Chiapas, Mexico," *Urban Anthropology* 27, no. 2 (1998): 165–95.

212. Bernard Ortiz de Montellano, "Empirical Aztec Medicine," *Science* 188, no. 4185 (1975): 215–20, argues that Aztec medicinal plants appear "effective if they are judged by Aztec standards." See also his *Aztec Medicine, Health and Nutrition*.

213. Interview with Esther "La Güera" Coronel, April 15, 1991, Cuernavaca, Morelos.

214. Ibid.

215. In the mid 1970s. Cristina Laurell calculated that almost 50 percent of the population practiced traditional medicine. See Cristina Laurell, "Medicina y Capitalismo en México," *Cuadernos Políticos* 5 (1975): 80–93.

216. Munch Galindo, *Etnología*, 212–13.

217. Dr. Jenaro Olea y Leyva, "Plan for the Regulation of Medical Practice in the State of Morelos," November 10, 1931, Box 39, Folder 65, AHEM.

218. Interviews with Joel Rogelio Sandoval, retired sanitary unit administrator, April 12, 1991, Cuernavaca, Morelos, and with Dr. Felipe García Sánchez, June 5, 1991, Mexico City.

219. Interview with Esther "La Güera" Coronel, April 15, 1991, Cuernavaca, Morelos. Coronel told me that one day, when she was a few months pregnant, she fell off her horse and had a miscarriage.

220. Interviews with Esther "La Güera" Coronel, April 15, 1991, Cuernavaca, Morelos, and with nurse and laboratory technician Lupita Serrano, April 12, 1991, Cuernavaca, Morelos.

221. Bailey to Ferrell, May 9, 1940, RG 1.1, Series 323, Box 20, Folder 165, RFA.

222. For more on Morelos fairs and rituals, see de la Peña, *Legacy of Promises*.

223. Bailey to Ferrell, May 9, 1940, RG 1.1, Series 323, Box 20, Folder 165, RFA.

224. Ferrell to Bailey, May 17, 1940, RG 1.1, Series 323, Box 20, Folder 165, RFA.

225. George Harrar diary, October 23 and 24, 1947, RG 12.1, Box 17, RFA.

226. Interview with Esther "La Güera" Coronel, April 15, 1991, Cuernavaca, Morelos.

227. Martha Grant, "Influencia de las Costumbres y Creencias Populares en los Servicios de un Centro de Salud," *Boletín de la Oficina Sanitaria Panamericana* 33, no. 4 (1952): 283–97. See also Kaja Finkler, *Physicians at Work, Patients in Pain: Biomedical Practice and Patient Response in Mexico* (Boulder, CO: Westview Press, 1991).

228. Some villagers, who refused to attend government clinics, had to be told that the health units *were* RF endeavors. Interview with Hermillo Espinoza Canales, April 15, 1991, Cuernavaca, Morelos.

229. To this day, medical graduates fulfilling their social service requirements in rural areas befriend *curanderos* in order to ensure a steady flow of patients. Interview with Dr. Héctor Gómez-Dantés, April 1991 and March 2000, Mexico City.

230. On labor, see, for example, Kevin J. Middlebrook, *The Paradox of Revolution: Labor, the State, and Authoritarianism in Mexico* (Baltimore: Johns Hopkins University Press, 1995); Javier Aguilar García, ed., *Historia de la CTM, 1936–1990: El Movimiento Obrero y el Estado Mexicano* (México, D.F.: Facultad de Ciencias Políticas y Sociales, Instituto de Investigaciones Sociales, Facultad de Economía, Universidad Nacional Autónoma de México, 1990). On rural agitation in Morelos, see Warman, *We Come to Object* Morales, *Morelos Agrario*; and de la Peña, *Legacy of Promises*. On Veracruz, see Fowler-Salamini, "Gender, Work, and Working-Class Women's Culture"; and Falcón and García Morales, *Semilla en el Surco*. More generally, see Blanca Rubio, *Resistencia Campesina y Explotación Rural en México* (México, D.F.: Ediciones Era, 1987); and Benjamin and Wasserman, *Provinces of the Revolution*.

231. Bailey to Ferrell, December 19, 1932, RG 1.1, Series 323, Box 17, File 141, RFA.

232. "Los Médicos Norteamericanos Recibidos en Salubridad," *El Universal*, March 28, 1933.

Chapter Four

1. With apologies to Leo Tolstoy.

2. See, for example, Gilbert M. Joseph and Daniel Nugent, eds., *Everyday Forms of State Formation: Revolution and the Negotiation of Rule in Modern Mexico* (Durham, NC: Duke University Press, 1994).

3. David Green, *The Containment of Latin America: A History of the Myths and Realities of the Good Neighbor Policy* (Chicago: Quadrangle, 1971); Ninkovich, *Diplomacy of Ideas*; Irwin F. Gellman, *Good Neighbor Diplomacy: United States Policies in Latin America, 1933-1945* (Baltimore: Johns Hopkins University Press, 1979); and Fredrick B. Pike, *FDR's Good Neighbor Policy: Sixty Years of Generally Gentle Chaos* (Austin, TX: University of Texas Press, 1992).

4. There is a vast bibliography on Cárdenas and the impact of his Presidency. Alan Knight's bibliographical essay, "The Rise and Fall of Cardenismo, c. 1930-c. 1946," in *Mexico since Independence*, ed. Leslie Bethell (Cambridge: Cambridge University Press, 1991), provides a comprehensive—though now dated—introductory survey. Hamilton's *Limits of State Autonomy* is still one of the best political syntheses of the era. Revised political biographies include the following: Adolfo Gilly, *El Cardenismo: Una Utopía Mexicana* (México, D.F.: Cal y Arena, 1994); Luis González y González, *Los Días del Presidente Cárdenas* (México, D.F.: Editorial Clío, 1997); and Enrique Krauze, *El Sexenio de Lázaro Cárdenas* (México, D.F.: Clío, 1999). More recently, a number of regional studies of Cardenismo have been published, such as Ben Fallaw, *Cárdenas Compromised: The Failure of Reform in Postrevolutionary Yucatán* (Durham, NC: Duke University Press, 2001); and Michael Snodgrass, *Deference and Defiance in Monterrey: Workers, Paternalism, and Revolution in Mexico, 1890-l950* (Cambridge: Cambridge University Press, 2003).

5. On educational developments, see Vaughan, *Cultural Politics in Revolution*, 30. On health developments, see Ana Maria Kapelusz-Poppi, "Rural Health and State Construction in Post-Revolutionary Mexico: The Nicolaita Project for Rural Medical Services," *The Americas* 58 (2001): 261-83. Eitan Ginzberg argues that Cárdenas's land redistribution effort in Michoacán was more centralized and corporatist than the simultaneous reforms under Governor Adalberto Tejeda's government in Veracruz, which sought to redistribute not just land but power to peasants. Eitan Ginzberg, "State Agrarianism versus Democratic Agrarianism: Adalberto Tejeda's Experiment in Veracruz, 1928-32," *Journal of Latin American Studies* 30 (1998): 341-72.

6. Julio Labastida, "De la Unidad Nacional al Desarrollo Estabilizador, 1940-1970," in *América Latina: Historia de Medio Siglo. Centroamérica, México y el Caribe*, vol. 2, ed. Pablo González Casanova (México, D.F.: Siglo XXI, 1981), 328-76; and Moisés González Navarro, *La Confederación Nacional Campesina* (México, D.F.: Costa-Amic, 1968).

7. See Medin, *Ideología y Praxis*; Arnaldo Córdova, *La Política de Masas del Cardenismo* (México D.F.: Serie Popular Era, 1974); and Eduardo Blanquel, "La Revolución Mexicana, 1921-1952," in *Historia Mínima de México*, ed. Daniel Cosío Villagas et al. (México, D.F.: Colegio de México, 1994), 147-56.

8. Comité Ejecutivo Nacional del Partido Nacional Revolucionario (PNR) *Plan Sexenal del PNR* (México, 1934), National Revolutionary Party, "Six-Year Plan, 1934-1940," English translation found with "Notes on Ferrell's Trip to Mexico, February 8-March 1, 1935," RG 2, Series 300, Box 559, Folder 3790, RFA.

9. "Plan Sexenal," Salubridad Pública, Partido Nacional Revolucionario, 1934, RG Lázaro Cárdenas, Folder 4255/18, Archivo General de la Nación, Mexico City, hereafter AGN.

10. The Six-Year Plan also advocated an improved judicial system, attention to crime, the development of adequate public welfare institutions, assistance to immigrants, and the reduction of gambling, prostitution, alcoholism, and obscenity. Work was to be used as a means to "reform delinquents."

11. Stated in a 1934 speech before the Querétaro Convention where the PNR's plan was developed. National Revolutionary Party, "Six-Year Plan, 1934–1940," English translation found with "Notes on Ferrell's Trip to Mexico, February 8–March 1, 1935," RG 2, Series 300, Box 559, Folder 3790, RFA.

12. Vaughan, *Cultural Politics in Revolution*. Also see José Vasconcelos, *La Raza Cósmica: The Cosmic Race: A Bilingual Edition*, trans. Didier T. Jaén (Baltimore: Johns Hopkins University Press, 1997).

13. "Plan Sexenal," Salubridad Pública, Partido Revolucionario Nacional, 1934, RG Lázaro Cárdenas, Folder 4255/18, AGN.

14. Hamilton, *Limits of State Autonomy*, 104–6.

15. Cole Blasier, *The Giant's Rival: The USSR and Latin America*, revised edition (Pittsburgh: University of Pittsburgh Press, 1987), 23; and Spenser, *Impossible Triangle*.

16. Report of interview of Charles A. Bailey by Wickliffe Rose, December 11, 1915, Boston, Biography File of Charles A. Bailey, RFA.

17. F. F. Russell to William Welch, April 11, 1924, Biography File of Charles A. Bailey, RFA.

18. Bailey to Ferrell, May 8, 1934, RG 2, Series 323, Box 100, Folder 789, RFA.

19. Bailey to Ferrell, August 4, 1934, RG 1.1, Series 323, Box 19, Folder 159, RFA.

20. Bailey to Ferrell, January 9, 1935, RG 1.1, Series 323, Box 19, Folder 160, RFA.

21. Bailey to Ferrell, May 8, 1934, RG 2, Series 323, Box 100, Folder 789, RFA.

22. Ibid.

23. Bailey to Ferrell, December 30, 1932, RG 1.1, Series 323, Box 19, Folder 157, RFA.

24. Bailey to Ferrell, May 8, 1934, RG 1.1, Series 323, Box 19, Folder 159, RFA.

25. Selskar Gunn to Max Mason, November 10, 1934, "Notes and Comments on a Visit to Mexico, September 2–November 15, 1934," RG 2, Series 323, Box 100, Folder 790, p. 3, RFA.

26. Joe C. Ashby, *Organized Labor and the Mexican Revolution under Lázaro Cárdenas* (Chapel Hill: University of North Carolina Press, 1963); Robert Alexander, *Labor Parties of Latin America* (New York: League for Industrial Democracy, 1942); Arturo Anguiano, *El Estado y la Política Obrera del Cardenismo*, Coleción Problemas de México (México, D.F.: Ediciones Era, 1975); Middlebrook, *Paradox of Revolution*; and Hamilton, *Limits of State Autonomy*, 108–41.

27. Debate on who and what Cárdenas was—socialist, opportunist, modernizer, reformist, Keynesian, or all of the above—continues to this day. He has been characterized variously as Mexico's true populist responding to the revolutionary demands of peasants and workers, as the popularly palatable representative of Mexico's new industrial and petit bourgeoisie, and as a people's man but one often mediated through powerful local, regional, and industrial caciques. See Alan Knight, "Cardenismo: Juggernaut or Jalopy?" *Journal of Latin American Studies* 26, no. 1 (1994): 73–107.

28. See Hamilton, *Limits of State Autonomy*, 142–83; and Josefina Zoraida Vázquez and Lorenzo Meyer, *The United States and Mexico* (Chicago: University of Chicago Press, 1985).

29. Ana María Carrillo, "Salud Pública y Poder durante el Cardenismo. México, 1934–1940," *Dynamis* 25 (2005): 145–78.

30. "Annual Report," 1935, Oficina Cooperativa de Especialización Sanitaria e Higiene Rural, Departamento de Salubridad Pública, RG 5, Series 3, Box 145, RFA.

31. Changes in the DSP budget reflected an overall increase in social spending under Cárdenas. Under the dictatorship of Porfirio Díaz, the government spent approximately

75 percent of its budget on administration; this dropped by 10 to 15 percent under President Obregón. Cárdenas held administrative costs to 40.5 percent of the budget, almost doubling expenditures on the economy to 37.4 percent, with 19.9 percent allotted to social expenditures (including health), a record that lasted until the 1960s. Solís Manjarrez, *Realidad Económica*.

32. Miguel Bustamante, "La Higiene en la República Mexicana," vol. 1, 1931–34, Servicio de Sanidad Federal en los Estados, DSP, RG Dr. Miguel E. Bustamante V, FCCBV. The National Commission for Food, Clothing, and Housing collaborated with the study. See Salvador González Herrejón, "Salubridad, Acción Médica y Economía," 1935, DSP, RG Cárdenas, Folder 425.5/18, AGN.

33. Siurob to Cárdenas, August 6, 1935, "Asuntos que se Someten a la Consideración del C. Presidente de la República," DSP, RG Public Health, Juridical Section, Box 44, Folder 7, AHSSA.

34. "Notes on Ferrell's Trip to Mexico, February 8–March 1, 1935," RG 2, Series 300, Box 559, Folder 3790, RFA.

35. Bailey to Ferrell, February 22, 1935, RG 2, Series 323, Box 119, Folder 907, RFA.

36. Manuel Carcamo Lardizábal, "El Departamento de Salubridad Pública como Institución Revolucionaria," July 10, 1935, RG Public Health, Juridical Section, Box 42, Folder 19, AHSSA.

37. Miguel E. Bustamante, "La Coordinación de los Servicios Sanitarios como Factor de Progreso Higiénico en México," in *La Atención Médica en el Medio Rural Mexicano, 1930–1980*, ed. Héctor Hernández Llamas (México, DF: Instituto Mexicano del Seguro Social, 1984), 35–90.

38. Bailey to Ferrell, May 8, 1934, RG 1.1, Series 323, Box 19, Folder 159, RFA.

39. Bailey to Ferrell, April 23, 1935, RG 1.1, Series 323, Box 19, Folder 160, RFA.

40. Warman, "*We Come to Object*"; Morales, *Morelos Agrario*; de la Peña, *Legacy of Promises*; Tobler, "Peasants and the Revolutionary State."

41. Bailey, "Public Health Cooperative Demonstration, State of Morelos and Supervised District," 1935, RG 1.1, Series 323, Box 20, Folder 161, RFA.

42. Ibid.

43. Bailey to Ferrell, May 13, 1935, RG 1.1, Series 323, Box 19, Folder 160, RFA.

44. Bailey, "Public Health Cooperative Demonstration, State of Morelos and Supervised District," 1935, RG 1.1, Series 323, Box 20, Folder 161, RFA.

45. Bailey to Ferrell, May 13, 1935, RG 1.1, Series 323, Box 19, Folder 160, RFA.

46. "Jefatura del Departamento de Salubridad Pública, Asuntos que se Someten a la Consideración del C. Presidente de la República," August 16, 1935, México, D.F. RG Public Health, Juridical Section, Box 42, Folder 17, AHSSA.

47. Bailey to Ferrell, May 13, 1935, RG 1.1, Series 323, Box 19, Folder 160, RFA.

48. Ibid.

49. Ferrell to Bailey, May 24, 1935, RG 1.1, Series 323, Box 19, Folder 160, RFA.

50. "Notes on Dr. Ferrell's Trip to Mexico, March 15–April 21, 1933," RG 2, Series 300, Box 553, Folder 3736, RFA.

51. Ferrell to Bailey, May 24, 1935, RG 1.1, Series 323, Box 19, Folder 160, RFA.

52. Bailey to Ferrell, June 7, 1935, RG 1.1, Series 323, Box 20, Folder 161, RFA.

53. Bailey to Ferrell, September 24, 1935, RG 1.1, Series 323, Box 20, Folder 161, RFA.

54. Antonio Pérez Alcocer to Abraham Ayala González, October 29, 1935, RG Public Health, Juridical Section, Box 42, Folder 7, AHSSA.

55. Ferrell to Bailey, October 29, 1935, RG 1.1, Series 323, Box 20, Folder 161, RFA.

56. Ibid.

57. Bailey to Ferrell, May 17, 1935 (including Ferrell's handwritten comments in the margin), RG 1.1, Series 323, Box 19, Folder 160, RFA.

58. Ferrell to Bailey, November 2, 1935, RG 1.1, Series 323, Box 20, Folder 161, RFA.

59. "Annual Report, 1935, Oficina Cooperativa de Especialización Sanitaria e Higiene Rural," DSP, RG 5, Series 3, Box 145, RFA.

60. Siurob to Cárdenas, December 20, 1935, "Asuntos que se Someten a la Consideración C. Presidente de la República," DSP, RG Public Health, A Presidential Section, Presidential Agreements Series, 1935, Book 2, AHSSA.

61. Siurob to Morelos Governor, June 13, 1936, RG Public Health, Presidential Section, Presidential Agreements Series, 1936, AHSSA.

62. Acuerdo Presidencial, June 12, 1936, RG Public Health, Presidential Section, Presidential Agreements Series, 1936, AHSSA.

63. Bailey to Ferrell, November 28, 1936, RG 1.1, Series 323, Box 20, Folder 162, RFA.

64. Bailey, "State of Morelos Project, Annual Report," 1936, Oficina de Especialización Sanitaria, RG 5, Series 3, Box 145, RFA.

65. Bailey to Ferrell, November 28, 1936, RG 1.1, Series 323, Box 20, Folder 162, RFA.

66. Bailey to Ferrell, "Summary of Preliminary Drafts of Budgets for Period January 1 to December 31, 1937," RG 1.1, Series 323, Box 20, Folder 162, RFA.

67. Bailey to Ferrell, November 28, 1936, RG 1.1, Series 323, Box 20, Folder 162, RFA.

68. "Asuntos que se Someten al Presidente," February 25, 1938, DSP, RG Public Health, Presidential Section, Presidential Agreements Series, AHSSA.

69. "Annual Report," 1937, Oficina de Especialización Sanitaria, RG 5, Series 3, Box 146, RFA.

70. "Public Health Administration, Program for 1937, U.S., Canada, Mexico," RG 5, Series 3, Box 19, Folder 154, RFA.

71. Ibid.

72. "Notes on Dr. Ferrell's Trip to Mexico March 15–April 21 1933," RG 2, Series 300, Box 553, Folder 3736; and Ferrell to Bailey, January 4, 1934, RG 1.1, Series 323, Box 100, Folder 789, RFA.

73. Excerpt from memorandum regarding Mexico and the IHD health program by Ferrell, February 12, 1935, RG 2, Series 300, Box 561, Folder 3814, RFA; and Ferrell to Josephus Daniels, November 6, 1936, RG 2, Series 300, Box 561, Folder 3814, RFA.

74. Siurob to U.S. Surgeon General Thomas Parran, June 9, 1937, RG 90, General Classified Records, Group VIII—Foreign Governments, 1936–44, Mexico, Box 474, File 0243, NARA.

75. Siurob, "Asuntos que se Someten a la Consideración del Presidente de la República," June 11, 1937, DSP, RG Public Health, Presidential Section, Presidential Agreements Series, 1937, AHSSA. For medical press coverage, see Salvador Iturbide Alvirez, "Panorama General de la Salubridad Pública en México," *Pasteur: Revista Mensual de Medicina*, 10, II, no. 4 (1937): 93–102.

76. For more details on maternal and child health programs, see Lauro Ortega, "Cómo Debe Entenderse en la Actualidad la Higiene Infantil," *Pasteur: Revista Mensual de Medicina* 10, II, no. 4 (1937): 129–33; and José Siurob, "La Sanidad en México" *Boletín de la Oficina Sanitaria Panamericana* 15, no. 12 (December 1936): 1148–53. The principles of maternal and child protection espoused by Siurob and his colleagues reflected such developments throughout the Americas in the 1930s. See Birn, "No More Surprising than a Broken Pitcher?" 17–46.

77. José Siurob, *Modern Tendencies of Public Health in the Republic of Mexico* (México, D.F.: DSP, 1936), 29. The cover depicts a muscular man with a serpent wrapped around him—an echo of the symbol of serpent and the shield—except that this man has gained control over the serpent, holding its head in his hands.

78. The average in 1934 was 1 nurse per 20,000 people. By 1937 it reached 1 nurse per 11,653 inhabitants.

79. Dr. General José Siurob, February 12, 1937, RG Public Health, Presidential Section, Presidential Agreements Series, 1937, AHSSA.

80. Ibid.

81. Celia A. de Reyes del Campillo, ¡*Hermana Campesina!* (México, D.F.: Departamento Autónomo de Prensa y Publicidad, 1938), especially 82–86.

82. Angel de la Garza Brito, "Progreso y Necesidades de la Higiene Rural," *Pasteur: Revista Mensual de Medicina* 10, II, no. 4 (1937): 146–56.

83. Alberto P. León, "Análisis Crítico de la Labor Desarrollada por la Oficina General de Epidemiología y Profilaxis de las Enfermedades Transmisibles de 1934 a 1938 en Relación con lo Estipulado por el Plan Sexenal," RG SSA/DSP, Box 20, Folder 34/034″938″/, AGN; José Siurob, "Resumen Sintético del Informe de Labores Realizadas por el Departamento de Salubridad Pública Cumpliendo los Mandatos del Plan Sexenal," May 18, 1937, DSP, RG Public Health, Presidential Section, Presidential Agreement, 1937, AHSSA.

84. José Siurob, "Resumen Sintético del Informe de Labores Realizadas por el Departamento de Salubridad Pública Cumpliendo los Mandatos del Plan Sexenal," May 18, 1937, DSP, RG Public Health, Presidential Section, Presidential Agreements, 1937, AHSSA.

85. Ignacio Belate to L. Cárdenas, August 26, 1938, RG Lázaro Cárdenas, File 425.5/127, AGN.

86. Presidente del Comisariado Ejidal en Imuris, Sonora, to Cárdenas, April 3, 1938, RG Lázaro Cárdenas, File 425.5/127, AGN.

87. Ronaldo Escamilla, Sindicato Chicleras El Zapote, to Lázaro Cárdenas, July 30, 1937, RG Lázaro Cárdenas, File 425.5/127, AGN.

88. Presidente del Comisariado Ejidal en Palizadas, Campeche, to Lázaro Cárdenas, June 26, 1938, RG Lázaro Cárdenas, File 425.5/127, AGN.

89. José Siurob, "Resumen Sintético del Informe de Labores Realizadas por el Departamento de Salubridad Pública Cumpliendo los Mandatos del Plan Sexenal," May 18, 1937, DSP, RG Public Health, Presidential Section, Presidential Agreements, 1937, AHSSA.

90. Ibid. Also see Pruneda, "Papel de México."

91. Office of Sanitary Specialization, "Annual Report 1937," RG 5, Series 3, Box 146, RFA.

92. U.S. Surgeon General Thomas Parran to Siurob, November 27, 1937, RG 90. General Classified Records, Group VIII—Foreign Governments, 1936–44 Mexico, Box 474, File 0243, NARA.

93. "Annual Report," 1937, Oficina de Especialización Sanitaria, RG 5, Series 3, Box 146, RFA.

94. José Siurob, "Resumen Sintético del Informe de Labores Realizadas por el Departamento de Salubridad Pública Cumpliendo los Mandatos del Plan Sexenal," May 18, 1937, DSP, RG Public Health, Presidential Section, Presidential Agreements, 1937, AHSSA. See also Siurob, "Sanidad en México."

95. Salvador Iturbide Alvírez to Secretario de Hacienda y Crédito Público, July 23, 1937, RG, DSP, Box 6, Folder 12/172.1/, AGN.

96. Primera Convención de Trabajadores de Salubridad, August 1–7, 1937, Mexico City, RG, DSP, Box 11, Folder 050(725.1)/2, AGN.

97. Wickliffe Rose memorandum, 1920, RG 1.2, Series 300, Box 2, File 14, RFA.

98. Wickliffe Rose "Scheme for the Promotion of Science on an International Scale," April 1923, Series 1, Box 5, Folder 100, RFA, as quoted in Robert E. Kohler, "Science and Philanthropy: Wickliffe Rose and the International Education Board," *Minerva* 23, no. 1 (Spring 1985): 76.

99. Kohler, "Science and Philanthropy," 75.

100. Miguel Bustamante's course of study was a notable exception to this policy even before the IHB was transformed into the IHD. International Health Division, *Fellowships to Mexico 1920–1944*; and *The Rockefeller Foundation Directory of Fellowship Awards, 1917–1950*, RG 1.2, Series 100, Box 32, Folder 239, RFA.

101. Vincent to Richard Pearce, August 27, 1918, RG 1.2, Series 100E, Box 29, Folder 217, RFA.

102. L. S. Rowe to Abraham Flexner, July 2, 1918, RG 1.2, Series 100E, Box 29, Folder 217, RFA.

103. J. A. Ryan to John D. Rockefeller Jr., November 6, 1922 and J. A. Ryan to George Vincent, December 1, 1922, RG 1.1, Series 323, Box 13, File 93, RFA.

104. International Health Division, *Fellowships to Mexico 1920–1944*; and *The Rockefeller Foundation Directory of Fellowship Awards, 1917–1950*, RG 1.2, Series 100, Box 32, Folder 239, RFA.

105. Table IIa, Public Health Fellowships and Nursing Fellowships for the Years 1917–1950, *The Rockefeller Foundation Directory of Fellowship Awards, 1917–1950*, RG 12, Series 100, Box 32, Folder 239, RFA.

106. Brazilian public health doctors comprised half of the first class at Johns Hopkins. See Fee, *Disease and Discovery*, 72–79.

107. Raymond Fosdick, ca. 1944, RG 1.2, Series 300, Box 1, Folder 7, RFA.

108. "Fellowships Policies and Programs" (Corrected January 29, 1929), RG 1.2, Series 100E, Box 29, Folder 218, RFA.

109. Lewis Hackett, "Notes for Volume 3," RG 3.1, Series 908, Box 4, Folder 20, RFA.

110. Bailey to Ferrell, April 23, 1935, RG 1.1, Series 323, Box 19, Folder 160, RFA.

111. Ferrell to Carr, January 31, 1930, RG 2, Series 323, Box 41, Folder 341, RFA.

112. According to Felipe García Sánchez, who worked at IHD health units for seven years before receiving a fellowship, the IHD preferred candidates with experience to avoid taking risks by accepting unknown individuals. Interview with Felipe García Sánchez, June 5, 1991, Mexico City.

113. Correspondence between Russell and Carr, February 1927, RG 5, Series 1.2, Box 296, File 3753, RFA.

114. Carr to Ferrell, February 12, 1930, RG 2, Series 323, Box 41, Folder 341, RFA.

115. H. Muench to Porter Crawford, January 29, 1942, RG 2, Series 300, Box 236, Folder 1632, RFA.

116. "Hopkins School of Hygiene Has Own League of Nations," Newspaper clipping found in February 1943, RG 2, Series 300, Box 252, Folder 1739, RFA.

117. Bustamante to William Howell, January 19, 1929, Alan Mason Chesney Medical Archives of the Johns Hopkins Medical Institutions, Baltimore, MD, RG JHU SHPH, Office of the Dean, Correspondence, Series 3A, Box 20, Folder Bru.

118. Bustamante to Reed, February 16, 1943, Alan Mason Chesney Medical Archives of the Johns Hopkins Medical Institutions, RG JHU SHPH, Office of the Dean, Correspondence, Series 3A, Box 20, Folder Buc-But.

119. Secretary-General to Bustamante, October 30, 1926, RG Dr. Miguel E. Bustamante V, Series Salud Pública/cursos, Box 2, Folder 3, FCCBV.

120. Carr to Russell, December 14, 1926, RG 5, Series 1.2, Box 257, File 3275, RFA.

121. H. Muench to Porter Crawford, January 29, 1942, RG 2, Series 300, Box 236, Folder 1632, RFA.

122. This request was made of Miguel Bustamante. De la Garza Brito to Bustamante, October 5, 1927, RG Dr. Miguel E. Bustamante V, Series Salud Pública/cursos, Box 2, Folder 3, FCCBV.

123. Interviews with Dr. Alberto P. León, April 10, 1991, and Dr. Felipe García Sánchez, June 5, 1991, Mexico City.

124. Ibid. Interview with Felipe García Sánchez, June 5, 1991, Mexico City. The theoretical perspective taught at Johns Hopkins and other schools powerfully shaped the views of students. My interview with García Sánchez took place at the height of the 1991 Peruvian cholera epidemic, which he viewed as easily amenable to technical intervention. For García Sánchez, there were no social causes of cholera, only biological factors. Likewise, he argued, with a few simple measures, in particular, isolating healthy carriers, the epidemic could be quickly combatted.

125. Interview with Luis Vargas, March 5, 1991, Mexico City.

126. Interview with Augusto Fujigaki Lechuga, May 31, 1991, Cuernavaca, Morelos. Dr. Fujigaki observed that the fellowships were the most important part of the RF's role in Mexico, because the returned fellows helped organize the national health system. He said that one could still see the influence of the RF through the training of second and third generations of physicians. Also see Armando Solórzano, "La Influencia de la Fundación Rockefeller en la Conformación de la Profesión Médica Mexicana, 1921–1949," *Revista Mexicana de Sociología* 58, no. 1 (1996): 173–203.

127. Juliana Martínez, "Policy Environments and Selective Emulation in the Making of Health Policies: Costa Rica, 1920–1997" (PhD diss., University of Pittsburgh, 1998).

128. Alberto P. León, "Análisis Crítico de la Labor Desarrollada por la Oficina General de Epidemiología y Profilaxis de las Enfermedades Transmisibles de 1934 a 1938 en Relación con lo Estipulado por el Plan Sexenal," RG, SSA/DSP, Box 20, Folder 34/034″938″/, AGN.

129. See Alberto P. León, "Cooperación de los Diversos Elementos Sociales en la Lucha contra las Enfermedades Transmisibles," *Pasteur: Revista Mensual de Medicina* 10, II, no. 4 (1937): 103–7.

130. Interview with Dr. Alberto P. León, April 10, 1991, Mexico City.

131. Torres Muñoz, "Cursos de Perfeccionamiento," 38–41.

132. DSP, Oficina Central de Higiene Rural y de Servicios Sanitarios en los Estados y Territorios. "Organización y Funcionamiento de los Servicios Sanitarios en los Estados y Territorios," Instructivo num. 10, México, D.F., February 1936, National Library of Medicine.

133. Angel de la Garza Brito, "El Presente y el Futuro de la Educación Higiénica Profesional en México," *Pasteur: Revista Mensual de Medicina* 14, I, no. 1 (1941): 14. His emphasis on U.S. models only increased over time. See Angel de la Garza Brito, "La Enseñanza de la Medicina Preventiva y de la Higiene, Factor en la Asistencia Médico Social," *Boletín de la Oficina Sanitaria Panamericana* 23, no. 7 (July 1944): 607–18. In the late 1930s, Mexican physicians began to shift their attention from France to the United States. See Gabriel Malda, "Visitando Rochester: La Clínica de los Hermanos Mayo," *Pasteur: Revista Mensual de Medicina* 10, I, no. 1 (1937): 12–20.

134. For example, see Miguel E. Bustamante, "Public Health and Medical Care in Mexico," *Annals of the American Academy of Political and Social Science* 208 (March 1940): 153–61; and works by Alberto León, Luis Vargas, and others in U.S. public health and tropical medicine journals.

135. Alberto P. León, "Análisis Crítico de la Labor Desarrollada por la Oficina General de Epidemiología y Profilaxis de las Enfermedades Transmisibles de 1934 a 1938 en Relación con lo Estipulado por el Plan Sexenal," RG, SSA/DSP, Box 20, Folder 34/034″938″/, AGN.

136. Charles Bailey, "List of IHD Fellowships to Mexico, Indicating Duration, School Attended, Assignments and Estimated Cost," 1935, RG 1.1, Series 323, Box 20, Folder 161, RFA.

137. "Cantidades Gastadas por la Fundación Rockefeller en su Cooperación con el Gobierno Mexicano de 1918 a 1938," RG Lázaro Cárdenas, Folder 534.1/1084, AGN.

138. Ferrell to Bailey, November 2, 1935, RG 1.1, Series 323, Box 20, Folder 161, RFA.

139. Bailey to Ferrell, Autumn, 1935, RG 1.1, Series 323, Box 20, Folder 161, RFA.

140. "Annual Report," 1937, Oficina de Especialización Sanitaria, RG 5, Series 3, Box 146, RFA.

141. George Payne to Ferrell, October 25, 1940, RG 1.1, Series 323, Box 20, Folder 165, RFA.

142. Ferrell to Payne, October 28, 1940, RG 1.1, Series 323, Box 20, Folder 165, RFA.

143. "Memorandum Concerning John A. Ferrell's Trip to Mexico April 21st–May 2nd, 1927," Diary Excerpt, May 19, 1927, RG 12.1, Box 19, RFA.

144. Charles V. Chapin, "Dirt, Disease, and the Health Officer," in *Papers of Charles V. Chapin, M.D.: A Review of Public Health Realities*, ed. Clarence L. Scamman (New York: The Commonwealth Fund, 1934), 21–22. See also Judith Walzer Leavitt, *Typhoid Mary. Captive*

to the Public's Health (Boston: Beacon Press, 1996), 23–26 and 262–63; and Cassedy, *Charles V. Chapin.*

145. Bailey to Ferrell, May 20, 1936, RG 2, Series 323, Box 134, Folder 1006, RFA.

146. "Los Resultados del Congreso Sanitario," *El Nacional,* May 18, 1936, RG 2, Series 323, Box 134, Folder 1006, RFA.

147. "Annual Report," 1936, Oficina Cooperativa de Especialización Sanitaria e Higiene Rural, Departamento de Salubridad Pública, RG 5, Series 3, Box 145, RFA.

148. Fellowship Recorder Cards, RG 10, IHB TG Mexico, RFA.; and "Travel and Training Grants International Health Division," RG 2, Series 300 E, Box 318, Folder 1522, RFA.

149. Carr to Ferrell, "Memorandum Regarding the Possibility of Establishing a Field Training Station in Mexico," August 23, 1931, RG 1.1, Series 323, Box 19, Folder 157, RFA.

150. Bailey, "Programa General de los Cursos en la Estación de Adiestramiento para Trabajadores de Salud Pública," November 1932, RG 1.1, Series 323, Box 19, Folder 157, RFA.

151. Bailey to Ferrell, September 21, 1932 and Ferrell to Bailey, December 1, 1932, RG 1.1, Series 323, Box 19, Folder 157, RFA.

152. Bailey to Ferrell, May 8, 1934, RG 1.1, Series 323, Box 19, Folder 159, RFA.

153. Ibid.

154. Bailey to Ferrell, January 3, 1935, RG 1.1, Series 323, Box 19, Folder 160, RFA.

155. Bailey, "Xochimilco Public Health Unit, Annual Report 1935," RG 5, Series 3, Box 145, RFA.

156. Ibid.

157. "Annual Report," 1939, Oficina de Especialización Sanitaria, RG 5, Series 3, Box 146, RFA.

158. In 1936, he left to head the DSP's new supervised sanitary district for the five states of Hidalgo, México, Michoacán, Morelos, and Tlaxcala accompanied by sanitary engineer Esteban Hoyo, also an IHD fellow. Hernández Lira to Bailey, June 1, 1936, "Annual Report," 1936, Oficina de Especialización Sanitaria, RG 5, Series 3, Box 145, RFA.

159. Miguel E. Bustamante, "Educación Sanitaria por Aplicación Práctica de los Conocimientos de Higiene," *Gaceta Médica de México* 68, no. 6 (1937): 652–53.

160. Ibid., 658–59.

161. Bailey to Ferrell, November 28, 1936, RG 1.1, Series 323, Box 20, Folder 162, RFA.

162. RF officers also complained about the revolution's influence on the medical schools' open admissions policy. "Proposed MEPH Program," April 17, 1956, RG 1.1, Series 323, Box 13, Folder 94, RFA.

163. McIntosh to Bailey, January 17, 1936, and Bailey to McIntosh January 25, 1936, RG 1.1, Series 323, Box 20, Folder 161, RFA.

164. Bailey to Ferrell, January 22, 1937, RG 1.1, Series 323, Box 20, Folder 163, RFA.

165. "Annual Report," 1936, Oficina Cooperativa de Especialización Sanitaria e Higiene Rural, Departamento de Salubridad Pública, RG 5, Series 3, Box 145, RFA.

166. Siurob, "Sanidad en México," 1145.

167. Bailey to Ferrell, April 23, 1935, RG 1.1, Series 323, Box 19, Folder 160, RFA. This attitude is contradicted by personal memoirs. See, for example, Mädy Fuerbringer Bermeo et al., "Lucrecia Lara Maldonado," in *Poblanas en la Salud Pública de México: Historias de Vida y Semblanzas* (Puebla, México: Honorable Ayuntamiento del Municipio de Puebla, 2001), 87–127.

168. "Mary Tennant's Diary from Trip to Mexico," February 11–March 11, 1936, p. 43, RG 2, Series 323, Box 135, Folder 1008, RFA.

169. Ibid., 42–43.

170. Ibid., p. 33.

171. I am grateful to Giulia El-Dardiry, who is studying the training of international nurses at the University of Toronto, for providing me with general background information. Also see Vessuri, "Enfermería de Salud Pública"; and Nunes Moreira, "Fundacão Rockefeller."

172. "Annual Report," 1939, Oficina de Especialización Sanitaria e Higiene Rural, DSP, RG 5, Series 3, Box 146, RFA; Hugh Smith as quoted in Andrew Warren's diary, April 23, 1945, RG 12.1, Officers' Diaries, Box 67, RFA.

173. Bailey to Ferrell, January 6, 1940, RG 1.1, Series 323, Box 20, Folder 165, RFA.

174. "Estimates, State Health Services, Tacuba Training Center and Demonstration Health Unit," 1948, 1949, RG 5, Series 3, Box 19, Folder 155, RFA.

175. Fee, *Disease and Discovery*, 184–204.

176. Bailey to Ferrell, September 4, 1939, RG 1.1, Series 323, Box 20, Folder 164, RFA.

177. "Additional Projects, Local Health Departments," 1943, RG 5, Series 3, Box 19, Folder 155, RFA.

178. Downs to Smith, June 28, 1948, RG 1.1, Series 323, Box 21, Folder 168, RFA.

179. Bailey to Ferrell, July 7, 1940, RG 2, Series 323, Box 199, Folder 1409, RFA.

180. Alfonso Pruneda, "Informe del Dr. D. Alfonso Pruneda, Secretario General del Departamento de Salubridad Pública de México en la Inauguración de la Escuela Anexa al Departamento de Salubridad," *Boletín de la Oficina Sanitaria Panamericana* 2 (1923): 305–9.

181. Instituto Nacional de Salud Pública, *Crónica de la Escuela de Salud Pública de México de 1922 a 2001. Relación de sus Protagonistas* (Cuernavaca, Morelos, México: Instituto Nacional de Salud Pública, 2002).

182. José Rodríguez Domínguez, "La Escuela de Salud Pública de México," *Salud Pública de México* 25, no. 5 (1983): 505–8.

183. Dr. Manuel Martínez Báez, "Memorandum, Escuela de Salubridad e Higiene," SSA, December 8, 1958, RG SSA, Section SubA (Subsecretariat of Assistance), Box 44, Folder 1, AHSSA.

184. "Escuela de Preparación y Adiestramiento," ca. 1935, DSP, RG DSP, Box 1, Folder/034/5, AGN.

185. Angel de la Garza Brito, "La Universidad en Relación con la Higiene Pública," *Pasteur: Revista Mensual de Medicina* 8, II, no. 1 (1935): 32–37.

186. Francisco Aguirre and Canuto Tavares to the Subsecretary of Health and Welfare, January 24, 1949, RG SSA, Section SubA, Box 44, Folder 1, AHSSA.

187. Dr. Manuel Martínez Báez, "Memorandum, Escuela de Salubridad e Higiene," SSA, December 8, 1958, RG SSA, Section SubA, Box 44, Folder 1, AHSSA; and de la Garza Brito, "Presente y el Futuro," 10–14.

188. Angel de la Garza Brito, "La Escuela de Salubridad e Higiene: Programas," *Salubridad y Asistencia* 7, no. 1 (1947): 117–21.

189. Fee, *Disease and Discovery*, 219–22.

190. Hugh Smith's diary, April 11, 1945, RG 12.1, Box 57, RFA.

191. "Excerpt from Confidential Trustees Bulletin," November 1943, RG 1.1, Series 323, Box 252, Folder 1739, RFA.

192. Lambert to Morones Prieto, August 25, 1947, RG SSA, Section Sub SyA (Subsecretariat of Health and Assistance) de SyA, Box 10, Folder 4, AHSSA.

193. "Proyecto de Reglamento de Becas de la Secretaría de Salubridad y Asistencia," RG SSA, Section SyA, Box 2, Folder 5, AHSSA.

194. See Alan Gregg, "Medical Education in Mexico," 1923, RG 1.1, Series 323, Box 13, Folder 95, RFA; Robert Lambert, "Medical Education in Mexico Survey," November 14–30, 1936, RG 1.1, Series 323, Box 13, Folder 95, RFA; and Robert Lambert, "Visit to Mexico," March 1–14, 1941, RG 1.1, Series 323, Box 13, Folder 95, RFA. For further analysis of these surveys, see Cueto, "Visions of Science and Development," 1–22.

195. J. J. Izquierdo to Gustavo Argil, December 8, 1943, Docket 425, Folder 2, Archivo Histórico de la Facultad de Medicina de la Universidad Nacional Autónoma de México.

196. Guy Hayes to John Bugher, April 7, 1956, RG 1.1, Series 323, Box 13, Folder 94, RFA.

197. See Smillie, "Salubridad"; and RF President J. G. Harrar, video, Dorothy Gordon Youth Program, 1963, RFA.

198. More recent scholarship suggests that the *ejidos* were not the anticapitalist alternatives portrayed by contemporaries but reflected Mexico's larger efforts in mixed economic development in the 1930s. See Dana Markiewicz, *The Mexican Revolution and the Limits of Agrarian Reform, 1915–1946* (Boulder, CO: Lynne Rienner Publishers, 1993), especially chapter 10, "The Ejido and the Legacy of Cardenismo," 113–18. Ginzberg, "State Agrarianism," agrees that the radical experiment of peasant-controlled *ejidos* under Adalberto Tejeda's watch in Veracruz was replaced with a corporativist, centralized model (which he believes ultimately doomed the viability of the *ejidos*).

199. See John Gledhill, *Casi Nada: A Study of Agrarian Reform in the Homeland of Cardenismo* (Albany: SUNY, 1991); and James Wilkie, *The Mexican Revolution: Federal Expenditure and Social Change since 1910* (Berkeley: University of California Press, 1967). Some foreign analysts also viewed the economic potential of ejidal development. See Eyler Simpson, *The Ejido: Mexico's Way Out* (Durham, NC: University of North Carolina Press, 1937).

200. Kapelusz-Poppi, "Physician Activists."

201. See Ana Maria Kapelusz-Poppi, "Morelia 1935: The First Conference for Rural Hygiene and the Program for State-Managed Medical Service" (paper presented at the XXIIth International Congress of the Latin American Studies Association, Miami, March 2000); and Pomposo Velásquez García, "Tesis para Obtener el Título de Médico Cirujano" (MD diss., Universidad Nacional de México, México, D.F. 1935). For a comprehensive perspective see Porter, *History of Public Health*; and Shula Marks, "South Africa's Early Experiment in Social Medicine: Its Pioneers and Politics," *American Journal of Public Health* 87, no. 3 (1997): 452–59.

202. González-Block, "Génesis."

203. Departamento de Salubridad Pública, *Rural Hygiene and Social Medicine Services of the Department of Public Health: Organization-Functions, Results Obtained until 1940* (México, D.F.: DSP, 1941), 7; Alvarez Amézquita et al., "Servicios Médicos."

204. José Siurob, *Social Medicine* (México, D.F.: Departamento de Salubridad Pública, 1940), 3.

205. "Primer Congreso de Higiene Rural Celebrado en Morelia, Michoacán," October 1935, RG SSA, Section Subsecretaría de Salubridad y Asistencia, Box 21, Folder 3, AHSSA.

206. Departamento de Salubridad Pública, *Rural Hygiene*, 6.

207. "Informe Concreto de Actividades Desarrolladas durante el Año Comprendido entre el 10 de Septiembre de 1935 y el 10 de Septiembre de 1936," RG DSP, Box 1, Folder/034/5, AGN.

208. Everardo Escárcega López and Escobar Toledo, *Historia de la Cuestión Agraria Mexicana*.

209. See Hansen, *The Politics of Mexican Development*.

210. Alvarez Amézquita et al., "Servicios Médicos," "Situación Sanitaria del Medio Ejidal," and "Servicios Cooperativos de Medicina Social e Higiene Rural," Programa de Labores, ca. 1946, Secretaría de Salubridad y Asistencia, RG Secretaría de Salubridad y Asistencia, Section Sub SyA, Box 23, Folder 6, AHSSA.

211. Siurob, *Social Medicine*; Departamento de Salubridad Pública, *Rural Hygiene* and Society of Friends, American Friends Service Committee, Students Peace Service, *Subjects Developed for the Coordinated Services of Rural Hygiene and Social Medical Services in the Laguna Region in the Conferences which are to Take Place from the 1st to the 6th of July 1939* México, D.F., Departamento de Salubridad Publica, 1940.

212. The IHD held from the beginning that public health should be a tax-funded service, but medical care was considered a separate matter. Many IHD staff became active in the strident 1930s debates over government's role in the organization and financing of medical care, when national health insurance was being considered as part of President

Franklin D. Roosevelt's Social Security Act of 1935. Eventually, the RF publicly supported national health insurance in the United States.

213. "Annual Report," 1936, Oficina Cooperativa de Especialización Sanitaria e Higiene Rural, DSP, RG 5, Series 3, Box 145, RFA.

214. Selskar Gunn to Max Mason, 10 November 1934, "Notes and Comments on a Visit to Mexico, September 2–November 15, 1934," RG 2, Series 323, Box 100, Folder 790, RFA.

215. Also see Vaughan, *State, Education, and Social Class*; and Vaughan, *Cultural Politics in Revolution*.

216. "Modelo de Carta (para Maestro Rural) de la Campaña de Saneamiento," Departamento de Salubridad Pública, ca, 1935, RG Secretaría de Salubridad y Asistencia, Section Sub SyA, Box 28, Folder 9, AHSSA; Alfonso Pruneda, "La Secretaría de Educación Pública de México y la Difusión de la Higiene," *Pasteur: Revista Mensual de Medicina* 2, I, no. 42 (1929): 52–54.

217. "Annual Report,"1936, Oficina Cooperativa de Especialización Sanitaria e Higiene Rural, Departamento de Salubridad Pública, RG 5, Series 3, Box 145, RFA.

218. See Siurob, *Social Medicine*; and *Rural Hygiene*. As is evidenced in the bibliography, the DSP published other articles and reports in English, but the pamphlets on the ejidal units were the only translated materials I found that examined a particular program rather than DSP activities as a whole.

219. See Kapelusz-Poppi, "Morelia 1935." Soviet developments in the 1920s may also have influenced ideas about rural service. In 1929, a National University of Mexico professor, Antonio Castro Leal, wrote a letter to Soviet Komissar of Education Lunacharskii, asking him for detailed information on so-called "Rabfak" (*rabochij fakul'tet* workers' schools, which prepared workers without any education for entering university), saying that he wanted to replicate them in Mexico. Lunacharskii sent him the information. RG 142 (Lunacharskii's collection), Series 1, Folder 779, 48–50. Rossiiskii Gosudarstvenny Arkhiv Sotsial' no-Politicheskoi Istorii (RGASPI), Russian State Archive of Socio-Political History, Moscow. I am grateful to Nikolai Krementsov for alerting me to this correspondence.

220. Jefe de la Oficina de Distribución de Médicos to municipalities, September 4, 1936, RG DSP, Box 12, Folder 173./1/, AGN.

221. See González y González, *Días del Presidente Cárdenas*, 237–39.

222. Bailey to Ferrell, January 11, 1936, RG 1.1, Series 323, Box 20, Folder 162, RFA.

223. Pilar Hernández Lira, "Necessity for Trained Personnel in Public Health Activity and Minimum Training Qualifications," Study Presented to the First National Congress of Rural Hygiene, Morelia, Michoacán, October 30, 1935, RG 2, Series 323, Box 119, Folder 907, RFA.

224. Gustavo Baz, speech given in September 1936, quoted in Fernando Benítez, *Lázaro Cárdenas y la Revolución Mexicana, III, El Cardenismo* (México, D.F.: Fondo de Cultura Económica, 1978), 114.

225. José Siurob, "Resumen Sintético del Informe de Labores Realizadas por el Departamento de Salubridad Pública Cumpliendo los Mandatos del Plan Sexenal," May 18, 1937, DSP, RG Public Health, Presidential Section, Presidential Agreements, 1937, AHSSA.

226. See, for example, Luis M. Arbona Medina, *Informe Médico-Social del Ejido Primero de Mayo, Campo 77, Valle del Yaqui, Sonora. Padecimientos Más Frecuentes en Sonora* (México, D.F.: UNAM, 1956); and Miguel E. Bustamante, "Papel del Médico Rural en la Investigación de las Enfermedades Tropicales en México," *Boletín de la Oficina Sanitaria Panamericana* 16, no. 2 (February 1937): 112–15.

227. Alfonso Pruneda, "El Servicio Médico-Social de la Universidad Nacional," *Gaceta Médica de México* 70, no. 2 (1940): 143–51.

228. George K. Strode's diary, 11 January 1947, RG 12.1, Box 61, RFA.

229. See Smith, *United States and Revolutionary Nationalism in Mexico*.

230. Bernardo Gastélum to F. F. Russell, May 20, 1925, RG 5, Series 3, Box 148, RFA.

231. The role of the oil companies in the RF's yellow fever campaign is discussed in Solórzano Ramos, *¿Fiebre Dorada o Fiebre Amarilla?*

232. Success was noted in 1925: "Apuntes para Mensaje Presidencial," September 1, 1925, Asuntos Técnicos de la Sección de Enfermedades Tropicales, RG Public Health, Section Presidential Secretariat, Box 9, Folder 15, AHSSA; but in 1930 conditions were once again appalling. See Ulises Valdés to Secretary-General of Health, October 6, 1930, RG, Public Health, Juridical Section, Box 22, Folder 16, AHSSA.

233. Daniel Yergin, *The Prize: The Epic Quest for Oil, Money, and Power* (New York: Touchstone, 1991), 272.

234. Dictamen 21, Servicio Jurídico, August 16, 1935, RG Public Health, Juridical Section, Box 42, Folder 16, AHSSA; "Convenio que Celebra el Departamento de Salubridad Pública por Conducto de la Jefatura de los Servicios Sanitarios Coordinados en el Estado de Nuevo León para los Efectos del Artículo 193 del Código Sanitario," Telésforo Chapa, signatory, August 31, 1935, RG Public Health, Juridical Section, Box 42, Folder 16, AHSSA.

235. "Informe de la Oficina Central del Servicio de Puertos y Fronteras," April 28, 1937, Section DSP, Box 11, Folder/033(13)/4, AGN.

236. Interview with Dr. Felipe García Sánchez, June 5, 1991, Mexico City.

237. "Annual Report," 1935, Oficina Cooperativa de Especialización Sanitaria e Higiene Rural, Departamento de Salubridad Pública, RG 5, Series 3, Box 145, RFA. At one point El Aguila withheld the salaries of Antilarval Service employees, accusing them of sympathizing with protesting oil workers. Dictamen 21, Servicio Jurídico, August 16, 1935, RG Public Health, Juridical Section, Box 42, Folder 16, AHSSA.

238. José Siurob and Companía Mexicana de Petróleo El Aguila, Agreement for the Coordination of Sanitary Services, May 1, 1936, RG Public Health, Juridical Section, Box 46, Folder 11, AHSSA.

239. Dr. A. de la Garza Brito to Oficina Jurídico-Consultiva, February 11, 1937, RG Public Health, Presidential Section, Presidential Agreements Series, 1937, AHSSA.

240. The oil industry's responsibility for larval control and other sanitary measures continued following the nationalization; by the 1950s, the national oil company PEMEX provided subsidies of over one million pesos a year (well over half a million 2004 dollars) for malaria control, local health units, and a tuberculosis treatment program. Bermúdez J. A., "Convenio entre la SSA y PEMEX," July 1956, México D.F., in RG SSA, National Malaria Campaign Section, Series 2, Box 2, Folder 1, 1956, AHSSA.

241. Lázaro Cárdenas, "Anunciación al Pueblo de la Expropriación de Petróleo," March 18, 1938, Palacio Nacional, reprinted in *Cuadernos Americanos* 30, no. 1 (1971): 105–8; Vázquez and Meyer, *United States and Mexico*; Salvador Mendoza, *La Doctrina Cárdenas* (México, D.F.: Ediciones Botas, 1939); Brown, *Oil and Revolution*; Frank Tannenbaum, *Mexico: The Struggle for Peace and Bread* (New York: Alfred A. Knopf, 1950); and Henry Justin Allen, *The Mexican Confiscations, Together with a Careful Survey of the Present Revolutionary Trends in Mexico* (New York, 1938).

242. Centro de Higiene Rural de Calmillo, Aguascalientes to Cárdenas, March 28, 1938, RG DSP, Box 5, File 12/130/25, AGN.

243. Telegram from Dr. Felipe Malo Juvera and fourteen others to Lázaro Cárdenas, March 21, 1938, RG DSP, Box 5, Folder 12/130/25, AGN.

244. Ferminte Díaz to Oficial Mayor, March 25, 1938, RG DSP, Box 5, Folder 12/130/25, AGN.

245. See González y González, *Los Días del Presidente Cárdenas.*

246. Dr. Alfonso Alarcón, Secretary-General, to DSP Personnel, April 12, 1938, RG Departamento de Salud Pública, Box 5, Folder 12/130/25, AGN.

247. Hamilton, *Limits of State Autonomy*, 240.

248. Ibid., chapters 7 and 8, especially 240–44.

249. Bailey to Ferrell, March 29, 1938, RG 1.1, Series 323, Box 20, Folder 164, RFA. When a meningitis epidemic struck Morelos, Cárdenas issued Bailey a special exception to

the spending freeze to control the outbreak. Ramón Acevedo to Charles Bailey, August 15, 1940, RG Public Health, Juridical Section, Box 54, Folder 4, AHSSA.

250. Bailey to Ferrell, December 4, 1938, RG 1.1, Series 323, Box 20, Folder 164, RFA.

251. Walter Earle to M. Watson, April 5, 1938, Correspondence between the RF and the DSP found in the library of the Department of Health and Preventive Medicine, Mexico City.

252. Ferrell to Bailey, April 1, 1938, RG 1.1, Series 323, Box 20, Folder 164, RFA.

253. Memorandum of John A. Ferrell's Conference: Vice President Henry Wallace, Raymond B. Fosdick, and John A. Ferrell, Regarding Mexico—Its Problems and Remedies," February 3, 1941, Senate Office Building, Washington, DC, RG 1.1, Series 323, Box 1, Folder 2, RFA; and interview with Esther "La Güera" Coronel, April 15, 1991, Cuernavaca, Morelos.

254. See, for example, Standard Oil of New Jersey, *Whose Oil Is It? The Question of Subsoil Rights in Mexico,* pamphlet issued in 1938 at 30 Rockefeller Plaza, New York, Cárdenas Microfilm, Role 9, Number 1, AGN.

255. Friedrich E. Schuler, *Mexico between Hitler and Roosevelt: Mexican Foreign Relations in the Age of Lázaro Cárdenas, 1934–1940* (Albuquerque: University of New Mexico Press, 1998).

256. Interview with Dr. Manuel Servín Massieu, Director, Institute of Hygiene, March 4, 1991.

257. Rodríguez de Romo, "Factores Determinantes," 93–101.

258. Wilson, *Ambassadors in White,* 41.

259. Cárdenas, "Agreement Concerning the DSP," July 5, 1935, RG Public Health, Juridical Section, Box 42, Folder 11, AHSSA.

260. Gellman, *Good Neighbor Diplomacy;* and Pike, *FDR's Good Neighbor Policy.*

261. Lorenzo Meyer, *México y Estados Unidos en el Conflicto Petrolero, 1917–1942* (México, D.F.: El Colegio de México, 1968); Yergin, *Prize;* Clayton R. Koppes, "The Good Neighbor Policy and the Nationalization of Mexican Oil: A Reinterpretation," *Journal of American History* 69 (1982): 62–81, argues that the 1942 agreement was only a "tactical interruption" in a State Department policy supportive of U.S. oil interests in Mexico that continued until 1950.

262. "Annual Report, 1935, Oficina Cooperativa de Especialización Sanitaria e Higiene Rural, DSP, RG 5, Series 3, Box 145, RFA.

263. Bailey to Ferrell, December 27, 1938, RG 1.1, Series 323, Box 20, Folder 164, RFA.

264. Ferrell to Bailey, February 2, 1939, RG 1.1, Series 323, Box 20, Folder 164, RFA.

265. Ferrell to Bailey, November 9, 1939, RG 1.1, Series 323, Box 20, Folder 164, RFA.

266. Bailey to Ferrell, April 26, 1940, RG 1.1, Series 323, Box 20, Folder 165, RFA.

267. "Memorandum para el Señor Presidente de la República," ca. 1938, RG Lázaro Cárdenas, Folder 534/1089, AGN; "Asuntos que se Someten al Presidente de la República," February 25, 1939, RG Public Health, Presidential Section, Presidential Agreements, 1939, AHSSA.

268. Gerard Colby with Charlotte Dennett, *Thy Will Be Done: The Conquest of the Amazon: Nelson Rockefeller and Evangelism in the Age of Oil* (New York: Harper Collins Publishers, 1995), 93–94.

269. Bailey to Ferrell, April 26, 1940, RG 1.1, Series 323, Box 20, Folder 165, RFA.

270. Bailey to Ferrell, October 23, 1939, RG 1.1, Series 323, Box 20, Folder 164, RFA.

271. Ferrell to Sawyer, July 18, 1940, RG 2, Series 323, Box 199, Folder 1409, RFA.

272. "Annual Report," 1938, Oficina de Especialización Sanitaria, RG 5, Series 3, Box 146, RFA.

273. "Annual Report," 1939, Oficina de Especialización Sanitaria, RG 5, Series 3, Box 146, RFA.

274. "Annual Report," Servicio de Higiene Rural, 1938, RG 5, Series 3, Box 145, RFA.

275. Bailey to Ferrell, April 26, 1940, RG 1.1, Series 323, Box 20, Folder 165, RFA.

276. "Mexico-Regional State and County Health Units, Extension of Designation," 1941, 1942, RG 5, Series 3, Box 19, Folder 154, RFA.

277. G. K. Strode's diary, January 11, 1947, RG 12.1, Box 61, RFA. Many Mexicans agreed with this assessment. Nurse Judith Castor believed that the Morelos service was "the best in the country" and served as a model for other states. Interview with Judith Castor, April 12, 1991, Cuernavaca, Morelos.

278. G. K. Strode's diary, January 11, 1947, RG 12.1, Box 61, RFA.

279. "Mexico—Annual Report," 1947, IHD, RG 5, Series 3, Box 146, RFA.

280. "Mexico-Regional Health District #3, Designation and Budget," December 18, 1942, RG 5, Series 3, Box 19, Folder 155, RFA.

281. Martínez Báez, "Instituto de Salubridad"; and Bustamante, "Papel del Médico Rural." Also see Ana Cecilia Rodríguez de Romo, "Manuel Martínez Báez, Congruencia Afortunada de Inteligencia e Integridad," *Revista de la Universidad Michoacana* 13 (1994): 115–25.

282. Martínez Báez, "Instituto de Salubridad."

283. See Rodríguez de Romo and Rodríguez Pérez, "Historia de la Salud Pública".

284. See Rodríguez de Romo, "Factores Determinantes"; Ana Cecilia Rodríguez de Romo, "Manuel Martínez Báez: Una Visión Muy Personal de Salud y Humanismo," in *La Cultura Científico-Tecnológica Nacional: Perspectivas Multidisciplinarias*, ed. Maria Luisa Rodríguez Sala, María Eugenia Cué, and Ignacio Gómezgil (México, D.F.: Instituto de Investigaciones Sociales, UNAM, 1992), 77–87; and Raúl Arreola Cortés, *Manuel Martínez Báez, Científico y Humanista* (Morelia, México: Universidad Michoacana de San Nicolás de Hidalgo, 1994).

285. "Annual Report," 1935, Oficina Cooperativa de Especialización Sanitaria e Higiene Rural, Departamento de Salubridad Pública, RG 5, Series 3, Box 145, RFA.

286. Bailey to Ferrell, July 23, 1935, RG 1.1, Series 323, Box 120, Folder 908, RFA.

287. "Annual Report," 1939, Oficina de Especialización Sanitaria, RG 5, Series 3, Box 146, RFA. Sawyer believed that U.S. scientists would not be willing to spend one year in Mexico and recommended that the institute wait until Mexicans had been trained overseas. Sawyer to Ferrell, January 27, 1939, RG 1.1, Series 323, Box 178, Folder 1289, RFA.

288. "Annual Report," 1939, Oficina de Especialización Sanitaria, RG 5, Series 3, Box 146, RFA.

289. Dimitra Giannuli, " 'Repeated Disappointment': The Rockefeller Foundation and the Reform of the Greek Public Health System, 1929–1940," *Bulletin of the History of Medicine* 72 (1998): 47–72.

290. Robert Lambert, "Visit to Mexico," March 1–14, 1941, RG 1.1, Series 323, Box 13, Folder 95, RFA.

291. Lambert to Fosdick, March 31, 1942, RG 1.1, Series 300, Box 1, Folder 2, RFA. G. K. Strode also believed that public health education "may have been our most significant contribution to Public Health," G. K. Strode, Memo for Scientific Directors' Meeting, October 26, 1944, as quoted by Lewis Hackett, Notes for Volume 3, RG 3.1, Series 908, Box 4, Folder 20, RFA. Even after other organizations began offering fellowships, Frederick Russell held that "Our fellowships are still more sought after than any others in Latin America. Our representatives protect them from political attack," as quoted by Lewis Hackett, Notes for Volume 3, RG 3.1, Series 908, Box 3, Folder 19, RFA.

292. The problem of duplication due to RF programs had been raised by Angel Brioso Vasconcelos as early as 1921. See chapter 1 and discussion in "Acta de la Sesión Celebrada por la Comisión Especial."

Chapter Five

1. See, for example, Patrick Marnham, *Dreaming with His Eyes Open: A Life of Diego Rivera* (New York: Alfred A. Knopf, 1998), 248–60. Other biographies include David Craven, *Diego Rivera: As Epic Modernist* (Boston: G. K. Hall, 1997); and Pete Hamill, *Diego Rivera* (New York: Harry N Abrams, 1999). Also see RG 2, Office of the Messrs Rockefeller, Business Interest Series, Box 94, Folder 706, and Box 93, Folder 704, Rockefeller Family Archives.

2. For Rivera's account, see Diego Rivera, *My Art, My Life: An Autobiography* (New York: Citadel Press, 1960).

3. "Mexico to Honor Rockefeller," *New York Times*, June 26, 1937, 15.

4. "Homenaje a Rockefeller," *El Universal*, September 19, 1937, 1.

5. Alfonso Pruneda, *La Fundación Rockefeller y su Obra en México* (Mexico, D.F.: Imprenta Mundial, 1937), OMR, RG 2, Series Senior Death Resolutions from Organizations #2 1937–38, Box 43, Folder 336, Rockefeller Family Archives.

6. "Mexico Honors Rockefeller," *St. Louis Post Dispatch*, September 19, 1937. Found in OMR, RG 2, Series Senior Death Resolutions from Organizations #2 1937–38, Box 43, Folder 336, Rockefeller Family Archives.

7. "Extract of the Address by Ambassador Daniels at the Unveiling of the Tablet to John D. Rockefeller at the Federal Health Department," September 18, 1937, OMR, RG 2, Series Senior Death Resolutions from Organizations #2 1937-8, Box 43, Folder 336, Rockefeller Family Archives.

8. "Homenaje a Rockefeller," 1.

9. Chernow, *Titan.*

10. González y González, *Días del Presidente Cárdenas*; Pere Foix, *Cárdenas* (México, D.F.: Editorial Trillas, 1971); and Enrique Krauze, *Lázaro Cárdenas: General Misionero* (México, D.F.: Fondo de Cultura Económica, 1987).

11. Examples of this view can be seen in Brown, "Public Health in Imperialism"; Quevedo et al., *Café y Gusanos*; and Solórzano Ramos, *¿Fiebre Dorada o Fiebre Amarilla?*

12. On this term see Walter Lippman, *Public Opinion* (New York: Macmillan, 1922); and Edward Herman and Noam Chomsky, *Manufacturing Consent: The Political Economy of the Mass Media* (New York: Pantheon, 1988).

13. See Williams, *Plague Killers*; and Hackett, "Once upon a Time," 105–15.

14. Fosdick, *Story of the Rockefeller Foundation.*

15. See, for example, Farley, *To Cast Out Disease.*

16. For comparative perspective on this point, see de Castro Santos, "Fundacão Rockefeller"; and Palmer, "Central American Encounters."

17. See Pyenson, "In Partibus Infidelium," 253–303.

18. Russell to Carr, May 19, 1927, RG 5, Series 1.2, Box 296, Folder 3753, RFA.

19. See Wilbur Sawyer's European diaries for these years. For example, Box 4 Diary Folder January 1–February 1, 1941, Wilbur Sawyer Manuscript Collection, History of Medicine Division, National Library of Medicine.

20. J. G. Harrar, "Mexican Agricultural Program: A Review of the First Six Years of Activities under the Joint Auspices of the Mexican Government and the Rockefeller Foundation," New York, 1950, RG 1.1, Series 323, Box 5, Folder 36, RFA.

21. By 1950, Weaver began complaining that "Mexico is not paying as much of the bill for this project as they ought," although he conceded that "all of the money involved is spent under the complete control of North Americans." He added, "they acquiesced, doubtless in part because of the prestige of the Rockefeller Foundation, and in part because it was, after all, a very good proposition which involved extremely little risk on their part. We were certainly in no position to expect, at that time, any different attitude on the part of the Mexicans. For one thing, we must remember that this was very frankly an experiment in our own minds, and that we were by no means certain that we were going to be able to accomplish anything important." Weaver to Chester Barnard, September 21, 1950, RG 1.1, Series 323, Box 3, Folder 21, RFA.

22. Weaver to Barnard, September 21, 1950, RG 1.1, Series 323, Box 3, Folder 21, RFA.

23. See Joseph Cotter, "The Rockefeller Foundation's Mexican Agricultural Project: A Cross-Cultural Encounter: 1943–1949," in *Missionaries of Science: The Rockefeller Foundation and Latin America*, ed. Marcos Cueto (Bloomington: Indiana University Press, 1994).

24. For further discussion of the Mexican Agricultural Program and its limitations, see Deborah Fitzgerald, "Exporting American Agriculture: The Rockefeller Foundation in Mexico, 1943–1953," *Social Studies of Science* 16 (1986): 457–83.

25. See "Memorandum of JAF of Conference: Vice President Wallace, Raymond B. Fosdick, and John A. Ferrell, regarding Mexico—Its Problems and Remedies," February 3, 1941, Senate Office Building, Washington, DC, RG 1.1, Series 323, Box 1, Folder 2, RFA.

26. "IHD Nutrition Program in Mexico," September 10, 1948, RG 1.1, Series 323, Box 12, Folder 83, RFA.

27. In its first year it was called the Office for Coordination of Commercial and Cultural Relations.

28. André Luiz Vieira de Campos, "The Institute of Inter-American Affairs and its Health Policies in Brazil during World War II," *Presidential Studies Quarterly*, 28, no. 3 (1998): 523–34, 524.

29. Programa Interamericano de Salud Pública, 1946, RG SSA, Section Sub SyA, Box 11, Folder 4, AHSSA; George G. Dunham, "The Cooperative Health Program of the American Republics," *American Journal of Public Health* 34, no. 8 (1944): 818–19; and Alfonso Pruneda, "La Salubridad y la Guerra," *Pasteur: Revista Mensual de Medicina* 18, I, no. 4 (1945): 69–74.

30. Sydnor Walker, interview with Laurence Duggan, Division of Latin American Affairs, Department of State, October 23, 1936, Washington, D.C., RG 2, Series 300, Box 133, Folder 997, RFA. Also see "Colegio de México Center for Historical Studies." RG 1.1, Series 323, Box 22, File 178, RFA.

31. Another war-related bilateral development that transpired in 1943 was the founding of the United States–Mexico Border Public Health Association, initially to maintain the health of the large concentration of troops on both sides of the border. See Humberto Romero Alvarez, *Health without Boundaries* (México, D.F.: United States–Mexico Border Public Health Association, 1975), 69–71.

32. The initial program expired on December 31, 1948 but was renewed under the auspices of the Truman Doctrine. See Dr. Gustavo Argil to Miguel Alemán, June 27, 1949, RG Miguel Alemán, Folder 577/8, AGN; and "Memorandum sobre Cooperación Económica Interamericana," June 30, 1947, Washington, DC, RG Miguel Alemán, Folder 565.4/190, AGN; Manuel Martínez Báez and Harold Hinman, "Allocation of Funds of Dirección de Cooperación Interamericana de Salubridad Pública," December 11, 1943, RG SSA, Section Sub SyA, Box 2, Folder 2, AHSSA; Alonzo Hardison to Ignacio Morones Prieto, April 12, 1948, RG SSA, Section Sub SyA, Box 11, Folder 4, AHSSA; and Honorary Brooks Hays, Representative of Arkansas, "The Republic of Mexico is Solving Economic and Social Problems," *Congressional Record—Appendix*, January 15, 1951, pp. A331–A332, RG 1.1, Series 323, Box 3, Folder 21, RFA.

33. See Victor Fernández Manero and Harold Hinman, Proyecto Mex-W2—Abastecimiento de Agua de Huajuapan, September 27, 1943, RG SSA, Section Sub SyA, Box 2, Folder 4, AHSSA; "Summary of Project Accomplishment," Project HC-1, Boca del Río, Veracruz, Health Center and Tropical Medicine Training Station, December 7, 1950, RG SSA, Section Sub SyA, Box 28, Folder 5, AHSSA; "Mexico Report on Cooperative Health Program of the Governments of Mexico and the United States, as of December 31, 1946," Health and Sanitation Division, Institute of Inter-American Affairs, Washington, DC, RG SSA, Section Sub SyA, Box 19, Folder 10, AHSSA; "Programa Interamericano de Salud Pública," 1946, RG SSA, Section Sub SyA, Box 11, Folder 4, AHSSA; and "La Dirección de Cooperación Interamericana de Salubridad Pública," *Salubridad y Asistencia* 7, no. 3 (1947): 259–61. Also see Hugh Smith's diary, March 26–April 4, 1948, p. 30, RG 12.1, Box 57, RFA.

34. These films, aimed at the "humble classes," had already been used in Bolivia, Peru, Paraguay, Ecuador, and Central America. Shown by teams of nurse-midwives, projectionists, and teachers (with salaries and equipment furnished by the U.S. government) the

films addressed issues such as stacking food on dirty floors in markets, washing dirty plates in cold water, spitting, and children crawling on dirty floors. Wyman Stone to Gustavo Baz, July 25, 1946, RG SSA, Section Sub SyA, Box 9, Folder 1, AHSSA. On U.S. film imperialism in Mexico in the 1940s, see Seth Fein, "Everyday Forms of Transnational Collaboration: U.S. Film Propaganda in Cold War Mexico," in *Close Encounters of Empire: Writing the Cultural History of U.S.–Latin American Relations,* ed. Gilbert Joseph, Catherine LeGrand, and Ricardo Salvatore (Durham, NC: Duke University Press, 1998), 400–450.

35. Hugh Smith's diary, March 26–April 4, 1948, p. 31, RG 12.1, Box 57, RFA.

36. All citations in this paragraph are from "Aid to Mexico, Memorandum from Ferrell to Fosdick," January 27, 1941, RG 2—Stacks, Box 561, Folder 3814, RFA.

37. Hugh Smith's Diary, March 26–April 4, 1948, p. 30, RG 12.1, Box 57, RFA.

38. Gustavo Baz, "La Fusión de los Servicios de Salubridad y Asistencia," in *Memoria, 1943–1944* (México, D.F.: Secretaría de Salubridad y Asistencia, 1944), 84–86; and Alberto P. León, "Secretaría de Salubridad y Asistencia," *Pasteur: Revista Mensual de Medicina* 14, I, no. 1 (1941): 1–6.

39. James Horn, "The Mexican Revolution and Health Care or the Health of the Mexican Revolution," *International Journal of Health Services* 15, no. 3 (1985): 485–99.

40. See Ana María Carrillo, "Pioneros de la Seguridad Social en México," *Boletín de la Sociedad Mexicana de Historia y Filosofía de la Medicina* 2 (2000): 26–32; and Carlos Mesa-Lago, *Social Security in Latin America: Pressure Groups, Stratification, and Inequality* (Pittsburgh: University of Pittsburgh Press, 1978), 220–21.

41. José Torres Torija, "El Seguro de Salud," *Pasteur: Revista Mensual de Medicina* 3, I, no. 3 (1930): 140–48.

42. See Anne-Emanuelle Birn, "Federalist Flirtations: The Politics and Execution of Health Services Decentralization for the Uninsured Population in Mexico, 1985–1995," *Journal of Public Health Policy* 20, no. 1 (1999): 81–108. Also see Milton Roemer, "Medical Care and Social Class in Latin America," *Milbank Memorial Fund Quarterly* 42 (part I, 1964): 54–64.

43. See Héctor Hernández Llamas, "Historia de la Participación del Estado en las Instituciones de Atención Médica en México, 1935–1980," in *Vida y Muerte del Mexicano,* ed. Federico Ortiz Quesada (México, D.F.: Folios Ediciones, 1982), 49–96; Cristina Laurell, "Crisis, Neoliberal Health Policy, and Political Processes in Mexico," *International Journal of Health Services* 21 (1991): 457–70; González-Block, "Génesis"; and Julio Frenk et al., "Medicina Liberal y Medicina Institucional en México," *Salud Pública de México* 18, no. 3 (1976): 481–93.

44. Until the 1960s, IMSS health services were located only in Mexico City.

45. G. K. Strode's diary, January 7, 1947, p. 5, RG 12.1, Box 61, RFA.

46. Samuel Benítez Armas, "Dirección de la Campaña Contra el Paludismo," 1947, RG SSA, Section SubA, Box 3, Folder 1, AHSSA.

47. "Meeting Regarding School of Public Health," March 18, 1949, RG SSA, Section SubA, Box 44, Folder 1, AHSSA.

48. Hugh Smith's diary, October 4 to October 13, 1950, RG 12.1, Box 57, RFA.

49. "Asuntos que se Someten a la Consideración del C. Presidente de la República," April 2, 1943, RG Public Health, Presidential Section, Series Presidential Agreement, 1943, AHSSA.

50. *Revista del Instituto de Salubridad y Enfermedades Tropicales* 10, no. 4 (December 1950): 195.

51. On the IHD's influence on the WHO, see Farley, *To Cast Out Disease,* 273–83.

52. Marcos Cueto, "International Health, the Rockefeller Foundation and Latin America during the 1940s," *Research Reports from the Rockefeller Archive Center* (Fall 2002): 17–20; and Paul Weindling, "Termination or Transformation? The Fate of the International Health Division as a Case Study in Foundation Decision-Making," *Research Reports from the Rockefeller Archive Center* (Fall 2002): 20–23.

53. Chester Barnard, "Some Miscellaneous Considerations Bearing on the IHD Future Program," 1950, RG 3.1, Series 908, Box 3, Folder 19, RFA.

54. José Luis Gómez Pimienta, "El Comité Nacional de Lucha contra la Tuberculosis," *Pasteur: Revista Mensual de Medicina* 14, I, no. 1 (1941): 7–9.

55. "Memorandum on the Principles of Administration of the IHD," W. Rose, 1922, RG 3.1, Series 908, Box 12, Folder 128, RFA.

56. Warren to Russell, March 16, 1926, and March 18, 1926, RG 5, Series 1.2, Box 258, File 3281, RFA. See Murard and Zylberman, "La Mission Rockefeller en France"; and David Barnes, *The Making of a Social Disease: Tuberculosis in Nineteenth-Century France* (Berkeley: University of California Press, 1995).

57. Russell to Warren, March 26, 1926, RG 5, Series 1.2, Box 258, File 3281, RFA.

58. Alvarez Amézquita et al., *Historia de la Salubridad*, 413–23.

59. Francisco de P. Miranda, "The Decrease of Tuberculosis in Mexico," *American Journal of Public Health* 21, no. 1 (1931): 37–42.

60. The local health unit collaboration—not a disease campaign per se—was an exception to this decision-making process, based on particular institutional and political developments in Mexico.

61. R. M. Moore to the RF, September 28, 1935, RG 2, Series 323, Box 120, Folder 908, RFA. Discussions of the prevalence, etiology, and control of onchocerciasis appeared frequently on the pages of Mexican medical journals such as *Pasteur*.

62. Bailey to Ferrell, May 8, 1934, RG 2, Series 323, Box 100, Folder 789, RFA.

63. Wilbur Sawyer to Ferrell, October 10, 1935, RG 2, Series 323, Box 120, Folder 908, RFA.

64. "Asuntos que se Someten al Presidente de la República," April 18, 1939, RG Public Health, Presidential Section, Presidential Agreements Series, 1939, AHSSA; Salvador González Herrejón, "Estado Actual del Problema de la Oncocercosis en la República Mexicana," *Boletín de la Oficina Sanitaria Panamericana* 15 (1936): 735–43.

65. "Memorandum" Presented by the Office of Technical Administration of the Campaign against Malaria and Other Parasitic Diseases of the Department of Public Health, to Be Considered by the President of the Republic, with the Approval of the Chief of the Department of Public Health," April 18, 1939, RG Public Health, Presidential Section, Presidential Agreements Series, 1939, AHSSA.

66. Bailey to Ferrell, April 26, 1940, RG 1.1, Series 323, Box 20, Folder 165, RFA.

67. *Bibliography of Onchocercosis*, Publication 242 (Washington, DC: Pan American Sanitary Bureau, 1947).

68. Manuel Gamio, "Exploración Económico-Cultural en la Región Oncocercosa de Chiapas," January 22, 1947, RG Miguel Alemán, File 425.5/5, AGN.

69. Interview with Dr. Felipe García Sánchez, former RF fellow and head of units in Veracruz, Morelos, and Xochimilco before becoming a high-level administrator in the DSP, June 5, 1991, Mexico City.

70. Secondary works on the RF's malaria efforts include the following: Marcos Cueto, "Una Reforma Fallida: La Fundación Rockefeller, la Malaria y la Salud Pública en el Peru, 1940–1949," *Revista Peruana de Ciencias Sociales* 2 (1990): 9–29; Uriel Kitron, "Malaria, Agriculture, and Development: Lessons from Past Campaigns," *International Journal of Health Services* 17 (1987): 295–326; Saúl Franco Agudelo, *El Paludismo en América Latina* (Guadalajara, México: Editorial Universidad de Guadalajara, 1990); and Harry Cleaver, "Malaria, the Politics of Public Health and the International Crisis," *Review of Radical Political Economics* 9 (1977): 81–103.

71. Birn, "Eradication, Control or Neither?"

72. The RF's first "serious" malaria survey did not take place until 1936, when half the population was found to live in endemic regions. See Darwin Stapleton, "The Dawn of DDT and its Experimental Use by the Rockefeller Foundation in Mexico, 1943–1952," *Parassitologia* 40, nos. 1–2 (1998): 149–58.

73. Russell to Carr, March 24, 1927, RG 5, Series 1.2, Box 296, File 3753, RFA.

74. See Rockefeller Foundation, *Annual Report* (New York: Rockefeller Foundation 1930–1937).

75. Galo Soberón y Parra, "Breves Apuntes acerca del Estado Actual de la Lucha contra el Paludismo," *Pasteur: Revista Mensual de Medicina* 10, II, no. 1 (1937): 17–22.

76. "Informe de Labores 1934–1935," DSP, RG Lázaro Cárdenas, Folder 425.5/18, AGN.

77. "Resources of the National Malaria Campaign," Autumn 1938, DSP, RG Cárdenas, Folder 433/290, AGN.

78. "Program of the National Malaria Campaign," Autumn 1938, DSP, RG Cárdenas, Folder 433/290, AGN. Also see Hector Gómez-Dantés and Anne-Emanuelle Birn, "Malaria and Social Movements in Mexico: The Last 60 Years," *Parassitologia* 42 (2000): 69–85.

79. Dr. General José Siurob, "DSP Informe de Labores Presidenciales, September 1, 1936–July 15, 1937," RG Public Health, Presidential Section, Presidential Agreements Series, 1937, AHSSA.

80. "Preliminary Conclusions, First Regional Convention of the National Malaria Campaign," 1938, DSP, RG, Cárdenas, Folder 433/290, AGN. On the RF's malaria effort in Italy, see Stapleton, "Success for Science or Technology?"

81. Siurob to Bailey, May 17, 1937, RG 1.1, Series 323, Box 18, Folder 145, RFA.

82. Rockefeller Foundation, *Annual Report* (New York: Rockefeller Foundation, 1939).

83. Gilberto Lavin to Abraham González Ayala, May 30, 1929, RG Public Health, Epidemiology Section, Box 53, Folder 6, AHSSA.

84. Manuel Rueda Magro to Chamber of Local Deputies, August 9, 1935, Antonio Pérez Alcocer to Bailey, January 23, 1936, RG Public Health, Epidemiology Section, Box 53, Folder 6, AHSSA.

85. Salvador Morales y Carbajal, "Informe Resumido de los Experimentos Realizados por la 'Campaña Contra el Paludismo' de la Dirección General de Epidemiología en el Estado de Morelos, hasta Diciembre de 1945, para Dominar el Anofelismo en los Cultivos de Arroz," *Salubridad y Asistencia* 7, no. 3 (1947): 313–24; and interview with Felipe García Sánchez, June 5, 1991, Mexico City.

86. Rates are not available for 1933, but population estimates suggest that Morelos's death rate would also rank it at fifteenth or sixteenth. Galo Soberón y Parra, "Lecciones de Malariología Elemental," Servicio de Sanidad Federal en los Estados, ca .1934, DSP, RG Public Health, Epidemiology Section, Box 53, Folder 6, AHSSA.

87. Interview with Luis Vargas, March 5, 1991, Mexico City.

88. Bailey to Ferrell, December 26, 1936, RG 1.1, Series 323, Box 20, Folder 162, RFA.

89. See J. W. Torres to Jesús González Gallo, August 4, 1942, RG Avila Camacho, Folder 423/2, AGN.

90. Bailey to Ferrell, July 7, 1940, RG 2, Series 323, Box 199, Folder 1409, RFA.

91. Bailey to Ferrell, April 26, 1940, RG 1.1, Series 323, Box 20, Folder 165, RFA.

92. In 1945 its budget was 820,000 pesos ($1.8 million in 2004 dollars). Pedro Miranda Sáyago, "Resumen del Movimiento de Ingresos y Egresos en la Oficina de la Campaña Contra el Paludismo en el Período del Primero de Enero al Once de Octubre de 1945," RG Avila Camacho, Folder 564.4/20, AGN, Campañas Sanitarias, 1948, RG SSA, Section SubA, Box 35, Folder 2, AHSSA.

93. See, for example, Liga Femenil de Acción y Lucha Social de San Bartolo, Tuxtepec, Oaxaca, to Manuel Avila Camacho, February 19, 1943, RG Avila Camacho, Folder 151.3/480, AGN; and Comité Pro-Lucha Antipalúdica to Miguel Alemán, March 1948, RG Miguel Alemán, Folder 425.5/73, AGN.

94. According to George Strode, the U.S. Army was cautious about employing DDT in louse control for U.S. soldiers so Strode offered an IHD field trial in Mexico. Lewis Hackett, interview with the Paynes, June 28, 1951, RG 3.1, Series 908, Box 4, Folder 20, RFA. The researchers involved in this trial were RF representative George Payne and the Mexican doctors and RF fellows Carlos Ortiz Mariotte and Felipe Malo Juvera. See Miguel Bustamante, "Hechos Sobresalientes en la Historia de la Secretaría de Salubridad y Asistencia," p. 24,

México, D.F., April 19, 1983, RG Dr. Miguel E. Bustamante V. FCCBV. For more on the DDT campaign in Mexico, see Stapleton, "Dawn of DDT," 149–58.

95. "The Rockefeller Foundation Health Commission: Mexico—Louse Control Studies—Allocation, November 14, 1942," RG 1.1, Series 323, Box 12, Folder 87, RFA.

96. James B. Gahan and George C. Payne, "Control de Anopheles Pseudopunctipennis con Pulveraciones Residuales de DDT Aplicadas en Edificios en México," *Salubridad y Asistencia* 6, no. 18 (1946): 71–76.

97. "The Mosquito-Killing Power of DDT," *Trustees Bulletin*, 1947, RG 1.1, Series 323, Box 17, Folder 144, RFA.

98. See Downs to Secretary of Health, March 10, 1947, RG SSA, Section SubA, Box 3, Folder 1, AHSSA; and *International Health Division Annual Report* (New York: Rockefeller Foundation, 1950), 50–51; and Gustavo Baz, *Memoria, 1943–1944* (México, D.F.: SSA, 1944).

99. Wilbur Downs, E. Bordas and A. Enríquez-Cháves, "El Control del Paludismo en la Región de Xochimilco, D.F.," *Revista del Instituto de Salubridad y Enfermedades Tropicales* 11 (1950): 99–103; Wilbur Downs et al., "Colonialización en el Laboratorio de Anopheles Aztecus Hoffmann," *Revista del Instituto de Salubridad y Enfermedades Tropicales* 9 (1948): 175–76; and Mark F. Boyd, "Estudios de Campo en el Paludismo," *Boletín del Departamento de Salubridad Pública* 6, no. 1 (1943): 39–42.

100. "Decreto Presidencial que Declara de Interés Público y de Beneficio Social la Campaña para Erradicar el Paludismo," *Diario Oficial*, December 17, 1955, vol. 213, no. 41, RG SSA, Presidential Section, Box 51, Folder 1, AHSSA.

101. Charles Nicolle, "Confidential Report to the French Minister of Foreign Affairs," August 12, 1931, Charles Nicolle papers, Folder 8, Archives of the Institut Pasteur, Paris (my translation). As cited in Ana Cecilia Rodríguez de Romo, "La Visita de Charles Nicolle a México en 1931," in *Estudios de Historia de la Medicina: Abordages e Interpretaciones*, ed. Ana Cecilia Rodríguez de Romo and Xóchitl Martínez Barbosa (México, D.F.: UNAM, 2001), 166. I am grateful to Ana Cecilia Rodríguez de Romo for bringing this report to my attention.

102. "Excerpt from Minutes of Officers' Conference," January 10, 1930, RG 3.2, Series 900, Box 60, Folder 332, RFA.

103. Ferrell to Bailey, March 4, 1935, RG 2, Series 323, Box 119, Folder 907, RFA.

104. Ferrell to Fosdick, "Memorandum on Aid to Mexico," January 27, 1941, RG 2, Box 561, Folder 3814, RFA.

105. In Brazil, the development of basic rural health outposts had accompanied a hookworm campaign in the late 1910s, but these posts were soon folded into a new National Department of Health with little RF involvement, leaving it to concentrate on its large-scale disease campaigns. See Hochman, *A Era do Saneamento* and Rosario Costa, *Lutas Urbanas e Controle Sanitario*.

106. Hugh Smith's diary, October 4 to October 13, 1950, RG 12.1, Box 57, RFA.

107. Frederick Russell's diary, June 28, 1923, RG 12.1, Box 53, Folder 1922–24, RFA.

108. Anne-Emanuelle Birn, "Buscando Desesperadamente la Descentralización: Las Políticas de Salud Mexicanas en Dos Epocas de Reforma (Los Años 20 y 30 y la Década de los 80)." *Dynamis* 25 (2005): 279–311; and Héctor Gómez-Dantés and Anne-Emanuelle Birn, "Malaria and Social Movements in Mexico: The Last 60 Years," *Parassitologia* 42 (2000): 69–85.

109. Julia Emilia Rodriguez, "The Failure of Public Health Philanthropy: The Rockefeller Foundation in Venezuela, 1926–1934" (MA diss., Columbia University, 1993).

110. Miguel E. Bustamante, "Problemas y Adquisiciones Recientes de la Higiene y la Medicina Preventiva," *Salubridad y Asistencia* 7, no. 2 (1947): 153–60.

111. Angel de la Garza Brito, "La Nueva Administración Pública," *Sociedad Mexicana de Higiene* (June 1950): 60–65.

112. "Organización de Una Campaña Sanitaria," 1948, RG SSA, Section SubA, Box 35, Folder 2, AHSSA.

113. See, for example, Dirección General de Salubridad Federal, "Informe Sintético de las Labores Desarrolladas Durante el Período Comprendido del 10 de Septiembre de 1941 al 30 de Junio de 1942," RG Public Health, Presidential Section, Box 15, Folder 3, AHSSA; Baz, *Memoria*; and "Plan Sexenal, 1940–1946," DSP, RG Public Health, Legal Section, Box 53, Folder 15, AHSSA.

114. Gastélum, *Memoria*. Also see Bernardo J. Gastélum *Días de Decisiones* (México, D.F.: Sociedad Mexicana de Historia y Filosofía de la Medicina, Monografías 1, 1976).

115. Jose Siurob, "Trabajo Sanitario en los Estados Unidos Mexicanos, 1934–1940" (México, D.F., DSP, April 26, 1940).

116. George Payne, interviewed by Lewis Hackett, ca. 1950, and Notes, vol. 1, RG 3.1, Series 908, Box 3, Folder 19, RFA.

117. In 1941, after the IHD had sponsored over forty fellows, the former Veracruz health officer who had worked closely with the hookworm campaign was aware of only half this number of RF fellows. Agustín Hernández Mejía, *Dieciocho Años de Trabajos Sanitarios en México* (Mexico, D.F., 1941).

118. See Martínez, "Policy Environments"; and Juliana Martínez, *Luces y Sombras: Formación y Transformación de las Políticas Sociales en América Latina* (San José, Costa Rica: Facultad Latinoamericana de Ciencias Sociales, 2000).

119. Interview with nurse and laboratory technician Lupita Serrano, April 12, 1991, Cuernavaca, Morelos.

120. Interview with Luis Vargas, March 5, 1991, Mexico City.

121. Carr to Strode, June 1, 1950, RG 3.1, Series 908, Box 14, Folder 148, RFA.

Epilogue

1. Cueto, *Valor de la Salud*. See also Basch, "Historical Perspective."

2. Weindling, *International Health Organisations*", especially Martin Dubin's chapter "The League of Nations Health Organization"; and Marta Balinska, *Une vie pour l'humanitaire: Ludwik Rajchman 1881–1965* (Paris: Editions la Découverte, 1995).

3. See, for example, Wilbur Sawyer's diary, Box 3, Diary # XXXI, December 30, 1940–May 31, 1944, pp. 207–11; and Box 4, Diary Folder January 10–February 1, 1941, February 2–17, 1941, and February 18–March 10, 1941, MS C 69, Wilbur A. Sawyer Papers, 1899–1952, History of Medicine Division, National Library of Medicine; and Weindling, "Philanthropy and World Health."

4. See David Arnold, *Science, Technology and Medicine in Colonial India* (Cambridge: Cambridge University Press, 2000); Myron Echenberg, *Black Death, White Medicine: Bubonic Plague and the Politics of Public Health in Colonial Senegal, 1914–1945* (Portsmouth, NH: Heinemann, 2002); Mark Harrison, *Public Health in British India: Anglo-Indian Preventive Medicine, 1859–1914* (Cambridge: Cambridge University Press, 1994); Daniel R. Headrick, *The Tentacles of Progress: Technology Transfer in the Age of Imperialism, 1850–1940* (New York: Oxford University Press, 1988); and William B. Cohen, "Malaria and French Imperialism," *Journal of African History* 24 (1983): 23–36.

5. Vicente Navarro, "The Underdevelopment of Health or the Health of Underdevelopment?: An Analysis of the Distribution of Human Health Resources in Latin America," International Journal of Health Services 4 (1974): 5–27.

6. Sawyer to Fosdick, August 31, 1949, RG 3.1, Series 908, Box 12, Folder 127, RFA. In 1963 on the occasion of the RF's fiftieth anniversary, RF President J. G. Harrar cited the founding of Johns Hopkins and the international fellowships as one of its greatest achievements, through which the RF "created the whole pattern of public health and medical education in this country and in 39 countries throughout the world." J. G. Harrar, video, Dorothy Gordon Youth Program, 1963, RFA.

7. John B. Grant, "International Trends in Health Care," presented to the IHD Scientific Directors, December 1947, RG 3.1, Series 900, Box 25, Folder 198, RFA. Also see John B. Grant, "International Trends in Health Care," *American Journal of Public Health* 38, no. 3 (1948): 381–97.

8. "Study of Efforts to Help Backward Peoples to Help Themselves," June 22, 1949, RG 3.2, Series 900, Box 60, Folder 332.

9. P. F. Russell, "Some Comments Regarding the IHD—Past and Future," November 3, 1950," p. 2 (A confidential memorandum written at the invitation of the director), RG 3.1, Series 908, Box 14, Folder 148, RFA.

10. See Löwy, *Virus, moustiques, et modernité.*

11. See, for example, C. L. Gonzalez, *Mass Campaigns and General Health Services,* Public Health Papers Number 29 (Geneva: World Health Organization, 1965), 15.

12. Gill Walt, "Global Cooperation in International Public Health," in *International Public Health: Diseases, Programs, Systems, and Policies,* ed. Michael Merson, Robert Black, and Anne Mills (Gaithersburg, MD: Aspen Publishers, 2001), 667–99.

13. "IHD and Other International Health Organizations" (MCB's memorandum, December, 1950), Lewis Hackett Notes—Vol. 3, RG 3.1, Series 908, Box 4, Folder 20, RFA.

14. Soper was perhaps best known for heading a successful campaign to eliminate *Anopheles gambiae* from Brazil and Egypt; his "faith in species eradication" guided his views on public health. See Fred L. Soper, *Building the Health Bridge: Selections from the Works of Fred L. Soper, M.D.* ed. J. Austin Kerr (Bloomington, IN: Indiana University Press, 1970); Soper, *Ventures in World Health*; and Malcolm Gladwell, "The Mosquito Killer," *New Yorker,* July 2, 2001, 42–51.

15. "IHD and Other International Health Organizations" (MCB's memorandum, December, 1950), Lewis Hackett Notes—Vol. 3, RG 3.1, Series 908, Box 4, Folder 20, RFA.

16. World Health Organization, *The First Ten Years of the World Health Organization* (Geneva: WHO, 1958).

17. Theodore M. Brown, Marcos Cueto, and Elizabeth Fee, "The World Health Organization and the Transition from 'International' to 'Global' Public Health," *American Journal of Public Health,* 96, no. 1 (2006): 62–72.

18. Department of State to the White House, 29 May 1953, *Foreign Relations of the United States,* vol. 3 (Washington, DC, 1979), 69.

19. As summarized by U.S. journalist Albert Deutsch, in *The World Health Organization: Its Global Battle against Disease* (New York: Public Affairs Committee, 1958), 9.

20. Yves Beigbeder, *L'Organisation Mondiale de la Santé* (Paris: Presses Universitaires de France, 1997), 105–8; Javed Siddiqi, *World Health and World Politics: The World Health Organization and the UN System* (Columbia. SC: University of South Carolina Press, 1995); and Norman Howard-Jones, "The World Health Organization in Historical Perspective," *Perspectives in Biology and Medicine* 24, no. 3 (1981): 467–82.

21. Cueto, *Valor de la Salud.*

22. Beigbeder, *L'Organisation Mondiale de la Santé,* 111–14.

23. *Ibid.,* 105–8; and Siddiqi, *World Health and World Politics.*

24. Beigbeder, *L'Organisation Mondiale de la Santé.*

25. Deutsch, *World Health Organization; Introducing WHO* (Geneva: WHO, 1976), 66.

26. Socrates Litsios, "The Long and Difficult Road to Alma-Ata: A Personal Reflection," *International Journal of Health Services* 32, no. 4 (2002): 709–32; Siddiqi, *World Health and World Politics*; and World Health Organization, *First Ten Years.*

27. See Siddiqi, *World Health and World Politics*; Randall Packard, "'No Other Logical Choice': Global Malaria Eradication and the Politics of International Health in the Postwar Era," *Parassitologia* 40, nos. 1 and 2 (June 1998): 217–30; Socrates Litsios, "Malaria Control, the Cold War, and the Postwar Reorganization of International Assistance," *Medical Anthropology* 17, no. 3 (May 1997): 255–78; Randall M. Packard and Peter J. Brown, "Rethinking Health, Development and Malaria: Historicizing a Cultural Model in

International Health," *Medical Anthropology* 17 (1997): 181–94; and Mary J. Dobson, M. Malowany, and R. W. Snow, "Malaria Control in East Africa: The Kampala Conference and the Pare-Taveta Scheme: A Meeting of Common and High Ground," *Parassitologia* 40, nos. 1 and 2 (June 1998): 149–66.

28. Dobson, Malowany, and Snow, "Malaria Control"; and World Health Organization, *The Second Ten Years of the World Health Organization, 1958–1967* (Geneva: WHO, 1968).

29. Beigbeder, *L'Organisation Mondiale de la Santé*, 128.

30. See Fenner et al., *Smallpox and Its Eradication* (Geneva: WHO, 1988), chapters 8 and 15.

31. Dmitry Venediktov, "Alma-Ata and After," *World Health Forum* 19 (1998): 79–86; and Dmitry Venediktov, interview July 2004, Moscow, Russia.

32. Donald A. Henderson, "Smallpox Eradication: A Cold War Victory," *World Health Forum* 19 (1998): 113–19.

33. See Paul Greenough, "Intimidation, Coercion and Resistance in the Final Stages of the South Asian Smallpox Eradication Campaign, 1973–1975," *Social Science and Medicine* 41, no. 5 (1995): 633–45; Sanjoy Bhattacharya, "Uncertain Victories: A Review of the Administration of the Final Phases of the Eradication of Smallpox in India, 1960–80," *American Journal of Public Health* 94, no. 11 (November 2004): 1875–83.

34. See "Declaration of Alma-Ata. International Conference on Primary Health Care, Alma-Ata, USSR, 6–12 September, 1978"; World Health Organization, "The Declaration of Alma-Ata," *World Health* (August/September 1988): 16–17; Venediktov, "Alma-Ata," 79–86; Litsios, "Long and Difficult Road," 709–32; and Marcos Cueto, "The Origins of Primary Health Care and Selective Primary Health Care," *American Journal of Public Health* 94 (2004): 1864–74.

35. Marcos Cueto, "The Promise of Primary Care," *Bulletin of the World Health Organization* 83, no. 5 (2005): 322.

36. Julia Walsh and Kenneth Warren, "Selective Primary Health Care: An Interim Strategy for Disease Control in Developing Countries," *New England Journal of Medicine* 301, no. 18 (1979): 967–74; and K. S. Warren, "The Evolution of Selective Primary Health Care," *Social Science and Medicine* 26, no. 8 (1988): 891–98.

37. See, for example, Kenneth Newell, "Selective Primary Health Care: The Counter Revolution," *Social Science and Medicine* 26 (1988): 903–6; David Werner and David Sanders, "Alma Ata and the Institutionalization of Primary Health Care," "Demise," and "Health Care as if People Mattered," in *Questioning the Solution: The Politics of Primary Health Care and Child Survival* (Palo Alto, CA: Healthwrights, 1997); and World Health Organization, *The Work of WHO, 1986–1987, Biennial Report of the Director-General to the World Health Assembly and to the United Nations* (Geneva: WHO, 1988).

38. Jennifer Prah Ruger, "Changing Role of the World Bank in Global Health in Historical Perspective," *American Journal of Public Health* 95, no. 1 (January 2005): 60–70; and Martha Finnemore, "Redefining Development at the World Bank," in *International Development and the Social Sciences: Essays on the History and Politics of Knowledge*, ed. F. Cooper and R. Packard (Berkeley: University of California Press, 1997), 203–27.

39. World Bank, *World Development Report 1993: Investing in Health* (Washington, DC: World Bank, 1993).

40. See A. Cristina Laurell and Oliva L. Arellano, "Market Commodities and Poor Relief: the World Bank Proposal for Health," *International Journal of Health Services* 26, no. 1 (1996): 1–18; and Debabar Banerji, "A Fundamental Shift in the Approach to International Health by WHO, UNICEF, and the World Bank: Instances of the Practice of 'Intellectual Fascism' and Totalitarianism in Some Asian Countries," *International Journal of Health Services* 29, no. 2 (1999): 227–59.

41. Martin McKee, Paul Garner, and Robin Stott, *International Co-operation in Health* (Oxford: Oxford University Press, 2001); and Mario Bronfman and Jorge Díaz Polanco, "La Cooperación Técnica Internacional y las Políticas de Salud," *Ciência e Saúde Coletiva* 8, no. 1 (2003): 227–41.

42. Fiona Godlee, "WHO in Retreat: Is It Losing Its Influence?" *British Medical Journal* 309 (1994): 1491–95, 1493; Fiona Godlee, "The World Health Organisation: WHO in Crisis," *British Medical Journal* 309 (1994): 1424–28; Fiona Godlee, "The World Health Organisation: WHO at Country Level: A Little Impact, No Strategy," *British Medical Journal* 309 (1994): 1636–39; and Gill Walt, "WHO under Stress: Implications for Health Policy," *Health Policy* 24 (1993): 125–44.

43. See Walt, "Global Cooperation"; and Ilona Kickbusch and Kent Buse, "Global Influences and Global Responses: International Health at the Turn of the Twenty-First Century," in *International Public Health: Diseases, Programs, Systems, and Policies*, ed. Michael Merson, Robert Black, and Anne Mills (Gaithersburg, MD: Aspen Publishers, 2001), 701–32.

44. Judith Justice, *Policies, Plans, and People: Foreign Aid and Health Development* (Berkeley: University of California Press, 1989); Catriona Waddington, "Does Earmarked Donor Funding Make It More or Less Likely that Developing Countries Will Allocate their Resources towards Programmes that Yield the Greatest Health Benefits?" *Bulletin of the World Health Organization* 82, no. 9 (September 2004): 703–6; Philip Musgrove, "Earmarking Could Be Beneficial: Cost Effectiveness Is Not the Only Criterion," *Bulletin of the World Health Organization* 82, no. 9 (September 2004): 706–7; Hilary Sunman, "Earmarked Funds and Sectorwide Approaches Can Encourage Harmonization," *Bulletin of the World Health Organization* 82, no. 9 (September 2004): 707; and Debabar Banerji, "Alma-Ata Showed the Route to Effective Resource Allocations for Health," *Bulletin of the World Health Organization* 82, no. 9 (2004): 707–8.

45. R. Bruce Aylward and David Heymann, "Can We Capitalize on the Virtues of Vaccines? Insights from the Polio Eradication Initiative," *American Journal of Public Health* 95, no. 5 (May 2005): 773–77.

46. See http://www.theglobalfund.org

47. Nancy Birdsall, preface to *Millions Saved: Proven Successes in Global Health*, by Ruth Levine and the What Works Working Group with Molly Kinder (Washington, D.C.: Center for Global Development, 2004).

48. See James Trostle, "International Health Research: The Rules of the Game," in *Global Health Policy, Local Realities: The Fallacy of the Level Playing Field*, ed. Linda Whiteford and Lenore Manderson (Boulder, CO: Lynne Rienner Publishers, 2000), 291–313.

49. Gill Walt, "Globalisation of International Health," *The Lancet* 351, no. 9100 (1998): 434–37. In 1990, external funding to developing countries constituted was only 2.9 percent of health expenditures, according to Catherine Michaud and Christopher Murray, "External Assistance to the Health Sector in Developing Countries: A Detailed Analysis, 1972–90," *Bulletin of the World Health Organization* 72, no. 4 (1994): 639–51. Also see L M Howard, "Public and Private Donor Financing for Health in Developing Countries," *Infectious Disease Clinics of North America* 5, no. 2 (June 1991): 221–34.

50. See http://www.dghonline.org/principles.html. (Doctors for Global Health)

51. See http://phmovement.org/. (People's Health Movement)

52. Some might argue that the RF principles of international health cooperation have persisted because they offer effective means of aiding host countries combat health problems and assuring donors that money is well spent. But this functionalist stance presumes that there is agreement on the approach and that the evaluation of effectiveness takes into account a complex understanding of health.

53. See, for example, Ilona Kickbusch, "The Development of International Health Policies: Accountability Intact?" *Social Science and Medicine* 51 (2000): 979–89; and Ulysses Panisset, *International Health Statecraft: Foreign Policy and Public Health in Peru's Cholera Epidemic* (Lanham, MD: University Press of America, 2000).

54. See Randall Packard, "Visions of Postwar Health and Development and their Impact on Public Health Interventions in the Developing World," in *International Development and the Social Sciences: Essays on the History and Politics of Knowledge*, ed. Frederick Cooper and Randall Packard (Berkeley: University of California Press, 1997), 93–115; Peter Hotez,

"Vaccine Diplomacy," *Foreign Policy* 124 (2001): 68–69; and Caroline Thomas, "Health of International Relations and International Relations of Health," *Review of International Studies* 15 (1989): 273–80.

55. Enormous investments by the United States and other industrialized countries in reproductive health certainly addressed important questions of birth spacing, women's health, and infant mortality reduction, albeit at times following the cultural agenda of Western feminists. But there were also accompanying political ends of reducing population pressures—to defuse revolutionary, potentially pro-Communist movements. See Betsy Hartmann, "Population Control I: Birth of an Ideology," and "Population Control II: The Population Establishment Today," *International Journal of Health Services* 27, no. 3 (1997): 523–57; and Peter J. Donaldson, "On the Origins of the United States Government's International Population Policy," *Population Studies* 44, no. 3 (1990): 385–99.

56. Jordan S. Kassalow, *Why Health Is Important to U.S. Foreign Policy* (Washington, DC: Council on Foreign Relations, 2001); and Daniel M. Fox and Jordan S. Kassalow, "Making Health a Priority of U.S. Foreign Policy," *American Journal of Public Health*, 91 (2001): 1554–56.

57. See, for example, Christine McMurray and Roy Smith, *Diseases of Globalization: Socioeconomic Transitions and Health* (London: Earthscan Publications, 2001); Meri Koivusalo and Eeva Ollila, *Making a Healthy World: Agencies, Actors and Policies in International Health* (London: Zed Press, 1997); Jonathan Mann et al., "Health and Human Rights," *Health and Human Rights*, 1, no. 1 (1994): 6–23; Ichiro Kawachi and Bruce Kennedy, *The Health of Nations: Why Inequality Is Harmful to your Health* (New York: New Press, 2002); Nancy Krieger, "Epidemiology and the Web of Causation: Has Anyone Seen the Spider?" *Social Science and Medicine* 39, no. 7 (1994): 887–903; Nancy Krieger and Elizabeth Fee, "Measuring Social Inequalities in Health in the United States: A Historical Review, 1900–1950," *International Journal of Health Services* 26, no. 3 (1996): 391–418; and Ana Diez-Roux, "Bringing Context Back into Epidemiology: Variables and Fallacies in Multi-Level Analysis," *American Journal of Public Health* 88, no. 2 (1998): 216–22.

58. For a fascinating account of the power struggle among international agencies in the area of vaccine development, see William Muraskin, *The Politics of International Health: The Children's Vaccine Initiative and the Struggle to Develop Vaccines for the Third World* (Albany: State University of New York Press, 1998).

59. Anne-Emanuelle Birn, "Gates's Grandest Challenge: Transcending Technology as Public Health Ideology," *The Lancet* 366 (2005): 514–519; and Martin Morse Wooster, "The Donors Are In: What Gates Can Learn from Rockefeller about Global Health," *Philanthropy Magazine*, August/September, 2001, http://www.philanthropyroundtable.org/magazines/2001/august/

60. Kyung M. Song, "Gates Doubles Health Vow," *Seattle Times*, May 17, 2005, http://seattletimes.nwsource.com/html/localnews/2002277559_gates17m.html. See also http://www.gatesfoundation.org

61. See Claudia Jardim, "Prevention and Solidarity: Democratizing Health in Venezuela" *Monthly Review* 56, no. 8 (2005), http://www.monthlyreview.org/ 0105jardim.htm; and Carles Muntaner, "Denunciation by Cliché: Is Chavez's Venezuela Populist or Socialist?" *Counterpunch*, May 5, 2005, http://www.counterpunch.org/ mutanero5052005.html

Bibliography

Books, Articles, and Dissertations

Abel, Christopher. "External Philanthropy and Domestic Change in Colombian Health Care: The Role of the Rockefeller Foundation, ca. 1920–1950." *Hispanic American Historical Review* 75, no. 3 (1995): 339–75.

Abir-Am, Pnina G. "The Rockefeller Foundation and the Rise of Molecular Biology." *Nature Reviews* 3 (January 2002): 5–10.

Acheson, Roy. *Wickliffe Rose of the Rockefeller Foundation: 1862–1914*. Cambridge, UK: Killycarn Press, 1992.

"Acta de la Sesión Celebrada por la Comisión Especial para la Campaña contra la Fiebre Amarilla, Octubre 19 de 1921, Presidencia del Sr. Dr. T. C. Lyster." In *Memoria de la Primera Convención de Fiebre Amarilla, Octubre 15–20 de 1921*, 155–63. México, D.F.: Departamento de Salubridad Pública, 1921.

Adams, Christine. "Maternal Societies in France: Private Charity Before the Welfare State." *Journal of Women's History* 17, no. 1 (2005): 87–111.

Agostoni, Claudia. "Médicos Científicos y Médicos Ilícitos en la Ciudad de México Durante el Porfiriato." In *Estudios de Historia Moderna y Contemporánea de México* 19 (2000): 13–31. México, D.F.: Universidad Nacional Autónoma de México (UNAM), 1999.

———. "Médicos y Parteras en la Ciudad de México Durante el Porfiriato." In *México en el Siglo XIX: Cuatro Estudios de Género*. Edited by Gabriela Cano and Georgette José Valenzuela, 71–95. México, D.F.: UNAM, 2001.

———. *Monuments of Progress. Modernization and Public Health in Mexico City, 1876–1910*. Calgary: University of Calgary Press; Denver: University Press of Colorado; México, D.F.: Instituto de Investigaciones Históricas, UNAM, 2003.

———. "Sanitation and Public Works in Late Nineteenth Century Mexico City." *Quipu: Revista Latinoamericana de Historia de las Ciencias y la Tecnologia* 12, no. 2 (1999): 187–201.

Agostoni, Claudia, and Elisa Speckman, eds. *Modernidad, Tradición, y Alteridad: La Ciudad de México en el Cambio de Siglo, XIX–XX*. México, D.F.: UNAM, 2001.

Agramonte, Aristides. "Some Observations upon Yellow Fever Profilaxis." In *Proceedings of the International Conference on Health Problems in Tropical America, Held at Kingston, Jamaica July 22 to August 1, 1924*. Edited by United Fruit Company, 201–27. Boston: United Fruit Company, 1924.

Aguayo, Sergio. *Myths and [Mis] Perceptions: Changing U.S. Elite Visions of Mexico.* Translated by Julián Brody. San Diego: Center for U.S.-Mexican Studies, University of California, 1998.

Aguilar Camín, Héctor, and Lorenzo Meyer. *In the Shadow of the Mexican Revolution: Contemporary Mexican History.* Translated by Luis Alberto Fierro. Austin: University of Texas Press, 1993.

Aguilar García, Javier, ed. *Historia de la CTM, 1936–1990: El Movimiento Obrero y el Estado Mexicano.* México, D.F.: Facultad de Ciencias Políticas y Sociales, Instituto de Investigaciones Sociales, Facultad de Economía, UNAM, 1990.

Aguirre Beltrán, Gonzalo. *Medicina y Magia: El Proceso de Aculturación en la Estructura Colonial.* México, D.F.: Instituto Nacional Indigenista (INI)/Secretaría de Educación Pública (SEP), 1980.

———. *Programas de Salud en la Situación Intercultural.* México, D.F.: Instituto Mexicano del Seguro Social (IMSS), 1980.

Agustín, José. *Tragicomedia Mexicana 1: La Vida en México de 1940 a 1970.* México, D.F.: Grupo Editorial Planeta, 1990.

Alchon, Suzanne Austin. *A Pest in the Land: New World Epidemics in a Global Perspective.* Albuquerque: University of New Mexico Press, 2003.

Alcina Franch, José. *Temazcalli: Higiene, Terapéutica, Obstetricia y Ritual en el Nuevo Mundo.* Sevilla, Spain: CSIC, 2000.

Alexander, Robert. *Labor Parties of Latin America.* New York: League for Industrial Democracy, 1942.

Allen, Henry Justin. *The Mexican Confiscations, Together with a Careful Survey of the Present Revolutionary Trends in Mexico.* New York: New York Herald-Tribune Newspaper Syndicate, 1938.

Alvarez, Adriana. "Resignificando los Conceptos de la Higiene. El Surgimiento de una Autoridad de las Primeras Instituciones Públicas de Salud. Buenos Aires 1880–1920." *História, Ciências, Saúde—Manguinhos* 6, no. 2 (1999): 293–314.

Alvarez Amézquita, José. "Influencia de la Salud Pública en el Desarrollo Social." In *Libro Conmemorativo del Primer Centenario.* Edited by Academia Nacional de Medicina, 630–40. México, D.F.: Comité Editorial de la Comisión Organizadora del Congreso del Centenario, 1964.

Alvarez Amézquita, José, Miguel E. Bustamante, Antonio L. Picazos, and F. Fernández del Castillo. *Historia de la Salubridad y de la Asistencia en México.* 4 vols. México, D.F.: Secretaría de Salubridad y Asistencia (SSA), 1960.

———. "Servicios Médicos Rurales Cooperativos en la Historia de la Salubridad y de la Asistencia en México." In *La Atención Médica en el Medio Rural Mexicano, 1930–1980.* Edited by Héctor Hernández Llamas, 93–107. México, D.F.: IMSS, 1984.

Anderson, Eric, and Alfred A. Moss, Jr. *Dangerous Donations: Northern Philanthropy and Southern Black Education, 1902–1930.* Columbia: University of Missouri Press, 1999.

Anderson, Warwick. "Colonial Pathologies: American Medicine in the Philippines, 1898–1921." PhD diss., University of Pennsylvania, 1992.

———. "Going through the Motions: American Public Health and Colonial 'Mimicry.'" *American Literary History* 14 (Winter 2002): 686–719.

———. "Immunities of Empire: Race, Disease, and the New Tropical Medicine, 1900–1920." *Bulletin of the History of Medicine* 70, no. 1 (Spring 1996): 94–118.

Angeles, Genaro. "Informe Rendido por el Delegado en la Ciudad de Córdoba, Ver." In *Memoria de la Primera Convención de Fiebre Amarilla, Octubre 15–20 de 1921*, 31. México, D.F.: Departamento de Salubridad Pública (DSP), 1921.

Anguiano, Arturo. *El Estado y la Política Obrera del Cardenismo*, Colección Problemas de México. México, D.F.: Ediciones Era, 1975.

Anzures y Bolaños, María del Carmen. *La Medicina Tradicional en México: Proceso Histórico, Sincretismos, y Conflictos.* México, D.F.: UNAM, 1983.

Apple, Rima D. *Mothers and Medicine: A Social History of Infant Feeding, 1890–1950.* Madison: University of Wisconsin Press, 1987.

Arbona Medina, Luis M. *Informe Médico-Social del Ejido Primero de Mayo, Campo 77, Valle del Yaqui, Sonora. Padecimientos Más Frecuentes en Sonora.* México, D.F.: UNAM, 1956.

Aréchiga, Hugo. "La Medicina en México." In *Un Siglo de Ciencias de la Salud en México.* Edited by Hugo Aréchiga and Luis Benítez-Bribiesca, 204–43. México, D.F.: Fondo de Estudios e Investigaciones Ricardo J. Zevada. Consejo Nacional para la Cultura y las Artes, Fondo de Cultura Económica, 2000.

Aréchiga Córdoba, Ernesto. "Dictadura Sanitaria, Educación, y Propaganda Higiénica en el México Revolucionario, 1917–1932." *Dynamis* 25 (2005): 117–44.

Arias, Patricia, and Lucía Bazán. *Demandas y Conflicto: El Poder Político en un Pueblo de Morelos.* México, D.F.: Editorial Nueva Imagen, 1979.

Armus, Diego, ed. *Entre Médicos y Curanderos: Cultura, Historia, y Enfermedad en la América Latina Moderna.* Buenos Aires: Grupo Editorial Norma, 2002.

———, ed. *Disease in the History of Modern Latin America: From Malaria to AIDS.* Durham, NC: Duke University Press, 2003.

Arnold, David. *Colonizing the Body: State Medicine and Epidemic Disease in Nineteenth-Century India.* Berkeley: University of California Press, 1993.

———. *Imperial Medicine and Indigenous Societies.* Manchester, UK: Manchester University Press, 1988.

———. *Science, Technology and Medicine in Colonial India.* Cambridge: Cambridge University Press, 2000.

Arnove, Robert, ed. *Philanthropy and Cultural Imperialism: The Foundations at Home and Abroad.* Boston: G. K. Hall and Co., 1980.

Arreola Cortés, Raúl. *Manuel Martínez Báez, Científico y Humanista.* Morelia, México: Universidad Michoacana de San Nicolás de Hidalgo, 1994.

Ashby, Joe C. *Organized Labor and the Mexican Revolution under Lázaro Cárdenas.* Chapel Hill: University of North Carolina Press, 1963.

Aylward, Bruce, and David Heymann. "Can We Capitalize on the Virtues of Vaccines? Insights from the Polio Eradication Initiative." *American Journal of Public Health* 95, no. 5 (May 2005): 773–77.

Ayora-Díaz, Steffan Igor. "Globalization, Rationality and Medicine: Local Medicine's Struggle for Recognition in Highland Chiapas, Mexico." *Urban Anthropology* 27, no. 2 (1998): 165–95.

Azize Vargas, Yamila, and Luis Alberto Avilés. "Participación de la Mujer en las Profesiones de Salud." *Puerto Rican Health Services Journal* 9 (April 1990): 9–16.

Azuela, Luz Fernanda. "Médicos y Farmacéuticos en las Sociedades Científicas Mexicanas del Siglo XIX." *Boletín Mexicano de Historia y Filosofía de Medicina* 5, no. 2 (2002): 15–20.

Azurdia, Roberto R, Raúl Paredes López, and Otto R. Menéndez. "La Salud como Necesidad Fundamental Para el Desarrollo Económico." *Salud Pública de México* 5 (1963): 517–21.

Bailey, David C. *¡Viva Cristo Rey! The Cristero Rebellion and the Church-State Conflict in Mexico.* Austin: University of Texas Press, 1974.

Baitenmann, Helga. "Rural Agency and State Formation in Postrevolutionary Mexico: The Agrarian Reform in Central Veracruz, 1915–1992." PhD diss., New School for Social Research, 1997.

Baldwin, Peter. *Contagion and the State in Europe, 1830–1930.* New York: Cambridge University Press, 1999.

Balinska, Marta. *Une vie pour l'humanitaire: Ludwik Rajchman, 1881–1965.* Paris: Editions la Découverte, 1995.

Banerji, Debabar. "Alma-Ata Showed the Route to Effective Resource Allocations for Health." *Bulletin of the World Health Organization* 82, no. 9 (2004): 707–8.

———. "A Fundamental Shift in the Approach to International Health by WHO, UNICEF, and the World Bank: Instances of the Practice of 'Intellectual Fascism' and Totalitarianism in Some Asian Countries." *International Journal of Health Services* 29, no. 2 (1999): 227–59.

Barnes, David. *The Making of a Social Disease: Tuberculosis in Nineteenth-Century France.* Berkeley: University of California Press, 1995.

Basalla, George. "The Spread of Western Science." *Science* 156 (1967): 611–22.

Basch, Paul F. "A Historical Perspective on International Health." *Infectious Disease Clinics of North America* 5 (1991): 183–96.

Baytelman, Bernardo. *De Enfermos y Curanderos: Medicina Tradicional en Morelos.* México, D.F.: Instituto Nacional de Antropología e Historia (INAH), 1986.

Baz, Gustavo. *Memoria, 1943–1944.* México, D.F.: SSA, 1944.

Bean, William B. *Walter Reed: A Biography.* Charlottesville: University Press of Virginia, 1982.

Behrens, Benedikt. *Ein Laboratorium der Revolution: Städtische Soziale Bewegungen und Radikale Reformpolitik im Mexikanischen Bundesstaat Veracruz, 1918–1932.* Frankfurt: Peter Lang AG, 2002.

Beigbeder, Yves. *L'Organisation Mondiale de la Santé.* Paris: Presses Universitaires de France, 1997.

Bell, Heather. *Frontiers of Medicine in the Anglo-Egyptian Sudan, 1899–1940.* Oxford: Oxford University Press, 1999.

Benchimol, Jaime L. *Dos Micróbios aos Mosquitos: Febre amarela e a Revolução Pasteuriana no Brasil.* Rio de Janeiro: Editora Fiocruz and Editora UFRJ, 1999.

———. *Febre Amarela: A Doença e a Vacina, uma História Inacabada.* Rio de Janeiro: Editora Fiocruz, 2001.

———. *Manguinhos do Sonho à Vida: A Ciência na Belle Epoque.* Rio de Janeiro: Casa de Oswaldo Cruz/Editora Fiocruz, 1990.

Benítez, Fernando. *Lázaro Cárdenas y la Revolución Mexicana, III, El Cardenismo.* México, D.F.: Fondo de Cultura Económica, 1978.

Benjamin, Thomas, and Mark Wasserman, eds. *Provinces of the Revolution: Essays on Regional Mexican History, 1910–1929.* Albuquerque: University of New Mexico Press, 1990.

Berlin, Elois Ann, and Brent Berlin. *Medical Ethnobiology of the Highland Mayas of Chiapas, Mexico: The Gastrointestinal Diseases.* Princeton, NJ: Princeton University Press, 1996.

Berliner, Howard. *A System of Scientific Medicine: Philanthropic Foundations in the Flexner Era.* New York: Tavistock, 1985.

Berlinguer, Giovanni. "Parasitoses and Development: Malaria and Echinococcosis." *Parassitologia* 33, no. 1 (1991): 1–10.

Berman, Edward H. *The Influence of the Carnegie, Ford, and Rockefeller Foundations on American Foreign Policy.* Albany: State University of New York Press, 1983.

Bethell, Leslie, ed. *Mexico since Independence.* Cambridge: Cambridge University Press, 1991.

Bhattacharya, Sanjoy. "Uncertain Victories: A Review of the Administration of the Final Phases of the Eradication of Smallpox in India, 1960–80." *American Journal of Public Health* 94, no. 11 (November 2004): 1875–83.

Birdsall, Nancy. Preface to *Millions Saved: Proven Successes in Global Health,* by Ruth Levine and the What Works Working Group with Molly Kinder. Washington, D.C.: Center for Global Development, 2004.

Birn, Anne-Emanuelle. "Buscando Desesperadamente la Descentralización: Las Políticas de Salud Mexicanas en Dos Epocas de Reforma (Los Años 20 y 30 y la Década de los 80)." *Dynamis* 25 (2005): 279–311.

———. "Dr. Miguel Bustamante." In *Doctors, Nurses, and Practitioners.* Edited by Lois Magner, 30–36. Westwood, CT: Greenwood Press, 1997.

———. "Eradication, Control or Neither? Hookworm vs. Malaria Strategies and Rockefeller Public Health in Mexico." *Parassitologia* 40, nos. 1–2 (1998): 137–47.

———. "Federalist Flirtations: The Politics and Execution of Health Services Decentralization for the Uninsured Population in Mexico, 1985–1995." *Journal of Public Health Policy* 20, no. 1 (1999): 81–108.

———. "Gates's Grandest Challenge: Overcoming Technology as Public Health Ideology." *The Lancet* 366 (August 6, 2005): 514–19.

———. "No More Surprising than a Broken Pitcher? Maternal and Child Health in the Early Years of the Pan American Sanitary Bureau." *Canadian Bulletin of Medical History* 19, no. 1 (2002): 17–46.

———. "A Revolution in Rural Health?: The Struggle over Local Health Units in Mexico, 1928–1940." *Journal of the History of Medicine and Allied Sciences* 53, no. 1 (1998): 43–76.

———. "Revolution, the Scatological Way: The Rockefeller Foundation's Hookworm Campaign in 1920s Mexico," in *Disease in the History of Modern Latin America: From Malaria to AIDS.* Edited by Diego Armus, 158–82. Durham: Duke University Press, 2003.

———. "Six Seconds Per Eyelid: The Medical Inspection of Immigrants at Ellis Island, 1892–1914." *Dynamis* 17 (1997): 281–316.

———. "Uruguay on the World Stage: How Child Health Became an International Priority." *American Journal of Public Health* 95, no. 9 (2005): 1506–1517.

———. "Wa(i)ves of Influence: Rockefeller Public Health in Mexico, 1920–1950." *Studies in History and Philosophy of Biological and Biomedical Sciences* 31 no. 3 (2000): 381–95.

Birn, Anne-Emanuelle, Raquel Pollero, and Wanda Cabella. "No Hay Que Llorar sobre Leche Derramada: El Pensamiento Epidemiológico y la Mortalidad Infantil en Uruguay, 1900–1940." *Estudios Interdisciplinarios de América Latina* 14 (2003): 35–65.

Birn, Anne-Emanuelle, and Armando Solórzano. "The Hook of Hookworm: Public Health and the Politics of Eradication in Mexico." In *Western Medicine as Contested Knowledge*. Edited by Andrew Cunningham and Bridie Andrews, 147–71. Manchester, UK: Manchester University Press/St. Martin's Press, 1997.

———. "Public Health Policy Paradoxes: Science and Politics in the Rockefeller Foundation's Hookworm Campaign in Mexico in the 1920s." *Social Science and Medicine* 49 (1999): 1197–1213.

Black, Victoria Lynn. "Taking Care of Baby: Chilean State-Making, International Relations and the Gendered Body Politic, 1912–1970." PhD diss., University of Arizona, 2002.

Blanquel, Eduardo. "La Revolución Mexicana, 1921–1952." In *Historia Mínima de México*. Edited by Daniel Cosío Villegas, Ignacio Bernal, Alejandra Moreno Toscano, Luis González, and Eduardo Blanquel, 147–56. México, D.F.: Colegio de México, 1994.

Blasier, Cole. *The Giant's Rival: The USSR and Latin America.* Revised edition. Pittsburgh: University of Pittsburgh Press, 1987.

Bliss, Katherine Elaine. *Compromised Positions: Prostitution, Public Health and Gender Politics in Revolutionary Mexico City.* University Park: Penn State University Press, 2001.

Blum, Ann S. "Children without Parents: Law, Charity, and Social Practice, Mexico City, 1870–1940." PhD diss., University of California, Berkeley, 1997.

———. "Conspicuous Benevolence: Liberalism, Public Welfare, and Private Charity in Porfirian Mexico City, 1877–1910." *The Americas* 58, 1 (2001): 7–38.

———. "Public Welfare and Child Circulation, Mexico City, 1877 to 1925." *Journal of Family History* 23, no. 3 (July 1998): 240–71.

Board of Governors of the Federal Reserve System. *Banking and Monetary Statistics.* Washington, DC: Board of Governors of the Federal Reserve System, 1943.

———. *Banking and Monetary Statistics, 1941–1970.* Washington, DC: Board of Governors of the Federal Reserve System, 1976.

Boccaccio, Mary. "Ground Itch and Dew Poison: The Rockefeller Sanitary Commission: 1909–1914." *Journal of the History of Medicine and Allied Sciences* 27 (1972): 30–53.

Bock, Gisela, and Pat Thane, eds. *Maternity and Gender Policies: Women and the Rise of the European Welfare States 1880s–1950s.* New York and London: Routledge, 1991.

Boli, John, and George M. Thomas, eds. *World Polity Formation since 1875: World Culture and International Non-Governmental Organizations.* Stanford, CA: Stanford University Press, 1999.

Bortz, Jeffrey L, and Stephen Haber. *The Mexican Economy, 1879–1930: Essays on the Economic History of Institutions, Revolutions, and Growth.* Stanford, CA: Stanford University Press, 2002.

Bowers, John. *Western Medicine in a Chinese Palace: Peking Union Medical College.* New York: Josiah Macy Jr. Foundation, 1972.

Boyd, Mark F. "Estudios de Campo en el Paludismo." *Boletín del Departamento de Salubridad Pública* 6, no. 1 (1943): 39–42.

Brannstrom, Christian. "Polluted Soil, Polluted Souls: The Rockefeller Hookworm Eradication Campaign in São Paulo, Brazil, 1917–1926." *Historical Geography* 25 (1997): 25–45.

Brieger, Gert H. "The Flexner Report: Revised or Revisited?" *Medical Heritage* 1 (1985): 24–34.

Brinkley, Garland L. "The Economic Impact of Disease in the American South, 1860–1940." *Journal of Economic History.* 55, no. 2 (June 1995): 371–73.

Bronfman, Mario, and Jorge Díaz Polanco. "La Cooperación Técnica Internacional y las Políticas de Salud." *Ciência e Saúde Coletiva* 8, no. 1 (2003): 227–41.

Brown, E. Richard. "Public Health in Imperialism: Early Rockefeller Programs at Home and Abroad." *American Journal of Public Health* 66, no. 9 (1976): 897–903.

———. "Rockefeller Medicine in China: Professionalism and Imperialism." In *Philanthropy and Cultural Imperialism: The Foundations at Home and Abroad.* Edited by Robert Arnove, 123–46. Boston: G. K. Hall and Co., 1980.

———. *Rockefeller Medicine Men.* Berkeley: University of California Press, 1979.

Brown, Jonathan C. *Oil and Revolution in Mexico.* Berkeley: University of California Press, 1993.

Brown, Peter. "Failure-as-Success: Multiple Meanings of Eradication in the Rockefeller Foundation Sardinia Project, 1946–1951." *Parassitologia* 40, nos. 1–2 (1998): 117–30.

———. "Malaria, Miseria, and Underpopulation in Sardinia: The 'Malaria Blocks Development' Cultural Model." *Medical Anthropology* 17 (1997): 239–54.

Brown, Theodore M. "Alan Gregg and the Rockefeller Foundation's Support of Franz Alexander's Psychosomatic Research." *Bulletin of the History of Medicine* 61, no. 2 (Summer 1987): 155–82.

Brown, Theodore M, Marcos Cueto, and Elizabeth Fee. "The World Health Organization and the Transition from 'International' to 'Global' Public Health," *American Journal of Public Health* 96, no. 1 (2006): 62–72.

Buhler-Wilkerson, Karen. "Bringing Care to the People: Lillian Wald's Legacy to Public Health Nursing." *American Journal of Public Health* 83 (1993): 1778–86.

Bullock, Mary. *An American Transplant: The Rockefeller Foundation and Peking Union Medical College.* Berkeley: University of California Press, 1980.

Bulman, Francisco, et al. "Dictamen Presentado a la Academia Nacional de Medicina, por la Comisión Encargada de Estudiar el Trabajo de Concurso Titulado: Tratamiento de la Uncinariasis, y Emparado por el Problema: Pro Aris et Focis Certare." *Gaceta Médica de México* 58, no. 6 (1927): 372–81.

Bulmer, Martin. "Philanthropic Foundations and the Development of the Social Sciences in the Early Twentieth Century: A Reply to Donald Fisher." *Sociology* 18 (1984): 572–79.

Bustamante, Miguel E. *Cinco Personajes de la Salud en México.* México, D.F.: Grupo Editorial Miguel Angel Porrúa, 1986.

———. "La Coordinación de los Servicios Sanitarios Federales y Locales Como Factor de Progreso Higiénico en México." *Gaceta Médica de México* 65 (1934): 179–228.

———. "La Coordinación de los Servicios Sanitarios Federales y Locales Como Factor de Progreso Higiénico en México." In *La Atención Médica en el Medio Rural Mexicano.* Edited by Héctor Hernández Llamas, 35–90. México, D.F.: IMSS, 1984.

Bustamante, Miguel E. "El Doctor Liceaga, Higienista." *Gaceta Médica de México* 70 (1940): 79–91.

————. "Distribución Geográfica de la Fiebre Amarilla en México de 1800 a 1923." *Revista del Instituto de Salubridad y Enfermedades Tropicales* 3, no. 2 (June, 1942): 93–105.

————. "Educación Sanitaria por Aplicación Práctica de los Conocimientos de Higiene." *Gaceta Médica de México* 68, no. 6 (1937): 651–63.

————. *La Fiebre Amarilla en México y su Origen en América.* México, D.F.: SSA, 1958.

————. "Hechos Sobresalientes en la Historia de la Secretaría de Salubridad y Asistencia." *Salud Pública de México* 25 (1983): 465–82.

————. "Higiene Municipal." *Revista Médica Veracruzana* 11 (1930): 81.

————. "Local Public Health Work in Mexico." *American Journal of Public Health* 21 (1931): 725–36.

————. "Mortalidad de Menores de un Año por Entidades Federales-México, 1923" 1941." *Revista del Instituto de Salubridad y Enfermedades Tropicales* 5 (1944): 101–15.

————. "Papel del Médico Rural en la Investigación de las Enfermedades Tropicales en México." *Boletín de la Oficina Sanitaria Panamericana* 16, no. 2 (February 1937): 112–15.

————. "Los Parásitos Intestinales y la Salud Pública." *Pasteur: Revista Mensual de Medicina* 6, II, no. 2 (1933): 29–34.

————. "Los Primeros Cincuenta Años de la Oficina Sanitaria Panamericana." *Boletín de la Oficina Sanitaria Panamericana* 33, no. 6 (1952): 471–531.

————. "Problemas y Adquisiciones Recientes de la Higiene y la Medicina Preventiva." *Salubridad y Asistencia* 7 (1947): 153–60.

————. "Public Health and Medical Care in Mexico." *Annals of the American Academy of Political and Social Science* 208 (March 1940): 153–61.

————. "La Situación Epidemiológica de México en el Siglo XIX." In *Ensayos Sobre la Historia de las Epidemias en México.* Edited by Enrique Florescano and Elsa Malvido, vol. 1, 37–66. México, D.F.: IMSS, 1982.

Bustamante, Miguel E, and Fernando Martínez Cortés. "Nota Sobre los Trabajos de Investigación en Salud Pública en México." *Salud Pública de México* 28 (1986): 191–97.

Bynum, William. "Policing Hearts of Darkness: Aspects of the International Sanitary Conferences." *History and Philosophy of the Life Sciences* 15 (1993): 421–34.

Caldwell, Bert W. "Informe de los Trabajos Efectuados en el Mes de Septiembre de 1921 Contra la Fiebre Amarilla en la Zona de Tampico-Túxpam." In *Memoria de la Primera Convención de Fiebre Amarilla, Octubre 15–20 de 1921,* 85–92. México, D.F.: DSP, 1921.

Cárdenas, Enrique, ed. *Historia Económica de México, Lecturas.* Vol. 3. México, D.F.: Fondo de Cultura Económica, 1992.

Cárdenas, Lázaro. "Anunciación al Pueblo de la Expropiación de Petroleo." Palacio Nacional, March 18, 1938. Reprinted in *Cuadernos Americanos* 30, no. 1 (1971): 105–8.

Cárdenas de la Peña, Enrique. *Medicina Familiar en México.* México, D.F.: IMSS, 1974.

Carmona y Valle, Manuel. *Leçons sur l'étiologie et la prophylaxie de la fièvre jaune, données à la fin de l'année 1884 aux élèves de clinique interne.* Mexico: Imp. du Ministère des Travaux Publiques, 1885.

Carnegie, Andrew. "The Gospel of Wealth." *North American Review* 148 (1889): 653–64, and 149 (1889): 682–98.

Carr, Henry P. "Conferencia Sobre la Uncinariasis Sustentada por el Doctor Henry Carr en el Departamento de Salubridad." *Salubridad* 3, nos. 3–4 (1932): 463–72.

———. "Lucha Contra la Uncinariasis." *Salubridad* 1 (1930): 175–82.

———. "Observations upon Hookworm Disease in Mexico." *American Journal of Hygiene* 6 (July Supplement, 1926): 42–61.

———. "Trabajos Desarrollados en la Lucha Contra La Uncinariasis." *Salubridad* 1, no. 3 (1930): 784–88.

———. "Trabajos Especiales del Servicio de Higiene Rural, a Cargo del Señor Dr. Henry P. Carr." *Salubridad* 3 (1932): 443–45.

Carrillo, Ana María. "Los Dificiles Caminos de la Campaña Antivariolosa en México." *Ciencias* 55–56 (July–December 1999): 18–25.

———. "Economía, Política, y Salud Pública en el México Porfiriano, 1876–1910." *História, Ciências, Saúde—Manguinhos* 9 (Supplement, 2002): 67–87.

———. "Epidemias, Saber Médico, y Salud Pública en el Porfiriato." PhD diss., UNAM, forthcoming.

———. "Estado de Peste o Estado de Sitio: Sinaloa y Baja California, 1902–1903." *Historia Mexicana* 54 (2005): 1049–1103.

———. "El Inicio de la Higiene Escolar en México: Congreso Higiénico Pedagógico de 1882." *Revista Mexicana de Pediatría* 66, no. 2 (March–April 1999): 71–74.

———. "Los Médicos Ante la Primera Campaña Antituberculosa en México." *Gaceta Médica de México* 137, no. 4 (2001): 361–69.

———. "Médicos del México Decimonónico: Entre el Control Estatal y la Autonomía Profesional." *Dynamis* 22 (2002): 351–75.

———. "Miguel E. Bustamante." In *Ciencia y Tecnología en México en el Siglo XX. Biografías de Personajes Ilustres.* Vol. 3, 143–58. México, D.F.: Secretaría de Educación Pública/Academia Mexicana de Ciencias/Consejo Consultivo de Ciencias de la Presidencia de la República/Consejo Nacional de Ciencia y Tecnología, 2003.

———. "Nacimiento y Muerte de una Profesión: Las Parteras Tituladas en México." *Dynamis* 19 (1999): 167–90.

———. "National and Imperial Interests in the American Public Health Association." Paper presented at the Latin American Perspectives on International Health symposium, University of Toronto, Toronto, Canada, May 5–7, 2005.

———. "La Patología del Siglo XIX y los Institutos Nacionales de Investigación Médica en México." *LABORAT-acta* 8, no. 1 (2001): 23–31.

———. "Physicians 'Who Know' and Midwives Who 'Need to Learn.'" In *Midwives in Mexico: Controversy and Change.* Edited by Robbie Davys-Floyd, Marcia Good-Maust, and Miguel Guernez. Austin: University of Texas Press, forthcoming.

———. "Pioneros de la Seguridad Social en México." *Boletín de la Sociedad Mexicana de Historia y Filosofía de la Medicina* 2 (2000): 26–32.

———. "Profesiones Sanitarias y Lucha de Poderes en el México del Siglo XIX." *Asclepio, Revista de Historia de la Medicina y de la Ciencia* 50, no. 2 (1998): 149–68.

———. "Salud Pública y Poder Durante el Cardenismo. México, 1934–1940." *Dynamis* 25 (2005): 145–78.

———. "Surgimiento y Desarrollo de la Participación Federal en los Servicios de Salud." In *Perspectiva Histórica de Atención a la Salud en México, 1902–2002.* Edited by Guillermo Fajardo Ortiz, Ana María Carrillo, and Rolando Neri Vela, 17–64. México, D.F.: Organización Panamericana de la Salud (OPS), 2002.

Carter, Henry Rose. *Yellow Fever: An Epidemiological and Historical Study of Its Place of Origin.* Baltimore: Williams and Wilkins, 1931.

Cassedy, James H. *Charles V. Chapin and the Public Health Movement.* Cambridge: Harvard University Press, 1962.

———. "The 'Germ of Laziness' in the South, 1900–1915: Charles Wardell Stiles and the Progressive, Paradox." *Bulletin of the History of Medicine* 45 (1971): 159–69.

Castañeda Camey, Xóchitl, Leonora Guzmán, and Ana Langer. "Una Alternativa para la Atención Perinatal: Las Parteras Tradicionales en el Estado de Morelos." *Ginecología y Obstetricia de México* 55 (December 1991): 353–57.

Castillo Nájera, Francisco. "Acta de la Tercera Sesión Plena, Octubre 18 de 1921." In *Memoria de la Primera Convención de Fiebre Amarilla, Octubre 15–20 de 1921,* 148. México, D.F.: DSP, 1921.

Cervera E. "Contestación al Trabajo del Nuevo Académico, Dr. Juan Solórzano Morfín." *Gaceta Médica de México* 58, no. 12 (1927): 760–64.

Cervera Andrade, Alejandro. "El Doctor Harald Seidelin." *Boletín Informativo de la Facultad de Medicina, Universidad de Yucatán* 1, no. 4 (1966): 34–36.

Chapin, Charles V. "Dirt, Disease, and the Health Officer." In *Papers of Charles V. Chapin, M.D.: A Review of Public Health Realities.* Edited by Clarence L. Scamman. New York: The Commonwealth Fund, 1934.

———. "State Health Organization." *Journal of the American Medical Association* 66, no. 10 (March 4, 1916): 699–703.

Chávez, Ignacio. *México en la Cultura Médica.* México, D.F.: El Colegio Nacional, 1947.

Chernow, Ron. *Titan: The Life of John D. Rockefeller, Sr.* New York: Random House, 1998.

Chomsky, Aviva. *West Indian Workers and the United Fruit Company in Costa Rica, 1870–1940.* Baton Rouge: Louisiana State University Press, 1996.

Cirillo, Vincent J. *Bullets and Bacilli: The Spanish-American War and Military Medicine.* New Brunswick, NJ: Rutgers University Press, 2004.

Cleaver, Harry. "Malaria, the Politics of Public Health, and the International Crisis." *Review of Radical Political Economics* 9 (1977): 81–103.

Cline, Howard F. *The United States and Mexico.* New York: Atheneum, 1966.

Cockroft, James. *Mexico's Hope: An Encounter with Politics and History.* New York: Monthly Review Press, 1998.

———. *Precursores Intelectuales de la Revolución Mexicana.* México, D.F.: Siglo XXI Editores, 1971.

"Código Sanitario de los Estados Unidos de México." *Boletín de la Oficina Sanitaria Panamericana* 5 (1926): 367–456.

Cohen, William B. "Malaria and French Imperialism," *Journal of African History* 24 (1983): 23–36.

Colby, Gerard, and Charlotte Dennett. *Thy Will Be Done: The Conquest of the Amazon: Nelson Rockefeller and Evangelism in the Age of Oil.* New York: Harper Collins Publishers, 1995.

Coleman, William. *Yellow Fever in the North: The Methods of Early Epidemiology.* Madison: University of Wisconsin Press, 1987.

Comité Ejecutivo Nacional del PNR, *Plan Sexenal del Partido Nacional Revolucionaro.* México, D.F.: 1934.

Connor M. E. "Acta de la Primera Sesión Plena, Octubre 15 de 1921." In *Memoria de la Primera Convención de Fiebre Amarilla, Octubre 15–20 de 1921*, 78. México, D.F.: DSP, 1921.

———. "Informe Preliminar Sobre la Campaña Contra la Fiebre Amarilla en Mérida, Yuc." In *Memoria de la Primera Convención de Fiebre Amarilla, Octubre 1–21 de 1921*, 21–25. México, D.F.: DSP, 1921.

Cook, Noble David. *Born to Die: Disease and New World Conquest, 1492–1650*. Cambridge: Cambridge University Press, 1998.

Cooper, Donald B. *Epidemic Disease in Mexico City, 1716–1813: An Administrative, Social, and Medical Study*. Austin: Institute of Latin American Studies, University of Texas Press, 1965.

Cooper, Donald C. "Brazil's Long Fight against Epidemic Disease, 1849–1917, with Special Emphasis on Yellow Fever." *Bulletin of the New York Academy of Medicine* 51 (1975): 672–96.

Córdova, Arnaldo. *La Ideología de la Revolución Mexicana*. México, D.F.: Ediciones Era, 1973.

———. *La Política de Masas del Cardenismo*. México D.F.: Serie Popular Era, 1974.

Cosío Villegas, Daniel. *A Compact History of Mexico*. México, D.F.: El Colegio de México, 1974.

———, ed. *Historia Moderna de México*. 8 vols. México, D.F.: Hermes, 1955–74.

Cosminsky, Sheila. "Childbirth and Change: A Guatemalan Study." In *Ethnography of Fertility and Birth*. Edited by Carol P. MacCormack, 205–29. New York: Academic Press, 1982.

———. "Midwifery and Medical Anthropology." In *Modern Medicine and Medical Anthropology in the United States–Mexico Border Population*. Edited by Boris Velimirovic, 116–26. Washington, DC: Pan American Health Organization (PAHO), Scientific Publication no. 359, 1978.

Cotter, Joseph. "The Rockefeller Foundation's Mexican Agricultural Project: A Cross-Cultural Encounter: 1943–1949." In *Missionaries of Science: The Rockefeller Foundation and Latin America*. Edited by Marcos Cueto, 97–125. Bloomington: Indiana University Press, 1994.

Crandon-Malamud, Libbet. *From the Fat of Our Souls: Social Change, Political Process, and Medical Pluralism in Bolivia*. Berkeley: University of California Press, 1991.

Craven, David. *Diego Rivera: As Epic Modernist*. Boston: G. K. Hall, 1997.

Crispín Castellanos, Margarito. "Hospital de Maternidad e Infancia. Una Perspectiva Histórica de un Centro de Beneficencia Pública de Fines del Siglo XIX." In *La Atención Materno Infantil: Apuntes para su Historia*. Edited by México, Secretaría de Salud, Dirección General de Atención Materno Infantil, 95–115. México, D.F.: Secretaría de Salud, 1993.

Croizier, Ralph. *Traditional Medicine in Modern China: Science, Nationalism, and the Tensions of Cultural Change*. Cambridge: Harvard University Press, 1968.

Crosby, Alfred W, Jr. *The Columbian Exchange: Biological and Cultural Consequences of 1492*. Westport, CT: Greenwood Press, 1972.

Cuarón, Alfredo. "Informe Presentado por el Delegado Sanitario Especial en Tampico." In *Memoria de la Primera Convención de Fiebre Amarilla, Octubre 15–20 de 1921*, 93–96. México, D.F.: DSP, 1921.

Cueto, Marcos. "The Cycles of Eradication: The Rockefeller Foundation and Latin American Public Health, 1918–1940." In *International Health Organisations and Movements, 1918–1939*. Edited by Paul Weindling, 222–43. Cambridge: Cambridge University Press, 1995.

———. "International Health, The Rockefeller Foundation and Latin America during the 1940s." *Research Reports from the Rockefeller Archive Center* (Fall 2002): 17–20.

———, ed. *Missionaries of Science: The Rockefeller Foundation and Latin America.* Bloomington: Indiana University Press, 1994.

———. "The Origins of Primary Health Care and Selective Primary Health Care." *American Journal of Public Health* 94 (2004): 1864–74.

———. "The Promise of Primary Care." *Bulletin of the World Health Organization* 83, no. 5 (2005): 322.

———. *El Regreso de las Epidemias. Salud y Sociedad en el Perú del Siglo XX.* Lima: Instituto de Estudios Peruanos (IEP), 1997.

———. "Una Reforma Fallida: La Fundación Rockefeller, La Malaria y la Salud Pública en el Peru, 1940–1949." *Revista Peruana de Ciencias Sociales* 2 (1990): 9–29.

———, ed. *Salud Cultura y Sociedad en América Latina: Nuevas Perspectivas Históricas.* Lima: IEP/OPS, 1996.

———. "Sanitation from Above: Yellow Fever and Foreign Intervention in Peru, 1919–1922." *Hispanic American Historical Review* 72, no. 1 (1992): 1–22.

———. *El Valor de la Salud: Una Historia de la Organización Panamericana de la Salud.* Washington DC: OPS, 2004.

———. "Visions of Science and Development: The Rockefeller Foundation and the Latin American Medical Surveys of the 1920s." In *Missionaries of Science: The Rockefeller Foundation and Latin America.* Edited by Marcos Cueto, 1–22. Bloomington: Indiana University Press, 1994.

Curti, Merle. "American Philanthropy and the National Character." *American Quarterly* 10 (1958): 420–37.

———. "Philanthropy." In *Dictionary of the History of Ideas.* Edited by Philip P. Wiener, 486–93. New York: Scribner, 1973–74.

Curtin, Philip D. *Disease and Empire: The Health of European Troops in the Conquest of Africa.* Cambridge: Cambridge University Press, 1998.

Darling, Samuel Taylor, Marshall Albert Barber, H. P. Hacker, and Robert Goldsmith. *Hookworm and Malaria Research in Malaya, Java, and the Fiji Islands: Report of the Uncinariasis Commission to the Orient.* New York: Rockefeller Foundation, International Health Board Publication No. 9, 1920.

de Campos, André Luiz Vieira. "The Institute of Inter-American Affairs and Its Health Policies in Brazil during World War II." *Presidential Studies Quarterly* 28, no. 3 (1998): 523–34.

de Castro Santos, Luiz A. "A Fundacão Rockefeller e o Estado Nacional: Historia e Politica de uma Missão Médica e Sanitaria no Brasil." *Revista Brasileira de Estudos de Populacão* 6, no. 1 (1989): 105–10.

———. "Os Primeiros Centros de Saúde nos Estados Unidos e no Brasil: Um Estudo Comparativo." *Teoria e Pesquisa* 40/41 (January–July, 2002): 137–81.

———. "Power, Ideology, and Public Health in Brazil, 1889–1930." PhD diss., Harvard University, 1987.

"The Declaration of Alma-Ata." *International Conference on Primary Care*, Alma-Ata, USSR, 6–12 September, 1978, World Health Organization.

Deeks, William E. *A Review of the Digestive Functions and Food Requirements for the Maintenance of Health with Particular Reference to the Tropics*. Boston: United Fruit Company, 1925.

de la Garza Brito, Angel. "La Enseñanza de la Medicina Preventiva y de la Higiene, Factor en la Asistencia Médico Social." *Boletín de la Oficina Sanitaria Panamericana* 23, no. 7 (July 1944): 607–18.

———. "La Escuela de Salubridad e Higiene: Programas." *Salubridad y Asistencia* 7, no. 1 (1947): 117–21.

———. "La Nueva Administración Pública." *Sociedad Mexicana de Higiene* (June 1950): 60–65.

———. "El Presente y el Futuro de la Educación Higiénica Profesional en México." *Pasteur: Revista Mensual de Medicina* 14, I, no. 1 (1941): 10–14.

———. "Progreso y Necesidades de la Higiene Rural." *Pasteur: Revista Mensual de Medicina* 10, II, no. 4 (1937): 146–56.

———. "La Universidad en Relación con la Higiene Pública." *Pasteur: Revista Mensual de Medicina* 8, II, no. 1 (1935): 32–37.

de la Peña, Guillermo. *A Legacy of Promises: Agriculture, Politics and Ritual in the Morelos Highlands of Mexico*. Austin: University of Texas Press, 1981.

Delaporte, François. *The History of Yellow Fever: An Essay on the Birth of Tropical Medicine*. Cambridge, MA: MIT Press, 1991.

del Castillo Troncoso, Alberto. "La Visión de los Médicos y el Reconocimiento de la Niñez en el Cambio del Siglo XIX al XX." *Boletín Mexicano de Historia y Filosofía de Medicina* 6, no. 2 (2003): 10–16.

Denoon, Donald. *Public Health in Papua New Guinea: Medical Possibility and Social Constraint, 1884–1984*. Cambridge: Cambridge University Press, 1989.

Departamento de Salubridad Pública. *Rural Hygiene and Social Medicine Services of the Department of Public Health: Organization-Functions, Results Obtained until 1940*. México, D.F.: DSP, 1941.

de Reyes del Campillo, Celia A. *Hermana Campesina*. México, D.F.: Departamento Autónomo de Prensa y Publicidad, 1938.

Despommier, Dickson D, Robert W. Gwadz, Peter J. Hotez, and Charles Knirsch. *Parasitic Diseases*. 4th ed. New York: Apple Tree, 2000.

Deutsch, Albert. *The World Health Organization: Its Global Battle against Disease*. New York: Public Affairs Committee, 1958.

Díaz Barriga Aguilar, Jesús, and José Quintín Olascoaga. "Lo que Come el Pueblo Mexicano y lo que Necesita Comer para Estar Bien Nutrido."*Salubridad y Asistencia* 1 (1949): 5–30.

Diez-Roux, Ana. "Bringing Context Back into Epidemiology: Variables and Fallacies in Multi-Level Analysis." *American Journal of Public Health* 88, no. 2 (1998): 216–22.

Dirección General de Estadística. *Cincuenta Años de Revolución Mexicana en Cifras*, México, D.F.: Nacional Financiera, S.A.. Subgerencia de Investigaciones Económicas, 1963.

"La Dirección de Cooperación Interamericana de Salubridad Pública." *Salubridad y Asistencia* 7, no. 3 (1947): 259–61.

Dirección General de Educación Pública. *Constitución Política de los Estados Unidos Mexicanos*. México, D.F.: Dirección General de Educación Pública, 1917.

Dobson, Mary J, M. Malowany, and R. W. Snow. "Malaria Control in East Africa: The Kampala Conference and the Pare-Taveta Scheme: A Meeting of Common and High Ground." *Parassitologia* 40, nos. 1 and 2 (June 1998): 149–66.

Donaldson, Peter. "Foreign Intervention in Medical Education: A Case Study of the Rockefeller Foundation's Involvement in a Thai Medical School." *International Journal of Health Services* 6 (1976): 251–70.

Donaldson, Peter J. "On the Origins of the United States Government's International Population Policy." *Population Studies* 44, no. 3 (1990): 385–99.

do Rosario Costa, Nilson. *Lutas Urbanas e Controle Sanitario: Origens das Políticas de Saúde no Brasil.* Petropolis, Brasil: Vozes & Abrasco, 1985.

Downs, Wilbur. "History of Epidemiological Aspects of Yellow Fever." *Yale Journal of Biology and Medicine* 55 (1982): 179–85.

Downs, Wilbur, E. Bordas, and A. Arizmende. "Colonialización en el Laboratorio de Anopheles Aztecus Hoffmann." *Revista del Instituto de Salubridad y Enfermedades Tropicales* 9 (1948): 175–76.

Downs, Wilbur, E. Bordas, and A. Enríquez-Chaves. "El Control del Paludismo en la Región de Xochimilco, D.F." *Revista del Instituto de Salubridad y Enfermedades Tropicales* 11 (1950): 99–103.

Doyal, Lesley. *The Political Economy of Health.* Boston: South End Press, 1979.

Dubin, Martin David. "The League of Nations Health Organisation," in Paul Weindling, ed., *International Health, Organisations, and Movements, 1918–1939:* 56–80. Cambridge: Cambridge University Press, 1995.

Duffy, John. *Sword of Pestilence: The New Orleans Yellow Fever Epidemic of 1853.* Baton Rouge: Louisiana State University Press, 1966.

———. "Yellow Fever in the Continental United States during the Nineteenth Century." *Bulletin of the New York Academy of Medicine* 54 (1968): 687–701.

Dunham, George G. "The Cooperative Health Program of the American Republics." *American Journal of Public Health* 34, no. 8 (1944): 818–19.

Duque, Luis Fernando. "The Future of Schools of Public Health in Latin America." In *Schools of Public Health in Latin America.* Report of a Macy Conference, Medellín, Colombia, November 17–19, 1974: 1–9. New York: Josiah Macy Jr. Foundation, 1974.

Dwork, Deborah. *War Is Good for Babies and Other Children: A History of the Infant and Child Welfare Movement in England, 1898–1918.* London: Tavistock, 1987.

Echenberg, Myron. *Black Death, White Medicine: Bubonic Plague and the Politics of Public Health in Colonial Senegal, 1914–1945.* Portsmouth, NH: Heinemann, 2002.

Ehrick, Christine. "Affectionate Mothers and the Colossal Machine: Feminism, Social Assistance and the State in Uruguay, 1910–1932." *The Americas* 58 (2001): 121–39.

———. "Madrinas and Missionaries: Uruguay and the Pan-American Women's Movement." *Gender and History* 10 (1998): 406–24.

Ellis, John H. *Yellow Fever and Public Health in the New South.* Lexington: University Press of Kentucky, 1992.

Enciclopedia de México. Vol. 5. México, D.F.: Enciclopedia de México, 1978.

"Epidemics in Mexico." *The Lancet* 140, no. 3616 (December 1892): 1404.

Erosa Barbachana, Arturo. "El Gobierno de Juárez y la Salud Pública de México." *Salud Pública de México* 19 (1977): 375–81.

Eroza Solana, Enrique, and Miguel Ángel Marmolejo. *El Agua en la Cosmovisión y Terapéutica de los Pueblos Indígenas de México.* México, D.F.: INI, 1999.

Escárcega López, Everardo, and Saúl Escobar Toledo. *Historia de la Cuestión Agraria Mexicana, 5. El Cardenismo: Un Parteaguas Histórico en el Proceso Nacional, 1934–1940.* México, D.F.: Siglo XXI Editores, 1990.

Espinosa Yunis, Leova. *Tradiciones y Costumbre del Sur de Veracruz: Recopilación y Rescate de las Raíces de Nuestra Identidad.* Guadalajara: Editorial Pandora, 2000.

Estrada Urroz, Rosalinda. "Control Sanitario o Control Social: La Reglamentación Prostibularia en el Porfiriato." *Boletín Mexicano de Historia y Filosofía de Medicina* 5, no. 2 (2002): 21–25.

Ettling, John. *The Germ of Laziness: Rockefeller Philanthropy and Public Health in the New South.* Cambridge, MA: Harvard University Press, 1981.

Eugenic News 22 (1937): 94.

Evans, Richard. *Death in Hamburg: Society and Politics in the Cholera Years 1830–1910.* Oxford: Oxford University Press, 1987.

"Extracto del Mensaje del General Alvaro Obregón, Presidente de los Estados Unidos de México." *Boletín de la Oficina Sanitaria Panamericana* 2 (1923): 301–4.

Fajardo Ortiz, Guillermo, Ana María Carrillo, and Rolando Neri Vela. *Perspectiva Histórica de Atención a la Salud en México, 1902–2002.* México, D.F.: OPS, 2002.

Falcón, Ojeda. "Apuntes Sobre el Ultimo Brote de Fiebre Amarilla Ocurrido en el Puerto de Veracruz, 1920–1921." *Boletín Epidemiológico* 19, no. 1 (1955): 71–77.

Falcón, Romana, and Soledad García Morales. *La Semilla en el Surco: Adalberto Tejeda y el Radicalismo en Veracruz, 1883–1960.* México, D.F.: El Colegio de México, 1986.

Fallaw, Ben. *Cárdenas Compromised: The Failure of Reform in Postrevolutionary Yucatán.* Durham, NC: Duke University Press, 2001.

Farley, John. *Bilharzia: A History of Imperial Tropical Medicine.* Cambridge: Cambridge University Press, 1991.

———. "The International Health Division of the Rockefeller Foundation: The Russell Years, 1920–1939." In *International Health Organisations and Movements, 1918–1939.* Edited by Paul Weindling, 203–43. Cambridge: Cambridge University Press, 1995.

———. *To Cast Out Disease: A History of the International Health Division of the Rockefeller Foundation, 1913–1951.* New York: Oxford University Press, 2004.

Faust, Ernest Carroll. *Human Helminthology: A Manual for Clinicians, Sanitarians, and Medical Zoologists.* Philadelphia: Lea and Febiger, 1929.

Fee, Elizabeth. *Disease and Discovery: A History of the Johns Hopkins School of Hygiene and Public Health, 1916–1939.* Baltimore: Johns Hopkins University Press, 1987.

———. "The Origins and Development of Public Health in the United States." In *Oxford Textbook of Public Health.* 3rd edition. Edited by Roger Detels, Walter Holland, James McEwen, and Gilbert S. Omenn, 33–54. Oxford: Oxford University Press, 1997.

———. "Public Health and the State: The United States." In *The History of Public Health and the Modern State.* Wellcome Series in the History of Medicine. Edited by Dorothy Porter, 224–75. Amsterdam: Rodopi, 1994.

Fee, Elizabeth, and Roy Acheson, eds. *A History of Education in Public Health: Health that Mocks the Doctors' Rules.* Oxford: Oxford University Press, 1991.

Fein, Seth. "Everyday Forms of Transnational Collaboration: U.S. Film Propaganda in Cold War Mexico." In *Close Encounters of Empire: Writing the Cultural History of U.S.-Latin American Relations*. Edited by Gilbert Joseph, Catherine LeGrand, and Ricardo Salvatore, 400–450. Durham, NC: Duke University Press, 1998.

Fenner F, D. A. Henderson, I. Arita, Z. Jezek, and I. D. Ladnyi. *Smallpox and Its Eradication*. Geneva: World Health Organization, 1988.

Ferguson, Mary. *China Medical Board and Peking Union Medical College: A Chronicle of Fruitful Collaboration, 1914–1951*. New York: The China Medical Board of New York, 1970.

Fernández del Castillo, Francisco. *Antología de los Escritos Histórico-Médicos del Doctor F. Fernández del Castillo*. México, D.F.: Facultad de Medicina, Universidad Nacional Autónoma de México, 1982.

Ficker, Sandra Kuntz. "The Export Boom of the Mexican Revolution: Characteristics and Contributing Factors." *Journal of Latin American Studies* 36 (2004): 267–96.

Fidler, David. "The Globalization of Public Health: The First 100 Years of International Health Diplomacy." *Bulletin of the World Health Organization* 79 (2001): 842–49.

Fildes, Valerie, Lara Marks, and Hilary Marland, eds. *Women and Children First: International Maternal and Infant Welfare, 1870–1945*. London: Routledge, 1992.

Finkler, Kaja. *Physicians at Work, Patients in Pain: Biomedical Practice and Patient Response in Mexico*. Boulder, CO: Westview Press, 1991.

———. *Spiritualist Healers in Mexico: Successes and Failures of Alternative Therapeutics*. New York: Praeger Publishers, 1985.

Finnemore, Martha. "Redefining Development at the World Bank." In *International Development and the Social Sciences: Essays on the History and Politics of Knowledge*. Edited by F. Cooper and R. Packard, 203–27. Berkeley: University of California Press, 1997.

Fisher, Donald. "Philanthropic Foundations and the Social Sciences: A Response to Martin Bulmer." *Sociology* 18 (1984): 580–87.

———. "Rockefeller Philanthropy and the British Empire: The Creation of the London School of Hygiene and Tropical Medicine." *History of Education* 7 (1978): 129–43.

———. "The Role of Philanthropic Foundations in the Reproduction and Production of Hegemony: Rockefeller Foundation and the Social Sciences." *Sociology* 17 (1983): 206–33.

Fitzgerald, Deborah. "Exporting American Agriculture: The Rockefeller Foundation in Mexico, 1943–1953." *Social Studies of Science* 16 (1986): 457–83.

Flexner, Abraham. *Medical Education in the United States and Canada*. New York: Carnegie Foundation for the Advancement of Teaching, Bulletin no. 4, 1910.

Flores, Francisco A. *Historia de la Medicina en México Desde la Epoca de los Indios Hasta el Presente*. México, D.F.: Oficina de la Secretaría de Fomento, 1886.

Flores Talavera, Rodolfo, and Miguel E. Bustamante. "Salud Pública y Desarrollo Económico y Social." *Salud Pública de México* 5 (1963): 777–91.

Foix, Pere. *Cárdenas*. México, D.F.: Editorial Trillas, 1971.

Fosdick, Raymond. *Adventure in Giving: The Story of the General Education Board*. New York: Harper and Row, 1962.

Fosdick, Raymond B. *The Story of the Rockefeller Foundation*. 2nd ed. New Brunswick, NJ: Transaction Publishers, 1989.

Foster, George M. "On the Origin of Humoral Medicine in Latin America." *Medical Anthropology Quarterly* 1 (1987): 355–99.

Fowler-Salamini, Heather. *Agrarian Radicalism in Veracruz, 1920–1938.* Lincoln: University of Nebraska Press, 1978.

———. "Gender, Work, and Coffee in Córdoba, Veracruz, 1850–1910." In *Women of the Mexican Countryside, 1850–1990: Creating Spaces, Shaping Transitions.* Edited by Heather Fowler-Salamini and Mary Kay Vaughan, 51–73. Tucson: University of Arizona Press, 1994.

———. "Gender, Work, and Working-Class Women's Culture in the Veracruz Coffee Export Industry, 1920–1945." *International Labor and Working-Class History* 63 (Spring, 2003):102–21.

———. "Women Coffee Sorters Confront the Mill Owners and the Veracruz Revolutionary State, 1915–1918." *Journal of Women's History* 14 (Spring 2002): 34–63.

Fox, Daniel M, and Jordan S. Kassalow. "Making Health a Priority of U.S. Foreign Policy." *American Journal of Public Health* 91 (2001): 1554–56.

Franco Agudelo, Saúl. *El Paludismo en América Latina.* Guadalajara: Editorial Universidad de Guadalajara, 1990.

———. "The Rockefeller Foundation's Antimalarial Program in Latin America: Donating or Dominating?" *International Journal of Health Services* 13 (1983): 51–67.

Frenk, Julio, Daniel López Acuña, José Luis Bobadilla, and Alejandro Alagón. "Medicina Liberal y Medicina Institucional en México." *Salud Pública de México* 18, no. 3 (1976): 481–93.

Friedlander, Judith. "Doña Zeferina Barreto: Biographical Sketch of an Indian Woman from the State of Morelos." In *Women of the Mexican Countryside, 1850–1990.* Edited by Heather Fowler-Salamini and Mary Kay Vaughan, 125–39. Tucson: University of Arizona Press, 1994.

Fuerbringer Bermeo, Mädy, Eugenia Barrientos González, Juana Rodríguez Velázquez, and Liliana González Fuerbringer. *Poblanas en la Salud Pública de México: Historias de Vida y Semblanzas.* Puebla, México: Honorable Ayuntamiento del Municipio de Puebla, 2001.

Gadelha, Paulo. "Conforming Strategies of Public Health Campaigns to Disease Specificity and National Contexts: The Rockefeller Foundation's Early Campaigns against Hookworm and Malaria in Brazil." *Parassitologia* 40, nos. 1–2 (1998): 159–75.

Gahan, James B, and George C. Payne. "Control de Anopheles Pseudopunctipennis con Pulveraciones Residuales de DDT Aplicadas en Edificios en México." *Salubridad y Asistencia* 6, no. 18 (1946): 71–76.

Gallager, Nancy Elizabeth. *Egypt's Other Wars: Epidemics and the Politics of Public Health.* Syracuse, NY: Syracuse University Press, 1990.

García Morales, Soledad. *La Rebelión Delahuertista en Veracruz.* Jalapa, México: Universidad Veracruzana, 1986.

Garner, Paul. *Porfirio Diaz: Del Héroe al Dictador: Una Biografía Política.* México, D.F.: Editorial Planeta, 2003.

Garrido, Luis Javier. *El Partido de la Revolución Institucionalizada (Medio Siglo de Poder Político en México): La Formación del Nuevo Estado, 1928–1945.* México, D.F.: Siglo XXI Editores, 1982.

Gastélum, Bernardo J. *Días de Decisiones.* México, D.F.: Sociedad Mexicana de Historia y Filosofía de la Medicina, Monografías 1, 1976.

Gastélum, Bernardo J. *Dos Años Seis Meses de Higiene en Sinaloa*. México, D.F.: DSP, 1934.
———. *Memoria de los Trabajos Realizados por el Departamento de Salubridad Pública 1925–1928*. Vol. I. México, D.F.: DSP, 1928.
Gellman, Irwin F. *Good Neighbor Diplomacy: United States Policies in Latin America, 1933–1945*. Baltimore: Johns Hopkins University Press, 1979.
Gershberg, Alec. "Fiscal Decentralization and Intergovernmental Relations: An Analysis of Federal versus State Education Finance in Mexico." *Review of Urban and Regional Development Studies* 7, 2 (1995): 119–42.
Giannuli, Dimitra. " 'Repeated Disappointment': The Rockefeller Foundation and the Reform of the Greek Public Health System, 1929–1940." *Bulletin of the History of Medicine* 72 (1998): 47–72.
Gillespie, James. "The Rockefeller Foundation, the Hookworm Campaign and a National Health Policy in Australia, 1911–1930." In *Health and Healing in Tropical Australia and Papua New Guinea*. Edited by Roy MacLeod and Donald Denoon, 64–87. Townsville, Australia: James Cook University, 1991.
Gilly, Adolfo. *El Cardenismo: Una Utopía Mexicana*. México, D.F.: Cal y Arena, 1994.
———. *La Revolución Interrumpida; México, 1910–1920: Una Guerra Campesina por la Tierra y el Poder*. México, D.F.: Ediciones El Caballito, 1971, repr. 1994.
Ginzberg, Eitan. "State Agrarianism versus Democratic Agrarianism: Adalberto Tejeda's Experiment in Veracruz, 1928–32." *Journal of Latin American Studies* 30 (1998): 341–72.
Glade, William P Jr, and Charles W. Anderson. *The Political Economy of Mexico*. Madison: University of Wisconsin Press, 1963.
Gladwell, Malcolm. "The Mosquito Killer." *New Yorker*, July 2, 2001, 42–51.
Gledhill, John. *Casi Nada: A Study of Agrarian Reform in the Homeland of Cardenismo*. Albany, NY: State University of New York, Institute for Mesoamerican Studies, 1991.
Glick, Thomas. "La Transferencia de las Revoluciones Científicas a Través de las Fronteras Culturales." *Ciencia y Desarrollo* 72 (1987): 77–89.
Godlee, Fiona. "WHO in Retreat: Is It Losing Its Influence?" *British Medical Journal* 309 (1994): 1491–95.
———. "The World Health Organisation: WHO at Country Level: A Little Impact, No Strategy." *British Medical Journal* 309 (1994): 1636–39.
———. "The World Health Organisation: WHO in Crisis, *British Medical Journal* 309 (1994): 1424–28.
Golden, Janet. *A Social History of Wet-Nursing in America: From Breast to Bottle*. Cambridge: Cambridge University Press, 1996.
Goldstein, Michael, and Peter Donaldson. "Exporting Professionalism: A Case Study of Medical Education." *Journal of Health and Social Behavior* 20 (1979): 322–37.
Gómez-Dantés, Héctor, and Anne-Emanuelle Birn. "Malaria and Social Movements in Mexico: The Last 60 Years." *Parassitologia* 42 (2000): 69–85.
Gómez-Dantés, Octavio. "Health Reform and Policies for the Poor in Mexico." In *Health Reform and Poverty in Latin America*, ed. P. Lloyd-Sherlock, 128–142. London: Institute of Latin American Studies, University of London, 2000.
Gómez-Galvarriato Freer, Aurora. "The Impact of Revolution: Business and Labor in the Mexican Textile Industry, Orizaba, Veracruz, 1900–1930." PhD diss., Harvard University, 1999.
Gómez Pimienta, José Luis. "El Comité Nacional de Lucha contra la Tuberculosis." *Pasteur: Revista Mensual de Medicina* 14, I, no. 1 (1941): 7–9.

Gonzalez, C. L. *Mass Campaigns and General Health Services.* Public Health Papers Number 29. Geneva: World Health Organization, 1965.

Gonzalez, Michael J. *The Mexican Revolution, 1910–1940.* Albuquerque: University of New Mexico Press, 2002.

González-Block, Miguel Angel. "Génesis y Articulación de los Principios Rectores de la Salud Pública de México." *Salud Pública de México* 32, no. 3 (1990): 337–51.

González Herrejón, Salvador. "Estado Actual del Problema de la Oncocercosis en la República Mexicana." *Boletín de la Oficina Sanitaria Panamericana* 15 (1936): 735–43.

González Navarro, Moisés. *La Confederación Nacional Campesina.* México, D.F.: Costa-Amic, 1968.

———. *História Moderna de México: El Porfiriato, La Vida Social.* México, D.F.: Editorial Hermes, 1957.

———. *Sociedad y Cultura en el Porfiriato.* México, D.F.: Cien de México, 1994.

González y González, Luis. *Los Días del Presidente Cárdenas.* México, D.F.: Editorial Clio, 1997.

Goodman, Neville. *International Health Organisations and their Work.* Edinburgh: Churchill Livingstone, 1971.

Gordon, Andrew J. "Mixed Strategies in Health Education and Community Participation: An Evaluation of Dengue Control in the Dominican Republic." *Health and Education Research: Theory and Practice* 3 (1988): 399–419.

Gorgas, William C. *Sanitation in Panama.* New York: Appleton, 1915.

Gould, Lewis L. *America in the Progressive Era, 1890–1914* New York: Longman, 2001.

Government Printing Office. *Foreign Relations of the United States 1924.* Vol 1. Washington, DC: Government Printing Office, 1939.

"Grandes Sabios Franceses que nos Visitan." *Pasteur: Revista Mensual de Medicina* 3, II, no. 2 (1930): 67.

Grant, John B. "International Trends in Health Care." *American Journal of Public Health* 38, 3 (1948): 381–97.

Grant, Martha. "Influencia de las Costumbres y Creencias Populares en los Servicios de un Centro de Salud." *Boletín de la Oficina Sanitaria Panamericana* 33, no. 4 (1952): 283–97.

Green, David. *The Containment of Latin America: A History of the Myths and Realities of the Good Neighbor Policy.* Chicago: Quadrangle, 1971.

Greenough, Paul. "Intimidation, Coercion and Resistance in the Final Stages of the South Asian Smallpox Eradication Campaign, 1973–1975." *Social Science and Medicine* 41, no. 5 (1995): 633–45.

Grey, Michael. *New Deal Medicine: The Rural Health Programs of the Farm Security Administration.* Baltimore: Johns Hopkins University Press, 1999.

Guadarrama L. "Informe de la Campaña Sanitaria contra la Fiebre Amarilla, en Túxpam, Ver. y Algunas Consideraciones sobre la Enfermedad." In *Memoria de la Primera Convención de Fiebre Amarilla, Octubre 15–20 de 1921,* 40–61. México, D.F.: DSP, 1921.

Guerra, Francisco. "Pre-Columbian Medicine: Its Influence on Medicine Today." In *Aspects of the History of Medicine in Latin America.* Edited by John Z. Bowers and Elizabeth F. Purcell, 1–15. New York: Josiah Macy Jr. Foundation, 1979.

Guiteras G. M. "Sanitary Work in Vera Cruz during the First Three Weeks of the American Occupation." *Public Health Reports* 29 (1914): 1619–23.

Gutiérrez A. "Informe de la Campaña Contra la Fiebre Amarilla que se ha Desarrollado en Papantla, Ver. desde el Mes de Noviembre de 1920 a la Fecha." In *Memoria de la Primera Convención de Fiebre Amarilla, Octubre 15–20 de 1921,* 108–111. México, D.F.: DSP, 1921.

Guy, Donna J. "The Pan American Child Congresses, 1916 to 1942: Pan Americanism, Child Reform, and the Welfare State in Latin America." *Journal of Family History* 23, no. 3 (July 1998): 272–91.

Hackett, Lewis. "Once upon a Time." *American Journal of Tropical Medicine and Hygiene* 9 (1960): 105–15.

Hale, Charles A. *The Transformation of Liberalism in Late Nineteenth Century Mexico.* Princeton, NJ: Princeton University Press, 1989.

Hall, Peter Dobkin. *Inventing the Nonprofit Sector and Other Essays on Philanthropy, Voluntarism, and Nonprofit Organizations.* Baltimore: Johns Hopkins University Press, 1992.

Hamill, Pete. *Diego Rivera.* New York: Harry N Abrams, 1999.

Hamilton, Nora. *The Limits of State Autonomy: Post-Revolutionary Mexico.* Princeton, NJ: Princeton University Press, 1982.

Hancock, Graham. *Lords of Poverty: The Power, Prestige and Corruption of the International Aid Business.* New York: Atlantic Monthly Press, 1989.

Hansen, Roger D. *The Politics of Mexican Development.* Baltimore: Johns Hopkins University Press, 1971.

Hanson, Henry. *The Pied Piper of Peru: Dr. Henry Hanson's Fight against "Yellow Jack" and Bubonic Plague in South America, 1919–1922.* Edited by Doris Hurnie. Jacksonville, FL: Convention Press, 1961.

Hardy, Anne. "Cholera, Quarantine and the English Preventive System, 1850–1895." *Medical History* 37 (1993): 250–69.

Harrison, Gordon. *Mosquitoes, Malaria, and Man: A History of the Hostilities since 1880.* New York: E. P. Dutton, 1978.

Harrison, Mark. *Climates and Constitutions: Health, Race, Environment and British Imperialism in India, 1600–1850.* Oxford: Oxford University Press, 1999.

———. *Public Health in British India: Anglo-Indian Preventive Medicine, 1859–1914.* Cambridge: Cambridge University Press, 1994.

Hart, John Mason. *Empire and Revolution: The Americans in Mexico since the Civil War.* Berkeley: University of California Press, 2002.

———. *Revolutionary Mexico: The Coming and Process of the Mexican Revolution.* Berkeley: University of California Press, 1987.

Hartmann, Betsy. "Population Control I: Birth of an Ideology" and "Population Control II: The Population Establishment Today." *International Journal of Health Services* 27, no. 3 (1997): 523–57.

Haynes, Keith Allen. "Orden y Progreso: The Revolutionary Ideology of Alberto J. Pani." In *Los Intelectuales y el Poder en México.* Edited by Roderic Camp, Charles Hale, and Josefina Zoraida Vásquez. México, D.F.: El Colegio de México, 1981.

Headrick, Daniel R. *The Tentacles of Progress. Technology Transfer in the Age of Imperialism, 1850–1940.* New York: Oxford University Press, 1988.

Hegner, Robert, and William Taliaferro. *Human Protozoology.* New York: MacMillan Company, 1924.

Heiser, Victor. *An American Doctor's Odyssey: Adventures in Forty-Five Countries.* New York: W. W. Norton and Company, Inc., 1936.

Henderson, Donald A. "Smallpox Eradication: A Cold War Victory." *World Health Forum* 19 (1998): 113–19.

Hendrick, Burton J. *The Life of Andrew Carnegie.* London: William Heinemann Ltd., 1933.

Herman, Edward, and Noam Chomsky. *Manufacturing Consent: The Political Economy of the Mass Media.* New York: Pantheon, 1988.

Hernández Lira, J. Pilar. "Distribución Geográfica y Patología de la Uncinariasis en la República Mexicana." *Boletín Epidemiológico* 8, no. 4 (1949): 111–15.

Hernández Llamas, Héctor, ed. *La Atención Médica en el Medio Rural Mexicano, 1930–1980.* México, D.F.: IMSS, 1984.

———. "Historia de la Participación del Estado en las Instituciones de Atención Médica en México, 1935–1980." In *Vida y Muerte del Mexicano.* Edited by Federico Ortiz Quesada, 49–96. México, D.F.: Folios Ediciones, 1982.

Hernández Mejía, Agustín. *Dieciocho Años de Trabajos Sanitarios en México.* México, D.F., 1941.

Hernández Sáenz, Luz María. *Learning to Heal: The Medical Profession in Colonial Mexico, 1767–1831.* New York: Peter Lang, 1997.

Hewa, Soma. *Colonialism, Tropical Disease and Imperial Medicine: Rockefeller Philanthropy in Sri Lanka.* Lanham, MD: University Press of America, 1995.

———. "The Hookworm Epidemic on the Plantations in Colonial Sri Lanka." *Medical History* 38 (1994): 73–90.

Hine, Darlene Clark. "Reflections on Nurse Rivers." Reprinted in *Tuskegee's Truths: Rethinking the Tuskegee Syphilis Study.* Edited by Susan M. Reverby, 386–95. Chapel Hill: University of North Carolina Press, 2000.

Hochman, Gilberto. *A Era do Saneamento: As Bases da Política de Saúde Pública no Brasil.* São Paulo: Editora Hucitec Anpocs, 1998.

Hochman, Gilberto, and Diego Armus, eds. *Cuídar, Controlar, Curar: Ensaios Históricos Sobre Saúde e Doença na América Latina e Caribe.* Rio de Janeiro: Editora Fiocruz, 2004.

Hofstadter, Richard. *The Age of Reform.* New York: Alfred A. Knopf, 1955.

Holland, William Robert. *Medicina Maya en los Altos de Chiapas: Un Estudio del Cambio Socio-Cultural.* Translated by Daniel Cazes. México, D.F.: Instituto Nacional Indigenista, 1963.

Horn, James. "The Mexican Revolution and Health Care or the Health of the Mexican Revolution." *International Journal of Health Services* 15, no. 3 (1985): 485–99.

Hotez, Peter. "Vaccine Diplomacy." *Foreign Policy* 124 (2001): 68–69.

Howard H. H. *The Control of Hookworm Disease by the Intensive Method.* New York: Rockefeller Foundation, International Health Board, Publication no. 8, 1919.

Howard L. M. "Public and Private Donor Financing for Health in Developing Countries." *Infectious Disease Clinics of North America* 5, no. 2 (June 1991): 221–34.

Howard-Jones, Norman. *The Pan American Health Organization: Origins and Evolution.* Geneva: World Health Organization, 1981.

———. *The Scientific Background of the International Sanitary Conferences, 1851–1938.* Geneva: World Health Organization, 1975.

Howard-Jones, Norman. "The World Health Organization in Historical Perspective." *Perspectives in Biology and Medicine* 24, no. 3 (1981): 467–82.

Huber, Brad R, and Alan R. Sandstrom, eds. *Mesoamerican Healers.* Austin: University of Texas Press, 2001.

Huberman, Leo. *We the People: The Drama of America.* Revised edition. New York: Monthly Review Press, 1960.

Huerta Jaramillo, Ana María Dolores. *Salut el Solatium: El Desarrollo de las Ciencias Médicas en Puebla Durante el Siglo XIX.* Puebla, México: Benemérita Universidad Autónoma de Puebla, Cuadernos del Archivo Histórico Universitario, 2000.

Humphreys, Margaret. "Kicking a Dying Dog: DDT and the Demise of Malaria in the American South, 1942–1950." *Isis* 87, no. 1 (March 1996): 1–17.

———. *Yellow Fever and the South.* New Brunswick, NJ: Rutgers University Press, 1992.

Instituto Nacional de Salud Pública. *Crónica de la Escuela de Salud Pública de México de 1922 a 2001. Relación de sus Protagonistas.* Cuernavaca, Morelos, México: Instituto Nacional de Salud Pública, 2002.

Iturbide Alvirez, Salvador. "Panorama General de la Salubridad Pública en México." *Pasteur: Revista Mensual de Medicina* 10, II, no. 4 (1937): 93–102.

Iturriaga, José E. *La Estructura Social y Cultural de México.* México, D.F.: Fondo de Cultura Económica, 1951.

Izquierdo, J. J. "Richard Mills Pearce Jr.: 1875–1930." *Gaceta Médica de México* 62 (1931): 38–39.

———. "Al Terminar los Estudios Médicos a Principios del Siglo." *Gaceta Médico de México* 95, no. 1 (1965): 91–96.

Jardim, Claudia. "Prevention and Solidarity: Democratizing Health in Venezuela." *Monthly Review* 56, no. 8 (2005), http://www.monthlyreview.org/0105jardim.htm

Jiménez, Christina. "Popular Organizing for Public Services: Residents Modernize Morelia Mexico, 1880–1920." *Journal of Urban History* 30, no. 4 (2004): 495–518.

Jones, Margaret. *Health Policy in Britain's Model Colony: Ceylon, 1900–1948.* New Delhi: Orient Longman, 2004.

———. "Infant and Maternal Health Services in Ceylon, 1900–1948: Imperialism or Welfare?" *Social History of Medicine* 15, no. 2 (2002): 263–89.

Joseph, Gilbert M, and Daniel Nugent, eds. *Everyday Forms of State Formation: Revolution and the Negotiation of Rule in Modern Mexico.* Durham, NC: Duke University Press, 1994.

Justice, Judith. *Policies, Plans, and People: Foreign Aid and Health Development.* Berkeley: University of California Press, 1989.

Kapelusz-Poppi, Ana Maria. "Morelia 1935: The First Conference for Rural Hygiene and the Program for State-Managed Medical Service." Paper presented at the XXII International Congress of the Latin American Studies Association, Miami, March, 2000.

———. "Physician Activists and the Development of Rural Health in Postrevolutionary Mexico." *Radical History Review* 80 (Spring 2001): 35–50.

———. "Rural Health and State Construction in Post-Revolutionary Mexico: The Nicolaita Project for Rural Medical Services." *The Americas* 58 (2001): 261–83.

Karl, Barry, and Stanley Katz. "Foundations and Ruling Class Elites." *Daedalus* 116 (1987): 1–40.

Kassalow, Jordan S. *Why Health Is Important to U.S. Foreign Policy.* Washington, DC: Council on Foreign Relations, 2001.

Katz, Friedrich. "Labor Conditions on Haciendas in Porfirian Mexico: Some Trends and Tendencies." *Hispanic American Historical Review* 54, no. 1 (1974): 1–47.

———. *The Life and Times of Pancho Villa.* Stanford, CA: Stanford University Press, 1998.

———. *Riot, Rebellion, and Revolution: Rural Social Conflict in Mexico.* Princeton, NJ: Princeton University Press, 1988.

———. *The Secret War in Mexico.* Chicago: University of Chicago Press, 1981.

Kavadi, Shirish. *The Rockefeller Foundation and Public Health in Colonial India, 1916–1945: A Narrative History.* Pune/Mumbai: Foundation for Research in Community Health, 1999.

———. " 'Wolves Come to Take Care of the Lamb.' " The Rockefeller Foundation's Hookworm Campaign in the Madras Presidency, 1920–1928." In *The Politics of the Healthy Life. An International Perspective.* Edited by Esteban Rodríguez-Ocaña, 89–111. Sheffield, UK: EAHMH Publications, 2002.

Kawachi, Ichiro, and Bruce Kennedy. *The Health of Nations: Why Inequality Is Harmful to Your Health.* New York: New Press, 2002.

Kay, Lily E. *The Molecular Vision of Life: Caltech, the Rockefeller Foundation, and the Rise of the New Biology.* New York: Oxford University Press, 1993.

———. "Rethinking Institutions: Philanthropy as a Historiographic Problem of Knowledge and Power." In "Philanthropy and Institution-Building in the Twentieth Century." *Minerva* 35, no. 3 (Autumn 1997): 283–93.

Kelly, Isabel. "An Anthropological Approach to Midwifery Training in Mexico." *Journal of Tropical Pediatrics* 1 (1956): 200–205.

Kemp, Amy. "The Rockefeller Foundation and the Faculdade de Medicina de São Paulo: A Case Study in Philanthropy as Policy." PhD diss., Indiana University, 2004.

Kemp, Amy, and Flavio Coelho Edler. "Medical Reform in Brazil and the U.S.: A Comparison of Two Rhetorics." *História, Ciências, Saúde—Manguinhos* 11, no. 3 (September/December, 2004): 569–85.

Kickbusch, Ilona. "The Development of International Health Policies: Accountability Intact?" *Social Science and Medicine* 51 (2000): 979–89.

———. "From Charity to Rights: Proposal for Five Action Areas of Global Health." *Journal of Epidemiology and Community Health* 58, no. 8 (August 2004): 630–31.

Kickbusch, Ilona, and Kent Buse. "Global Influences and Global Responses: International Health at the Turn of the Twenty-First Century." In *International Public Health: Diseases, Programs, Systems, and Policies.* Edited by Michael Merson, Robert Black, and Anne Mills, 701–32. Gaithersburg, MD: Aspen Publishers, 2001.

King, Charles R. *Children's Health in America: A History.* New York: Twayne Publishers, 1993.

Kiple, Kenneth F, ed. *The Cambridge World History of Human Disease.* Cambridge: Cambridge University Press, 1993.

———. *The Caribbean Slave: A Biological History.* Cambridge: Cambridge University Press, 1984.

Kitron, Uriel. "Malaria, Agriculture, and Development: Lessons from Past Campaigns." *International Journal of Health Services* 17 (1987): 295–326.

Klaus, Alisa. *Every Child a Lion: The Origins of Maternal and Infant Health Policy in the United States and France, 1890–1920.* Ithaca, NY: Cornell University Press, 1993.

———. "Depopulation and Race Suicide: Maternalism and Pronatalist Ideologies in France and the United States." In *Mothers of a New World.* Edited by Seth Koven and Sonya Michel, 188–212. New York: Routledge, 1993.

Knaut, Andrew L. "Yellow Fever and the Late Colonial Public Health Response in the Port of Veracruz." *Hispanic American Historical Review* 77 (1997): 619–44.

Knight, Alan. "Cardenismo: Juggernaut or Jalopy?" *Journal of Latin American Studies* 26, no. 1 (1994): 73–107.

———. *The Mexican Revolution.* 2 vols. Cambridge: Cambridge University Press, 1986.

———. "The Mexican Revolution: Bourgeois? Nationalist? Or Just a 'Great Rebellion'?" *Bulletin of Latin American Research* 4, no. 2 (1985): 1–37.

———. "Popular Culture and the Revolutionary State in Mexico, 1910–1940." *Hispanic American Historical Review* 74, no. 3 (1994); 393–444.

———. "The Rise and Fall of Cardenismo, c. 1930–c. 1946." In *Mexico since Independence.* Edited by Leslie Bethell, 241–320. Cambridge: Cambridge University Press, 1991.

———. *U.S. Mexican Relations, 1910–1940: An Interpretation.* San Diego: University of California, San Diego, Centre for U.S.-Mexican Studies, 1987.

Kobrin, Frances E. "The American Midwife Controversy: A Crisis of Professionalization." *Bulletin of the History of Medicine* 40 (1966): 350–63.

Kocyba, Henryk Karol. "La Medicina y la Religión entre los Mayas Prehispánicos." In *Historia de la Salud en México,* 13–26. México, D.F.: INAH, 1996.

Kohler, Robert E. *Partners in Science: Foundations and Natural Scientists, 1900–1945.* Chicago: University of Chicago Press, 1991.

———. "Science and Philanthropy: Wickliffe Rose and the International Education Board." *Minerva* 23 (Spring 1985): 75–95.

Koivusalo, Meri, and Eeva Ollila. *Making a Healthy World: Agencies, Actors and Policies in International Health.* London: Zed Press, 1997.

Koppes, Clayton R. "The Good Neighbor Policy and the Nationalization of Mexican Oil: A Reinterpretation." *Journal of American History* 69 (1982): 62–81.

Koven, Seth, and Sonya Michel, eds. *Mothers of a New World: Maternalist Politics and the Origins of Welfare States.* New York: Routledge, 1993.

Kraut, Alan. *Goldberger's War: The Life and Work of a Public Health Crusader.* New York: Hill and Wang, 2003.

Krauze, Enrique. *El Sexenio de Lázaro Cárdenas.* México, D.F.: Clío, 1999.

———. *Lázaro Cárdenas: General Misionero.* México, D.F.: Fondo de Cultura Económica, 1987.

Krieger, Nancy. "Epidemiology and the Web of Causation: Has Anyone Seen the Spider?" *Social Science and Medicine* 39, no. 7 (1994): 887–903.

Krieger, Nancy, and Elizabeth Fee. "Measuring Social Inequalities in Health in the United States: A Historical Review, 1900–1950." *International Journal of Health Services* 26, no. 3 (1996): 39–418.

Kuhnke, LaVerne. *Lives at Risk: Public Health in Nineteenth-Century Egypt.* Berkeley: University of California Press, 1990.

Kunitz, Stephen J. "Hookworm and Pellagra: Exemplary Diseases in the New South." *Journal of Health and Social Behavior* 29 (1988): 139–48.

Labastida, Julio. "De la Unidad Nacional al Desarrollo Estabilizador, 1940–1970." In *América Latina: Historia de Medio Siglo. Centroamérica, México y el Caribe.* Vol. 2. Edited by Pablo González Casanova, 328–76. México: Siglo XXI, 1981.

Ladd-Taylor, Molly, ed. *Raising a Baby the Government Way: Mothers' Letters to the Children's Bureau, 1915–1932.* New Brunswick, NJ: Rutgers University Press, 1986.

———. "Why Does Congress Wish Women and Children to Die?" In *Women and Children First: International Maternal and Infant Welfare, 1870–1945.* Edited by Valerie Fildes, Lara Marks, and Hilary Marland, 121–32. London: Routledge, 1992.

Lagemann, Ellen C. *Philanthropic Foundation: New Scholarship, New Possibilities.* Bloomington: Indiana University Press, 1999.

———. *Private Power for the Public Good: A History of the Carnegie Foundation for the Advancement of Teaching.* Middletown, CO: Wesleyan University Press; Scranton, PA: Harper & Row, 1983.

Langfeld, Millard. *Introduction to Infectious and Parasitic Diseases Including Their Cause and Manner of Transmission.* Philadelphia: P. Blakiston, 1907.

Lanning, John Tate. *The Royal Protomedicato: The Regulation of the Medical Profession in the Spanish Empire.* Durham, NC: Duke University Press, 1985.

Laurell, Cristina. "Crisis, Neoliberal Health Policy, and Political Processes in Mexico." *International Journal of Health Services* 21 (1991): 457–70.

———. "Medicina y Capitalismo en México." *Cuadernos Políticos* 5 (1975): 80–93.

Laurell, Cristina, and Oliva L. Arellano. "Market Commodities and Poor Relief: The World Bank Proposal for Health." *International Journal of Health Services* 26, no. 1 (1996): 1–18.

Lavrin, Asunción. *Women, Feminism, and Social Change in Argentina, Chile, and Uruguay.* Lincoln and London: University of Nebraska Press, 1995.

Lear, John. *Workers, Neighbors, and Citizens: The Revolution in Mexico City.* Lincoln: University of Nebraska Press, 2001.

Leavitt, Judith Walzer. *Typhoid Mary. Captive to the Public's Health.* Boston: Beacon Press, 1996.

Lefaucheur, Nadine. "La puériculture d'Adolphe Pinard." In *Darwinisme et société.* Edited by Patrick Tort, 413–46. Paris: Presses Universitaires de France, 1992.

León, Alberto P. "Cooperación de los Diversos Elementos Sociales en la Lucha Contra las Enfermedades Transmisibles." *Pasteur: Revista Mensual de Medicina* 10, II, no. 4 (1937): 103–7.

———. "Secretaría de Salubridad y Asistencia." *Pasteur: Revista Mensual de Medicina* 14, I, no. 1 (1941): 1–6.

León, Nicolas. *La Obstetricia en México.* México, D.F.: Tipografía de la viuda de F. Díaz de León, sucrs. 1910.

Lewis, Oscar. *Life in a Mexican Village: Tepoztlán Restudied.* Urbana: University of Illinois Press, 1963.

Liceaga, Eduardo. *Memoria Leida en la Reunión de la Asociación Americana de Salubridad Pública Verificada en Boston, Mass., E.U.A., del 25 al 29 de Septiembre de 1905.* México, D.F.: A. Carranza y Compañía, Impresores, 1905.

———. *Mis Recuerdos de Otros Tiempos.* México, D.F., 1949.

Link, William A. " 'The Harvest Is Ripe, but the Laborers Are Few': The Hookworm Crusade in North Carolina, 1909–1915." *North Carolina Historical Review* 67 (January 1990): 1–27.

———. "Privies, Progressivism, and Public Schools: Health Reform and Education in the Rural South, 1909–1920." *Journal of Southern History* 54 (1988): 623–42.

Lipp, Frank J. *The Mixe of Oaxaca: Religion, Ritual, and Healing.* Austin: University of Texas Press, 1991.

Lippman, Walter. *Public Opinion.* New York: Macmillan, 1922.

Litsios, Socrates. "The Long and Difficult Road to Alma-Ata: A Personal Reflection." *International Journal of Health Services* 32, no. 4 (2002): 709–32.

———. "Malaria Control, the Cold War, and the Postwar Reorganization of International Assistance." *Medical Anthropology* 17, no. 3 (May 1997): 255–78.

López Sánchez, José. *Finlay: El Hombre y la Verdad Científica.* La Habana, Cuba: Editorial Científico-Técnica, 1986.

Löwy, Ilana. *Virus, moustiques, et modernité: La fièvre jaune au Brésil entre science et politique.* Series histoire des sciences, des techniques et de la médecine. Paris: Éditions des Archives Contemporaines, 2001.

———. "What/Who Should Be Controlled: Opposition to Yellow Fever Campaigns in Brazil, 1900–1939." In *Contested Knowledge: Reactions to Western Medicine in the Modern Period.* Edited by Andrew Cunningham and Bridie Andrews, 124–46. Manchester, UK: Manchester University Press, 1997.

Loyo, Mauro. "Informe de los Trabajos Efectuados en el Puerto de Veracruz, con el Objeto de Dominar el Brote de Fiebre Amarilla que Comenzó en Junio de 1920." In *Memoria de la Primera Convención de Fiebre Amarilla, Octubre 15–20 de 1921,* 128–31. México, D.F.: DSP, 1921.

Lozoya, Xavier, and Carlos Zolla, eds. *La Medicina Invisible: Introducción al Estudio de la Medicina Tradicional de México.* México, D.F.: Folios Ediciones, 1983.

Ludmerer, Kenneth M. *Learning to Heal: The Development of American Medical Education.* New York: Basic Books, 1985.

Lyons, Maryinez. *The Colonial Disease: A Social History of Sleeping Sickness in Northern Zaire, 1900–1940.* Cambridge: Cambridge University Press, 1992.

Lyster, Theodore C. "Informe del Director de la Comisión Especial Contra la Fiebre Amarilla." In *Memoria de la Primera Convención de Fiebre Amarilla, Octubre 15–21 de 1921,* 11–20. México, D.F.: DSP, 1921.

———. "Plan de Campaña, 12 de diciembre de 1920." Reprinted in *Memoria de la Primera Convención de Fiebre Amarilla, Octubre 15–20 de 1921,* 13–16. México, D.F.: DSP, 1921.

Ma, Qiusha. "The Rockefeller Foundation and Modern Medical Education in China, 1915–1951." PhD diss., Case Western Reserve University, 1995.

Macías, Anna. *Against All Odds: The Feminist Movement in Mexico to 1940.* Westport, CT: Greenwood Press, 1982.

MacLeod, Roy, and Milton Lewis, eds. *Disease, Medicine, and Empire: Perspectives on Western Medicine and the Experience of European Expansion.* London: Routledge, 1988.

Madsen, Claudia. *A Study of Change in Mexican Folk Medicine.* New Orleans: Tulane University Middle American Research Institute, 1965.

Maglen, Krista. " 'The First Line of Defence': British Quarantine and the Port Sanitary Authorities in the Nineteenth Century." *Social History of Medicine* 15, no. 3 (December 2002): 413–28.

Malda, Gabriel. "Sesión Plena del 20 de Octubre de 1921, Alocución de Clausura." In *Memoria de la Primera Convención de Fiebre Amarilla, Octubre 15–20 de 1921*, 168. México, D.F.: DSP, 1921.

———. "Visitando Rochester: La Clínica de los Hermanos Mayo." *Pasteur: Revista Mensual de Medicina* 10, I, no. 1 (1937): 12–20.

Malvido, Elsa, and Miguel Ángel Cuenya. "La Pandemia de Cólera de 1833 en la Ciudad de Puebla." In *El Cólera de 1833: Una Nueva Patología en México. Causas y Efectos*. Edited by Miguel Ánguel Cuenya et al., 11–45. México, D.F.: INAH, 1992.

Malvido, Elsa, and Maria Elena Morales, eds. *Historia de la Salud en México*. México, D.F.: INAH, 1996.

Manderson, Lenore. *Sickness and the State: Health and Illness in Colonial Malaysia, 1870–1940*. Cambridge: Cambridge University Press, 1996.

Mann, Jonathan, Larry Gostin, Sofia Gruskin, Troyen Brennan, Zita Lazzarini, and Harvey V. Fineberg, "Health and Human Rights." *Health and Human Rights* 1, no. 1 (1994): 6–23.

Marinho, Maria G. S. M. C. *Norte-Americanos no Brasil: Uma História da Fundação Rockefeller na Universidade de São Paulo, 1934–1952*. Campinas, Brasil: Editora Autores Associados, 2001.

Markiewicz, Dana. *The Mexican Revolution and the Limits of Agrarian Reform 1915–1946*. Boulder, CO: Lynne Rienner Publishers, 1993.

Marks, Shula. "South Africa's Early Experiment in Social Medicine: Its Pioneers and Politics." *American Journal of Public Health* 87, no. 3 (1997): 452–59.

Marnham, Patrick. *Dreaming with His Eyes Open: A Life of Diego Rivera*. New York: Alfred A. Knopf, 1998.

Márquez, Patricio V, and Daniel J. Joly. "A Historical Overview of the Ministries of Public Health and the Medical Programs of the Social Security Systems in Latin America." *Journal of Public Health Policy* 7 (1986): 378–94.

Márquez Morfin, Lourdes. *La Desigualdad ante la Muerte en la Ciudad de México*. México, D.F.: Siglo XXI, 1994.

Martin, Percy Alvin, ed. *Who's Who in Latin America: A Biographical Dictionary of the Outstanding Living Men and Women of Spanish America and Brazil*. Palo Alto, CA: Stanford University Press, 1935.

Martínez, Juliana. *Luces y Sombras: Formación y Transformación de las Políticas Sociales en América Latina*. San José, Costa Rica: Facultad Latinoamericana de Ciencias Sociales, 2000.

———. "Policy Environments and Selective Emulation in the Making of Health Policies: Costa Rica, 1920–1997." PhD diss., University of Pittsburgh, 1998.

Martínez, Pedro Daniel. "Planeación de la Salud Pública Como Factor de Desarrollo Nacional." *Salud Pública de México* 5 (1963): 621–26.

Martínez Báez, Manuel. "El Instituto de Salubridad y Enfermedades Tropicales." *Anales de la Sociedad Mexicana de Historia de la Ciencia y de la Tecnología* 1 (1969): 146.

Martínez Cortés, Fernando. "La Historia de la Salubridad en México." *Médico Moderno* 38, no. 2 (1999): 7–95.

Mazzaferri, Anthony. "Public Health and Social Revolution in Mexico: 1870–1930." PhD diss., Kent State University, 1968.

McBride, David. *Missions for Science: U.S. Technology and Medicine in America's Africa World*. New Brunswick, NJ: Rutgers University Press, 2002.

McCaa, Robert. "Spanish and Nahuatl Views on Smallpox and Demographic Catastrophe in the Conquest of Mexico." *Journal of Interdisciplinary History* 25, no. 3 (Winter 1995): 397–431.

McCusker, John J. *How Much Is That in Real Money? A Historical Price Index for Use as a Deflator of Money Values in the Economy of the United States.* Worcester, MA: American Antiquarian Society, 1992.

McKee, Martin, Paul Garner, and Robin Stott. *International Co-operation in Health.* Oxford: Oxford University Press, 2001.

McLeod, James Angus. "Public Health, Social Assistance and the Consolidation of the Mexican State: 1877–1940." PhD diss., Tulane University, 1990.

McMurray, Christine, and Roy Smith. *Diseases of Globalization: Socioeconomic Transitions and Health.* London: Earthscan Publications, 2001.

Meade, Teresa, and Mark Walker, eds. *Science, Medicine and Cultural Imperialism.* New York: St. Martin's Press, 1991.

Mears, J. Ewing. *The Triumph of American Medicine in the Construction of the Panama Canal.* 3rd ed. Philadelphia: William J. Dornan, 1913.

Meckel, Richard A. *Save the Babies: American Public Health Reform and the Prevention of Infant Mortality, 1850–1929.* Baltimore: Johns Hopkins University Press, 1990.

Medin, Tzvi. *Ideología y Praxis Política de Lázaro Cárdenas.* México, D.F.: Siglo XXI, 1982.

———. *El Minimato Presidencial: Historia Política del Maximato, 1928–1935.* México D.F.: Ediciones Era, 1982.

Melosh, Barbara. *"The Physician's Hand": Work Culture and Conflict in American Nursing.* Philadelphia: Temple University Press, 1982.

Melville, Roberto. *Crecimiento y Rebelión: El Desarrollo Económico de las Haciendas Azucareras en Morelos, 1880–1910.* México, D.F.: Editorial Nueva Imagen, 1979.

Memoria de la Primera Convención de Fiebre Amarilla, Octubre 15–20 de 1921. México, D.F.: DSP, 1921.

Méndez, Marciano Netzhualcoyotzi. "La Influenza de 1918 en Tlaxcala: Mortandad y Efectos Sociales." *Boletín Mexicana de Historia y Filosofía de Medicina* 6, no. 1 (2003): 23–31.

Mendiola Gómez, Jaime. "Historical Synthesis of Medical Education in Mexico." In *Aspects of the History of Medicine in Latin America.* Edited by John Bowers and Elizabeth Purcell, 88–96. New York: Josiah Macy Jr. Foundation, 1979.

Mendoza, Salvador. *La Doctrina Cárdenas.* México, D.F.: Ediciones Botas, 1939.

Menéndez, Eduardo. *Poder, Estratificación Social y Salud. Análisis de las Condiciones Sociales y Económicas de la Enfermedad en Yucatán.* México, D.F.: La Casa Chata, 1981.

Mercado, Ulises. "The Traditional Midwife in Mexico." *Scalpel and Tongs* (January–February 1994): 11.

Mesa-Lago, Carlos. *Social Security in Latin America: Pressure Groups, Stratification, and Inequality.* Pittsburgh: University of Pittsburgh Press, 1978.

Meyer, Jean A. *The Cristero Rebellion: The Mexican People between Church and State, 1926–1929.* Cambridge: Cambridge University Press, 1976.

———. *La Revolution Mexicaine, 1910–1940.* Paris: Calmann-Levy, 1973.

———. "Mexico in the 1920s." in Leslie Bethell, ed., *Mexico since Independence* (Cambridge: Cambridge University Press, 1991): 218–27.

Meyer, John W, John Boli, and George M. Thomas. "World Society and the Nation-State." *American Journal of Sociology* 103, no. 1 (1997): 144–81.

Meyer, Lorenzo. *México y Estados Unidos en el Conflicto Petrolero, 1917–1942*. México, D.F.: El Colegio de México, 1968.

Michaud, Catherine, and Christopher Murray. "External Assistance to the Health Sector in Developing Countries: A Detailed Analysis, 1972–90." *Bulletin of the World Health Organization* 72, no. 4 (1994): 639–51.

Middlebrook, Kevin J. *The Paradox of Revolution: Labor, the State, and Authoritarianism in Mexico*. Baltimore: Johns Hopkins University Press, 1995.

Milkis, Sidney M, and Jerome M. Mileur, eds. *Progressivism and the New Democracy*. Amherst: University of Massachusetts Press, 1999.

Miller, Francesca. *Latin American Women and the Search for Social Justice*. Hanover, NH: University Press of New England, 1991.

Miranda, Francisco de P. "The Decrease of Tuberculosis in Mexico." *American Journal of Public Health* 21, no. 1 (1931): 37–42.

———. "Evolución de la Sanidad en México." *Boletín de la Oficina Sanitaria Panamericana* 9 (1930): 233–40.

———. "The Public Health Department in Mexico City." *American Journal of Public Health* 20 (1930): 1125–28.

Mitchell B. R. *International Historical Statistics: The Americas 1750–1993*. 4th ed. New York: Stockton Press, 1998.

Moll, Aristides. "The Pan American Sanitary Bureau: Its Origin, Development and Achievements: A Review of Inter-American Cooperation in Public Health, Medicine, and Allied Fields." *Boletín de la Oficina Sanitaria Panamericana* 19 (1940): 1219–34.

Molyneux, Maxine. *Women's Movements in International Perspective: Latin America and Beyond*. Basingstoke, UK, and New York: Palgrave, 2001.

Montalvo, Victoriano. "Informe Presentado por el Delegado Sanitario en Puerto México, Ver." In *Memoria de la Primera Convención de Fiebre Amarilla, Octubre 15–20 de 1921*, 132–35. México, D.F.: DSP, 1921.

Morales, Marcel. *Morelos Agrario: La Construcción de una Alternativa*. México, D.F.: Plaza y Valdés, 1994.

Morales y Carbajal, Salvador. "Informe Resumido de los Experimentos Realizados por la 'Campaña Contra el Paludismo,' de la Dirección General de Epidemiología en el Estado de Morelos, Hasta Diciembre de 1945, para Dominar el Anofelismo en los Cultivos de Arroz." *Salubridad y Asistencia* 7, no. 3 (1947): 313–24.

Moreno Corral, Marco Arturo. *Odisea 1874 o el Primer Viaje Internacional de Científicos Mexicanos*. México, D.F.: Fondo de Cultura Económica, 1986.

Moreno Cueto, Enrique, Julio Miguel Viveros, Miguel A. Díaz de Sandi, Martha E. García Ugarte, and Eduardo Césarman Vitis. *Sociología Histórica de las Instituciones de Salud*. México, D.F.: IMSS, 1982.

Moscoso Pastrana, Prudencio. *La Medicina Tradicional de los Altos de Chiapas*. San Cristóbal de las Casas, México: Editorial Tradición, 1982.

Moulin, Anne Marie. "Patriarchal Science: The Network of Overseas Pasteur Institutes." In *Science and Empires: Historical Studies about Scientific Development and European Expansion*. Edited by Patrick Petitjean, Catherine Jami, and Anne Marie Moulin, 307–20. Boston Studies in the Philosophy of Science, Dordrecht, Netherlands: Kluwer Academic Press, 1992.

Mullan, Fitzhugh. *Plagues and Politics: The Story of the United States Public Health Service*. New York: Basic Books, 1989.

Munch Galindo, Guido. *Etnología del Istmo Veracruzano.* México, D.F.: UNAM, 1983.

Muntaner, Carles. "Denunciation by Cliché: Is Chavez's Venezuela Populist or Socialist?" *Counterpunch,* May 5, 2005, http://www.counterpunch.org/mutanero5052005. html

Murard, Lion, and Patrick Zylberman. "Les fondations indestructibles: La santé publique en France et la Fondation Rockefeller." *Médicine/Sciences* 18, no. 5 (2002): 625–32.

———. *L'hygiene dans la république: La santé publique en France, ou l'utopie contrariée, 1870–1918.* Paris: Fayard, 1996.

———. "La Mission Rockefeller en France et la creation du Comité National de Defense contre la Tuberculose, 1917–1923." *Revue d'histoire moderne et contemporaine* 34 (April–June 1987): 257–81.

———. "Seeds for French Health Care: Did the Rockefeller Foundation Plant the Seeds between the Two World Wars?" *Studies in the History and Philosophy of Biological and Medical Sciences* 31, no. 3 (2000): 463–75.

Muraskin, William. *The Politics of International Health: The Children's Vaccine Initiative and the Struggle to Develop Vaccines for the Third World.* Albany: State University of New York Press, 1998.

Muriel, Josefina. *Hospitales de la Nueva España.* 2 vols. México, D.F.: UNAM/Cruz Roja Mexicana, 1991.

Musgrove, Philip. "Earmarking Could Be Beneficial: Cost Effectiveness Is Not the Only Criterion." *Bulletin of the World Health Organization* 82, no. 9 (September 2004): 706–7.

Navarro, Vicente, ed. *Imperialism, Health and Medicine.* Farmingdale, NY: Baywood Publishers, 1981.

———. "The Underdevelopment of Health or the Health of Underdevelopment." *International Journal of Health Services* 4 (1974): 5–27.

"Necrología." *Gaceta Médica de México* 58 (1927): 632.

Newell, Kenneth. "Selective Primary Health Care: The Counter Revolution." *Social Science and Medicine* 26 (1988): 903–6.

Ninkovich, Frank. *The Diplomacy of Ideas: U.S. Foreign Policy and Cultural Relations, 1938–1950.* Cambridge: Cambridge University Press, 1981.

———. "The Rockefeller Foundation, China, and Cultural Change." *Journal of American History* 70 (1984): 799–820.

Norvell, Elizabeth Jean. "Syndicalism and Citizenship: Postrevolutionary Worker Mobilizations in Veracruz." In *Border Crossings: Mexican and Mexican-American Workers.* Edited by John Mason Hart, 93–116. Wilmington, DE: Scholarly Resources, 1998.

Novo, Salvador. *Breve Historia y Antología Sobre la Fiebre Amarilla.* México, D.F.: La Prensa Médica Mexicana, 1964.

Nunes Moreira, Martha C. "A Fundação Rockefeller e a Construção da Identidade Profissional de Enfermagem no Brasil na Primeira República." *História, Ciências, Saúde—Manguinhos* 5 (November 1998–February 1999): 621–45.

Núñez Becerra, Fernanda. *La Prostitución y su Represión en la Ciudad de México (Siglo XIX): Prácticas y Representaciones.* Barcelona: Biblioteca Latinoamericana de Pensamiento, 2002.

Obregón, Alvaro. "Acuerdo del C. Presidente de los Estados Unidos Mexicanos, por el que se Crea 'La Comisión Especial para la Campaña Contra la Fiebre Amarilla.'" In *Historia de la Salubridad y de la Asistencia en México.* Edited by José Alvarez Amézquita, Miguel E. Bustamante, Antonio L. Picazos, and F. Fernández del Castillo, 154. México, D.F.: SSA, 1960.

———. "Extracto del Mensaje del General Alvaro Obregón, Presidente de los Estados Unidos de México." *Boletín de la Oficina Sanitaria Panamericana* 2 (1923): 301–4.

Ocaranza, Fernando. *Historia de la Medicina en México.* México, D.F.: Laboratorios Midy, 1934.

O'Connor, Alice. *Poverty Knowledge: Social Science, Social Policy, and the Poor in Twentieth-Century U.S. History.* Princeton, NJ: Princeton University Press, 2001.

O'Connor F. W. "Concern of the United States with Tropical Diseases." *American Journal of Public Health and The Nation's Health* 25 (1935): 1–10.

Office International d'Hygiène Publique. *Vingt-cinq ans d'activité de l'Office International d'Hygiène Publique, 1909–1933.* Paris: Office International d'Hygiène Publique, 1933.

Ojeda Falcón, Ramón. "Apuntes Sobre el Ultimo Brote de Fiebre Amarilla Ocurrido en el Puerto de Veracruz, 1920–1921." *Boletín Epidemiológico* 19, no. 1 (1955): 71–77.

Oliver, Lilia. "El Cólera en los Barrios de Guadalajara." In *Salud, Cultura y Sociedad en América Latina: Nuevas Perspectivas Históricas.* Edited by Marcos Cueto, 87–109. Lima: IEP y OPS, 1996.

———. "La Pandemia de Cólera Morbus: El Caso de Guadalajara." In *Ensayos Sobre la Historia de las Epidemias en México.* Vol. 2. Edited by Enrique Florescano and Elsa Malvido, 565–81. México, D.F.: IMSS, 1982.

Ornelas, Carlos. *La Descentralización de la Educación en México.* Santiago, Chile: Comisión Económica para la América Latina y el Caribe, 1997.

Ortega, Lauro. "Cómo Debe Entenderse en la Actualidad la Higiene Infantil." *Pasteur: Revista Mensual de Medicina* 10, II, no. 4 (1937): 129–33.

Ortiz de Montellano, Bernard. *Aztec Medicine, Health and Nutrition.* New Brunswick, NJ: Rutgers University Press, 1990.

———. "Empirical Aztec Medicine." *Science* 188, no. 4185 (1975): 215–20.

Ortiz Quesada, Federico, ed. *Vida y Muerte del Mexicano.* México, D.F.: Folios Ediciones, 1982.

Osornio, Enrique. "Nota Presentada por el Jefe del Cuerpo Médico Militar." In *Memoria de la Primera Convención de Fiebre Amarilla, Octubre 15–20 de 1921,* 105–7. México, D.F.: DSP, 1921.

Packard, Randall M. "'No Other Logical Choice': Global Malaria Eradication and the Politics of International Health in the Postwar Era." *Parassitologia* 40, nos. 1 and 2 (June 1998): 217–30.

———. "Visions of Postwar Health and Development and their Impact on Public Health Interventions in the Developing World." In *International Development and the Social Sciences: Essays on the History and Politics of Knowledge.* Edited by Frederick Cooper and Randall Packard, 93–115. Berkeley: University of California Press, 1997.

Packard, Randall M. *White Plague, Black Labor: Tuberculosis and the Political Economy of Health and Disease in South Africa.* Berkeley, CA: University of California Press, 1989.

Packard, Randall M, and Peter J. Brown. "Rethinking Health, Development and Malaria: Historicizing a Cultural Model in International Health." *Medical Anthropology* 17 (1997): 181–94.

Packard, Randall M, and P. A. Gadelha. "A Land Filled with Mosquitoes: Fred L. Soper, the Rockefeller Foundation, and the *Anopheles gambiae* Invasion of Brazil." *Parassitologia* 36, nos. 1–2 (1994): 197–213.

Palmer, Steven. "Central American Encounters with Rockefeller Public Health, 1914–1921." In *Close Encounters of Empire: Writing the Cultural History of U.S.-Latin American Relations.* Edited by Gilbert Joseph, Catherine LeGrand, and Ricardo Salvatore, 311–32. Durham, NC: Duke University Press, 1998.

———. *From Popular Medicine to Medical Populism, Doctors, Healers, and Public Power in Costa Rica 1800–1940.* Durham, NC: Duke University Press, 2003.

Pan American Health Organization. *Health Services Research: An Anthology.* Washington, DC: PAHO, 1992.

Pan American Sanitary Bureau. *Bibliography of Onchocercosis. Publication 242.* Washington, DC: PASB, 1947.

———. *Transactions of the Seventh Pan American Sanitary Conference of the American Republics, held in Havana, Cuba, November 5 to 15, 1924.* Washington, DC: PASB, 1924.

Pan American Union. *Transactions of the Fourth International Sanitary Conference of the American Republics, held in San José, Costa Rica, December 25, 1909 to January 3, 1910.* Washington, DC: Pan American Union, 1910.

Pani, Alberto. *Hygiene in Mexico: A Study of Sanitary and Educational Problems.* Translated by Ernest L. de Gogorza. New York and London: Knickerbocker Press, 1917.

Panisset, Ulysses. *International Health Statecraft: Foreign Policy and Public Health in Peru's Cholera Epidemic.* Lanham, MD: University Press of America, 2000.

"Las Parasitósis Intestinales de México." *Boletín de la Oficina Sanitaria Panamericana* 7 (1928): 575–79.

Parks, Lois, and Gustave Nuremberger. "The Sanitation of Guayaquil." *Hispanic American Historical Review* 23 (1943): 197–221.

Parra, Pilar Alicia. "Midwives in the Mexican Health System." *Social Science and Medicine* 37, no. 11 (1993): 1321–29.

Patterson, K. David. *Health in Colonial Ghana: Diseases, Medicine and Socio-Economic Change, 1900–1955.* Waltham, MA: Crossroads Press, 1981.

Peard, Julyan. *Race, Place, and Medicine: The Idea of the Tropics in Nineteenth-Century Brazil.* Durham, NC: Duke University Press, 1999.

———. "Tropical Disorders and the Forging of a Brazilian Medical Indentity," *Hispanic American Historical Review* 77, no. 1 (1997): 1–45.

Pemberton, Rita. "A Different Intervention: The International Health Commission/ Board, Health, Sanitation in the British Caribbean, 1914–1930." *Caribbean Quarterly* 49, no. 4 (2003): 87–103.

Penfield, Wilder. *The Difficult Art of Giving: The Epic of Alan Gregg.* Boston: Little, Brown and Company, 1967.

Peregrina Pellón, Luis. "La Enseñanza de la Salud Pública en América Latina." *Educación Médica y Salud* 6 (1976): 9–18.

Pernick, Martin S. "Politics, Parties, and Pestilence: Epidemic Yellow Fever in Philadelphia and the Rise of the First Party System." In *Sickness and Health in America: Readings in the History of Medicine and Public Health*. Edited by Judith Walzer Leavitt and Ronald Numbers, 356–71. Madison: University of Wisconsin Press, 1985.

Perrín, Tomás. "¿Virus, o Leptospiras?" *Pasteur: Revista Mensual de Medicina* 3, II, no. 1 (1930): 11–13.

Pike, Fredrick B. *FDR's Good Neighbor Policy: Sixty Years of Generally Gentle Chaos*. Austin: University of Texas Press, 1992.

Pimenta Rocha, Heloísa H. *A Higienização dos Costumes: Educação Escolar e Saúde no Projeto do Instituto de Higiene de São Paulo, 1918–1925*. Campinas, Brazil: Mercado das Letras, 2003.

Plesset, Isabel R. *Noguchi and His Patrons*. Rutherford, NJ: Fairleigh Dickinson University Press, 1980.

Porter, Dorothy. *Health, Civilization, and the State: A History of Public Health from Ancient to Modern Times*. London: Routledge, 1999.

———, ed. *The History of Public Health and the Modern State*. Wellcome Institute for the History of Medicine. Amsterdam: Rodopi, 1994.

Potthast, Barbara, and Eugenia Scarzanella, eds. *Mujeres y Naciones en América Latina: Problemas de Inclusión y Exclusión*. Frankfurt: Iberoamericana Vervuert, 2001.

Power, Helen J. *Tropical Medicine in the Twentieth Century: A History of Liverpool School of Tropical Medicine*. London: Kegan Paul International, 1999.

Pressman, Jack. "Human Understanding: Psychosomatic Medicine and the Mission of the Rockefeller Foundation." In *Greater than the Parts: Holism in Biomedicine, 1920–1950*. Edited by Christopher Lawrence and George Weisz, 189–208. New York: Oxford University Press, 1998.

Preston, Samuel H, and Michael R. Haines. *Fatal Years: Child Mortality in Late Nineteenth-Century America*. Princeton, NJ: Princeton University Press, 1991.

Prieto I, *The Supreme Board of Health of Mexico: Its History*. México, D.F.: Consejo Superior de Salubridad, 1903.

Pruneda, Alfonso. "Informe del Dr. D. Alfonso Pruneda, Secretario General del Departamento de Salubridad Pública de México en la Inauguración de la Escuela Anexa al Departamento de Salubridad." *Boletín de la Oficina Sanitaria Panamericana* 2 (1923): 305–9.

———. "El Papel de México en la Cooperación Sanitaria Interamericana." *Boletín de la Oficina Sanitaria Panamericana* 23, no. 9 (September 1944): 780–85.

———. "La Salubridad y la Guerra." *Pasteur: Revista Mensual de Medicina* 18, I, no. 4 (1945): 69–74.

———. "La Secretaría de Educación Pública de México y la Difusión de la Higiene." *Pasteur: Revista Mensual de Medicina* 2, I, no. 42 (1929): 52–54.

———. "El Servicio Médico-Social de la Universidad Nacional." *Gaceta Médica de México* 70, no. 2 (1940): 143–51.

Purnell, Jennie. *Popular Movements and State Formation in Revolutionary Mexico: The Agraristas and Cristeros of Michoacán*. Durham, NC: Duke University Press, 1999.

Pyenson, Lewis. "In Partibus Infidelium: Imperialist Rivalries and Exact Sciences in Early Twentieth Century Argentina." *Quipu* 1 (1984): 253–303.

Quevedo, Emilio, Catalina Borda, Juan Carlos Eslava, Claudia Mónica García, María Del Pilar Guzmán, Paola Mejía, and Carlos Ernesto Noguera. *Café y Gusanos, Mosquitos y Petróleo: El Tránsito desde la Higiene hacia la Medicina Tropical y la Salud Pública en Colombia, 1873–1953.* Bogotá: Universidad Nacional de Colombia, Facultad de Medicina, Instituto de Salud Pública, 2004.

Quezada, Noemí. *Enfermedad y Maleficio: El Curandero en el México Colonial.* México, D.F.: UNAM, 1989.

Quijano, Narezo M. "México en las Relaciones Internacionales de Salud." *Salud Pública de México* 25 (1983): 519–23.

Quintín Olascoaga, José. "Datos para la Historia de la Nutriología en México." *Salubridad y Asistencia* 8 (1948): 305–15.

Ramer, Samuel C. "Feldshers and Rural Health Care in the Early Soviet Period." In *Health and Society in Revolutionary Russia.* Edited by Susan G. Solomon and John F. Hutchinson, 121–45. Bloomington: Indiana University Press, 1990.

Ramírez de Arellano, Annette B. "The Politics of Public Health in Puerto Rico: 1926–1940." *Revista de Salud Pública de Puerto Rico* 3 (1981): 35–58.

Ramos, Pedro, Jorge Díaz González, José Manuel Alvarez Manilla, and Juan Alvarez Tostado. *Proyección Social del Médico.* México, D.F.: Manuel Casas, 1965.

Ramos Galván, Rafael. "Normas Aceptadas para Juzgar la Normalidad de los Aportes Alimenticios." *Salubridad y Asistencia* 1 (1944): 23–35.

Ramos Pioquinto, Donato, ed. *Salud y Tradiciones Reproductivas en la Sierra Norte de Oaxaca: Un Estudio de Caso.* Oaxaca: Secretaría Académica, 1998.

Redfield, Robert. *Tepoztlán: A Mexican Village.* Chicago: University of Chicago Press, 1930.

Reverby, Susan M. *Ordered to Care: The Dilemma of American Nursing, 1850–1945.* Cambridge: Cambridge University Press, 1987.

———. "Rethinking the Tuskegee Syphilis Study: Nurse Rivers, Silence, and the Meaning of Treatment." In *Tuskegee's Truths: Rethinking the Tuskegee Syphilis Study.* Edited by Susan M. Reverby, 365–85. Chapel Hill: University of North Carolina Press, 2000.

Revista del Instituto de Salubridad y Enfermedades Tropicales 10, no. 4 (December 1950): 195.

Riley, James. *The Eighteenth-Century Campaign to Avoid Disease.* London: Macmillan Press Ltd., 1987.

Rivera, Diego. *My Art, My Life: An Autobiography.* New York: Citadel Press, 1960.

Rockefeller Foundation. *Annual Reports, 1915–1960.* New York: Rockefeller Foundation.

———. *International Health Division Annual Report.* New York: Rockefeller Foundation, 1950.

Rodrigues de Faria, Lina. "A Fundação Rockefeller e os Serviços de Saúde em São Paulo, 1920–1930: Perspectivas Históricas." *História, Ciências, Saúde—Manguinhos* 9, no. 3 (September–December 2002): 561–90.

Rodriguez, Julia Emilia. "The Failure of Public Health Philanthropy: TheRockefeller Foundation in Venezuela, 1926–1934." MA diss., Columbia University, 1993.

Rodríguez, Martha Eugenia. "Las Juntas de Sanidad en la Nueva España, Siglos XVIII y XIX." *Revista de Investigación Clínica* 53, no. 3 (May–June, 2001): 276–80.

Rodríguez, Martha Eugenia. "Legislación Sanitaria y Boticas Novohipanas." *Estudios Historicos Novohispanos* 17 (1997): 151–69.

Rodríguez, Martha Eugenia, and Ana Cecilia Rodríguez de Romo. "Asistencia Médica e Hygiene Ambiental en la Ciudad de México, Siglos XVI–XVIII." *Gaceta Médica de México* 135, no. 2 (1999): 189–98.

Rodríguez de Romo, Ana Cecilia. "La Ciencia *Pasteuriana* A Través de la Vacuna Antirrábica." *Dynamis* 16 (1996): 291–316.

————. "Factores Determinantes en el Origen y Desarrollo de un Político-Científico Mexicano: Manuel Martínez Báez." In *Enfoques Multidisciplinarias de la Cultura Científico-Tecnológica en México*. Edited by Maria Luisa Rodríguez Sala, and José Omar Moncada Maya, 93–101. México, D.F.: Instituto de Investigaciones Sociales, UNAM, 1994.

————. "Manuel Martínez Báez: Congruencia Afortunada de Inteligencia e Integridad." *Revista de la Universidad Michoacana* 13 (1994): 115–25.

————. "Manuel Martínez Báez: Una Visión Muy Personal de Salud y Humanismo." In *La Cultura Científico-Tecnológica Nacional: Perspectivas Multidisciplinarias*. Edited by Maria Luisa Rodríguez Sala, María Eugenia Cué, and Ignacio Gómezgil, 77–87. México, D.F.: Instituto de Investigaciones Sociales, UNAM, 1992.

————. "La Visita de Charles Nicolle a México en 1931." In *Estudios de Historia de la Medicina: Abordages e Interpretaciones*. Edited by Ana Cecilia Rodríguez de Romo, and Xóchitl Martínez Barbosa, 159–72. México, D.F.: UNAM, 2001.

————. "Los Médicos Como Gremio de Poder en el Porfiriato." *Boletín Mexicano de Historia y Filosofía de Medicina* 5, no. 2 (2002): 4–9.

Rodríguez de Romo, Ana Cecilia, and Martha Eugenia Rodríguez Pérez. "Historia de la Salud Pública en México: Siglos XIX y XX." *História, Ciências, Saúde— Manguinhos* 2 (1998): 293–310.

Rodríguez Domínguez, José. "La Escuela de Salud Pública de México." *Salud Pública de México* 25, no. 5 (1983): 505–8.

Rodríguez Ocaña, Esteban. "Foreign Expertise, Political Pragmatism, and Professional Elite: The Rockefeller Foundation in Spain, 1919–39." *Studies in History and Philosophy of Biological and Biomedical Sciences* 31, no. 3 (2000): 447–61.

————. "La Salud Pública en la España de la Primera Mitad del Siglo XX." In *El Centro Secundario de Higiene Rural de Talavera de la Reina y la Sanidad Española de su Tiempo*. Edited by Juan Atenza y José Martínez, 21–42. Toledo, Junta de Comunidades de Castilla la Mancha, 2001.

Roemer, Milton. "Medical Care and Social Class in Latin America." *Milbank Memorial Fund Quarterly* 42 (part I, 1964): 54–64.

Rojas Aguilar, Gil. "Informe del Delegado Sanitario en Yucatán." In *Memoria de la Primera Convención de Fiebre Amarilla, Octubre 15–20 de 1921*, 143–46. México, D.F.: DSP, 1921.

Rollet, Catherine. "La lutte contre la mortalité internationale infantile dans le passé: Essai de comparaison internationale," *Santé publique* 2 (1993): 4–20.

Romero Alvarez, Humberto. *Health without Boundaries*. México, D.F.: United States–Mexico Border Public Health Association, 1975.

Ronzón, José. *Sanidad y Modernización en los Puertos del Alto Caribe 1870–1915*. México, D.F.: Universidad Autónoma Metropolitana, Unidad Azcapotzalco/Grupo Editorial Miguel Angel Porrúa, 2004.

Rosen, George. *A History of Public Health.* New York: MD Publications, 1958.

Rosenberg, Emily. *Spreading the American Dream: American Economic and Cultural Expansion, 1890–1945.* New York: Hill and Wang, 1982.

Rosenzweig, Fernando. "El Comercio Exterior." In *Historia Moderna de México.* Vol. 7. Edited by Daniel Cosío Villegas, 635–729. México, D.F.: Hermes, 1965.

Rubel, Arthur J, Carl W. O'Neil, and Rolando Collado-Ardon. *Susto, A Folk Illness.* Berkeley: University of California Press, 1984.

Rubio, Blanca. *Resistencia Campesina y Explotación Rural en México.* México, D.F.: Ediciones Era, 1987.

Ruger, Jennifer Prah. "Changing Role of the World Bank in Global Health in Historical Perspective." *American Journal of Public Health* 95, no. 1 (January 2005): 60–70.

Saavedra, Alfredo. "Historia del Movimiento Eugenésico en México." *Pasteur: Revista Mensual de Medicina* 8, I, no. 1 (1935): 19–26.

Sainsbury, Diane. *Gender Equality and Welfare States.* Cambridge: Cambridge University Press, 1996.

Santas, Andrés. "Schools of Public Health in Latin America." In *Schools of Public Health: Present and Future.* Edited by John Bowers and Elizabeth Purcell, 134–43. New York: Josiah Macy Jr. Foundation, 1974.

Saralegui, José. *Historia de la Sanidad Internacional.* Montevideo: Imprenta Nacional, 1958.

Scarzanella, Eugenia. "Proteger a las Mujeres y los Niños. El Internacionalismo Humanitario de la Sociedad de las Naciones y las Delegadas Sudamericanas." In *Mujeres y Naciones en América Latina: Problemas de Inclusión y Exclusión.* Edited by Barbara Potthast and Eugenia Scarzanella. Frankfurt: Iberoamericana Vervuert, 2001.

Schell, Patience A. *Church and State Education in Revolutionary Mexico City.* Tucson: University of Arizona Press, 2003.

———. "Nationalizing Children through Schools and Hygiene: Porfirian and Revolutionary Mexico City." *The Americas* 60, no. 4 (April 2004): 558–87.

Schendel, Gordon. *Medicine in Mexico: From Aztec Herbs to Betatrons.* Austin: University of Texas Press, 1968.

Schneider, William H. "The Men Who Followed Flexner: Richard Pearce, Alan Gregg, and the Rockefeller Foundation Medical Division, 1919–1951." In *Rockefeller Philanthropy and Modern Biomedicine: International Initiatives from World War I to the Cold War.* Edited by William H. Schneider, 7–60. Bloomington and Indianapolis: Indiana University Press, 2002.

———. "Puericulture and the Style of French Eugenics." *History and Philosophy of the Life Sciences* 8 (1986): 265–77.

———, ed. *Rockefeller Philanthropy and Modern Biomedicine: International Initiatives from World War I to the Cold War.* Bloomington and Indianapolis: Indiana University Press, 2002.

Schuler, Friedrich E. *Mexico between Hitler and Roosevelt: Mexican Foreign Relations in the Age of Lázaro Cárdenas, 1934–1940.* Albuquerque: University of New Mexico Press, 1998.

Sealander, Judith. *Private Wealth and Public Life: Foundation Philanthropy and the Reshaping of American Social Policy from the Progressive Era to the New Deal.* Baltimore: Johns Hopkins University Press, 1997.

Secretaría de la Economía Nacional. *El Café. Aspectos Económicos de su Producción y Distribución en México y en el Extranjero.* México, D.F.: Secretaría de la Economía Nacional, 1933.

Servicio Antilarvario, Departamento de Salubridad Pública. "Sumario Sobre el Informe de los Trabajos Realizados en 1924 en Vera Cruz, México." *Boletín de la Oficina Sanitaria Panamericana* 4 (1925): 168–73.

Servín Massieu, Manuel. *Microbiología, Vacunas, y el Rezago Científico de México a Partir del Siglo XIX.* México, D.F.: Plaza y Valdés Editores, 2000.

Sesto, Julio. *A Través de América: El México de Porfirio Díaz.* 2nd ed. Illustrated. México, D.F.: F. Sempere y Cia, Editores, 1910.

Shaplen, Robert. *Toward the Well-Being of Mankind: Fifty Years of the Rockefeller Foundation.* New York: Doubleday and Company, Inc., 1964.

Shein, Max. *El Niño Precolombino.* Mexico, D.F.: Editorial Villicaña, S.A., 1986.

Siddiqi, Javed. *World Health and World Politics: The World Health Organization and the UN System.* Columbia, SC: University of South Carolina Press, 1995.

Silva, Rafael. "The Health Problem in Mexico." *American Journal of Public Health* 21, no. 1 (1931): 31–36.

Silva Herzog, Jesús. *Breve Historia de la Revolución Mexicana.* México, D.F.: Fondo de Cultura Económica, 1960.

———. "Cárdenas en la Presidencia." *Cuadernos Americanos* 30 (1971): 91–104.

———. "México a 50 Años de su Revolución." *Cuadernos Americanos* 23 (1964): 7–30.

Simpson, Eyler. *The Ejido: Mexico's Way Out.* Durham: University of North Carolina Press, 1937.

Siurob, José. *Modern Tendencies of Public Health in the Republic of Mexico.* México, D.F.: DSP, 1936.

———. "La Sanidad en México." *Boletín de la Oficina Sanitaria Panamericana* 15, no. 12 (December 1936): 1148–53.

———. *Social Medicine in Mexico.* México, D.F.: DSP, 1940.

———. *Trabajo Sanitario en los Estados Unidos Mexicanos, 1934–1940.* México, D.F.: DSP, April 26, 1940.

Skirius, John. "Railroad, Oil and Other Foreign Interests in the Mexican Revolution, 1911–1914." *Journal of Latin American Studies* 35 (2003): 25–51.

Sklar, Kathryn Kish. "The Historical Foundations of Women's Power in the Creation of the American Welfare State, 1830–1930." In *Mothers of a New World: Maternalist Politics and the Origins of Welfare States.* Edited by Seth Koven and Sonya Michel, 43–93. New York: Routledge, 1993.

Skocpol, Theda. *Protecting Soldiers and Mothers: The Political Origins of Social Policy in the United States.* Cambridge, MA: Belknap Press of Harvard University Press, 1992.

Smillie, Wilson G. "The Results of Hookworm Disease Prophylaxis in Brazil." *American Journal of Hygiene* 2, no. 1 (1922): 77–94.

———. "La Salubridad en Latino América." *Boletín de la Oficina Sanitaria Panamericana* 29, no. 2 (1950): 171–80.

Smith, Frances E. "Medicine in Mexico." *The Lancet* 208, no. 5373 (1926): 413.

Smith, Hugh H. *Life's A Pleasant Institution: The Peregrinations of a Rockefeller Doctor.* Tucson, AZ: self-published, 1978.

Smith, Margaret Charles, and Linda Janet Holmes. *Listen to Me Good: The Life Story of an Alabama Midwife.* Columbus: Ohio State University Press, 1996.

Smith, Robert Freeman. *The United States and Revolutionary Nationalism in Mexico, 1916–1932.* Chicago: University of Chicago Press, 1972.

Smith, Susan L. *Sick and Tired of Being Sick and Tired: Black Women's Health Activism in America, 1890–1950.* Philadelphia: University of Pennsylvania Press, 1995.

Snodgrass, Michael. *Deference and Defiance in Monterrey: Workers, Paternalism, and Revolution in Mexico, 1890–1950.* Cambridge: Cambridge University Press, 2003.

Soberón y Parra, Galo. "Breves Apuntes Acerca del Estado Actual de la Lucha contra el Paludismo." *Pasteur: Revista Mensual de Medicina* 10, II, no. 1 (1937): 17–22.

Society of Friends, American Friends Service Committee, and Students Peace Service. *Subjects Developed for the Coordinated Services of Rural Hygiene and Social Medical Services in the Laguna Region in the Conferences Which Are to Take Place from the 1st to the 6th of July 1939.* México, D.F.: DSP, 1940.

Solís Manjarrez, Leopoldo. *La Realidad Económica Mexicana: Retrovisión y Perspectivas.* México, D.F.: Siglo XXI Editores, 1970.

Solomon, Susan G. "Knowing the 'Local': Rockefeller Foundation Officers' Site Visits to Russia in the 1920s." *Slavic Review* 62, no. 4 (Winter 2003): 710–32.

Solomon, Susan G, and John F. Hutchinson, eds. *Health and Society in Revolutionary Russia.* Bloomington: Indiana University Press, 1990.

Solomon, Susan G, and Nikolai Krementsov. "Giving and Taking across Borders: The Rockefeller Foundation and Soviet Russia, 1919–1928." *Minerva* 3 (2001): 265–98.

Solórzano, Armando. "La Influencia de la Fundación Rockefeller en la Conformación de la Profesión Médica Mexicana, 1921–1949." *Revista Mexicana de Sociología* 58, no. 1 (1996): 173–203.

———. "The Rockefeller Foundation in Mexico: Nationalism, Public Health, and Yellow Fever, 1911–1924." PhD. diss., University of Wisconsin–Madison, 1990.

———. "The Rockefeller Foundation in Revolutionary Mexico: Yellow Fever in Yucatan and Veracruz." In *Missionaries of Science: The Rockefeller Foundation and Latin America.* Edited by Marcos Cueto, 52–71. Bloomington: Indiana University Press, 1994.

———. "Sowing the Seeds of Neo-imperialism: The Rockefeller Foundation's Yellow Fever Campaign in Mexico." *International Journal of Health Services* 22 (1992): 529–54.

Solórzano Morfín, Juan. "Algunos Datos para el Estudio de las Parasitosis Intestinales de México." *Gaceta Médica de México* 58, no. 12 (1927): 742–59.

———. "Tratamiento de la Uncinariasis." *Gaceta Médica de México* 58 (1927): 329–71.

Solórzano Ramos, Armando. *¿Fiebre Dorada o Fiebre Amarilla? La Fundación Rockefeller en México, 1911–1924.* Guadalajara: Universidad de Guadalajara, 1997.

Somolinos d'Ardois, Germán. *Capítulos de Historia Médica Mexicana.* México, D.F.: Sociedad Mexicana de Historia y Filosofía de la Medicina, 1978.

Soper, Fred L. *Building the Health Bridge: Selections from the Works of Fred L. Soper, M.D.* Edited by J. Austin Kerr. Bloomington: Indiana University Press, 1970.

———. *Ventures in World Health: The Memoirs of Fred Lowe Soper.* Edited by John Duffy. Washington, DC: PAHO, 1977.

Soper, Fred L, Bruce D. Wilson, Servulo Lima, and Valdemar Sa Antunes. *The Organization of Permanent Nation-Wide Anti-Aedes Aegypti Measures in Brazil.* New York: Rockefeller Foundation, 1943.

Soto, Shirlene Ann. *Emergence of the Mexican Woman: Her Participation in Revolution and Struggle for Equality, 1910–1940.* Denver, CO: Arden Press, Inc., 1990.

Soustelle, Jacques. *Daily Life of the Aztecs on the Eve of the Spanish Conquest.* Stanford, CA: Stanford University Press, 1970.

Spenser, Daniela. *Impossible Triangle: Mexico, Soviet Russia, and the United States in the 1920s.* Durham, NC: Duke University Press, 1998.

Stapleton, Darwin H. "The Dawn of DDT and Its Experimental Use by the Rockefeller Foundation in Mexico, 1943–1952." *Parassitologia* 40, nos. 1–2 (1998): 149–58.

———. "Lessons of History? Anti-malaria Strategies of the International Health Board and the Rockefeller Foundation from the 1920s to the Era of DDT." *Public Health Reports* 119 (March–April 2004): 205–15.

———. "A Success for Science or Technology? The Rockefeller Foundation's Role in Malaria Eradication in Italy, 1924–1935." *Medecina nei Secoli* 6, no. 1 (1994): 213–28.

Starr, Paul. *The Social Transformation of American Medicine.* New York: Basic Books, 1982.

Stepan, Nancy. *Beginnings of Brazilian Science: Oswaldo Cruz, Medical Research and Policy, 1890–1920.* New York: Science History Publications, 1981.

———. *"The Hour of Eugenics": Race, Gender, and Nation in Latin America.* Ithaca, NY: Cornell University Press, 1991.

———. "The Interplay between Socio-Economic Factors and Medical Science: Yellow Fever Research, Cuba and the United States." *Social Studies of Science* 8 (1978): 397–423.

Stern, Alexandra M. "Eugenics beyond Borders: Science and Medicalization in Mexico and the U.S. West, 1900–1950." PhD diss., University of Chicago, 1999.

———. "Responsible Mothers and Normal Children: Eugenics, Nationalism, and Welfare in Post-Revolutionary Mexico, 1920–1940." *Journal of Historical Sociology* 12, no. 4 (1999): 369–97.

———. "From Mestizophilia to Biotypology: Racialization and Science in Mexico, 1920–1960." In *Race and Nation in Modern Latin America.* Edited by Nancy Appelbaum, Anne S. Macpherson, and Karin Alejandra Rosemblatt, 187–210. Chapel Hill: University of North Carolina Press, 2003.

———. "Unraveling the History of Eugenics in Mexico." *Mendel Newsletter.* August 1999: 1–10.

Stern, Alexandra M, and Howard Markel. "International Efforts to Control Infectious Diseases, 1851 to the Present." *JAMA* 292 (2004): 1474–79.

Stoll, N. R. "Investigations on the Control of Hookworm Disease. XV. An Effective Method of Counting Hookworm Eggs in Feces." *American Journal of Hygiene* 3, no. 2 (1923): 59–70.

———. "Investigations on the Control of Hookworm Disease. XVIII. On the Relation between the Number of Eggs Found in Human Feces and the Number of Hookworms in the Host." *American Journal of Hygiene* 3 (1923): 156–79.

Strode, George, ed. *Yellow Fever.* New York: McGraw Hill, 1951.

Studies in History and Philosophy of Science Part C: Studies in History and Philosophy of Biological and Biomedical Sciences 31, no. 3 (September 2000), special issue on Medicine as a Social Instrument, Rockefeller Foundation, 1913–45.

Sunman, Hilary. "Earmarked Funds and Sectorwide Approaches Can Encourage Harmonization." *Bulletin of the World Health Organization* 82, no. 9 (September 2004): 707.

Sutton, Francis X. "The Ford Foundation: The Early Years." *Daedalus* 116 (1987): 41–91.

Sweezy, Paul M. "A Great American." *Monthly Review* 41 (1989): 37–44.

Szreter, Simon. "Economic Growth, Disruption, Deprivation, Disease and Death: On the Importance of the Politics of Public Health for Development." *Population Development Review* 23 (1997): 693–728.

Tannenbaum, Frank. *Mexico: The Struggle for Peace and Bread.* New York: Alfred A. Knopf, 1950.

———. *Peace by Revolution, An Interpretation of Mexico.* New York: Columbia University Press, 1933.

Taussig, Michael. *The Devil and Commodity Fetishism.* Chapel Hill: University of North Carolina Press, 1980.

Thomas, Caroline. "Health of International Relations and International Relations of Health." *Review of International Studies* 15 (1989): 273–80.

Tobler, Hans Werner. "Peasants and the Revolutionary State, 1910–1940." In *Riot, Rebellion, and Revolution: Rural Social Conflict in Mexico.* Edited by Frederich Katz, 487–518. Princeton, NJ: Princeton University Press, 1988.

———. *La Revolución Mexicana: Transformación Social y Cambio Político, 1876–1940.* Mexico City: Alianza Editorial, 1994.

Torres Muñoz, Adrián. "Los Cursos de Perfeccionamiento en París." *Pasteur: Revista Mensual de Medicina* 8, II, no. 2 (1935): 38–41.

Torres Torija, José. "El Seguro de Salud." *Pasteur: Revista Mensual de Medicina* 3, I, no. 3 (1930): 140–48.

Transactions of the Fourth International Sanitary Conference of the American Republics, held in San José, Costa Rica, December 25, 1909 to January 3, 1910. Washington, DC: Pan American Union, 1910.

Trostle, James. "International Health Research: The Rules of the Game." In *Global Health Policy, Local Realities: The Fallacy of the Level Playing Field.* Edited by Linda Whiteford and Lenore Manderson, 291–313. Boulder, CO: Lynne Rienner Publishers, 2000.

Trueba, Guadalupe. "Birth in Pre-Hispanic Mexico." *International Midwife* 7 (Winter 1997): 45–47.

Tuñon, Julia. *Mujeres en México: Una Historia Olvidada.* México, D.F.: Editorial Planeta, 1987.

Turshen, Meredith. *The Politics of Public Health.* New Brunswick, NJ: Rutgers University Press, 1989.

United Fruit Company, ed. *Proceedings of the International Conference on Health Problems in Tropical America, Held at Kingston, Jamaica, July 22 to August 1, 1924.* Boston: United Fruit Company, 1924.

Vasconcelos, Angel Brioso. "Acta de la Segunda Sesión Plena Octubre 17 de 1921." In *Memoria de la Primera Convención de Fiebre Amarilla, Octubre 15–20 de 1921,* 120. México, D.F.: DSP, 1921.

———. "El Vocal del Consejo: Casos Registrados de Junio 8 a Diciembre 28 de 1920, 11 de octubre de 1921." In *Memoria de la Primera Convención de Fiebre Amarilla, Octubre 15–20 de 1921,* 18. México, D.F.: DSP, 1921.

Vasconcelos, José. *La Raza Cósmica: The Cosmic Race: A Bilingual Edition.* Translated and annotated by Didier T. Jaén, afterword by Joseba Gabilondo. Baltimore: Johns Hopkins University Press, 1997.

Vaughan, Mary Kay. *Cultural Politics in Revolution: Teachers, Peasants, and Schools in Mexico, 1930–1940.* Tucson: University of Arizona Press, 1997.

———. "Modernizing Patriarchy: State Policies, Rural Households and Women in Mexico 1930–1940." In *Hidden Histories of Gender and the State in Latin America.* Edited by Elizabeth Dore and Maxine Molyneux, 194–214. Durham, NC, and London: Duke University Press, 2000.

———. *The State, Education, and Social Class in Mexico, 1880–1928.* DeKalb: Northern Illinois University Press, 1982.

Vaughan, Megan. *Curing their Ills: Colonial Power and African Illness.* Oxford: Polity Press, 1991.

Vázquez, Josefina Zoraida, and Lorenzo Meyer. *The United States and Mexico.* Chicago: University of Chicago Press, 1985.

Velásquez García, Pomposo. "Tesis para Obtener el Título de Médico Cirujano." MD diss., Universidad Nacional de México, 1935.

Venediktov, Dmitry. "Alma-Ata and After." *World Health Forum* 19 (1998): 79–86.

Vera Estañol, Jorge. *La Revolución Mexicana: Orígenes y Resultados.* México, D.F.: Grupo Editorial Miguel Angel Porrúa, 1957.

Vernon, Raymond. *The Dilemma of Mexico's Development: The Role of the Private and Public Sector.* Cambridge, MA: Harvard University Press, 1963.

Vessuri, Hebe. "Enfermería de Salud Pública, Modernización, y Cooperación Internacional: El Proyecto de la Escuela Nacional de Enfermeras, 1936–1950." *História, Ciências, Saúde—Manguinhos* 8, no. 3 (September–December, 2001): 507–39.

Viesca Treviño, Carlos. "Eduardo Liceaga y la Participación Mexicana en la Fundación de la Organización Panamericana de la Salud." *Revista Cubana de Salud Pública* 24, no. 1 (1998): 11–18.

———. "La Medicina Novohispana." In *Un Siglo de Ciencias de la Salud en México.* Edited by Hugo Aréchiga and Luis Benitez Bribiesca, 56–99. México, D.F.: Fondo de Estudios e Investigaciones Ricardo J. Zevada, Consejo Nacional para la Cultura y las Artes, Fondo de Cultura Económica, 2000.

———. *Medicina Prehispánica de México: El Conocimiento Médico de los Nahuas.* México, D.F.: Panorama Editorial, 1986.

Villanueva, Aquilino. "Los Problemas Fundamentales en México en Materia de Salubridad." *Boletín de la Oficina Sanitaria Panamericana* 8 (1929): 1194–96.

Vincent, George. "The Work of the Rockefeller Foundation: Health as an International Bond." Speech given at the Empire Club, Toronto, March 9, 1920. In *The Empire Club of Canada Speeches, 1920.* Edited by the Empire Club of Canada, 126–45. Toronto: Empire Club of Canada, 1921.

Viniegra Osorio, Gustavo. "Consideraciones Generales Sobre la Salubridad en México." *Salubridad y Asistencia* 6 (1946): 89–101.

von Pettenkofer, Max. *The Value of Health to a City: Two Popular Lectures.* Translated with an introduction by Henry E. Sigerist. Baltimore: Johns Hopkins University Press, 1941.

Waddington, Catriona. "Does Earmarked Donor Funding Make It More or Less Likely that Developing Countries Will Allocate their Resources towards Programmes that Yield the Greatest Health Benefits?" *Bulletin of the World Health Organization* 82, no. 9 (September 2004): 703–6.

Walker, M. E. M. *Pioneers of Public Health: The Story of Some Benefactors of the Human Race.* Edinburgh: Oliver & Boyd, 1930.

Wall, Joseph Frazier. *Andrew Carnegie.* New York: Oxford University Press, 1970.

Walsh, Julia, and Kenneth Warren. "Selective Primary Health Care: An Interim Strategy for Disease Control in Developing Countries." *New England Journal of Medicine* 301, no. 18 (1979): 967–74.

Walt, Gill. "Globalisation of International Health." *The Lancet* 351, no. 9100 (1998): 434–37.

———. "Global Cooperation in International Public Health." In *International Public Health: Diseases, Programs, Systems, and Policies.* Edited by Michael Merson, Robert Black, and Anne Mills, 667–99. Gaithersburg, MD: Aspen Publishers, 2001.

———. "WHO under Stress: Implications for Health Policy." *Health Policy* 24 (1993): 125–44.

Warman, Arturo. *"We Come to Object": The Peasants of Morelos and the National State.* Translated by Stephen K. Ault. Baltimore: Johns Hopkins University Press, 1980.

Warren, Kenneth S. "The Evolution of Selective Primary Health Care." *Social Science and Medicine* 26, no. 8 (1988): 891–98.

———. "Tropical Medicine or Tropical Health: The Heath Clark Lectures, 1988." *Reviews of Infectious Diseases* 12 (1990): 142–56.

Washburn B. E. "The Economic Value of a Hookworm Campaign." In *Proceedings of the International Conference on Health Problems in Tropical America, Held at Kingston, Jamaica July 22 to August 1, 1924,* 613–22. Boston: United Fruit Company, 1924.

Washburn Benjamin E. *As I Recall.* New York: Rockefeller Foundation, 1960.

Watkins, Susan Cotts. "Social Networks and Social Science History." *Social Science History* 19, no. 3 (Fall 1995): 295–311.

Watson, Irving. *Sanitary Authorities of the United States of America, the Dominion of Canada, and the Republic of Mexico.* Washington, DC: American Public Health Association, 1894.

Weindling, Paul, ed. *International Health Organisations and Movements, 1918–1939.* Cambridge: Cambridge University Press, 1995.

———. "Philanthropy and World Health: The Rockefeller Foundation and the League of Nations Health Organization." *Minerva* 35, no. 3 (Autumn 1997): 269–81.

———. "Public Health in Germany." In *The History of Public Health and the Modern State.* Wellcome Series in the History of Medicine. Edited by Dorothy Porter, 119–31. Amsterdam: Rodopi, 1994.

———. "Termination or Transformation? The Fate of the International Health Division as a Case Study in Foundation Decision-Making." *Research Reports from the Rockefeller Archive Center* (Fall 2002): 20–23.

Werner, David, and David Sanders. *Questioning the Solution: The Politics of Primary Health Care and Child Survival.* Palo Alto, CA: Healthwrights, 1997.

Wheatley, Steven C. *The Politics of Philanthropy: Abraham Flexner and Medical Education.* Madison: University of Wisconsin Press, 1989.

White, Joseph H. "Epidemiologia y Profilaxis de la Fiebre Amarilla." *Boletín de la Oficina Sanitaria Panamericana* 3 (1924): 5–9.

Wiebe, Robert. *The Search for Order, 1877–1920.* New York: Hill & Wang, 1967.

Wilkie, James. *The Mexican Revolution: Federal Expenditure and Social Change since 1910.* Berkeley: University of California Press, 1967.

Wilkinson, Lise. "Burgeoning Visions of Global Public Health: The Rockefeller Foundation, the London School of Hygiene and Tropical Medicine, and the 'Hookworm Connection.'" *Studies in History and Philosophy of Biological and Biomedical Sciences* 31, no. 3 (2000): 397–407.

Wilkinson, Lise, and Anne Hardy. *Prevention and Cure: The London School of Hygiene and Tropical Medicine.* London: Kegan Paul, 2001.

Williams, Greer. *The Plague Killers.* New York: Charles Scribner's Sons, 1969.

Williams, Steven C. "Nationalism and Public Health: The Convergence of Rockefeller Foundation Technique and Brazilian Federal Authority during the Time of Yellow Fever, 1925–1930." In *Missionaries of Science: The Rockefeller Foundation and Latin America.* Edited by Marcos Cueto, 23–51. Bloomington: Indiana University Press, 1994.

Wilson, Charles Morrow. *Ambassadors in White: The Story of American Tropical Medicine.* New York: Henry Holt and Company, 1942.

Winslow, Charles E. A. *Lo que Cuesta la Enfermedad y lo que Vale la Salud.* Washington, DC: PASB, 1955.

Womack, John. "The Mexican Revolution, 1910–1920." In *Mexico since Independence.* Edited by Leslie Bethell, 125–200. Cambridge: Cambridge University Press, 1991.

———. *Zapata and the Mexican Revolution.* New York: Knopf, 1969.

Wood, Andrew. "Close Encounters of Empire? The Rockefeller Foundation and the Battle against Yellow Fever in Veracruz, Mexico." Unpublished manuscript, 2000.

———. *Revolution in the Street: Women, Workers, and Urban Protest in Veracruz, 1870–1920.* Wilmington, DE: Scholarly Resources, 2001.

Wooster, Martin M. "The Donors Are In: What Gates Can Learn from Rockefeller About Global Health." *Philanthropy Magazine,* August/September 2001, http://www.philanthropyroundtable.org/magazines/2001/august/

———. *The Foundation Builders: Brief Biographies of Twelve Great Philanthropists.* Washington, DC: The Philanthropy Roundtable, 2001.

Worboys, Michael. "The Emergence of Tropical Medicine: A Study in the Establishment of a Scientific Specialty." In *Perspectives on the Emergence of Scientific Disciplines.* Edited by Gerard Lemaine, Roy MacLeod, Michael Mulkay, and Peter Weingart, 75–98. The Hague: Mouton & Co., 1976.

World Bank. *World Development Report 1993: Investing in Health.* Washington, DC: World Bank, 1993.

World Health Organization. "The Declaration of Alma-Ata." *World Health* (August/September 1988): 16–17.

———. *The First Ten Years of the World Health Organization.* Geneva: World Health Organization, 1958.

———. *The Second Ten Years of the World Health Organization, 1958–1967.* Geneva: World Health Organization, 1968.

———. *The Work of WHO, 1986–1987, Biennial Report of the Director-General to the World Health Assembly and to the United Nations.* Geneva: World Health Organization, 1988.

Yergin, Daniel. *The Prize: The Epic Quest for Oil, Money, and Power.* New York: Touchstone, 1991.

Yip, Ka-che. *Health and National Reconstruction in Nationalist China: The Development of Modern Health Services, 1928–1937*. Ann Arbor, MI: Association for Asian Studies, Inc., 1995.

———. "Health and Society in China: Public Health Education for the Community, 1912–1937." *Social Science and Medicine* 16 (1982): 1197–1205.

Young, James Clay. *Medical Choice in a Mexican Village*. New Brunswick, NJ: Rutgers University Press, 1981.

Zárate Campos, María Soledad. "De Partera a Matrona. Los Inicios de la Profesionalización del Cuidado de la Madre y de los Hijos en Chile, 1870–1920." *Revista Colegio de Matronas* 7, no. 2 (1999): 13–18.

———. "Proteger a las Madres: Origen de un Debate Público, 1870–1920." *Revista Nomadías—Serie Monográfica* 1 (1999): 163–82.

Zea, Leopoldo. *El Positivismo en México*. México, D.F.: Biblioteca del Instituto Nacional de Estudios Históricos de la Revolución Mexicana, 1953.

Zinsser, Hans. "The Perils of Magnanimity: A Problem in American Education." *Atlantic Monthly* 139 (1927): 246–50.

Zolla, Carlos and Virginia Mellado. *La Medicina Tradicional de los Pueblos Indígenas de México*. México, D.F.: INI, 1994.

Personal Interviews

Bustamante, Juan. May 8, 1991, Oaxaca, Oaxaca.

Castor, Judith. April 12, 1991, Cuernavaca, Morelos.

Chávez, Adolfo. April 30, 1991, Mexico City.

Coronel, Esther "La Güera" and husband. April 15, 1991, Cuernavaca, Morelos.

Espinoza Canales, Hermillo. April 15, 1991, Cuernavaca, Morelos.

Frausto, Guadalupe. May 31,1991, Cuernavaca, Morelos.

Fujigaki Lechuga, Augusto. May 31, 1991, Cuernavaca, Morelos.

Galván Sánchez, Carmen Eugenia. April 11, 1991, Cuernavaca, Morelos.

García Sánchez, Felipe. June 5, 1991, Mexico City.

Gomez-Dantés, Hector. April 1991 and March 2000, Mexico City and Cuernavaca, Morelos.

González, Inés. April 12,1991, Cuernavaca, Morelos.

Guzmán de Alfaro, Martita. April 12, 1991, Cuernavaca, Morelos.

Hoffmann, Anita. June 4,1991, Mexico City.

Horn, James. April 11, 1991, Cuernavaca, Morelos.

Laurell, Cristina. April 16, 1991, Mexico City.

León, Alberto P. April 10, 1991, Mexico City.

Pérez Laredo, Luz. June 3, 1991, Mexico City.

Román García, José Guadalupe. April 15, 1991, Cuernavaca, Morelos.

Sandoval, Joel Rogelio. April 12, 1991, Cuernavaca, Morelos.

Serrano, Lupita. April 12, 1991, Cuernavaca, Morelos.

Serrano, Margarita. April 12, 1991, Cuernavaca, Morelos.

Serrano Cruz, Maria Guadalupe. April 11, 12, and 15, 1991, Cuernavaca, Morelos.

Servín Massieu, Manuel. March 4, 1991, Mexico City.

Soberón, Guillermo. April 30, 1991, Mexico City.
Vargas, Luis. March 5, 1991, Mexico City.
Venediktov, Dmitry. July 2004, Moscow, Russia.
Zarzosa, Jaime. April 11, 1991, Cuernavaca, Morelos.

Libraries, Archives, and Manuscript Sources

Alan Mason Chesney Archives of the Johns Hopkins Medical Institutions, Baltimore, MD.
    Record Group Johns Hopkins University School of Hygiene and Public Health, Office of the Dean—Correspondence.
Archivo General de la Nación, Mexico City. (AGN)
    Presidential Record Groups for Plutarco Elías Calles, Emilio Portes Gil, Pascual Ortiz Rubio, Abelardo Rodríguez, Lázaro Cárdenas, Manuel Avila Camacho, and Miguel Alemán.
    Record Groups Departamento de Salubridad Pública and Secretaría de Salubridad y Asistencia.
Archivo General del Estado de Oaxaca, Oaxaca, Oaxaca.
Archivo General del Estado de Yucatán, Mérida, Yucatán.
Archivo Histórico del Estado de Jalisco, Guadalajara, Jalisco.
Archivo Histórico del Estado de Morelos, Cuernavaca, Morelos. (AHEM).
Archivo Histórico del Estado de Veracruz, Jalapa, Veracruz.
Archivo Histórico de la Facultad de Medicina de la Universidad Nacional Autónoma de México.
Archivo Histórico de la Secretaría de Salud, Mexico City. (AHSSA)
    Record Groups Salud Publica (Public Health), Secretaria de Salubridad y Asistencia (SSA).
Archivo Histórico de la Universidad Nacional Autónoma de México, Mexico City.
Archivo Histórico de Relaciones Exteriores, Mexico City.
Archivo Histórico Municipal, Oaxaca, Oaxaca.
Archivo Municipal de Guadalajara, Guadalajara, Jalisco.
Biblioteca del Colegio de México, Mexico City.
Biblioteca del Instituto Nacional de Salud Pública, Secretaría de Salud, Cuernavaca, Morelos.
Biblioteca del Instituto de Salubridad y Enfermedades Tropicales, Mexico City.
Biblioteca de la Academia Nacional de Medicina de México, Mexico City.
Biblioteca de la Dirección General de Epidemiología, Secretaría de Salud, Mexico City.
Biblioteca Miguel Bustamante, Departamento de Salud Pública, Facultad de Medicina, Universidad Nacional Autónoma de México, Mexico City.
Biblioteca Nacional de México, Mexico City.
Biblioteca y Hemeroteca de la Secretaría de Salud, Mexico City.
Centro de Estudios de História de México CONDUMEX, Mexico City.
Fundación Cívico-Cultural Bustamante Vasconcelos, Oaxaca, Oaxaca. (FCCBV)
    Record Group Dr. Miguel E. Bustamante V.

Instituto Nacional de la Nutrición Salvador Zubiran, Mexico City.

Instituto Nacional de Salud Pública, Cuernavaca, Morelos.

Library of Congress, Washington, DC.

National Archives and Record Administration, College Park, MD. (NARA)
Record Group SA. General Records of the Department of State. Record Group
90. Records of the Public Health Service 1912–1968. Microfilm Division, State
Department Decimal File, M 274 Roll 135—Public health, vital statistics, hygiene,
and sanitation.

National Library of Medicine, History of Medicine Division, Bethesda, MD.
Book, Pamphlet, and Manuscript Collection.

New York Academy of Medicine, New York City.

New York Public Library, New York City.

Rockefeller Archive Center, Sleepy Hollow, NY.
Rockefeller Foundation Archives. (RFA) Rockefeller Family Archives.

Index

Page numbers followed by f, t, or n refer to figures, tables, and notes respectively.

In January 1921, after a decade of bloody warfare, Mexico's new government found an unlikely partner in its struggle to fulfill the Revolution's promises to the populace. An ambitious philanthropy, born of the wealth of America's most notorious capitalist, made its way into Mexico by offering money and expertise to counter a looming public health crisis. Why did the Rockefeller Foundation and Revolutionary Mexico get together, and how did their relationship last for thirty-plus years amidst binational tensions, domestic turmoil, and institutional soul-searching?

Transcending standard hagiographic accounts as well as simplistic arguments of cultural imperialism, *Marriage of Convenience* offers a nuanced analysis of the interaction between the foundation's International Health Division and Mexico's Departamento de Salubridad Pública as they jointly promoted public health through campaigns against yellow fever and hookworm disease, organized cooperative rural health units, and educated public health professionals in North American universities and Mexican training stations. Drawing from a wealth of archival sources in both Mexico and the United States, Anne-Emanuelle Birn uncovers the complex give-and-take of this early experience of international health cooperation.

Though it was far from love at first sight, Mexico and the Rockefeller Foundation managed to live with one another through moments of productive cooperation, borrowings back and forth, mutual disdain, outright hostility, and bona fide accomplishments that shaped the development of public health ideologies, practices, and institutions. In tracing the challenges of health cooperation between the Rockefeller Foundation and Revolutionary Mexico, Birn provides historical insights into the policies, paradigms, and practices of the global health field today.

Anne-Emanuelle Birn is Canada research chair in international health at the University of Toronto.

Printed and bound by CPI Group (UK) Ltd, Croydon, CR0 4YY

27/10/2024

14580347-0003